Foot and Ankle Surgery in Children and Adolescents

Johannes Hamel

Foot and Ankle Surgery in Children and Adolescents

Springer

Johannes Hamel
Centre for Foot and Ankle Surgery
Schoen Clinic München Harlaching
Munich
Germany

ISBN 978-3-030-58107-7 ISBN 978-3-030-58108-4 (eBook)
https://doi.org/10.1007/978-3-030-58108-4

Based on the translation from the German language edition: Operative Behandlung von Fuß und Sprunggelenk im Kindes- und Jugendalter by Johannes Hamel Copyright © Springer-Verlag GmbH Deutschland 2019. All Rights Reserved. ISBN 978-3-662-56591-9.

This Springer imprint is published by the registered company Springer Nature Switzerland AG
The registered company address is: Gewerbestrasse 11, 6330 Cham, Switzerland

Preface

This book is an extended version of a German text published in 2019. It attempts to fill a gap between the almost unmanageable literature in journals in recent decades; older and in some instances very comprehensive works such as those of Coleman or Tachdjian; and a recently published book by Mosca, which is strongly based on principles. The ways to treat juvenile/adolescent and neurogenic deformities of the foot and ankle have changed considerably in the last 20 years, and so an attempt to present a summary of them seemed to make sense.

This book deals with propaedeutic aspects but only insofar as they are of direct consequence for therapy. The main focus is on surgical treatment; conservative therapeutic aspects are presented in detail in the case of congenital contract deformities, otherwise they are less thoroughly considered. Surgical techniques are described, but the book is not a surgical manual; a lot of knowledge is presumed. The aspect of indications and differential indications is partially discussed in detail (as Mercer Rang stated, "the decision is more important than the incision"). In this context, imaging diagnostics and pedographic functional diagnostics, which have hardly been used in practice for foot deformities in children and adolescents so far, are given extensive coverage. All the sequelae of idiopathic clubfoot, management of neglected clubfoot in less developed countries, use of arthroereisis and osteotomy techniques in flexible and rigid planovalgus deformities, principles for the treatment of neurogenic and especially cavovarus deformities are discussed in detail. The current literature is taken into account but without any claim of completeness and only insofar as it contributes to understanding. In particular, however, numerous case studies and treatment courses are presented for illustrative purposes, as monitoring of the course of treatment is indispensable, especially during growth.

This book reflects the experiences of a single author, with all of the limitations that this entails, but has been developed over many years of discussion and exchange with numerous specialist colleagues. To name but a few, I would like to mention the long-standing co-lecturers of the Children's Foot Workshop—which I have been holding regularly since 1999 as part of the German Ankle and Foot Society (D.A.F.) Foot Surgery Certificate—Dr. Erica Lamprecht, PD Eberhardt, Dr. Döderlein, Dr. de Pellegrin, Dr. Helmers, and Prof. Raab; colleagues in the Children's Orthopedics Department in Vienna-Speising; and many others. I want to give special thanks to Prof. V. Mosca for many discussions, Dr. Schraml of the Feuerkinder Project in Tanzania, and Prof. M. Walther and his departmental team in Munich, where I have been able to contribute some of the experience described here since 2017.

Mr. Kühn for the German version and recently Mr. Himmelhan (Figs. 1.99a, b; 3.2b; 4.43a, b; 4.52; 4.56; 5.53a–d; 7.24; 10.2a, b; and 10.16a–c) have made significant contributions to this book with their numerous high-quality drawings. I would also like to thank the employees of the Springer Nature publishing house for their attentive supervision of this book project and Mrs. B. Steffan for the translation. Dr. Kalpen of the Novel Company provided very substantial support in the processing of the pedographs.

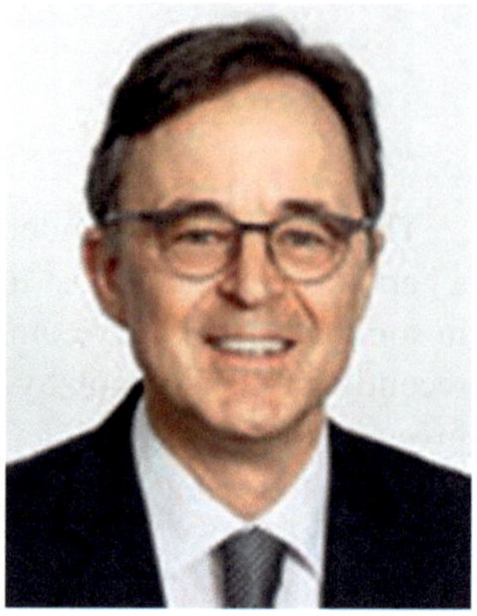

Munich, Germany, October 2020 Johannes Hamel

Contents

The Idiopathic Clubfoot

1

Contents

1.1 Introduction

Idiopathic clubfoot (Fig. 1.1) is the most frequent of the congenital, contracted deformities in Central Europe with a prevalence of about about 1–2 promille and occurs more frequently in the male sex. As a rule, it is now already detected prenatally by sonography (Pullinger et al. 2014), so that the first orthopedic consultation of the pregnant mother usually takes place at this time. If there are no further malformations or syndromal diseases, the expectant parents can and should be informed about the necessary therapy and the generally very favorable prognosis today and thus also be reassured. In most cases the expectant parents appreciate the early information. Unlike in the

J. Hamel, *Foot and Ankle Surgery in Children and Adolescents*, https://doi.org/10.1007/978-3-030-58108-4_1

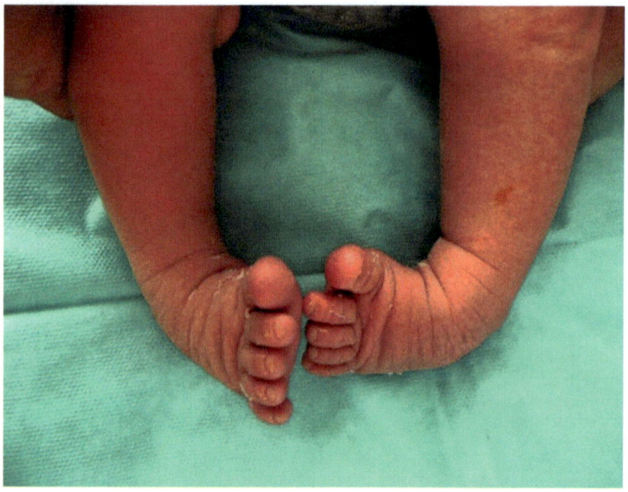

Fig. 1.1 Untreated bilateral clubfoot of the newborn child

past, treatment then begins without urgency during the first 2 weeks of life.

The extensive literature on idiopathic clubfoot is hardly manageable. Much of what was published in the years before about 2000 has lost its direct significance for today's therapists in so far as, with the propagation of the Ponseti method, the perspective on therapeutic questions and thus the relevance of published results have completely changed in many respects. In addition to specifically selected literature references in the text, the following works in particular are recommended for further basic information:

Recommended Monographs and Manuals on the Idiopathic Clubfoot

- Döderlein L et al (1999) Der Klumpfuß—Extensive, lexical work with a broad representation of history as well (German language)
- Ponseti IV (1996) Congenital clubfoot—fundamentals of treatment—Presentation of the Ponseti concept with all its propaedeutics
- Mosca V (2014) Principles and management of pediatric foot and ankle deformities—Describes not the clinical entity in a comprehensive form, but principles of indication and treatment
- Ricco Al, Richards BS, Herring JA (2014) Disorders of the foot (Chapter 23). In: Tachdjian's pediatric orthopaedics. Elsevier Saunders, Philadelphia—Comprehensive description

1.2 Therapeutically Relevant Pathomorphology/Pathophysiology

The literature on the pathomorphology of idiopathic clubfoot is extensive (see bibliography for some important papers, e.g. Ippolito 1995, Shapiro and Glimcher 1979, Ippolito and Ponseti 1980, Mc Kay 1982) and almost all anatomical structures have been proven to show changes compared to the normal foot (see box "Structural disorders"). With all pathomorphological findings, the question can be asked to what extent these are primary deviations or secondary phenomena, which can be at least partially reversible by suitable therapeutic measures.

Structural Disorders of the Idiopathic Clubfoot

– Dysplasia of the tarsal skeletal elements (especially the talus).
– Contracture of the tarsal joint capsules and soft tissues medial, plantar, and dorsal.
– Shortening of the flexor and invertor muscles.
– Overstretching and weakness of the evertor musculature.
– Deviating muscle fiber composition.
– Creases and indentations of the skin.
– Partly vascular anomalies.
– Partly neural aberrations.

At the beginning of the pathomorphological chain there seems to be a ***fibrotic process during the intrauterine development in the medial talonavicular region*** (Fig. 1.2) with an *inversion contracture of the peritalar complex* (Fig. 1.3). The deformation especially of the talus and calcaneus (see

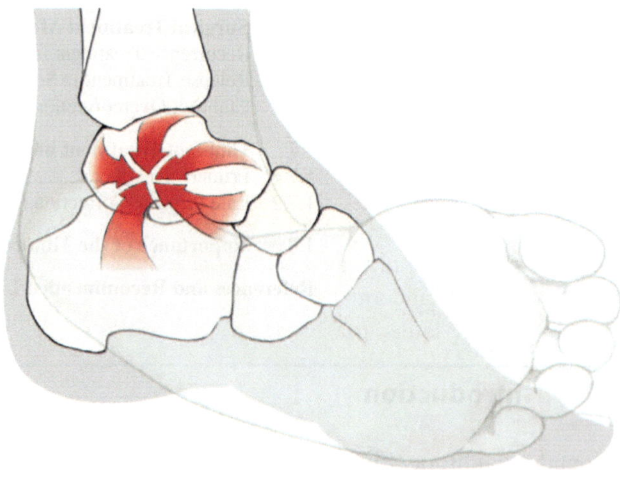

Fig. 1.2 Assumption of a fibrotic process as a starting point for the development of the idiopathic clubfoot

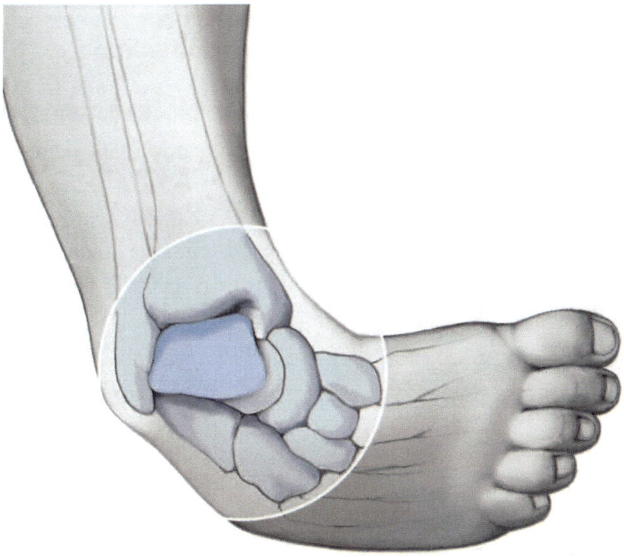

Fig. 1.3 Inversion contracture of the peritalar complex

below) and other skeletal elements seem to be of a secondary nature and partially reversible after successful treatment of the contracture. Soft tissue contractures are also present dorsally and plantar. In addition, there is a considerable *muscular imbalance* in the congenital clubfoot, the primary or secondary character of which is also questionable (see box "Main pathomorphological phenomena").

Main Pathomorphological Phenomena of the Idiopathic Clubfoot

- *Inversion contracture* of the peritalar complex
  - Talonavicular region/calcaneocuboid joint/tibiotalar joint.
- *Muscular imbalance*
  - Contracture of the flexing and inverting muscles.
  - Overstretching and weakness of the peroneal muscles.
  - Altered muscle mechanics due to misalignment.

Anatomical alterations can be found throughout the whole tarsal region with abnormal shape and size of the skeletal elements and the joint surfaces. Only the "regions of interest," which are of direct importance for the treatment and how they present to the primary therapist in the newborn clubfoot, will be discussed in more detail here. Sonographic imaging of these regions of interest each documents the condition of the predominantly still cartilaginous skeleton in infancy.

1.2.1 Talonavicular Region

In the medial talonavicular region, inversion contracture of the peritalar complex shows the most pronounced anatomical changes (Figs. 1.4 and 1.54a), and here the (hypothetically) intrauterine fibrotic process (Fig. 1.2) can be assumed:

- Deformity of the talar head/neck region with shortening of the talus (Figs. 1.4c, d and 1.15).
- Soft tissue contracture with strongly thickened connective tissue structures of the medial talonavicular joint capsule and the tibionavicular ligamentous tissue.
- Medial dislocation of the navicular, whose medial pole is in close vicinity to the medial malleolus (Figs. 1.4b, 1.5 and 1.54); this is an expression of the peritalar rotational malalignment with displacement of the anterior section of the calcaneus under the talus.
- Shortening of the posterior tibial tendon.

1.2.2 Calcaneocuboid Region

The calcaneocuboid region shows an angulation of the anterior part of the calcaneus with medial deviation of the joint surface (Simons 1993; Grayhack et al. 1995; Pirani et al. 2001) (Figs. 1.6 and 1.54b). Only in very severe cases additionally a "subluxation" with steplike alignment can be observed, as often assumed earlier due to the radiological aspect (Fig. 1.7b). This is of direct importance for the treatment to be applied: A true subluxation might require a surgical release for reduction as it was recommended earlier, whereas a deformity of the anterior calcaneal region can be treated by applying correcting forces by manipulation. Realignment can thus be achieved by plastic transformation of the soft cartilaginous tissue as it is developed in the newborn.

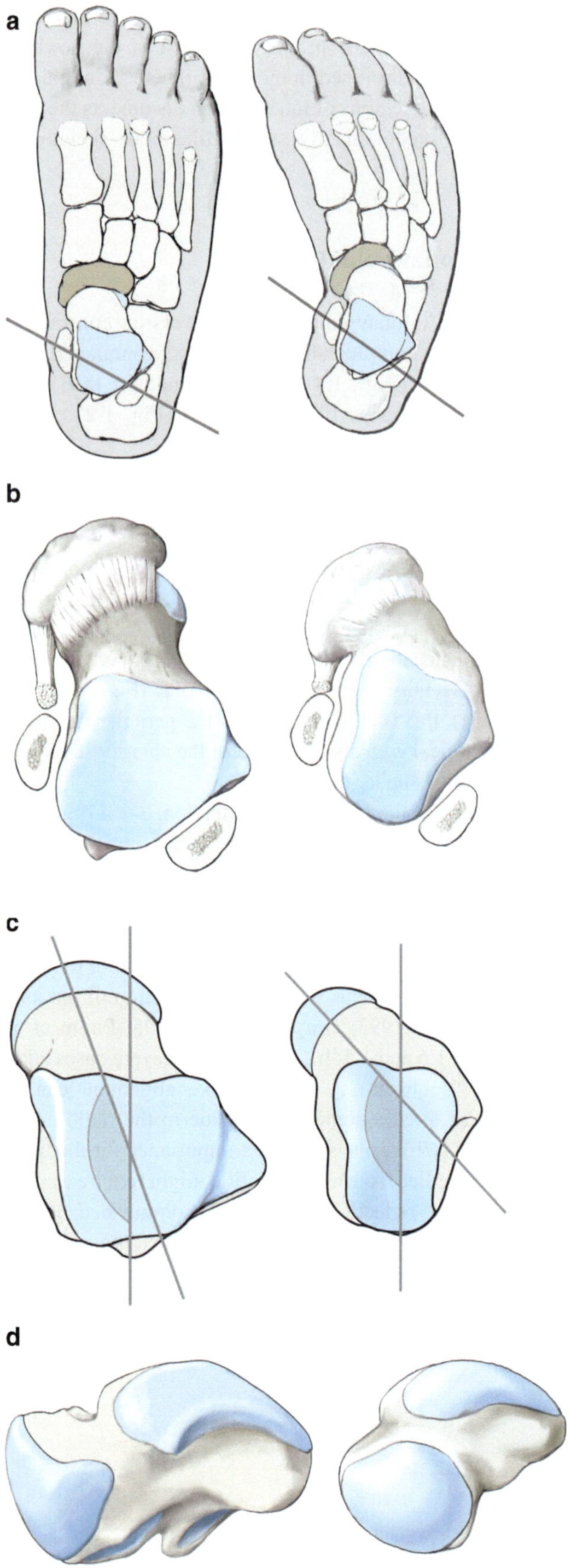

Fig. 1.4 The illustrations show the typical clubfoot findings in comparison to the normal foot in the transverse plane of the foot. The entire foot is shown with the peritalar inversion and outward rotation of the malleolar region (**a**), the talonavicular joint with the navicular dislocated far medially (**b**) and the talus itself with deformity of the head-neck region and shortening in the view from above (**c**) and from the medial side (**d**)

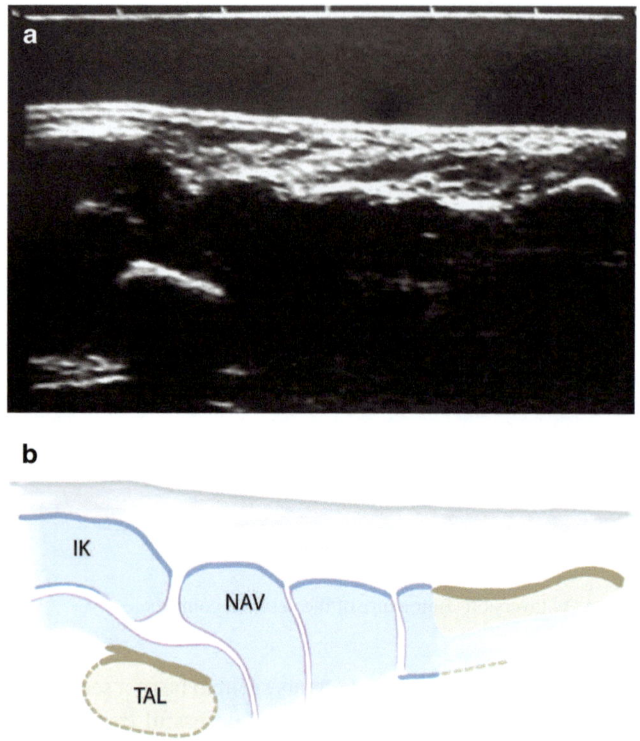

Fig. 1.5 Sonographic transverse section (**a**) of the medial talonavicular region in a 5-month-old child with insufficiently pretreated clubfoot and explaining drawing (**b**). The still complete inversion of the hindfoot can be recognized by the talonavicular malposition. The medial navicular pole (NAV) is directly adjacent to the medial malleolus (IK); the bony contour of the talar ossific nucleus (TAL) is located deeply in the foot

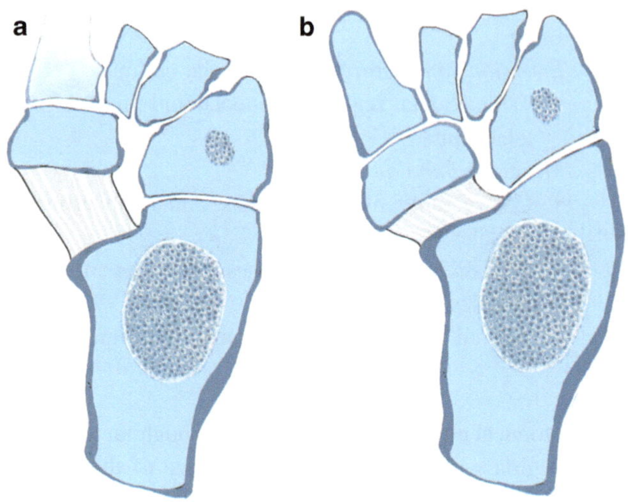

Fig. 1.6 Section through the calcaneocuboid region in the transverse plane of a normal foot of a newborn (**a**) and in the idiopathic clubfoot with medial angulation of the cartilaginous parts of the processus anterior calcanei (**b**)

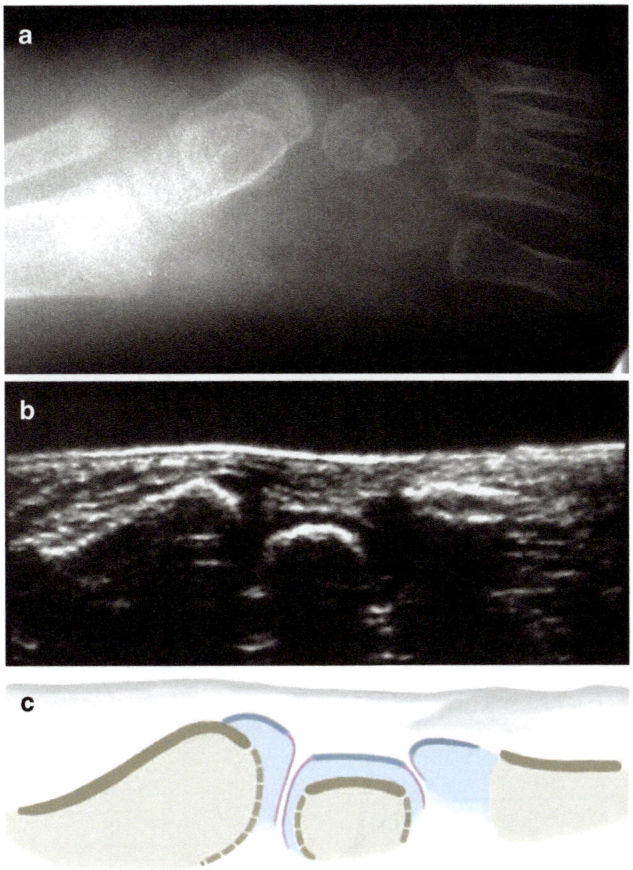

Fig. 1.7 Dorsoplantar X-ray (**a**) and lateral sonographic transverse section of the calcaneocuboid region (**b** and **c**) in a 6-month-old child with severe clubfoot. The calcaneocuboid malposition with slight subluxation is clearly visible

1.2.3 Tibiotalar Joint and Distal Lower Leg

The upper ankle joint is in contracted plantar flexion with distinct shortening and differently pronounced fibrotic thickening of the dorsal capsule and other soft tissue structures (calf muscles with Achilles tendon, peroneal tendon sheaths, posterior parts of the deltoid ligament, ligamentum fibulocalcaneare, and long toe flexors). Before the Ponseti technique was widely used, contracture of the dorsal capsular structures in the clubfoot of the newborn were considered to be more or less resistant to corrective forces and surgical release, therefore would be mandatory. However, this can no longer be maintained with the experience of the Ponseti technique, because percutaneous tenotomy of the Achilles tendon is sufficient in most cases. The equinus contracture is associated with a slight anterior displacement of the talus, and the dorsal tibial base is located close to the calcaneus (Figs. 1.8 and 1.9). Mitchell et al. (2018) found abnormalities in the anterior ankle region by MRI studies, which they described as a decrease in talar neck depth as the main reason of persisting equinus deformity after posterior soft tissue release.

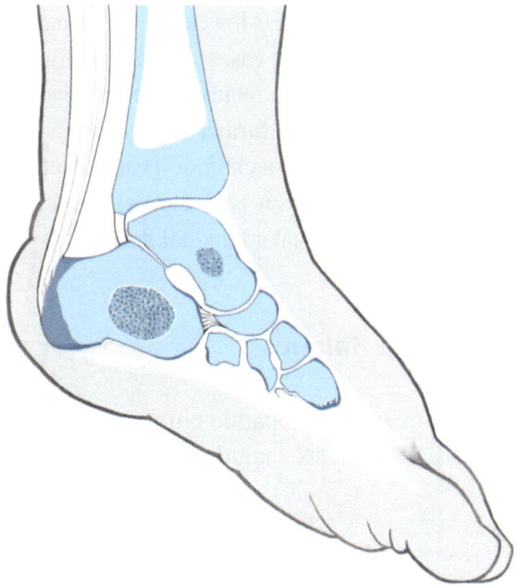

Fig. 1.8 Equinus deformity of the foot in the newborn. The ossific nuclei of talus and calcaneus are still small and eccentrically located at this early age

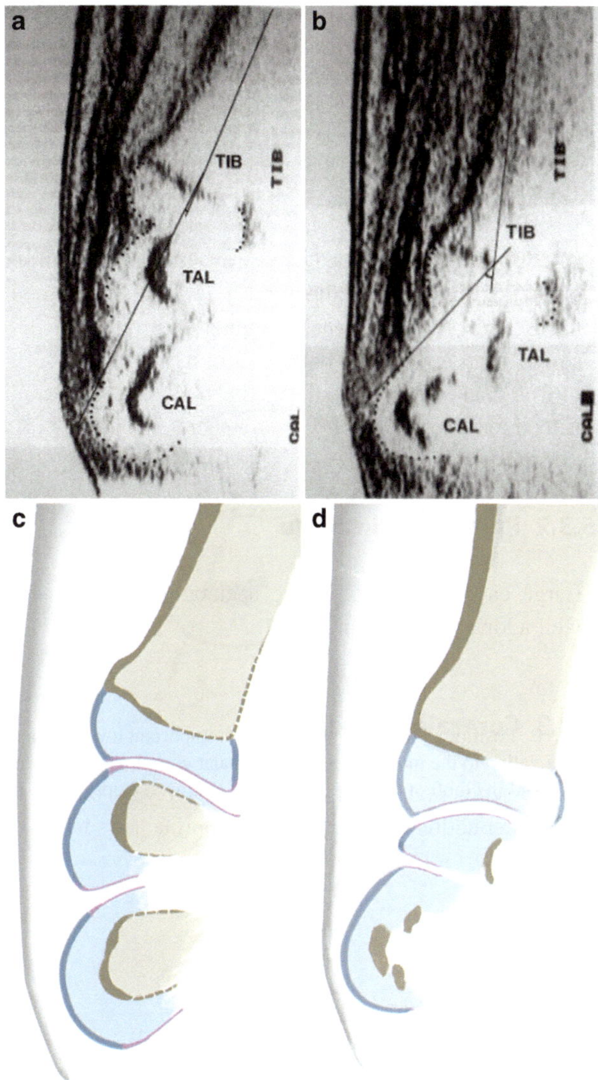

Fig. 1.9 Posterior longitudinal section in the widest possible dorsal extension in a 6-month-old child with unilateral clubfoot (**b** and **d**) compared to the unaffected side (**a** and **c**) after redressive plaster treatment and before tenotomy. *TIB* tibia, *TAL* talus, *CAL* calcaneus

The rotational profile of the lower leg is estimated differently in the literature. In most cases, there is a slight outward rotation of the malleolar region relative to the knee joint motion axis (Fig. 1.4a), which can be further increased by redression, especially with an imprecise technique (Farsetti et al. 2012). Supramalleolar inward rotation is rarely observed (Fig. 1.75) but can be simulated by subtalar residual deformity.

1.2.4 Muscular Balance

The muscle status in the idiopathic clubfoot is characterized by shortened calf muscles including the flexors (Mm. tib. posterior, hallucis longus, and digitorum longus), overstretched and weakened peroneal muscles, and a functional change of the anterior tibial muscle, which has a strong supinatory and less of a dorsal extending effect due to the malposition (Fig. 1.10). Even after tarsal realignment, a relative weakness of the peroneal muscles of varying degrees remains, which is an essential factor for relapse development (Gelfer et al. 2014). Recent MRI examinations show the high extent of persistent changes in the lower leg muscles (Moon et al. 2014). Especially persistent disbalance of antagonistic effects of M. tibialis anterior versus M. peroneus longus and M. tibialis posterior versus M. peroneus brevis is of major importance.

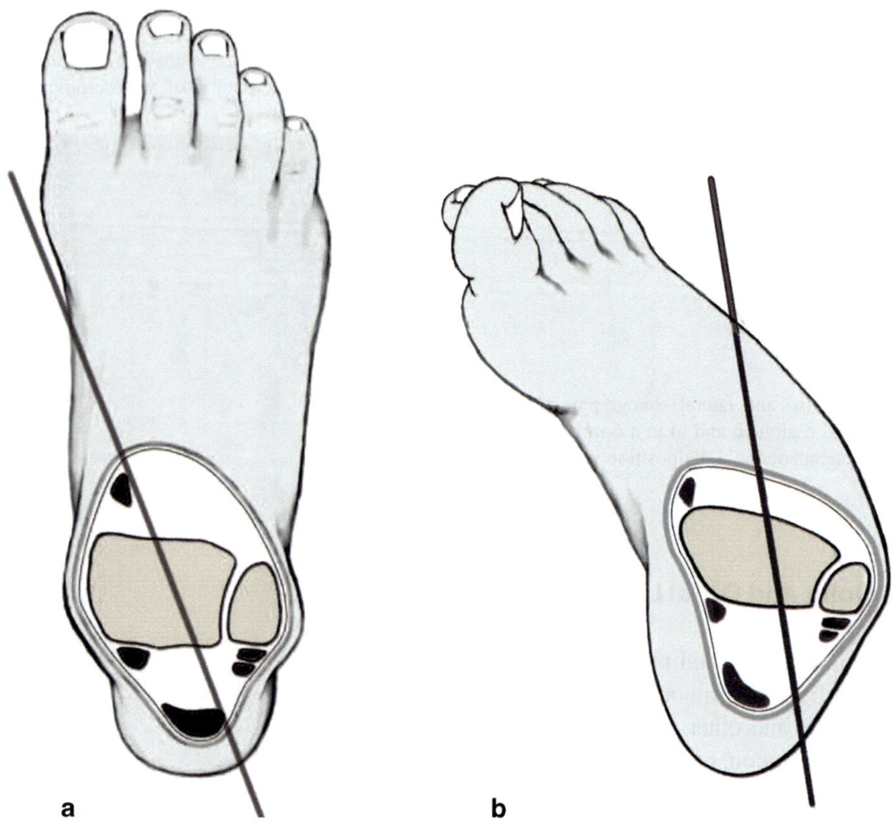

Fig. 1.10 Position of the tendons of the most important lower leg muscles in relation to the motion axis of the subtalar complex in the normal foot (**a**) and in clubfoot (**b**). The anterior tibial muscle in particular has a strong supinating effect on the clubfoot, since its tendon insertion is located far medial to the subtalar motion axis

1.3 Clinical Diagnostics and Follow-Up

Especially in the case of changing therapists and in training situations, it is important to document the findings before, during, and after the redression phase. Thereby the progress of treatment can be demonstrated but also a "plateau phase" with no further correction as well as a relapse.

Parameters Suitable for Monitoring Progress

- Dimeglio score (Fig. 1.11)
- Pirani score (Fig. 1.13)
- Rotational position of the foot in the cast (Fig. 1.32)
- Sonographic alignment (Sect. 1.4.2)

1.3.1 Examination in Infancy

During the examination of the newborn's clubfoot, particularly the *extent of deformity, rigidity, and formation of skin creases* are assessed. The malposition in spontaneous posture consists of five components: Equinus deformity contracture, hindfoot varus, peritalar inversion, midfoot and forefoot adduction, and midfoot pronation (cavus). For each singular component, it is possible to describe how far the deformity deviates from the normal position during the manual correction attempt. According to the *classification system of Dimeglio et al. (*1995*)*, point values (from 0 to 20 points) can be assigned for this, and thus the extent of deformity and rigidity can be assessed semi-quantitatively (Fig. 1.11).

During *palpation and manual examination* of the clubfoot, these findings are particularly noticeable: In all cases, the Achilles tendon is tightly tensed with shortened calf muscles, the lateral malleolus is palpated far dorsally, and the talar head is prominent at the anterolateral tarsal region. The fact that the mid- and forefoot complex is *pronated* in relation to the rear foot (Fig. 1.12) is confusing for the less experienced examiner, but of particular therapeutic importance. Although the entire

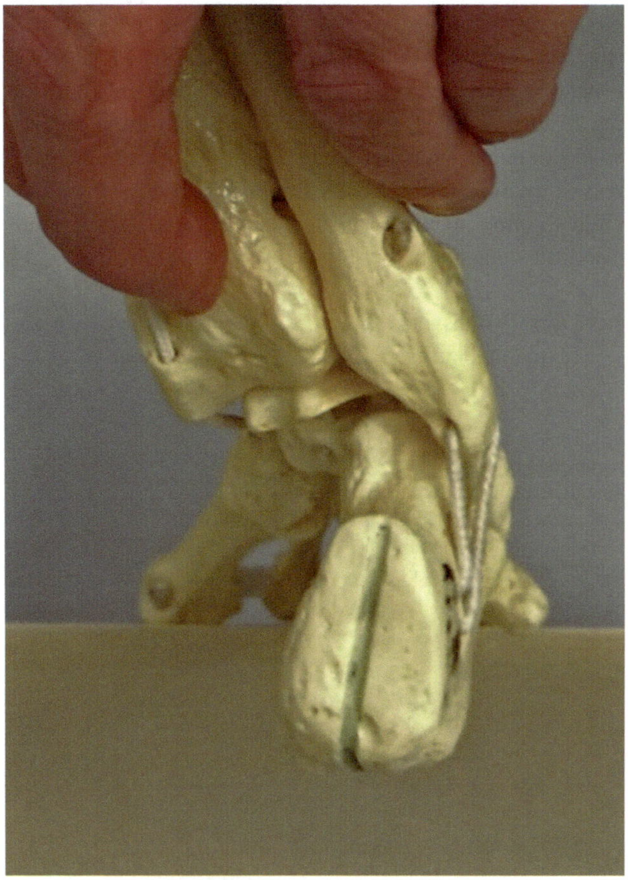

Fig. 1.12 (By O. Eberhardt) Pronation of the forefoot in relation to the rear foot, recognizable by the plantarized metatarsal I with clear inversion of the rear foot

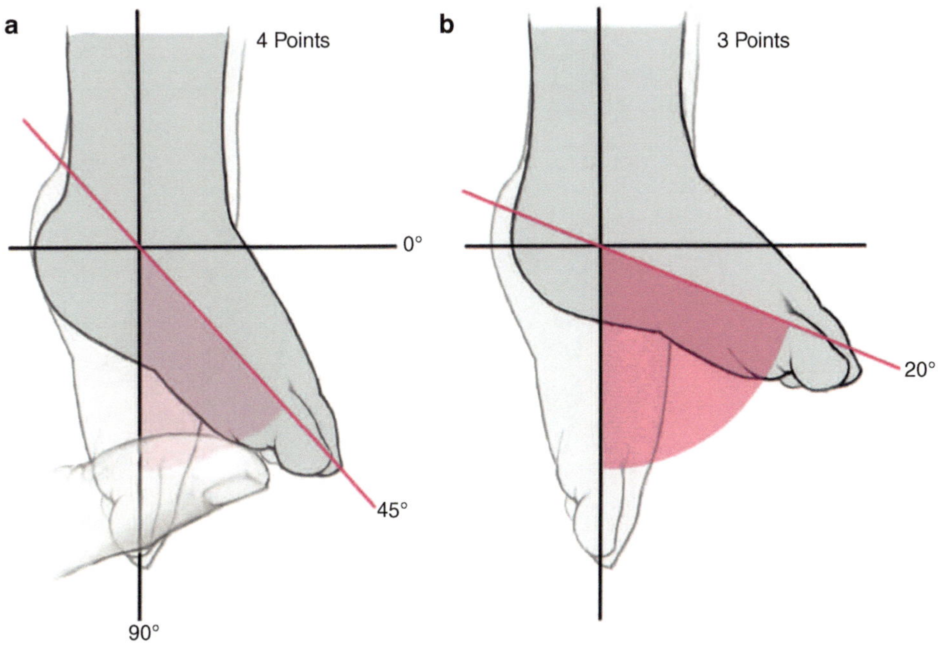

Fig. 1.11 Evaluation of the equinus component according to the Dimeglio classification. If an equinus deformity contracture of more than 45° (**a**) exists, 4 points are assigned, at 20°–45° 3 points, etc. (**b**). Similarly, the other components of malposition are recorded semi-quantitatively

foot appears supinated and the soles of both feet face each other in the case of bilateral clubfoot (Fig. 1.1), the forefoot is pronated. This mid- and forefoot pronation is synonymous with the cavus component of the medial column.

In connection with Ponseti primary therapy, the semi-quantitative Pirani score (Fig. 1.13) has worked satisfactorily, in which six individual criteria are tested and each evaluated with 0–1 point, so that severe clubfeet primarily reach up to 6 points. Repeated evaluation during the first weeks of redressment makes it possible to measure the progress of treatment. Figure 1.94 shows an example of an older child's course of treatment documented with Pirani score. The following singular criteria are evaluated:

(a) Dorsal transverse crease above the tuber calcanei (explained in Fig. 1.13a).
(b) Curved shape of the lateral foot rim (explained in Fig. 1.13b).
(c) Medial crease formation (explained in Fig. 1.13c).
(d) Laterally palpable talar head as an expression of the talonavicular malposition. Talonavicular joint palpatorily completely (0 points) or partially (0.5 points) repositionable or fixed subluxated (1 point).
(e) "Empty" heel, i.e., a cranially positioned Tuber calcanei not palpable in the heel fat pad. Tuber calcanei from plantar well palpable (0 points) or in heel cushion from plantar not palpable (1 point).
(f) The extent of the equinus contracture. Dorsal extension clearly above 0° (0 points), to neutral (0.5 points), or less than neutral (1 point).

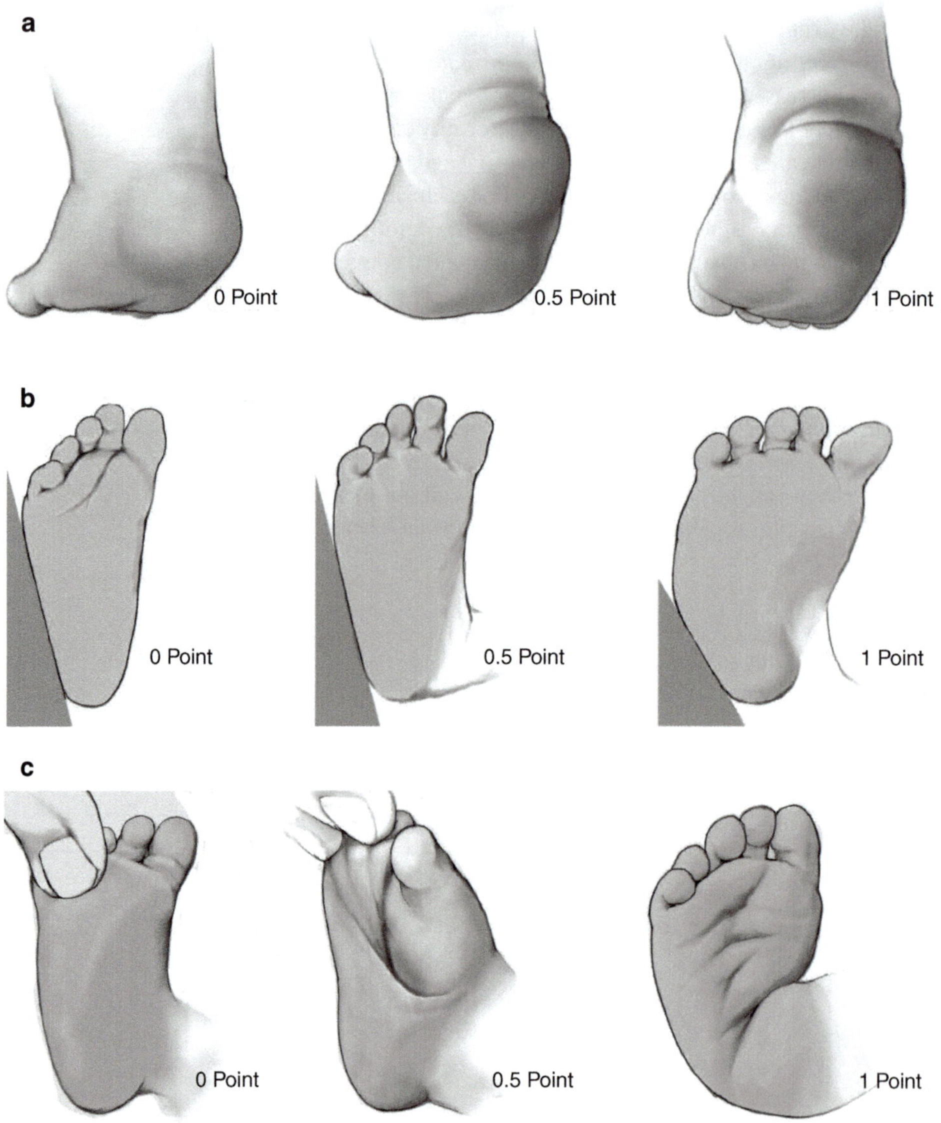

Fig. 1.13 Three of six parameters of the semi-quantitative clinical Pirani score (see text) (Pirani 2004). Dorsal crease (**a**), lateral foot rim (**b**), medial crease (**c**)

1.3.2 Assessment After Infancy

The clinical evaluation and documentation of findings during follow-up checks—mostly of pre-treated patients—in infants and schoolchildren must be carried out in the same way as described under Sect. 1.3.1. Dimeglio classification and Pirani score are also applicable. In addition, however, the foot position while standing is also assessed and a visual gait analysis is carried out. Of particular importance are:

- *Exact monitoring of the dorsal extension.* If the mobility decreases, there is a need for action. Hypermobility of the Chopart joints can simulate good mobility of the upper ankle joint. Recurrence is usually initiated by a gradual decrease in dorsal extension.
- *Assessment of the rotational profile of the lower extremity.* The foot progression angle observed in the clinical gait analysis (i.e., the orientation of the foot in relation to the gait direction) may appear normal if a still existing inversion contracture of the hindfoot is compensated by the hip joint as the complementary joint of the subtalar complex, recognizable by a laterally turned orientation of the patella. The medial and lateral malleolus (intermalleolar axis) are palpated to estimate the rotational conditions. This imaginary line connecting the malleoli is evaluated in relation to the transverse knee joint bending axis (cf. Fig. 1.75). Normally there is an outward rotation of the intermalleolar axis of not more than about 20°–25° (Fig. 1.4a).
- *The activity and effect of the anterior tibial muscle* can be closely observed during the active lifting of the foot and in the swing phase of gait. A film recording with slow-motion function is very helpful. A strong supinatory effect of this muscle due to a lack of evertor activity means a risk for relapse (see Fig. 1.56).

Numerous clinical and mixed clinical-radiological scores have been described for the evaluation of results (see Sect. 1.5.6) after clubfoot treatment (overview in: Döderlein et al. 1999; Krauspe et al. 2006). However, the significance appears limited, and the evaluation can vary greatly depending on the score that has been applied.

1.4 Diagnostic Imaging and Gait Analysis

No diagnostic imaging is required to constitute the diagnosis of idiopathic clubfoot. The significance of imaging techniques—which is not uniformly viewed in the literature—lies in the presentation of therapeutically important details in the course of treatment, in the quantification of the extent of the deformity, and in the evaluation of treatment outcome. The use of X-ray diagnostics, sonographic evaluation of tarsal alignment and pedography will be presented here, as these techniques have proven their validity to the author. An MRI, CT, or DVT (Fig. 1.24) examination is reserved for special questions.

1.4.1 X-Ray Diagnostics

Each radiographic image of the clubfoot requires a standardized adjustment technique to assess the positional relationship of the skeletal elements. False rotations or an image taken in a random spontaneous posture does not permit a meaningful evaluation.

1.4.1.1 X-Ray Diagnostics in Infancy

Since the tarsus is only partly ossified in infancy (Fig. 1.14) and the ossification nuclei are often not located centrally in the cartilaginous structures (Fig. 1.15), the informative value of X-ray images is fundamentally limited. Moreover, any attempt at radiographic imaging of the clubfoot only makes sense if the farthest possible corrected foot position is recorded.

X-ray diagnostics before the second to third month of life is practically never necessary. Before and about 4 weeks after

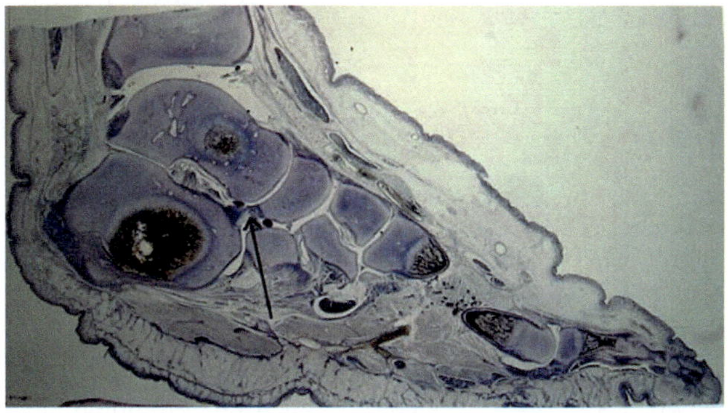

Fig. 1.14 Anatomical longitudinal section of the foot of a stillborn fetus without deformity at the age of 8 months of development. The still minimally developed ossification state and the acentric position of the osseous nuclei are visible. In contrast, the ligaments (the ligamentum bifurcatum is shown) are already clearly formed

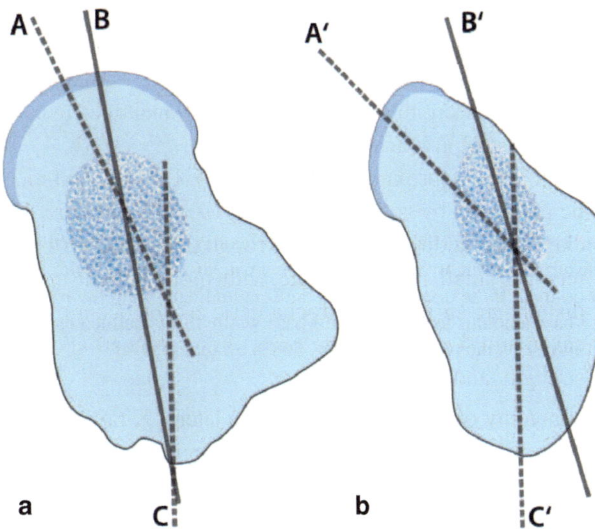

Fig. 1.15 (According to Shapiro and Glimcher 1979) Transversal cross-section through a healthy newborn talus (**a**) and a clubfoot talus with an eccentrically located osseous nucleus (**b**). The osseous nucleus axis (B and B′) describes neither the longitudinal axis of the corpus tali (C and C′) nor that of the talar neck axis (A and A′)

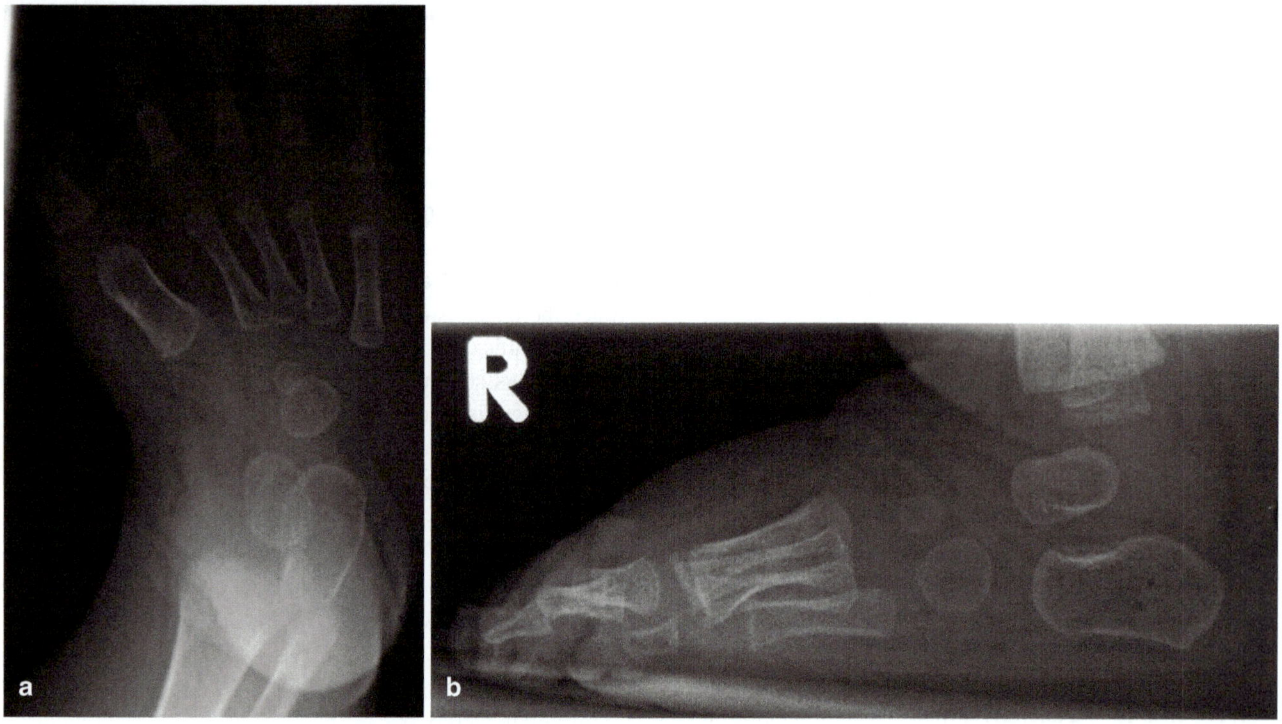

Fig. 1.16 5-week-old patient with idiopathic clubfoot, plaster redression since first week of life (tenotomy 3 weeks later). The typical signs of clubfoot can still be seen to a moderate extent, especially in the dorsoplantar image (**a**): talus-metatarsal-I-basis relationship "-2" (cf. Fig. 1.17), clear calcaneocuboid malposition. In the lateral projection, the talocalcaneal angle appears reduced (**b**)

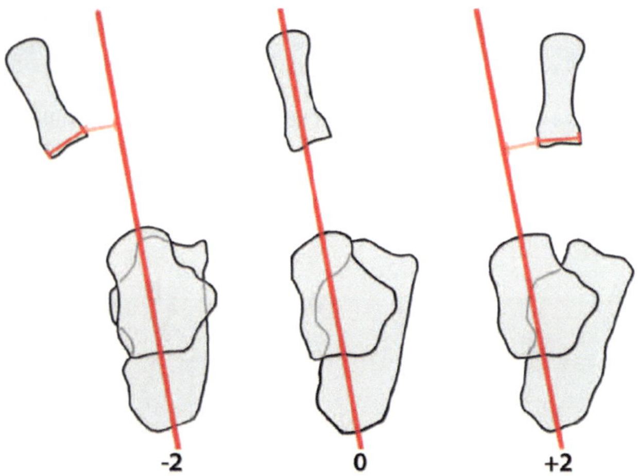

Fig. 1.17 (Indirect) assessment of the talonavicular positional relationship according to Simons (1978) in a patient who's navicular is not yet ossified. If the distance of the talar longitudinal axis to the metatarsal I base amounts to a metatarsal I base width, this is defined as "−2"; if it intersects the metatarsal I base, this is evaluated as "0"

the tenotomy of the Achilles tendon, a lateral X-ray can confirm the indication and success of the tenotomy (Fig. 1.34). This can be important in the further course (Figs. 1.20, 1.44 and 1.47) and is therefore used by the author at least in clinically ambiguous cases. Kang and Park (2015) were able to show that a lateral X-ray image with maximum dorsal extension is clearly superior to a purely clinical evaluation of the indication for tenotomy.

Still from the era of primary surgical clubfoot treatment, radiographic evaluation of tarsal alignment and assessment of findings according to Simons (1978) has generally become established, provided there is an indication for radiological imaging: a strictly lateral radiograph with a plantar support of a small wooden board in the widest possible dorsal extension for simulating an image under load is combined with a dorsoplantar image, in which the widest possible corrected position is also recorded (Fig. 1.16). These images should be taken in the rare cases of surgical correction in the first year of life and then also intraoperatively. The information obtained from the dorsoplantar image can, however, also be obtained by sonographic transverse sections (Sect. 1.4.2).

The following parameters for the description of the tarsal malposition have proven to be particularly valuable:

- *Talus-metatarsal-I-base relationship in dorsoplantar image (Fig. 1.17).*
- *Talocalcaneal angles (TC angle ap and TC angle lat.) in both planes (Figs. 1.18 and 1.19), the TC-index according to Beatson and Pearson (1966) as the sum of both talocalcaneal angles is much more meaningful than the single angles.*
- *Anterior tibio-calcaneal angle (ATC angle) to describe the equinus component in the lateral projection (Fig. 1.19).*
- *Talus-metatarsal I angle in the lateral projection (TMT-I angle lat.) to describe the cavus component (cf., e.g., Fig. 1.44a).*

Normal Values of Tarsal X-Ray Parameters
- TC angle ap (>20°)
- TC angle lat (>25°)
- TC index (>40°)
- ATC angle (<75°–80°)
- TMT-I angle lat (<+10°)
- Talus-metatarsal I base relationship ("0" to "+2")

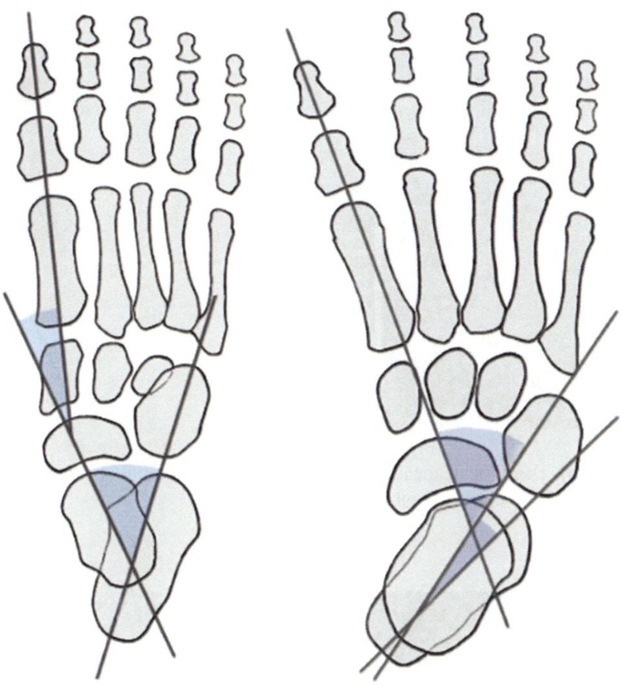

Fig. 1.18 Determination of the TC angle ap and the TMT-I angle ap for normal foot with negative values (**a**) and club foot with positive values (**b**). With the TMT-I angle ap, the hindfoot inversion and the mid-foot forefoot adduction are recorded in combination

1.4.1.2 X-Ray Diagnostics After Infancy

Even in toddlers and schoolchildren, the use of X-ray diagnostics is only necessary for a given special indication. Whenever possible, X-rays should be carried out while the patient is standing. When positioning for the lateral image, particular attention should be paid to any remaining malpositioning components: The medial and lateral malleolus should be adjusted by rotating the foot so that their connecting line (intermalleolar axis) is not rotated more than about 20°–25° outwards from the knee joint motion axis ("hind-foot-centered" imaging technique; see Sect. 7.3). Indications for X-ray diagnostics include, among others:

- Insufficient or regressive dorsal extension of the upper ankle joint after tenotomy to assess heel position (Fig. 1.53).
- Before and after each surgical correction for indication and outcome documentation. Minor, but already functionally effective malpositions are often radiologically with-

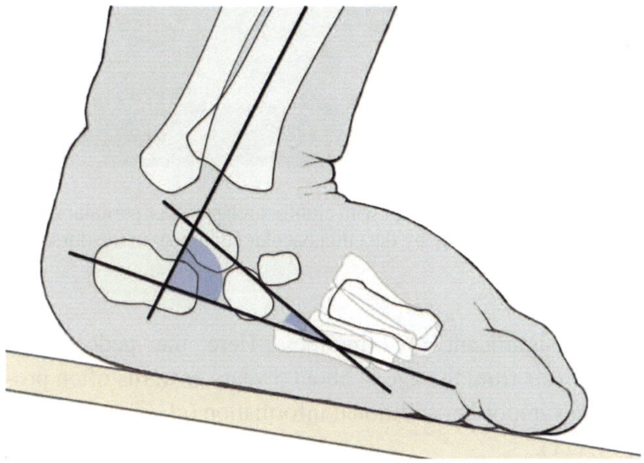

Fig. 1.19 Determining the ATC angle (anterior tibio-calcaneal angle) and the TC angle lat. The lateral projection is taken in a simulated weight-bearing position with a wooden board below the foot

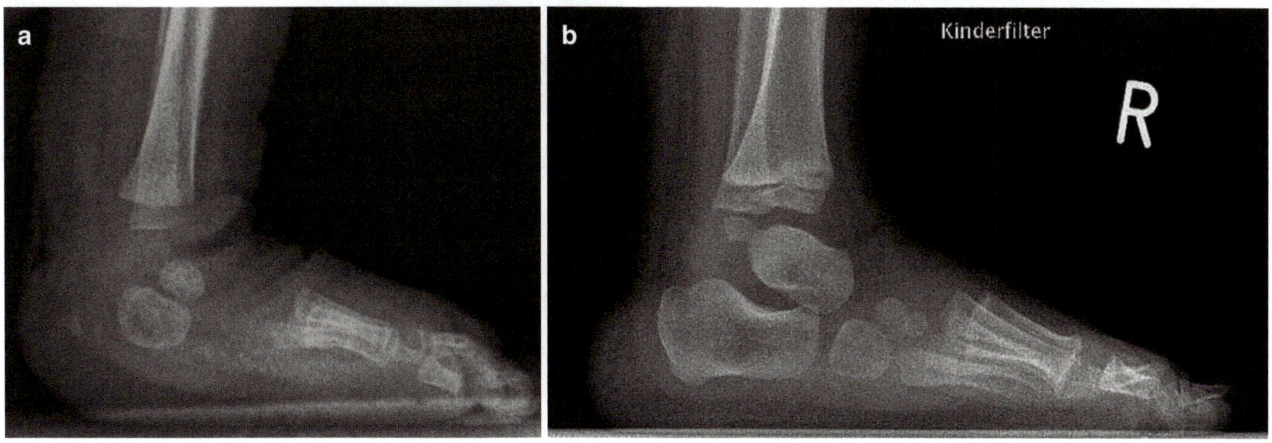

Fig. 1.20 Lateral X-ray projection of an idiopathic clubfoot in a newborn (**a**). The ATC angle is over 90°, thus a clear indication for tenotomy (see Sect. 1.5.2). In this image also, the contours of the cartilaginous shape of the calcaneus can be observed. With 1.5 years (**b**) acceptable corrected position, however, with still significantly increased ATC angle and reduced calcaneal pitch angle (requires observation)

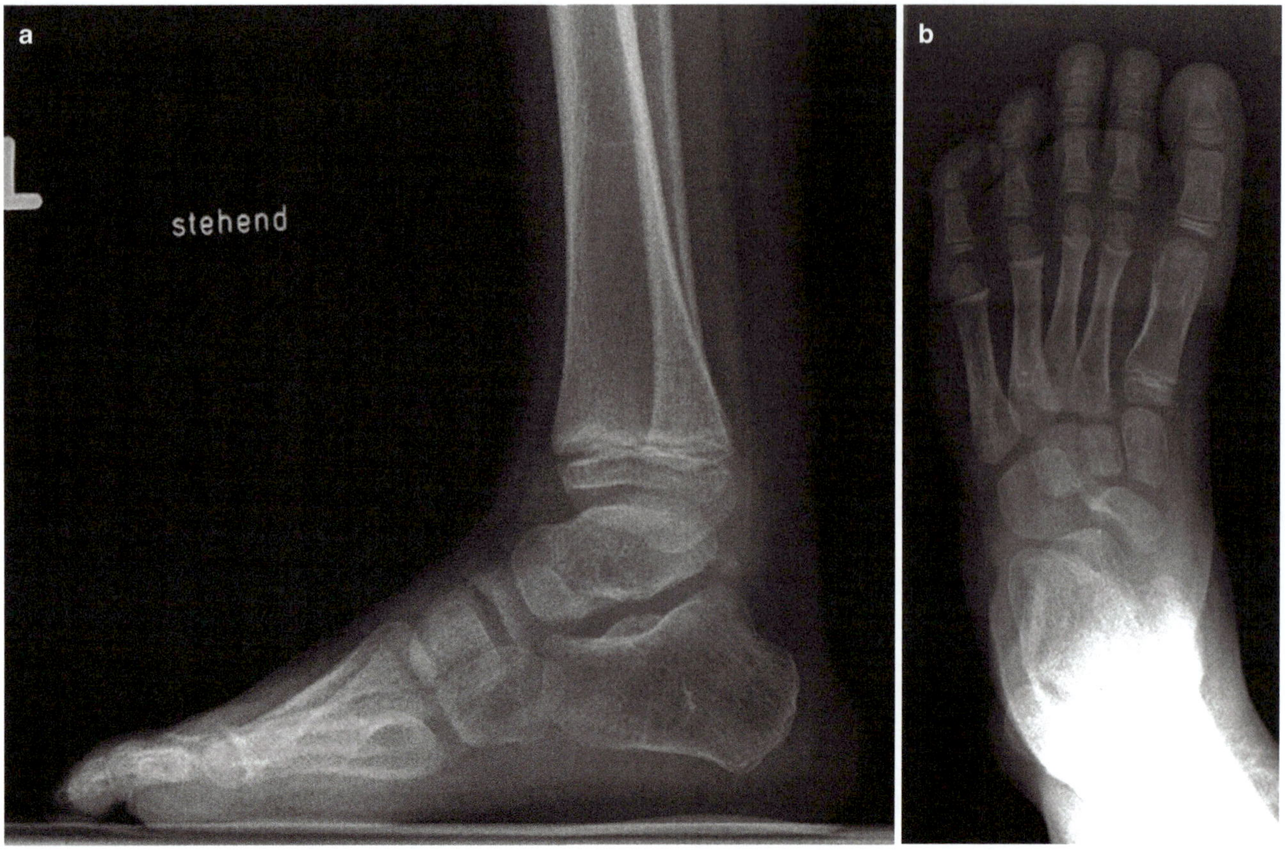

Fig. 1.21 5-year-old patient with clubfoot relapse after peritalar release (**a** and **b**). The talocalcaneal-navicular complex is incompletely corrected, recognizable especially by the talonavicular alignment in the dorsoplantar image (**b**); a new surgical intervention is planned

out significant abnormalities. Here the pedographic analysis from the age of about 5 years onwards often provides important additional information (cf. Figs. 1.69 and 1.111).

- Talonavicular alignment in the dorsoplantar projection (Fig. 1.21), but due to the late ossification of the os naviculare not directly assessable before about the age of 4–5 years (sonography in younger children superior!)
- Suspicion of significant shape disorders of individual skeletal elements (e.g., flat top talus (Fig. 1.22), navicular malformation, upper ankle joint valgus deformity, lack of slope (inclination of the joint surface) of the tibial base in the lateral projection). The "Anterior Talar Motion Segment" (Fig. 1.23) measures the capacity of the ankle joint for dorsal extension and remains reduced even in treated clubfeet with otherwise overall good results.
- Preoperative planning in severe deformities can be facilitated by 3-D reconstruction (Fig. 1.24).

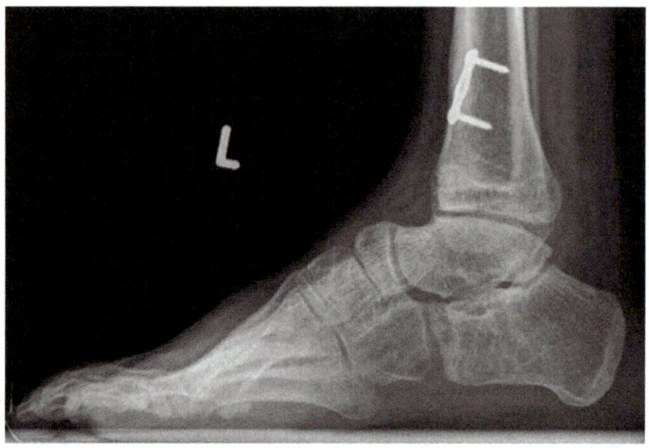

Fig. 1.22 15-year-old clubfoot patient with a peritalar release performed externally and further previous operations. The extreme flattening of the trochlea tali ("flat top talus") is well recognizable and decisive for the planning and success prospects of further surgical measures

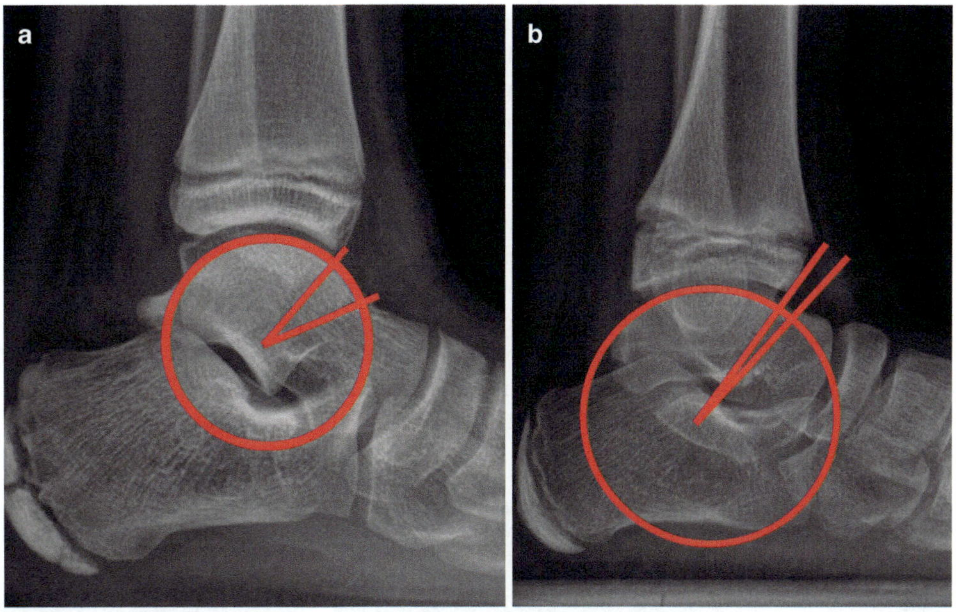

Fig. 1.23 The "Anterior Talar Motion Segment" of a normal foot (**a**) in comparison to a clubfoot (**b**). The radius of the trochlea tali is increased and the available range of motion for dorsal extension of the ankle joint is diminished in clubfeet

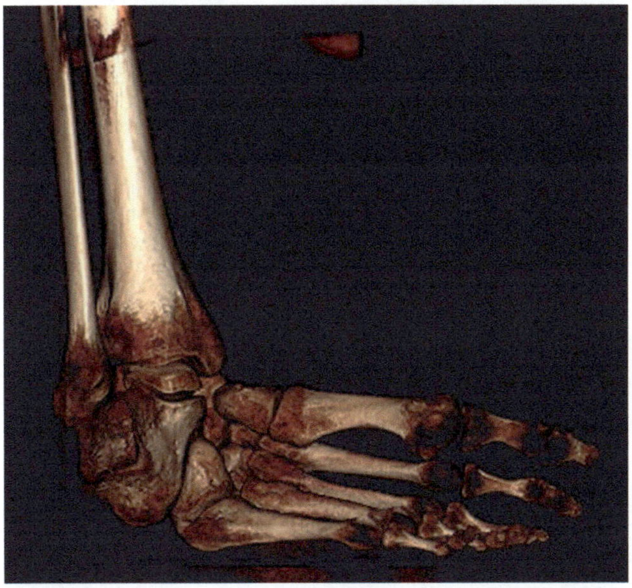

Fig. 1.24 Digital Volume Tomogram (DVT) with 3-D reconstruction in a weight-bearing position of a severe neglected clubfoot of an 18-year-old patient. The marked peritalar dislocation can be evaluated precisely and appropriate surgical correction can be planned thereby

1.4.2 Sonographic Assessment of Tarsometatarsal Alignment

Since the foot skeleton—and in particular the os naviculare—is still predominantly cartilaginous in infancy and only partly ossified in early childhood, sonography seems to be especially useful for the depiction of the positional conditions like in the child's hip joint. In the literature since the 1990s, there have been several suggestions for technique and assessment, all of which have not yet been widely used. The author's technique will be presented, since it has proven itself in routine practice and furthermore allows a more precise understanding of the tarsal deformity and its correction effects already in infancy (Hamel and Becker 1996). It can largely replace dorsoplantar X-rays and is superior to them in some respects. The examiner can be sure, for example, that the maximum corrected position has actually been recorded.

With sonographic alignment assessment, the "regions of interest" described in Sect. 1.2 can be dynamically represented in the widest possible corrected position. For the tibiotalar joint and the calcaneocuboid region, examples can be found in Figs. 1.7 and 1.9. In practice however, the representation of the medial talonavicular region (see Sect. 1.2.1) in an *oblique transverse section* (Fig. 1.26), which can also be evaluated quantitatively, has proved particularly effective. This allows the center of the hindfoot inversion (with shortened and deformed talus as well as the talonavicular subluxation and false correction effects at the naviculo-cuneiforme joint) and thus of the clubfoot as a whole to be recorded. This is possible alternatively only by magnetic resonance imaging (Pirani et al. 2001), however, without the advantage of dynamic examination.

During the examination in infancy and early childhood, the child is examined sitting on the mother's lap, and the mother turns the thigh of the leg strongly inwards so that the examiner can use one hand to position the foot in maximum eversion. A 7.5 mHz transducer with a transducer width of preferably approx. 5–6 cm is placed on the medial foot margin using a silicone pad for better coupling (Fig. 1.25), and the medial malleolus, talar head-neck region, the cartilaginously formed medial navicular pole, the likewise cartilaginous structure of the medial cuneiform, and the metatarsal I base are presented with the greatest possible manual correction of the clubfoot deformity. Due to the coupling problems of the transducer in the newborn, this is often only possible after one or two phases of redressive plaster casts but then allows the talonavicular malalignment to be precisely determined. It is not uncommon to find discrepancies with the clinical impression. Ponseti's view, which the complete talonavicular reduction is always clinically well recognizable, cannot be fully agreed to from sonographic experience. The findings gained from the application of sonographic alignment diagnostics in the follow-up of Ponseti-treated children are summarized in Sect. 1.5.6.2. Sonography can also be used in preoperative diagnostics (cf. Fig. 1.52).

For the quantification of inversion contracture, two proposals have been described in the recent literature on sonographic alignment diagnostics: Measurement of the distance of the medial malleolus/medial navicular pole (depending on the foot size) according to Aurell et al. (2005) and angle measurement of the talonavicular region (independent of the foot size) according to Hamel and Becker (1993, 1996), adopted, e.g., also by Suda et al. (2006) and Desai et al. (2008). The determination of the TnC_E angle (Fig. 1.26) and its derivation are explained in more detail (see box "The TnC_E angle"). Figures 1.27 and 1.28 show comparative examples of both feet in unilateral clubfoot of different ages with drawn TnC_E angles.

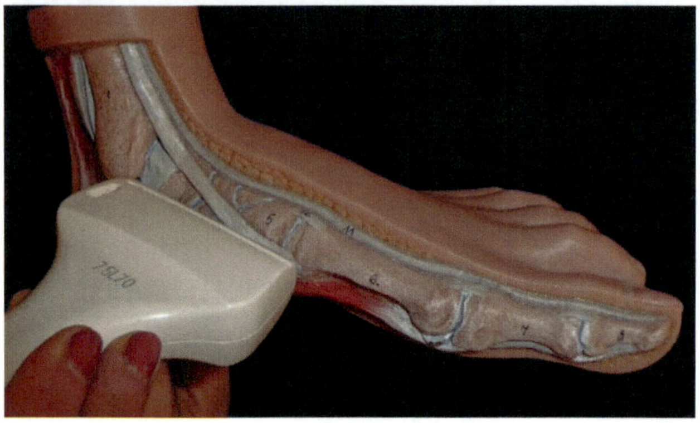

Fig. 1.25 Positioning of the transducer for the oblique medial transverse section (the required silicone pad is not shown)

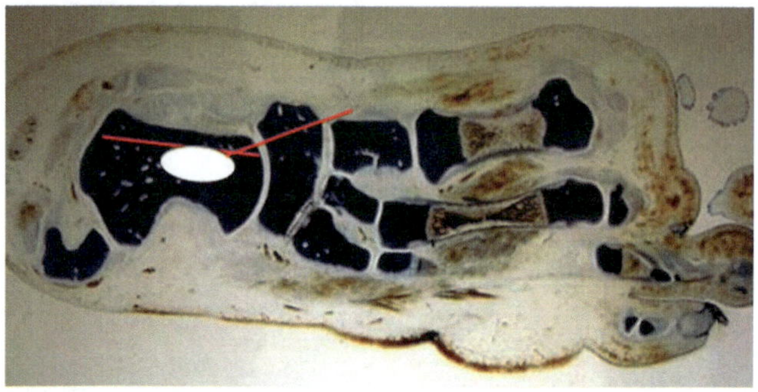

Fig. 1.26 Transverse section through a foot from the eighth month of prenatal development in the sectional plane corresponding to the sonographic transverse section. A talar nucleus (not yet present at this age, but appearing later) and the TnC_E angle were drawn in

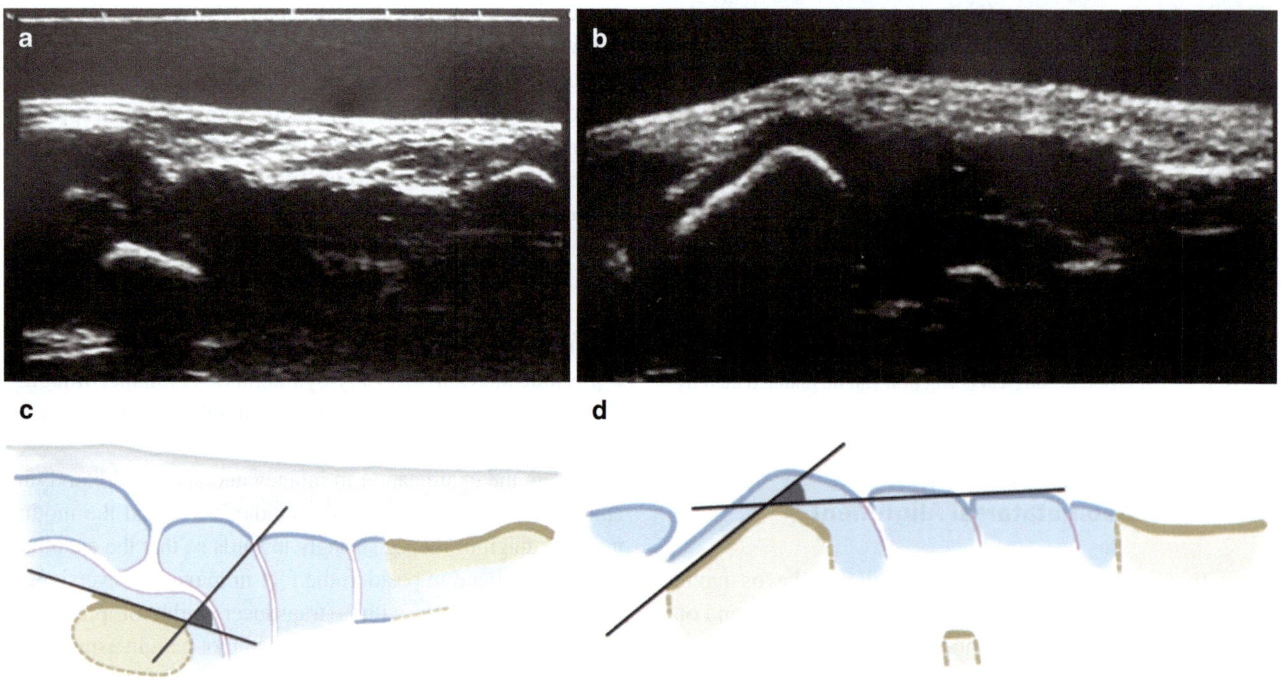

Fig. 1.27 Sonographic transverse section of an uncorrected clubfoot at the age of 5 months (**a** and **c**) with a TnC_E angle of approx. +75° and a healthy opposite side (**b** and **d**) with a TnC_E angle of approx. −30°

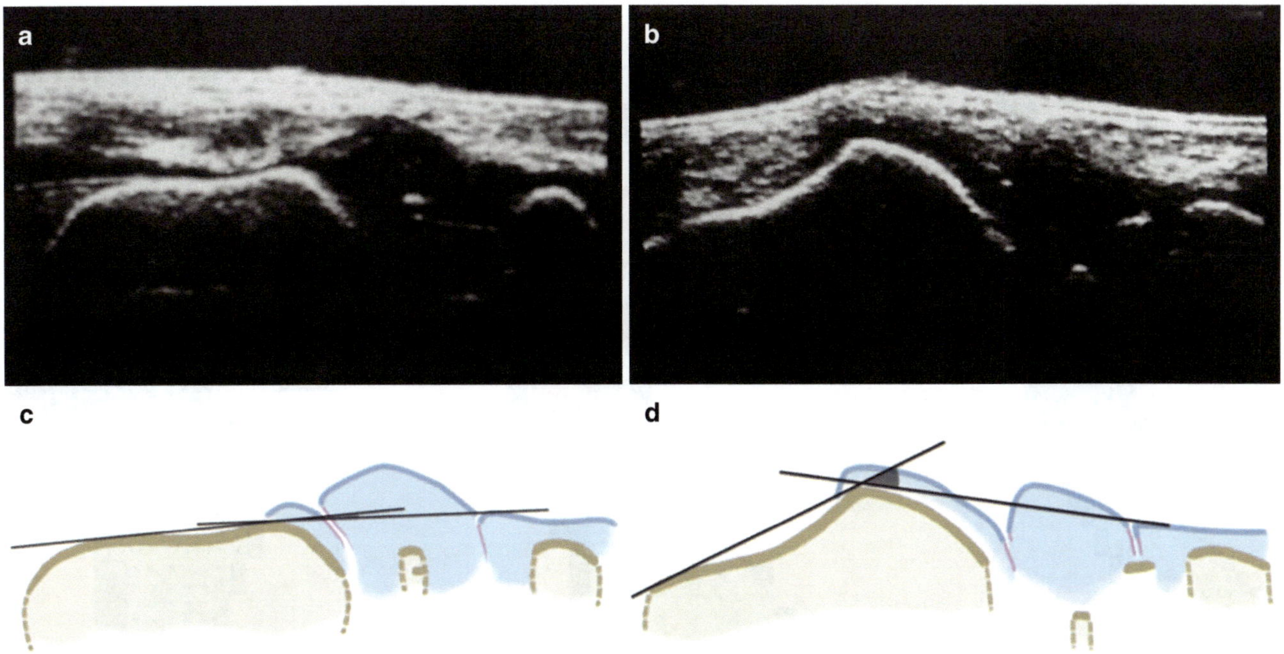

Fig. 1.28 Sonographic transverse section in a 4-year-old child with unilateral clubfoot, Ponseti pretreatment with clinically good results (**a** and **c**), TnC_E angle just below 0°. The normalization of the talar shape and the good talonavicular alignment are visible. In comparison to the healthy opposite side (**b** and **d**), however, the mobility of the hindfoot (eversion) remains clearly limited, as can be seen from the TnC_E angle of −28°

The TnC_E Angle (After Hamel and Becker 1993) as a Measure of the Peritalar Inversion (cf. Fig. 1.26)

- Tangent to the longitudinal axis of the medial contour of the talar osseous nucleus ("Tn").
- Line between the point at which the bone contour of the talus deviates laterally and the most medial point of the (cartilaginous) contour of the medial cuneiform structure ("C").
- The widest possible correction in eversion ("E") should be recorded.
- The medial navicular pole itself is not suitable as a landmark because it shows great individual differences.
- The normal range of the TnC_E angle is about −20° to −30° and is largely constant in the first years of life; for severe untreated clubfeet, initial values of up to +60° to +90° are measured.

1.4.3 Pedography

Pedography, as a common gait-analytic procedure, is of practical value for the assessment of the functional condition of clubfoot subsequent states from the age of about 5 years, especially in the context of follow-up examinations. Examples are presented in Sect. 1.6. Wallace et al. (2016) provide an overview of the literature on pedographic analyses of the normal and deformed child's foot. Among the numerous, also quantitative information that a pedographic analysis provides, it is first of all the maximum pressure image with recording of the center of pressure progression line, which permits information about the foot function during the stance phase and is preferably used in the treatment examples presented here. A color scale marks the measured peak pressures clearly and semi-quantitatively, which are also indicated as numbers in each field of the measuring plate (ascending from low to high peak pressure as black, dark blue, light blue, green, yellow, red, or violet; see Fig. 1.29c). The gait line ("center of pressure progression," COPP-line) indicates the position of the body's center of gravity, how and in what chronological sequence it moves over the loaded area during the stance phase of gait in marked sections of 10 ms. The treatment examples presented in Sect. 1.6, in particular, clearly show that pedography can provide valuable additional information compared to X-ray diagnostics, for example. For the clubfoot therapist, there are essentially four practical areas of application:

1. Analysis and documentation of clubfoot (relapse) conditions. Pedographic characteristics of the (recurrent) clubfoot are, among others, the high load on the lateral metatarsus with extensive lack of load transmission of the hindfoot and medial metatarsal ray with lateralization of the center of pressure progression line (e.g., Fig. 1.29b).
2. Diagnosis of severe functional changes in clubfoot overcorrection (Hamel 2011; Hamel and Nell 2016). The load pattern that deviates significantly from the normal with a

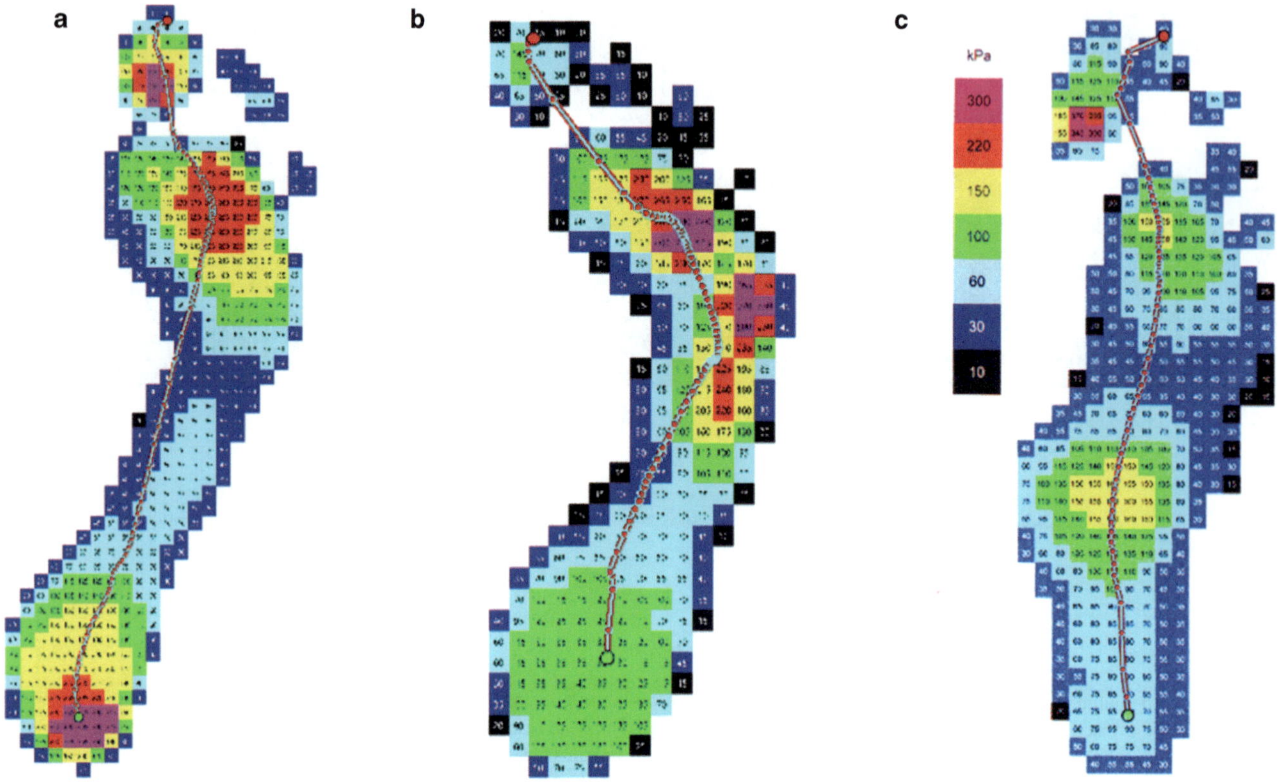

Fig. 1.29 Typical examples of a pedographic maximum pressure recording of a normal juvenile foot (**a**), a 6-year-old patient with clubfoot relapse (**b**, see text) and a severe clubfoot overcorrection (**c**)

lack of indentation and overloading in the middle foot segment with reduced peak pressures in the forefoot area, compensated by increased use of toe flexors, are typical pedographic signs of overcorrection (e.g., Fig. 1.29c).

3. Evaluation of the therapeutic effects of secondary interventions. Pedographically, the functional changes achieved in schoolchildren and adolescents can be represented, including remaining unphysiological load distributions (e.g., Fig. 1.76d).
4. Pedography reveals to be the most sensitive method for detecting slight functional abnormalities. In the evaluation of healing results according to different forms of primary treatment, pedography proves to be the most accurate method with which even minor deviations from the normal can be recorded. For example, the more recent literature reports pedographically documented functional deviations even with favorable outcome results after Ponseti primary therapy (Sinclair et al. 2009; Kelly et al. 2017), which may be important for the further refinement of clubfoot primary therapy (cf. also Fig. 1.42c). One of the main characteristics in clubfeet treated according to the Ponseti concept with good clinical results is the altered load transmission at the metatarsals with a shift from medial to lateral compared to normal feet (Sinclair et al. 2009). Huber and Dutoit (2004) found a correlation between preserved hindfoot pronation at the early stance phase of walking, detected pedographically by a short medial deviation of the center of pressure line immediately after heel strike, and a better long-term prognosis in surgically treated clubfeet.

1.5 Treatment Concepts for Clubfoot Primary Therapy

1.5.1 Therapy Change in the Last Decades

Every clubfoot therapy concept consists of three treatment phases—*reposition, (surgical) release, and retention.* In recent decades, three main concepts have been widespread in Central Europe:

- The *Imhäuser concept* (Imhäuser 1984) with redression plaster phase after the three-point correction principle similar to Kite's method (including "Kite's error"), limited purely dorsal release (Achilles tendon and dorsal capsule) at the age of about 3–4 months and long-time splinting follow-up treatment.
- The *peritalar release* (McKay 1983a, b) with extended capsulolysis for single-stage subtalar derotation at the age of about 4–10 months after preparatory plaster redression and with subsequent splint retention, widely used in the 1990s.

- The *Ponseti treatment concept* (Ponseti 1992, 1996), which has prevailed since about the year 2000 in Central Europe (and worldwide), is today the method of choice (Zionts et al. 2012) and will be discussed here in detail. It does not differ from the previously customary peritalar release in that it also strives for subtalar derotation, but it does so in a non-surgical way. The superiority of the Ponseti concept over the peritalar release is now well documented in the literature (e.g., Ippolito et al. 2003; Smith et al. 2014).

1.5.2 Primary Treatment According to the Ponseti Concept

The Ponseti concept envisages the correction of the idiopathic clubfoot in three treatment steps: Subtle redressive plaster technique according to pathomorphologically justified principles of subtalar derotation with weekly change of the long-leg cast, percutaneous tenotomy of the Achilles tendon, and retention in a foot abduction orthosis up to the age of 4.

In the first treatment step, the middle-forefoot pronation is first corrected by one or two redressive plaster dressings (Fig. 1.30a). This is done by raising the medial foot ray and placing the medial forefoot in correct relation to the hindfoot. After this redression step, the entire sole of the foot appears still inclined, facing the contralateral foot.

Only then is the inversion contracture of the peritalar complex addressed (subtalar derotation). For this purpose, the mid-forefoot segment including the calcaneus is rotated in an outward direction in relation to the talus, fixed by smooth counter-pressure at the talar head-neck region. Thereby a successive derotation of the subtalar foot plate with respect to the talus occurs (Figs. 1.30b and 1.31). Here, the calcaneus is not touched by the therapist's redressive hands. It corrects itself spontaneously in such a way that the tuber calcanei moves medially and the hindfoot varus component (cf. Fig. 1.12) is transferred to a physiological valgus position (Fig. 1.31b, c). No (forced) attempt is made to correct the equinus component. With increasing correction of the peritalar complex, the equinus component is also spontaneously reduced to a certain degree. In the respective best possible position, the foot is fixed in the long-leg cast, which is changed weekly. Clinically, the increasing correction can be seen in the progressive external rotation of the foot in relation to the longitudinal axis of the thigh up to 70° (Figs. 1.31 and 1.32).

a

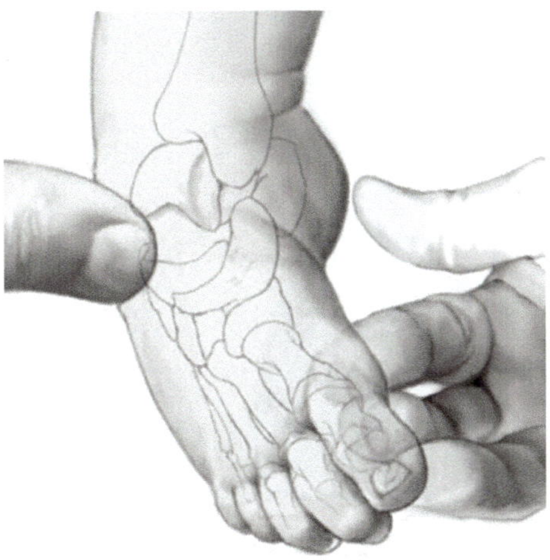

b

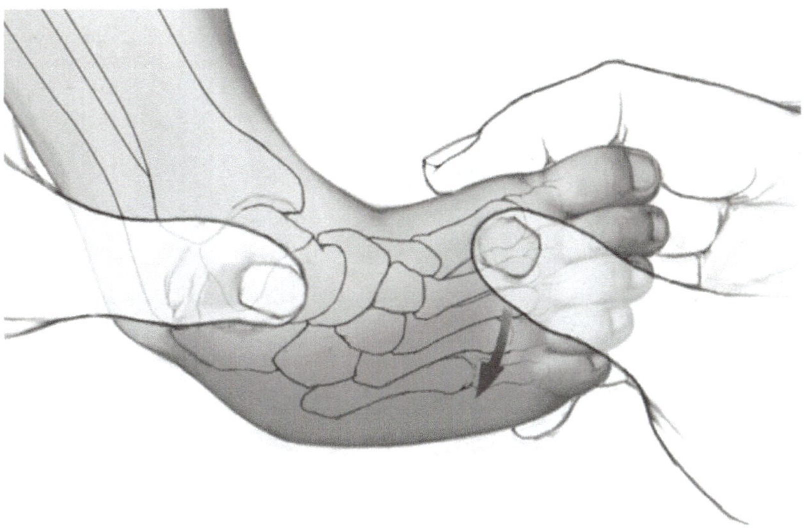

Fig. 1.30 In the first step of redression, the cavus component of the medial ray is corrected (**a**), only then is the peritalar complex corrected with stepwise reduction of the inversion contracture (**b**) by rotation of the subtalar foot plate outwards against the talus fixed by manual counter-pressure at the talar head-neck region

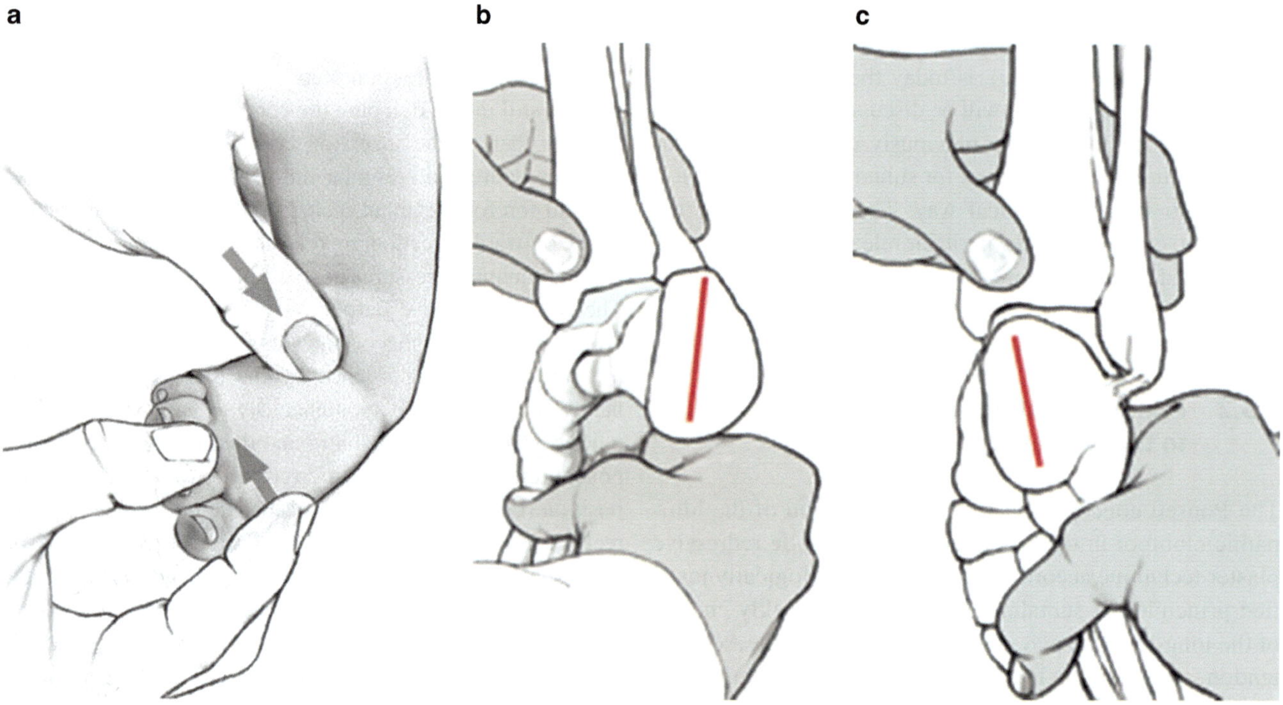

Fig. 1.31 In a later stage of redressment, the foot is clearly rotated outwards (**a**). The dorsal view shows how the hindfoot varus (**b**) also corrects itself within the subtalar derotation and the tuber calcanei moves medially, so that the fibulocalcaneal ligament comes under tension (**c**)

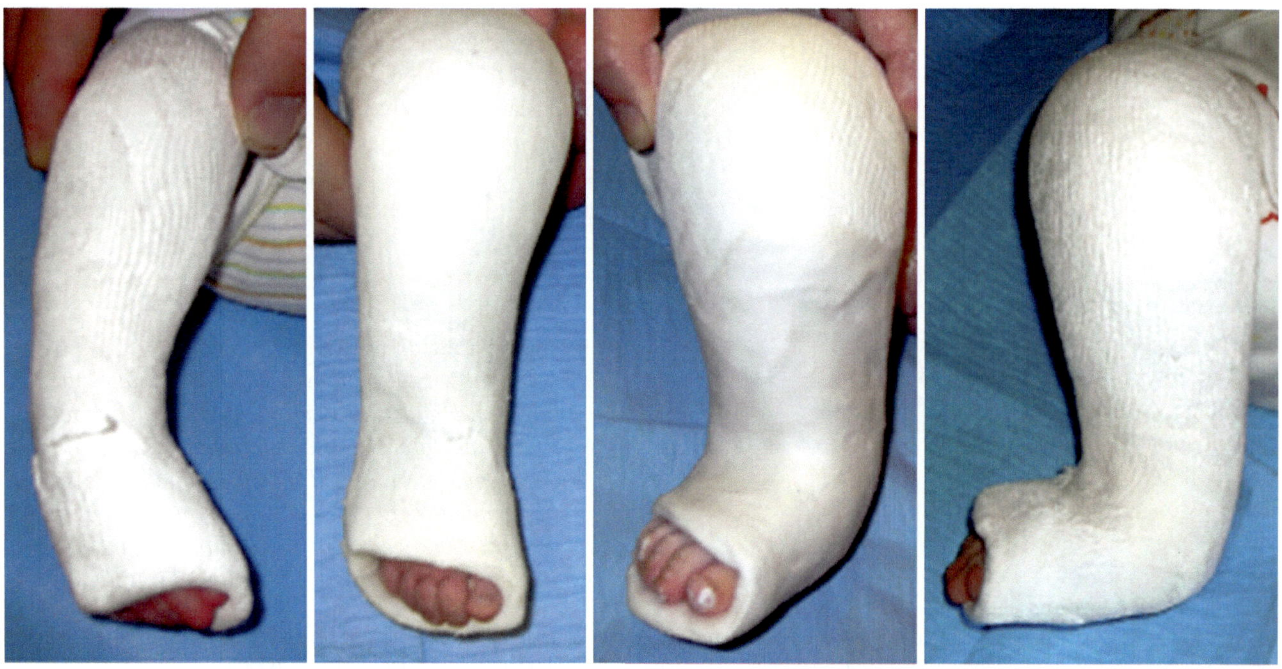

Fig. 1.32 (Picture by O. Eberhardt) Sequence of redressive cast dressings with increasing correction. The foot is outward rotated up to 70° in relation to the thigh in the final cast

The proceeding correction should be documented with the semi-quantitative clinical Pirani score (Sect. 1.3.1 and Fig. 1.94). Monitoring of the process of increasing reduction of the talonavicular joint is possible by sonography. Follow-up ultrasound observations show that the skeletal correction process is often not completed until months later, when the retention splint is already being used (Sect. 1.5.3).

Plaster Technique
- Cotton wool padding only one to two layers (stocking optional).
- No paper.
- Plaster of Paris (approx. two 6 cm rolls at newborn age).
- Soft cast is possible alternatively, but correction will be less precise.
- In difficult cases, plastering in two stages (first up to the middle of the lower leg).
- Thigh included up to the groin.
- 90° knee flexion.
- Forming of a supracondylar undercut against slipping.

After usually about 5–7 redressive cast dressings and according to clinical criteria, full correction of the hindfoot inversion and plateau phase in the Pirani score, a percutaneous tenotomy of the Achilles tendon is performed followed by immobilization for another 3–4 weeks in the long-leg cast dressing in clear abduction and about 15°–20° dorsal extension. It is an absolute exception if this tenotomy does not seem necessary in mild cases. In case of doubt, the tenotomy should be performed, as it is associated with hardly any risks and considerably facilitates further treatment. In borderline cases, a lateral X-ray (anterior tibio-calcaneal angle >75°–80°) shows more precisely than the clinical assessment, whether the calcaneus position is acceptable (Kang and Park 2015). As a rule, continuity of the Achilles tendon can be well palpated again approx. 6 weeks after tenotomy. It is important that a dorsal extension of at least 15°–20° is achieved clinically after the tenotomy, if necessary after a second manipulation and cast change 1 week after tenotomy. Otherwise, the probability of further later interventions is high (Hosseinzadeh et al. 2015).

Primary correction is achieved with the Ponseti treatment in experienced hands in about 95% of cases. A tenotomy is recommended in almost all cases and also facilitates the subsequent splint treatment. Radler et al. (2007) found a reduction of the anterior tibio-calcaneal angle of 16.9° by the tenotomy on average (see Fig. 1.34). In some cases, in which percutaneous tenotomy had to be followed later by open surgery, there was hardly any obvious scarring in the area of the previously tenotomized Achilles tendon.

Tenotomy (Fig. 1.33)
- *Up to the age of about 6 months usually without anesthesia (Emla patch, paracetamol suppository, possibly also local anesthetics, but then, the tendon is more difficult to palpate).*
- *Mother (father) lying or half-sitting on the examination table, child lying in close physical contact with mother (father).*
- *Palpate tendon above calcaneus well and several times, mark if necessary.*
- *Let the assistant hold the thigh well fixed.*
- *Therapist holds the foot with one hand in dorsal extended position of the ankle.*
- *Double skin disinfection.*
- *A single-use 15 mm scalpel is inserted medial of the Achilles tendon about 1 cm above the calcaneus in the longitudinal direction (caution: calcaneus can be positioned high up!).*
- *The scalpel is rotated 90° and the tendon is cut from inside out without damaging the skin; a distinct loss of resistance can be felt, sometimes even heard.*
- *The incision is covered in sterile way, suture or steri-strips are not necessary.*
- *After the tenotomy 3–4 weeks of long-leg cast in 60°–70° abduction and the widest possible dorsal extension, if the primary dorsal extension of approx. 15°–20° is not reached, a cast change with remanipulation is scheduled.*

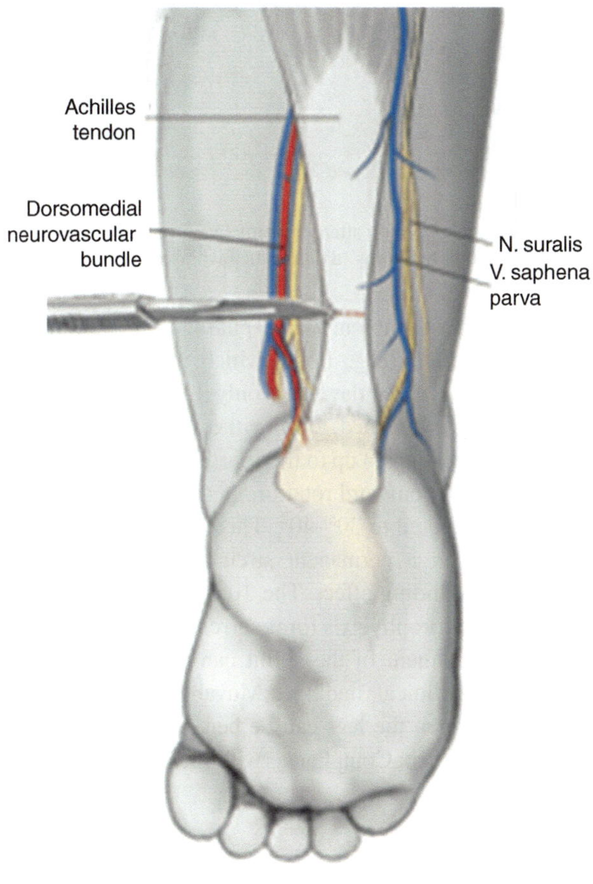

Fig. 1.33 Percutaneous tenotomy of the Achilles tendon. The scalpel is inserted at the medial edge of the Achilles tendon, and the tendon is completely severed from inside to outside

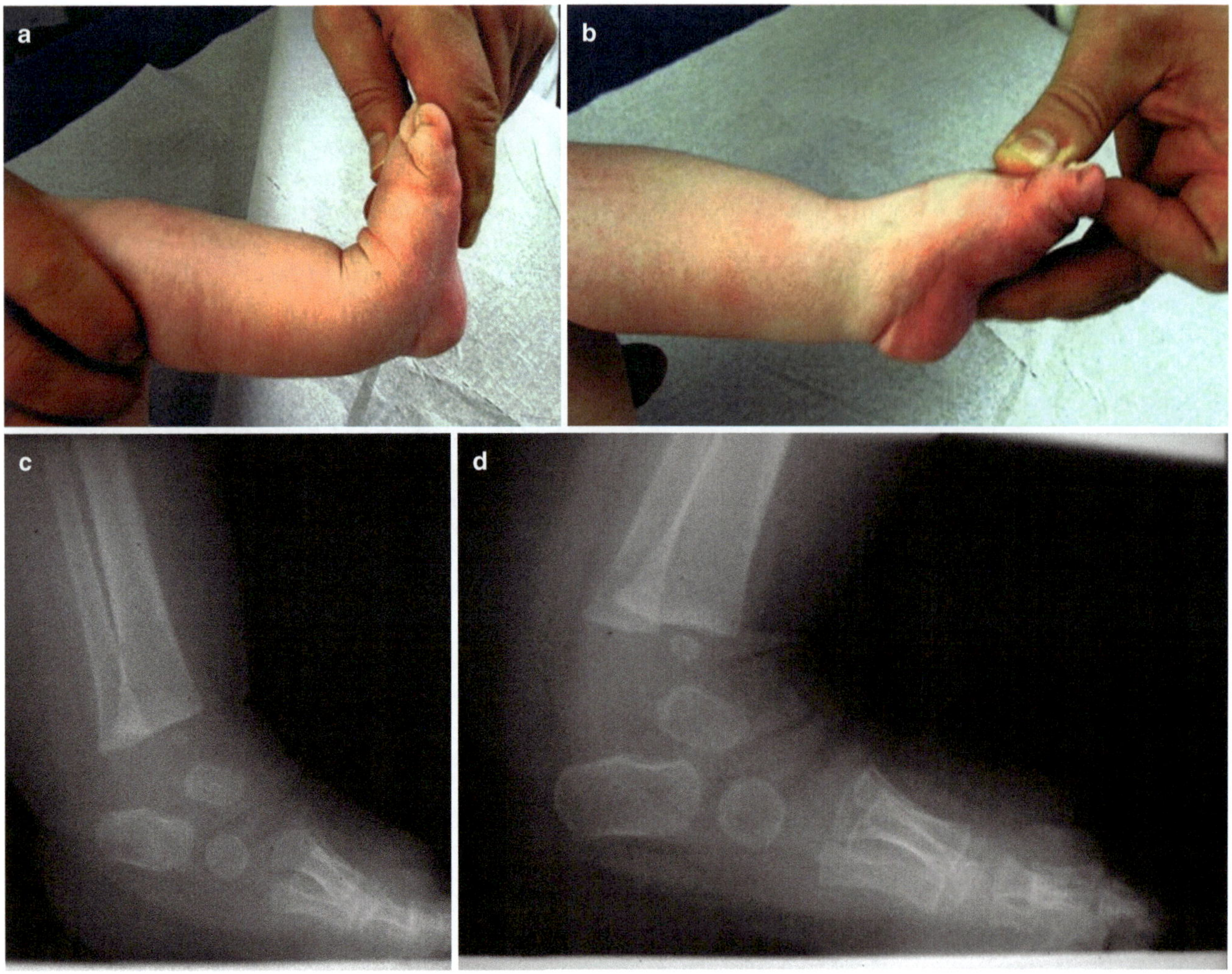

Fig. 1.34 Range of motion after tenotomy in a 5-month-old child (external pretreatment) with almost free mobility (**a** and **b**). X-ray examination before (**c**) and after tenotomy (**d**) show the favorable skeletal realignment with a clear effect on the ATC angle in the lateral projection

After the post-tenotomy cast phase, a foot abduction orthosis is applied (Fig. 1.35), which must be worn for 3 months for 23 h per day, then only 15 h per day (target value not always reached) during the sleep phases of the child ("night and naps") up to the fourth birthday. The splint is adjusted to 70° outward rotation, in the case of the opposite side not affected to 30°–40°. This keeps the soft tissues dorsomedially in a permanent stretching position with a strong growth-guiding effect. The 10°–15° dorsal extension setting provides prophylaxis for recurrence of equinus deformity. The adjustment of the splint can be easily modified depending on clinical findings. Movable splints are also available, in which the legs can be bent and stretched individually in the knee. Compliance with these orthoses is better, but the dorsal extension is sometimes less consistently preserved, depending on the posture of the child.

The initiation of brace treatment is one critical phase of Ponseti treatment and compliance problems are not uncommon. The slipping of the foot out of the orthosis is closely associated with pressure sores in the heel area and on the dorsum of the foot. These problems are to be expected, especially if the dorsal extension is not significantly more than 10°. Once the brace treatment has been successfully initiated, there are hardly any problems to be expected in the following months. From the end of the second year of life however, brace problems can occur more frequently, especially if the splint management is not completely consistent and "ritualized" by the parents or if initial recurrences are

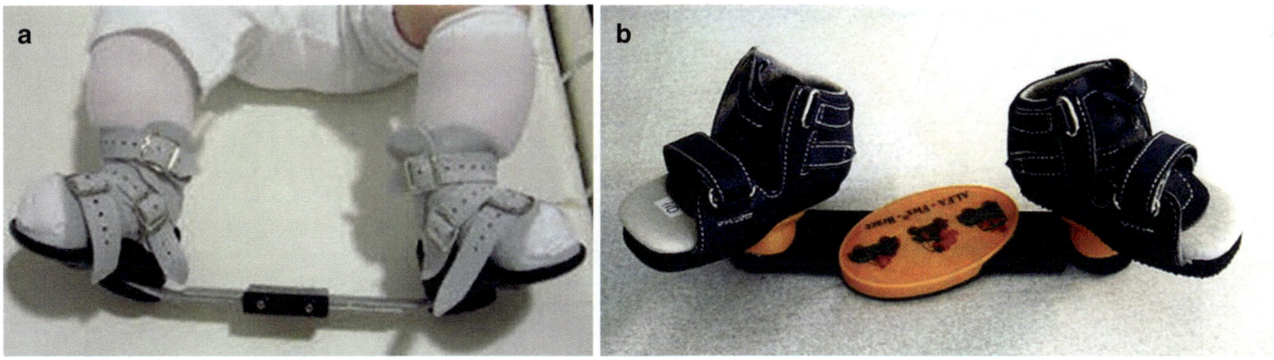

Fig. 1.35 Two models (**a** and **b**) of the Denis Browne foot abduction Brace (FAB)

overlooked. In this phase, it is the therapist's task to repeatedly and urgently explain to the parents the importance of a sufficiently long duration of wear, even if the correction seems successful.

Treatment with Foot Abduction Orthosis (Denis Browne Splint)

- The orthosis is applied directly after cast removal 3–4 weeks after tenotomy.
- Detailed instruction of the parents, especially about the possible problem of slipping out of the orthosis.
- Regular control of the skin by the parents.
- During the first few days, the technician and doctor must be available for the parents.
- Problems with the splint are to be treated as "emergencies."
- The doctor checks that the splint is fitted correctly a few days after it has been applied.
- The orthosis is placed for 3 months for 23 h a day, then only 15 h during the child's resting periods.

1.5.3 Treatment Examples (Course)

The typical course of correction in two girls treated from birth with severe clubfoot (initial Pirani score 6, TnC_E angle before start of treatment +75° or 80°) will be illustrated exemplarily:

Case 1 (Fig. 1.36) After eight redressive plaster dressings and clinically complete correction, percutaneous tenotomy was performed at the age of 10 weeks. After further immobilization for 4 weeks, the abduction splint was retained for 23 h per day for 3 months, followed by 15 h per day during resting periods until the fourth birthday. As the sonographic course shows, the complete correction in the talonavicular region is only achieved sonographically at about 8 months. This has also been observed in many other cases and shows that further skeletal correction can still be expected during the splint phase.

Clinically functionally, the patient in infancy showed a very good correction result with strong active plantar flexion (Fig. 1.36k). From the age of 5 years on, the girl practiced very intensive dancing. Sonographically, a very slight decrease in correction could be observed at 6.5 years after discontinuation of the abduction splint at the age of 4 years (Fig. 1.36j) with a slightly false correction in the naviculo-cuneiforme line. A magnetic resonance tomogram made due to short-term complaints—which could never be completely clarified and did not occur later—shows a certain talonavicular residual deformity in spontaneous posture (Fig. 1.36l).

Case 2 (Fig. 1.37) In this case of severe initial deformity, complete correction was observed in the course of the first year of life by redressive plaster treatment, tenotomy at the age of 8 weeks, and subsequent retention in the foot abduction brace. An anterior tibial tendon transfer was necessary at the age of 5, followed by further clinically and radiological favorable development.

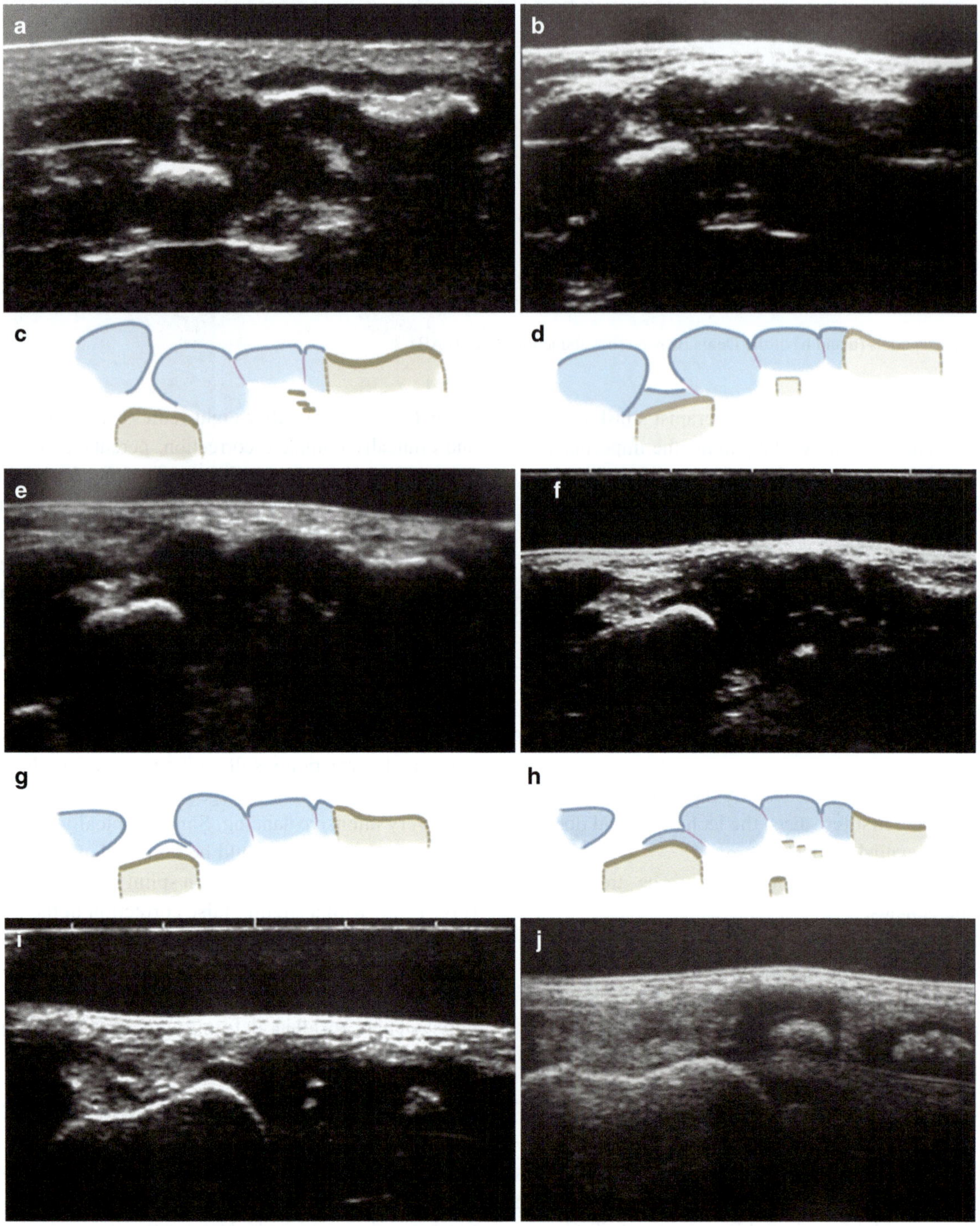

Fig. 1.36 (Case 1) Severe clubfoot during primary treatment: At the age of 2 weeks (**a** and **c**), 8 weeks (**b** and **d**), 14 weeks (after tenotomy, **e** and **g**), and 8 months (**f** and **h**). Primary complete contact of medial navicular pole and medial malleolus with TnC_E angle of approx. +80°. Correction to about +10° after 8 months. Very good functional result in the further course, as the photo at the age of 2 years shows (**k**). Complete correction at 4 years of age with negative TnC_E angle (**i**), but after removal of the splint at 6.5 years, a slight decrease in correction with clubfoot-typical talonavicular inversion (**j**). The MRI at the age of 9 years (due to subsequently decreasing complaints) too shows a moderate talonavicular malposition in spontaneous posture with clinically still good correction position (**l**). At age 14 years, tarsal bones are well developed with slight typical changes (**m** and **n**)

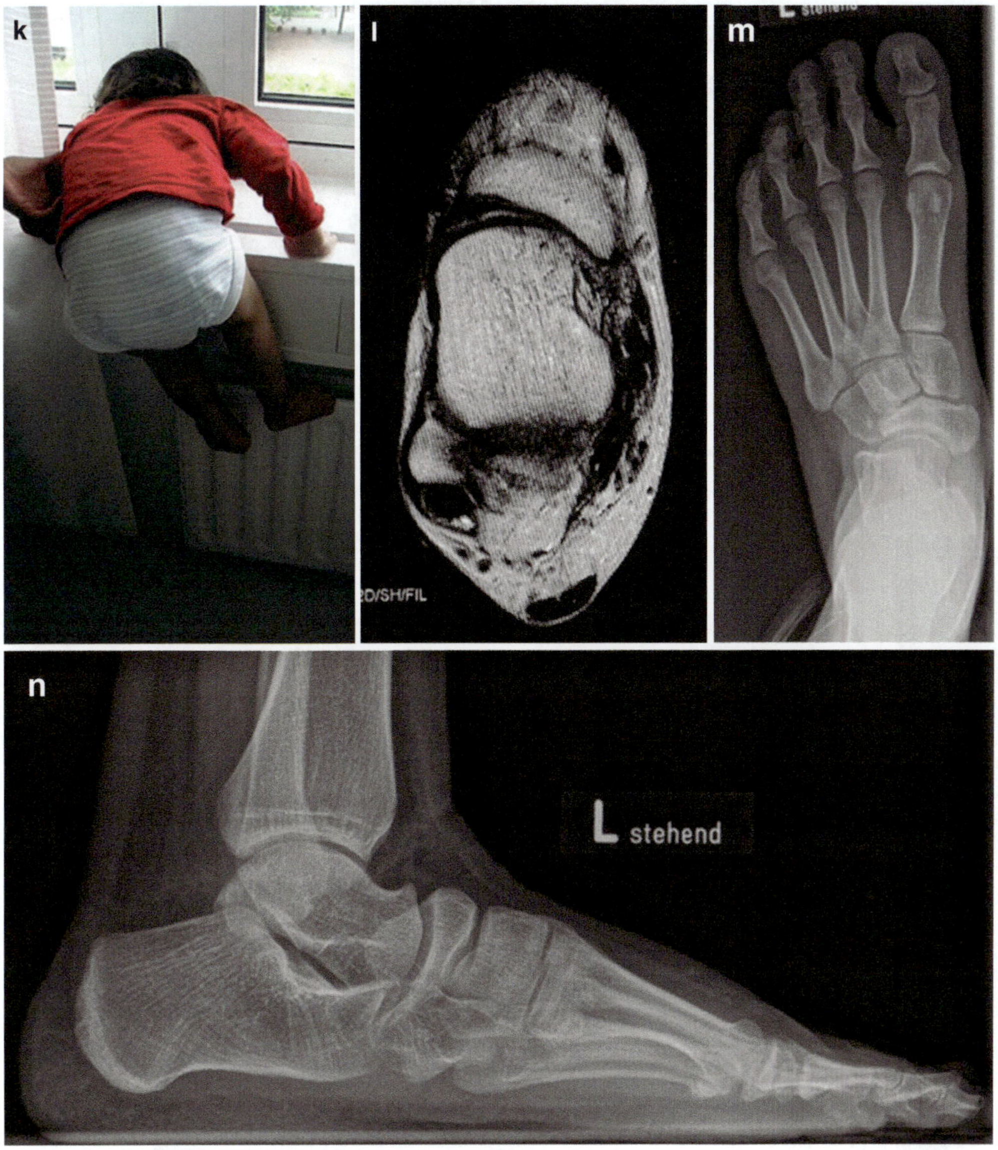

Fig. 1.36 (continued)

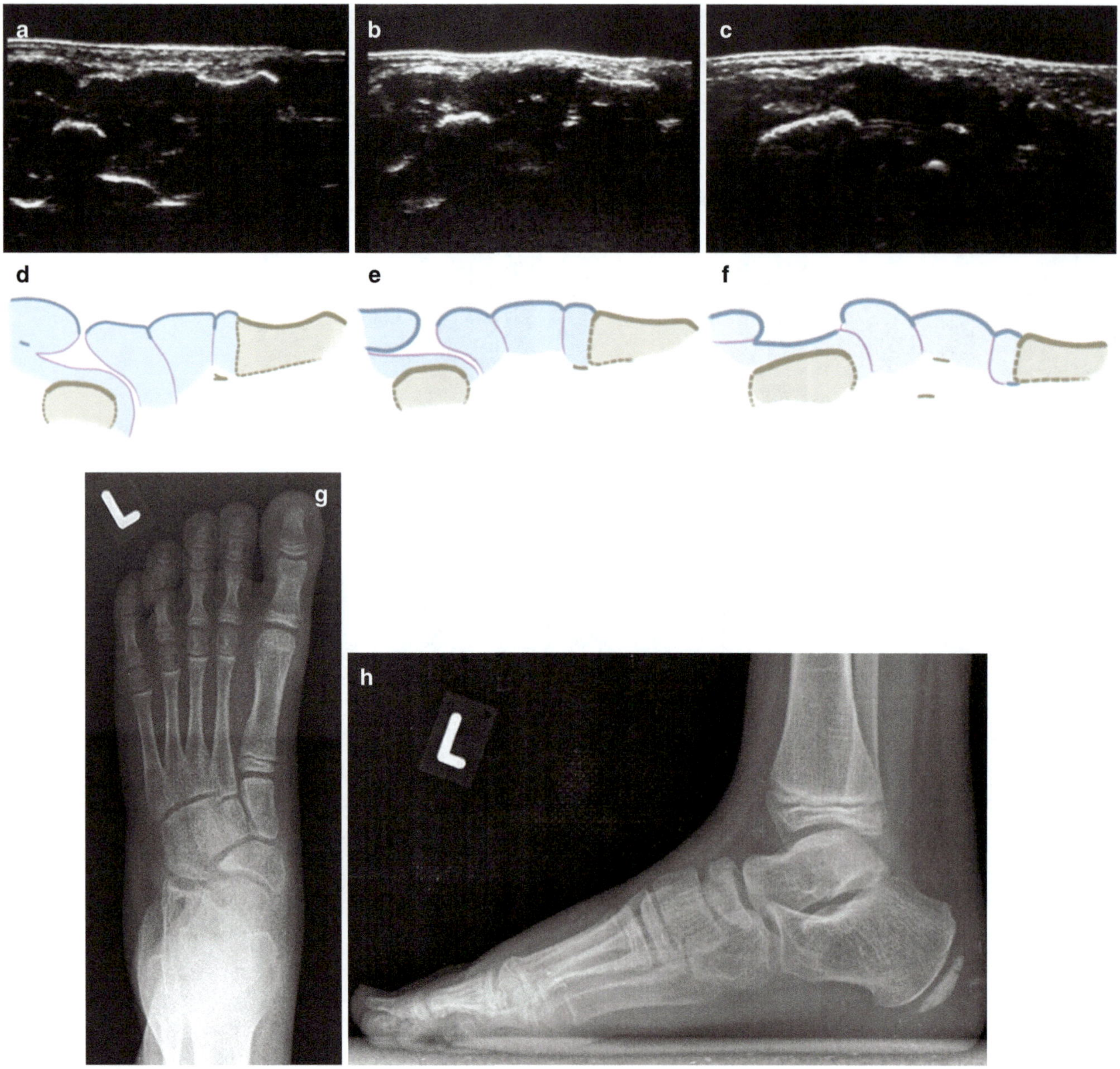

Fig. 1.37 (Case 2) Correction process during the redressive phase in the medial sonographic section at the age of 3 weeks (**a** and **d**), 8 weeks (**b** and **e**), and 12 months (**c** and **f**) with severe initial findings (TnC_E at +75°). The progressive correction was monitored sonographically. At the age of 10 years (**g** and **h**), very good radiological development of the tarsal skeleton with slight flattening of the lateral os naviculare, typical for treated clubfeet (**g**)

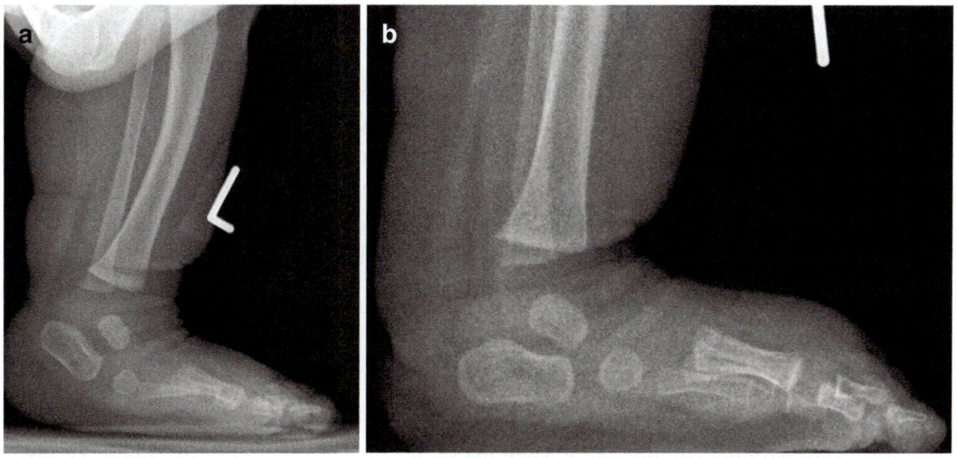

Fig. 1.38 5-month-old clubfoot patient, pretreated externally, tenotomy urgently indicated with clear development of a rocker bottom deformity (**a**), 5 weeks after tenotomy (**b**), anterior tibio-calcaneal angle improved in this case. If the tarsal joints are significantly destabilized, the heel correction can often remain incomplete despite the tenotomy

1.5.4 Possible Errors and Complications of Ponseti Primary Therapy

Optimum results with Ponseti primary treatment can only be expected if the treatment guidelines developed by Ponseti are followed very closely. Modifications should only be made with extreme restraint. The **most common problems and errors** in Ponseti primary therapy are the following (Ponseti (1997)):

Redressive Plaster Treatment

- *Treatment with lower leg cast.*
- *Insufficient casting technique (excessive padding, insufficient fit).*
- *The foot slips back in the cast (caution! "emergency": remove cast!).*
- *Insufficient cavus correction at start of redression.*
- *Inadequate counter-pressure at talar head-neck region.*
- *Redression too forced with false correction in the tarsometatarsal region ("horizontal breach"), inadequate trial to improve dorsal extension without tenotomy (rocker bottom deformity) (Fig. 1.38a)*

Tenotomy

- *Execution of the tenotomy before complete subtalar correction.*
- *Omission of tenotomy despite indication (in case of doubt perform tenotomy!).*
- *Tenotomy too distal (injury of the calcaneus).*
- *Incomplete tenotomy.*
- *Traumatizing tenotomy (venous bleedings described in literature).*
- *Omission of a second tenotomy although indicated.*

Splint Treatment

- *Underestimation of the importance of retention treatment (wearing time!).*
- *Insufficient parent education.*
- *Splint treatment without complete correction.*

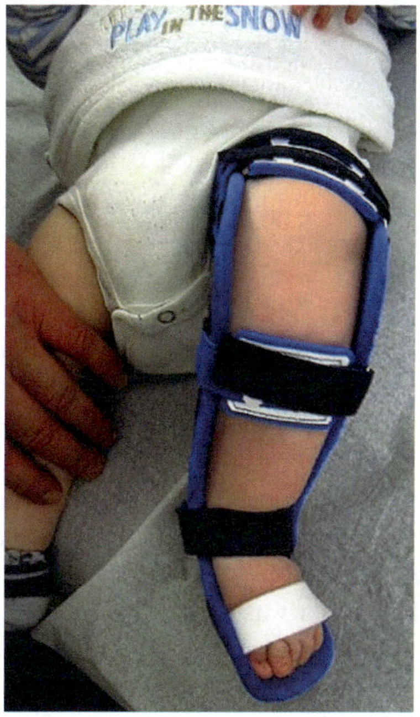

Fig. 1.39 Long-leg brace for retention after clubfoot correction as an alternative, if the foot abduction brace cannot be applied. The fixation strips are mounted from inside of the brace to increase the effect. The foot should be rotated outwards even more than shown here

- *Foot slipping out of the splint.*
- *Pressure sores (mostly in combination with slipping out of the splint).*

If possible, deviations from the intended concept should not be made but are often requested by the parents. For logistic reasons and only very rarely for medical reasons, it may be necessary to change the treatment method completely, e.g., to a primary surgical procedure. There may also be reasons to perform the tenotomy under anesthesiological conditions and in the sense of an open procedure. In case of pressure sores during the retention phase, a new cast phase may have to be interposed until the pressure sores have healed. Complete interruption of the retention should be avoided. In very rare cases, especially in the case of unilateral clubfoot, it may be necessary to switch to a long-leg-splint treatment (Fig. 1.39), with outward rotation of the foot similar to the foot abduction brace. However, this is only rarely necessary in exceptional cases and is significantly less effective than the Denis Browne brace (George et al. 2011).

1.5.5 Cooperation with Parents

The Ponseti treatment is only possible in close coordination and coworking with the parents. Only when the sequence of the treatment steps has been explained to the parents in detail, will they be prepared to cooperate even in difficult cases. The following measures have proved very effective:

- Longer conversation before birth (reassurance and establishing a relationship of trust).
- Appropriate written information (brochure or similar), the Internet often creates confusion.
- Use of cast changes for information about the next treatment step.
- No deviation from the concept (especially with changing therapists).
- Prompt availability (by phone) of the therapist.

Depending on the possibilities of the parents, regular stretching treatment is of great value and should be stimulated and demonstrated by the therapist without overtaxing the family. The author was able to observe individual cases in which anterior tibial tendon transfer that seemed necessary could be avoided in the further course thereby.

1.5.6 Results of Ponseti Primary Treatment

The result of a clubfoot treatment can be described with the following parameters, which are also elements of many scores:

Criteria for Outcome Evaluation of Treated Clubfeet

1. Overall clinical alignment.
2. Muscular balance of the foot.
3. Radiologic alignment and shape of skeletal structures.
4. Mobility, in particular of the ankle complex.
5. Long-term absence of pain and arthritic changes.
6. Subjective patient satisfaction.
7. Function in everyday life and during (sportive) activities.
8. Ability to wear normal shoes.

Some further comments on this:

1. It seems no longer sufficient to merely demand a "plantigrade foot"; a foot can be plantigrade and still exhibit significant abnormalities in weight distribution during the stance phase of gait (cf. Fig. 1.76d). Therefore, a good alignment includes physiological adaption to the ground. Obvious intoeing was seen frequently in clubfeet treated in former times and seems to be less frequent after Ponseti primary treatment (Mindler et al. 2014).
2. Distribution and amount of muscular forces play an important role for normal or near normal function, especially in the late stance and swing phase of gait. Special emphasis should be given to the function of the evertors and to the amount of activity or overactivity of the M. tibialis anterior.
3. The shape of the talus in later childhood allows certain conclusions to be drawn about the result achieved (see Sect. 1.8). The closer the talar shape comes to normal and recovers from its initial deformity (Sect. 1.2.1) (e.g., radius of curvature of the trochlea tali (Fig. 1.23), talar length, angulation of the head-neck region), the better the overall functional result. Late results after Ponseti therapy (Ponseti et al. 1981; Cooper and Dietz 1995) often show slightly false correction effects in the area of the naviculo-cuneiforme joint line ("horizontal breach") and a laterally flattened contour of the os naviculare (e.g., Figs. 1.37g and 1.40). Both phenomena can compensate for an incomplete talonavicular reposition and are apparently compatible with a functionally good result.
4. The mobility of the hindfoot joints should be as unrestricted as possible, but at least about 10°–0°–25° at the ankle joint so that all everyday activities can be performed unhindered. A certain restriction of ankle dorsiflexion will remain in nearly all cases. Richards et al (2008) found slight advantages for the Ponseti primary treatment in this regard over another conservative treatment concept. Even the flexibility of the talocalcaneonavicular complex never reaches normal values in the idiopathic clubfoot, as shown in particular by functional sonographic examinations (Fig. 1.28), but partial mobility is of great importance for more differentiated functions.
5. Justifiably, clinical and radiological long-term results are demanded for the Ponseti concept, some of which are already available (Laaveg and Ponseti 1980; Cooper and Dietz 1995; Ippolito et al. 2003). Smith et al. (2014) found a superiority of Ponseti-treated children over primarily surgically treated patients in the long run.

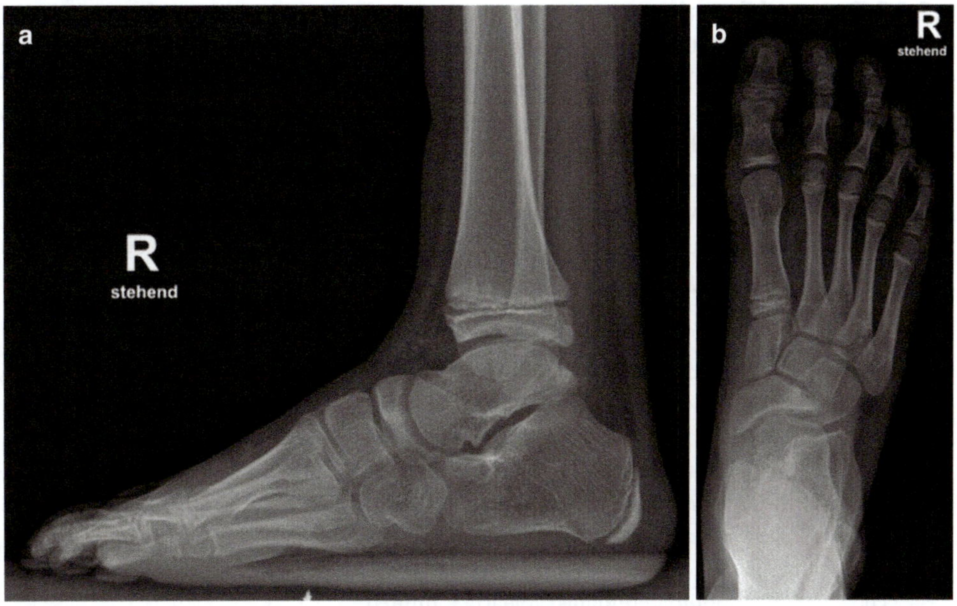

Fig. 1.40 12-year-old boy with severe clubfoot, treated according to the Ponseti concept (**a** and **b**). This case shows more apparent tarsal disorder, especially talonavicular residual malalignment (**b**), compensated at the lesser tarsal bones

6. Of course, one basic criteria for a good result should be the patient's own estimation. It can be observed, however, that subjective patient judgment and objective findings often differ widely, especially in childhood (e.g., Alkar et al. 2017). Therefore, the subjective satisfaction—considered separately—is only of limited conclusiveness.
7. Today, instrumental gait analysis allows a more precise assessment of the function, for example, when walking. Pedographic studies after clubfoot treatment (Lampe et al. 2017) and especially clubfoot patients treated according to the Ponseti concept (Kelly et al. 2017) are increasingly being published. There are still considerable differences between treated clubfeet and age-appropriate normal findings. Even with the "good results" after Ponseti treatment, there are clear differences to the normal, an indication of the high sensitivity of this procedure. However, it must be emphasized that such severe functional disturbances as in the case of clubfoot overcorrection, observed frequently after surgical peritalar release (Sect. 1.6.3), have not been seen in patients treated according to Ponseti.
8. It is of great subjective importance for the patient to be able to wear normal shoes.

1.5.6.1 Results of the Ponseti Therapy in Literature

In the last two decades, extensive literature has been published on the results, problems, and singular aspects of the Ponseti treatment emerged, which can be summarized approximately as follows:

Experiences with Ponseti Primary Therapy in the Literature

- Primary correction achievable in 90–100%.
- Tenotomy in about 60–100% required.
- Compliance problem with the abduction splint is widespread, usually between 20% and 50%.
- Recurrence rate at approx. 30–40% (strong correlation with compliance problems).
- TAT rate 20–40%.
- Good results in early childhood, but measurable differences to normal feet.
- Long-term results after completion of growth only available to a limited extent.

With the results of the instrumental gait analysis, further statements on the functional treatment results are possible at least up to the early schoolchild age (Kelly et al. 2017), which, however, still have to be pursued in higher age groups.

Typical Pedographic Findings After Ponseti Therapy (According to Kelly et al. 2017)

- Shortened temporal heel load.
- The maximum force is usually already reached in the middle stance phase.
- Slightly reduced force development of the forefoot in the late stance phase.
- Slight transfer of load to the lateral metatarsus.
- Reduced load on the medial metatarsal ray (cf. Fig. 1.42c).

1.5.6.2 Personal Experiences

After adopting the Ponseti concept, the author prospectively observed a group of 25 consecutive severe clubfeet from 2004 to 2009 clinically, sonographically, and radiographically up to school age (Hamel 2012) and later. The sonographically documented correction occurred in all cases, on average, the TnC_E angle was reduced from +52.3° to −5.4°, in some cases during the first weeks, in other cases it took months until the TnC_E angle reached values around 0°.

> **Essential Observations from the Sonographic Follow-Up Examination**
> - Sufficient tarsal correction occurred in all cases.
> - Complete correction was observed in several cases only after 8–12 months (Sect. 1.5.3).
> - Slightly false correction is localized in the naviculo-cuneiforme line.
> - The tarsal mobility remains clearly limited (Fig. 1.28).
> - The talar shape is recovering well.

The indication for a later anterior tibial tendon transfer (Sect. 1.6.1.3) due to slight or impending recurrence or overactivity of the anterior tibial muscle was observed in 9 out of the 25 cases (36%). As a rule, it was performed after previous plaster redression and partly in combination with limited dorsal release at age 5–7. In also nine cases (partial overlapping), a dynamic lower leg night splint with continuous dorsal extending effect on the ankle (Fig. 1.41) had to be used temporarily, due to reduction of the dorsal extension below 10°. In most cases, this resulted in a limited increase in dorsal extension. This form of dynamic night splinting, which is not part of the original Ponseti concept, now is considered routinely in those cases with loss of dorsal extension. Similar experience and recommendation was published by Mitchell et al. (2018). Long-term experience after Ponseti primary treatment shows that further controls and, in many cases, therapy up to the completion of growth are necessary. In individual cases, the high value of regular daily stretching treatment by the parents could be observed, although this is usually difficult to accomplish for longer periods.

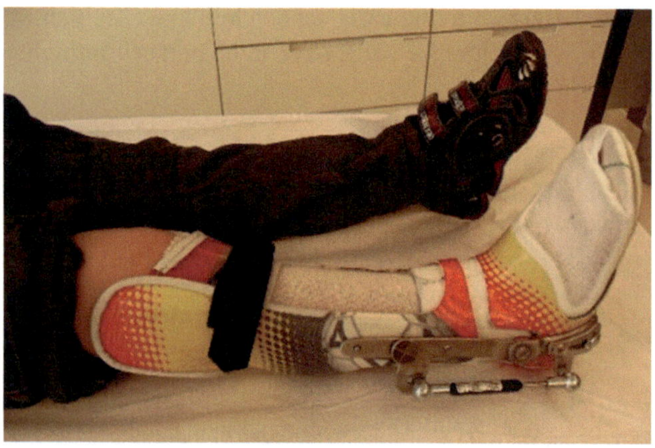

Fig. 1.41 Dynamic lower leg night support splint to improve or maintain dorsal extension. The knee condyles are included to control rotation and a continuous slight dorsal extending force is applied

Twenty-two out of the group of 25 severe clubfeet that were observed from newborn age could be examined with standardized X-rays in adolescent age (10–15 years, 12.0 years in the average) and compared to age-matched normal feet (prepared for publishing). Talar length was 95.5% of the normal group, and there was no significant difference in the radius of the trochlea tali, but in the radius-length quotient. Marked difference was found in the Anterior Talar Motion Segment (Fig. 1.23), that was reduced to about one-half of the values of the normal group. Residual slight talonavicular malalignment in the transversal plane was frequently observed, compensated at the lesser tarsus in the majority of cases. Figure 1.40 shows one of the most distinctive cases of this group; another one seems close to normal in tarsal bone shape and alignment (Fig. 1.42). Supramalleolar valgus deformity, that is described in literature as a quite common finding in surgically treated clubfeet (Sect. 1.8 and Chap. 8), developed only in one special case (Fig. 1.47), which had to be treated by a posterior release in the second year of life because of persisting equinus due to an aberrant soleus muscle. To summarize these radiologic findings, deviations in talar skeletal development seem to be less severe after Ponseti primary treatment in comparison to surgically treated clubfeet. Especially cases of severe flat top talus like in Figs. 1.69 and 1.84 were not observed in patients observed according to Ponseti.

The special advantages of the Ponseti treatment are according to the previous own experiences: Avoidance of internal scarring, dislocations, talar necrosis, and severe overcorrections. Due to the very early correction of the equinus component, the trochlea tali can form better (Fig. 1.42a), a decisive factor for the later ankle function (cf. Sect. 1.8). Pedographically, a load distribution close to the normal load pattern was observed in most of the cases (Fig. 1.42c).

In the education of the parents however, despite these overall favorable results, it continues to be important to point out remaining unavoidable slight deficits from the beginning:

> **Unavoidable Consequences of Idiopathic Clubfoot**
> - Weakening of the calf muscles with a measurable deficit of at least 1–2 cm in relation to the non-affected opposite side in unilateral cases.
> - Slight shortening of the foot (up to 1 cm, in extreme cases 1.5 cm) and rarely of the affected leg.
> - Moderate limitation of ankle and peritalar joint mobility.

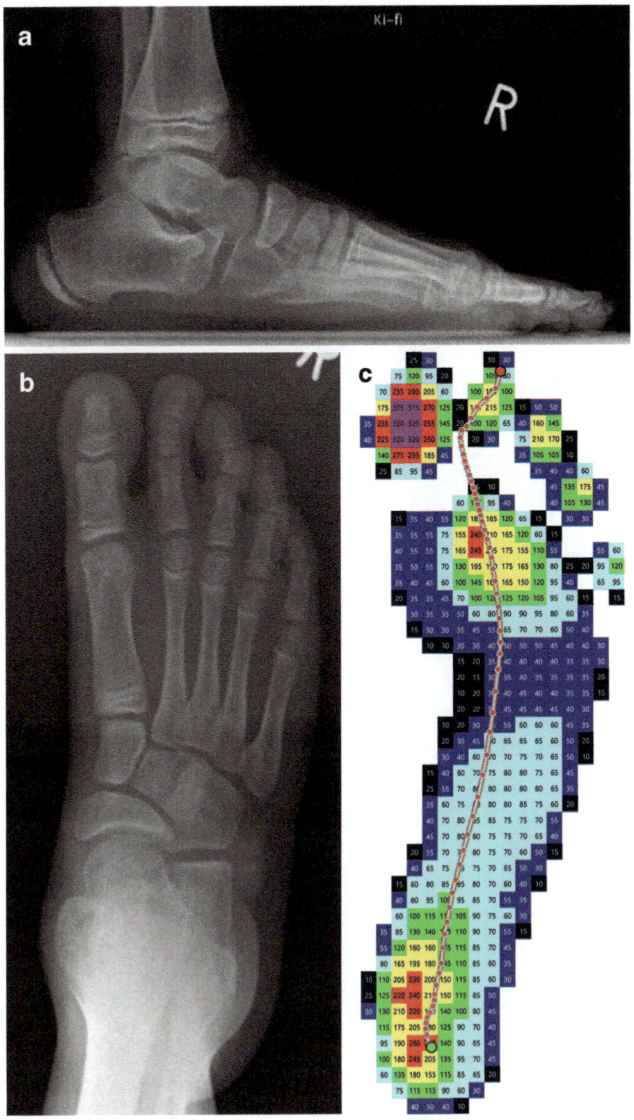

Fig. 1.42 10-year-old boy, treated from the first week of life according to the Ponseti concept with severe idiopathic clubfoot (initial findings: TnC_E angle +56°) with clinically and radiological good development (**a** and **b**). The upper ankle joint showed a mobility of 15°–0°–25°. Pedographically almost normal load distribution (**c**) with reduced peak pressure below metatarsal I, presumably corresponding to a persistent weakness of the peroneus longus muscle

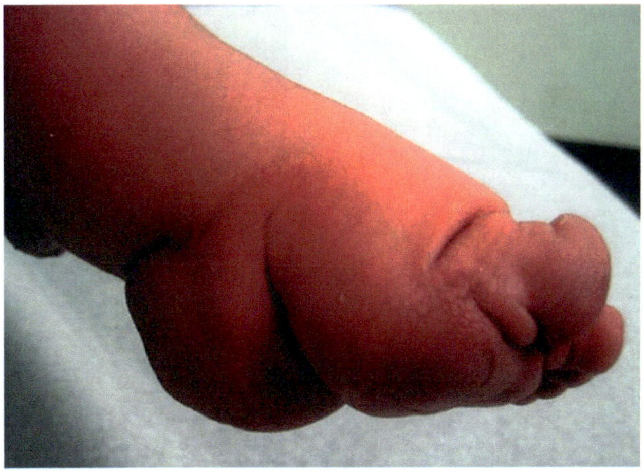

Fig. 1.43 Atypical clubfoot in newborn age

1.5.7 Special Forms of Congenital Clubfoot (Atypical Clubfoot, Arthrogryposis, MMC)

The "atypical clubfoot" is a special form. It is an often very "fleshy," compact foot with strong transverse and plantar creases, and conspicuously (seemingly) short medial foot ray (Fig. 1.43). The extent of the inversion contracture itself often appears to be less pronounced with a particularly marked cavus component. Such deformities may occur iatrogenically after faulty redressive plaster treatment, and this severe complication may be the foremost frequent etiology. A prolonged redressive treatment is necessary with often strongly prolonged cavus correction phase by so-called Ponseti II technique (Fig. 1.45), in which the cavus component is specifically addressed by stretching the plantar soft tissues. Long and difficult redression phases must be expected with these feet. Figure 1.44 shows such a course of treatment. However, the results can be similarly favorable for atypical clubfoot as for normal clubfoot when treated properly.

Arthrogrypotic clubfeet (Fig. 1.46), which often show very high rigidity similar to meningomyelocele, are also treated with Ponseti primary therapy (Boehm et al. 2008; Gerlach et al. 2009). However, primary correction often cannot be achieved in pronounced cases, so that many of these children have to undergo surgical release. Nevertheless, an extended therapy trial with redressive plaster is justified in any case (Eberhardt et al. 2012). In such deformities, it may be useful to reduce an extreme equinus component before the complete tarsal correction by a tenotomy in order to enable further redression.

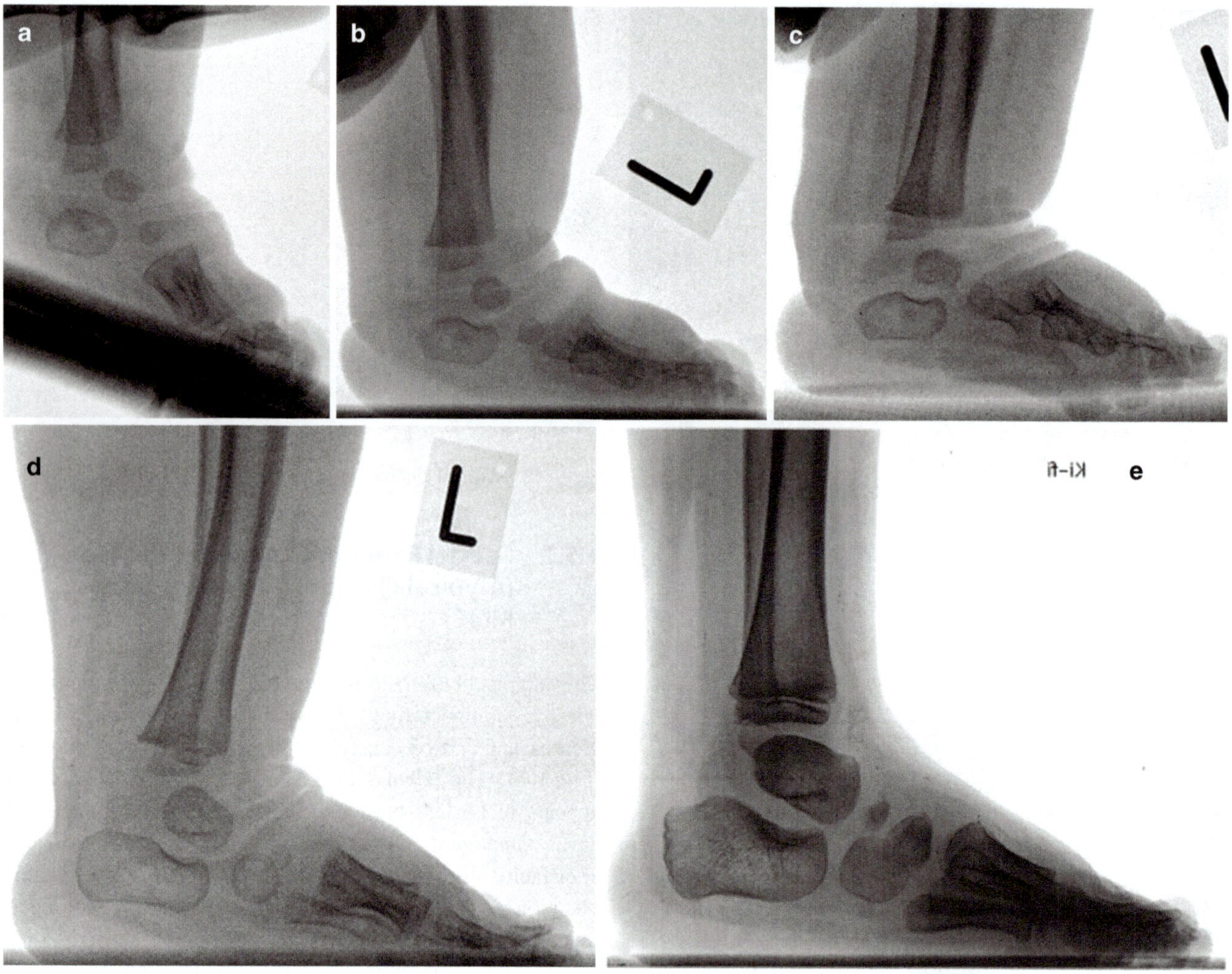

Fig. 1.44 Atypical clubfoot after redressive plaster treatment with 6 weeks of age (**a**), tenotomy not yet performed, but further plaster redression (Ponseti II technique, Fig. 1.45), with 12 weeks of age significantly improved cavus component (**b**), satisfactory heel development with 16 weeks after tenotomy (**c**), further course with 15 months (**d**) and in fifth year of life (**e**) still to be observed

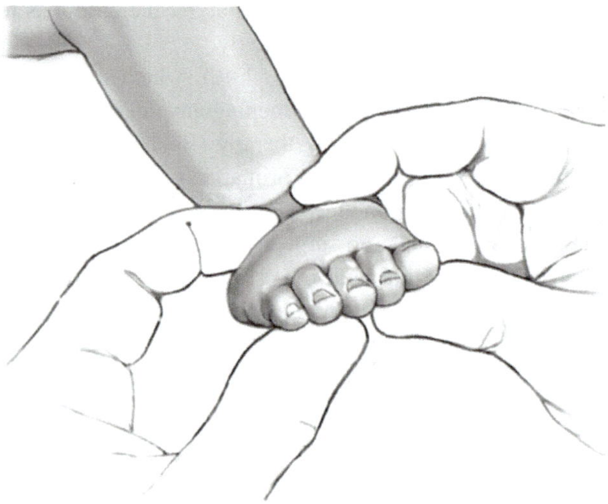

Fig. 1.45 Ponseti II redression technique for correcting the cavus component in atypical clubfeet. The plantar soft tissue structures are stretched with both hands of the therapist

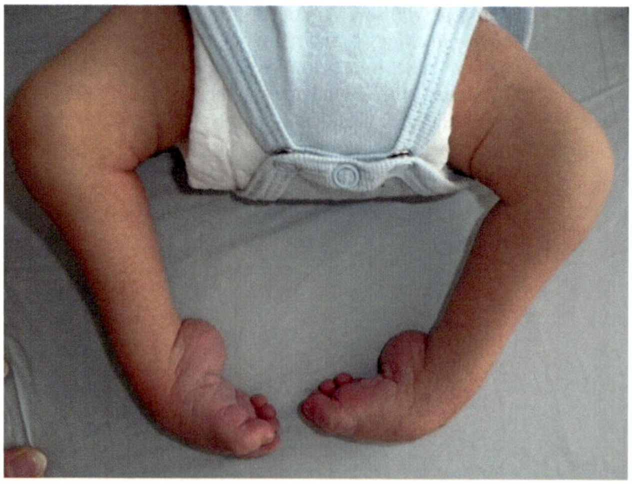

Fig. 1.46 Bilateral arthrogrypotic clubfeet with pronounced rigidity and marked cavus deformity component

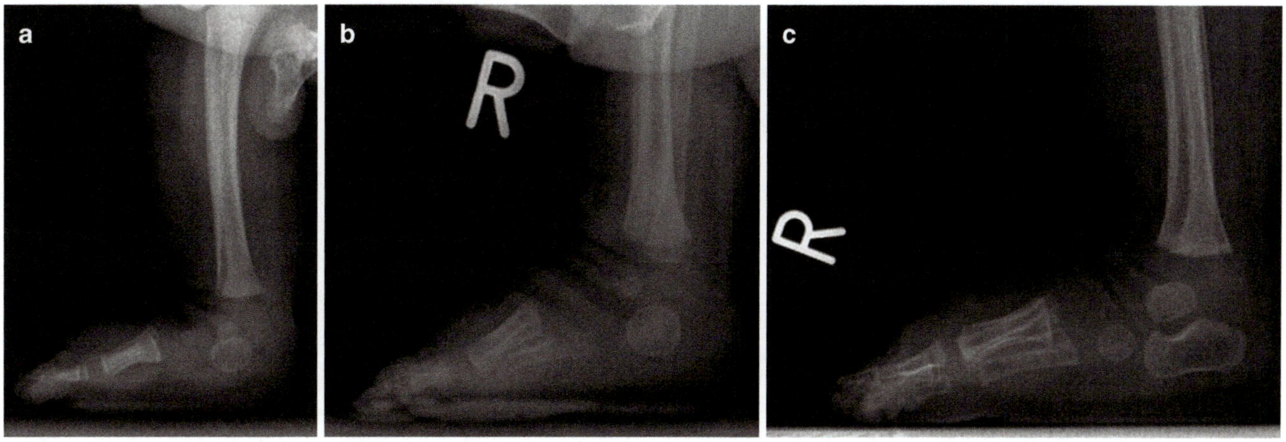

Fig. 1.47 Severe clubfoot (sonographic TnC_E angle primarily +70°), radiological aspect with 6 weeks before tenotomy (**a**). Three months after tenotomy, insufficient correction of the calcaneus position with still very low ossification status of the tarsal bones (**b**), with 15 months still equinus deformity (**c**). In the context of an open posterior release, an accessory soleus muscle was observed and resected, which retrospectively explains the inadequate effect of the tenotomy. In the further course, considerable flattening of the trochlea tali and supramalleolar valgus deformity was observed (cf. Fig. 1.108)

1.5.8 Surgical Primary Treatment

A surgical release beyond the percutaneous tenotomy of the Achilles tendon is not necessary in most cases during the first year of life and is generally associated with the risk of postoperative scar contractures. Ponseti therefore generally advised against opening the joint capsules. However, there are special circumstances in which surgical treatment may already be indicated at an early age (Jauregui et al. 2017):

- Particularly severe initial findings that do not respond adequately to Ponseti primary treatment.
- Insufficient effect of percutaneous tenotomy, e.g., in the presence of accessory muscles (Fig. 1.47).
- Incompliance of parents or non-feasibility of Ponseti treatment due to external circumstances.
- Special parental request.

1.5.8.1 Limited Posterior Release

An open posterior release similar to the one described earlier by Imhäuser (1984) is indicated if a once or twice performed percutaneous tenotomy could only inadequately correct the equinus contracture (heel elevation) (e.g., also with accessory musculature; see Fig. 1.47). Significant persisting inversion contracture of the peritalar complex should be absent.

Technique

The procedure is performed in the prone position using a 3–4 cm long horizontal incision ("Mini-Cincinnati"). The dorsomedial neurovascular bundle and the sural nerve are localized for better orientation and to prevent any violation. The Achilles tendon is severed in a Z-shaped form for later suturing with controlled lengthening, leaving the medial part of the calcaneal attachment intact. Other possible soft tissue resistances such as accessory muscles are released or resected. If a dorsal extension of about 15° is not achieved afterwards, capsulolysis is performed (Fig. 1.48). After the dorsal capsule of the upper ankle has been visualized, it is completely split up to the medial and lateral malleolus, so that the dorsal talar parts can be easily seen when the foot is dorsally extended. The tendon of the flexor hallucis longus muscle must be protected. The peroneal tendon sheaths and the ligamentum fibulocalcaneare can also be optionally included in the release procedure (Fig. 1.48c). A toe flexion contracture can be released supramalleolar by intramuscular or Z-shaped tenotomy, but more easily by percutaneous tenotomy at the metatarsophalangeal joint level (Mosca 2014). According to Jauregui et al. (2017), the gain in dorsal extension achieved by such a limited dorsal release can generally be maintained in the further course. If sufficient dorsal extension cannot be achieved by posterior release as described above, the shape of the talar neck region with low offset is the most likely reason (Mitchell et al. 2018).

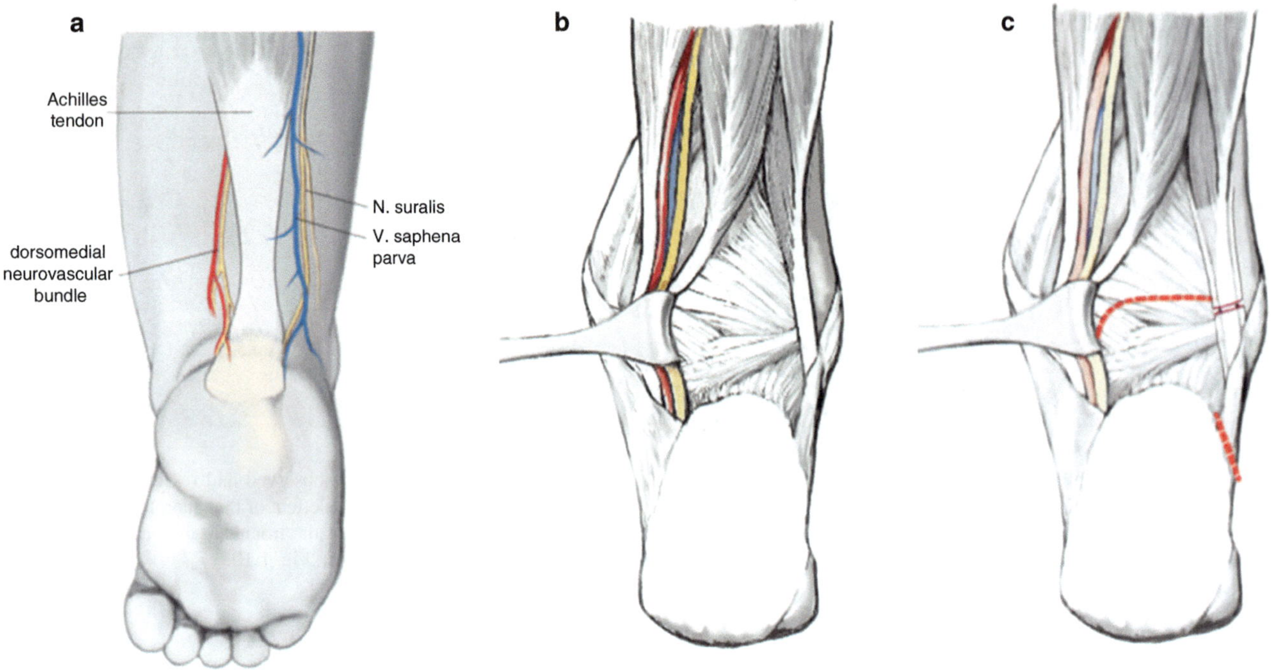

Fig. 1.48 Limited posterior release preserving the neurovascular structures (**a**) with Z-shaped lengthening of the Achilles tendon (not shown) and splitting of the capsule of the upper ankle joint with protection of the FHL tendon (**b**) as well as release of the peroneal tendon sheath and the ligamentum fibulocalcaneare at its calcaneal attachment (**c**)

1.5.8.2 Peritalar Release

The aim of a peritalar release is the subtalar derotation of the talocalcaneal-navicular joint complex similar to the conservative Ponseti method (McKay 1983a, b; Simons 1985; Krauspe and Parsch 1995; Ricco et al. 2014). A surgical peritalar release is indicated at the age of about 4 months to 5 years, if a significant inversion contracture of the talocalcaneal-navicular complex cannot be corrected by redressive plaster treatment or if this is not possible or desired for logistical reasons. Particularly well proven is the cosmetically favorable transverse Cincinnati skin incision (Crawford et al. 1982), whereby all structures that should be addressed are easily accessible. A partial "a la carte" peritalar release is also possible (Fig. 1.52).

Technique

The procedure is performed in prone position. The incision extends from the medial navicular pole via the Achilles tendon slightly proximal to the dorsal transverse skin crease up to the level of the lateral malleolus and can be extended as required (Figs. 1.49 and 1.50). The dorsomedial and dorsolateral neurovascular structures are carefully visualized and slung on. After the Achilles tendon has been severed in a Z-shaped form for subsequent suturing under controlled lengthening, a thorough posterior release of the tibiotalar joint is performed (see Sect. 1.5.8.1). This is supplemented by a successive capsulotomy of the posterior, medial (including talonavicular joint), and lateral subtalar joint. Inframalleolar, the posterior tibial tendon serves as a guiding structure for locating the talonavicular joint after a Z-shaped severing for subsequent suturing with slight lengthening. With a sufficient release, it is possible to achieve the required subtalar derotation and thus also to completely correct severe peritalar malpositions. In the desired position, the talocalcaneal and talonavicular joints are fixed with K-wires for 4–6 weeks. After 6 weeks of immobilization in the long-leg-cast, physiotherapeutic mobilization is performed and a relapse prophylaxis by night splinting in a long-leg-splint.

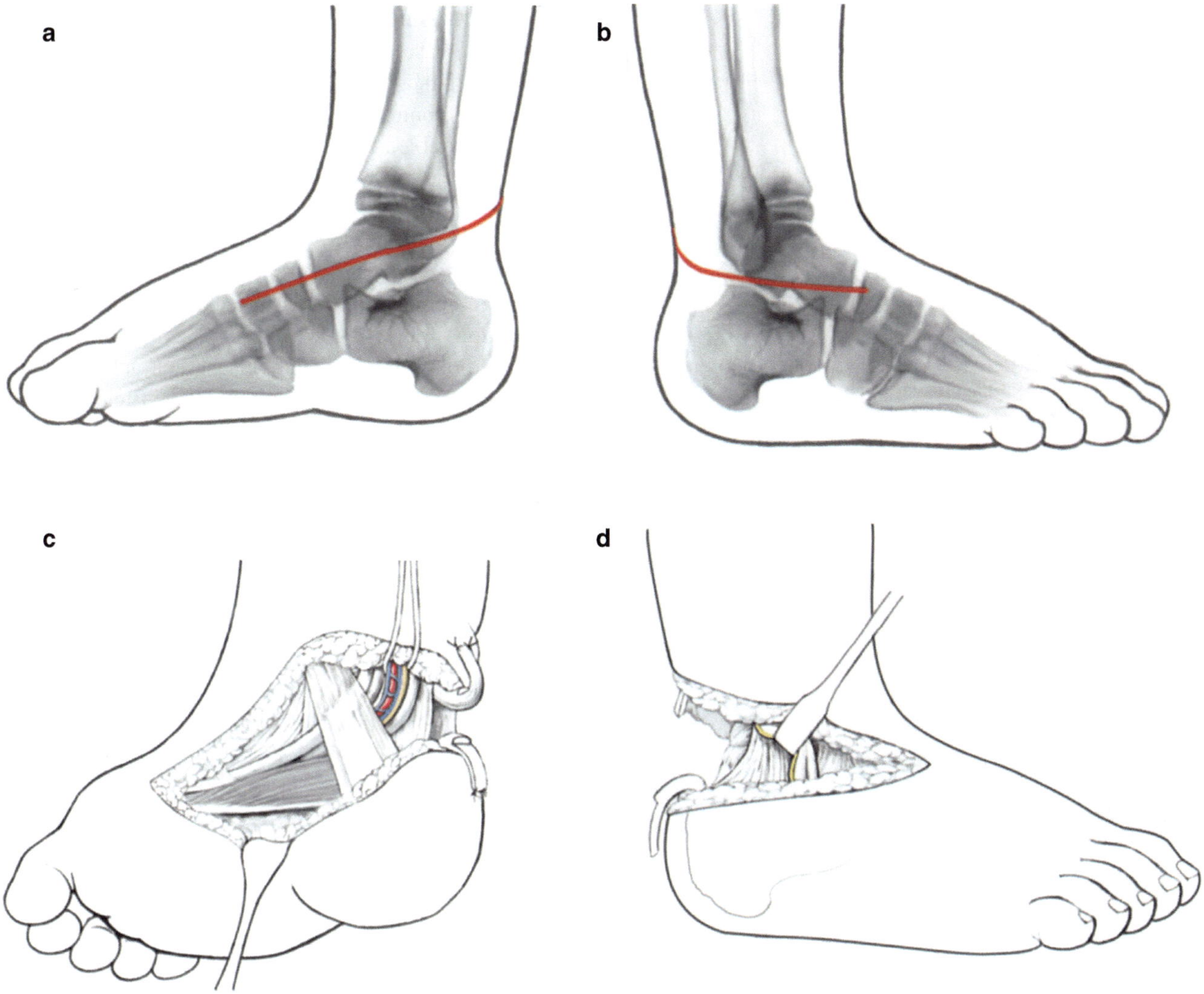

Fig. 1.49 Cincinnati skin incision medial (**a**) and lateral (**b**) as access for a complete peritalar release. After presentation of the dorsomedial (**c**) and dorsolateral (**d**) structures, the talocalcaneo-navicular complex is subjected to a capsular release, thus enabling subtalar derotation. In (**c**) the laciniate ligament has not yet been severed

Peritalar Release

Obligatory Soft Tissue Structures to Be Released

- *Achilles tendon (Z-shaped)*
- *Posterior ankle joint capsule*
- *Peroneal tendon sheaths*
- *Lig. calcaneofibulare*
- *Lig. laciniatum (including visualization of neuro-vascular structures)*
- *Posteromedial subtalar capsule*
- *Talonavicular joint capsule (medial)*
- *Posterior tibial tendon (Z-shaped cut at the infra-malleolar level)*

Optional Soft Tissue Structures to Be Included

- *Plantar fascia*
- *M. abductor hallucis—origin*
- *Lateral subtalar capsule*
- *Lateral talonavicular capsule (Lig. bifurcatum)*
- *Calcaneocuboid joint capsule*
- *Long toe flexors (intramuscular or Z-shaped)*

Ligament Structures to Be Preserved with Caution

- *Deep medial delta ligament (upper ankle joint)*
- *Talocalcaneal interosseous ligamentous connections*

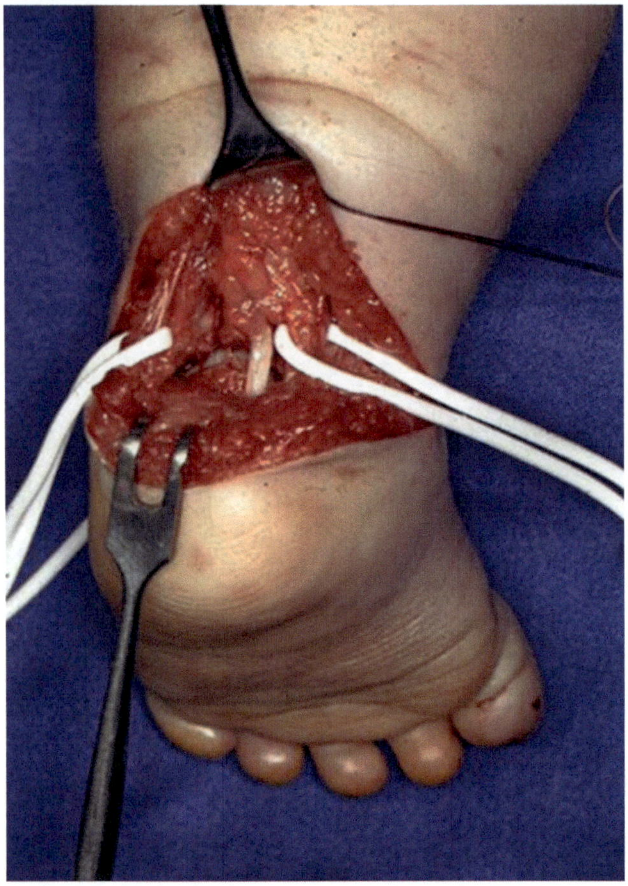

Fig. 1.50 Operative situs at peritalar release. The Achilles tendon was severed, the dorsomedial neurovascular bundle and nervus suralis with V. saphena parva are secured and protected, and the flexor hallucis longus tendon is well visible

The early results after peritalar release are generally very good in case of technically optimal performance in experienced hands (cf. Figs. 1.51 and 1.52). However, scarring and contracture of the peritalar joint complex remains inevitable. Skeletal malalignments, e.g., at the talonavicular joint, will persist permanently and often become apparent only later. The main problem is the danger of overcorrection, which may manifest itself years later (Sect. 1.6.3). Iatrogenic muscular insufficiencies due to over-lengthening or scar formation around the posterior tibial tendon, for example, can also contribute to this. Overall, although the peritalar release can achieve favorable long-term results, the line between sufficient correction and overcorrection (Fig. 1.77) is quite narrow. Ippolito et al. (2003) and Dobbs et al. (2006), for example, described unfavorable results in comparison with patients treated according to Ponseti. Alkar et al. (2017) described a high proportion of poor results 22 years after dorsomedial release, however, surprisingly with high patient satisfaction.

Two treatment examples with favorable results from the author's transition period from standardized peritalar release to the Ponseti concept will be presented (Figs. 1.51 and 1.52). In both cases, the Ponseti concept would have been applied today.

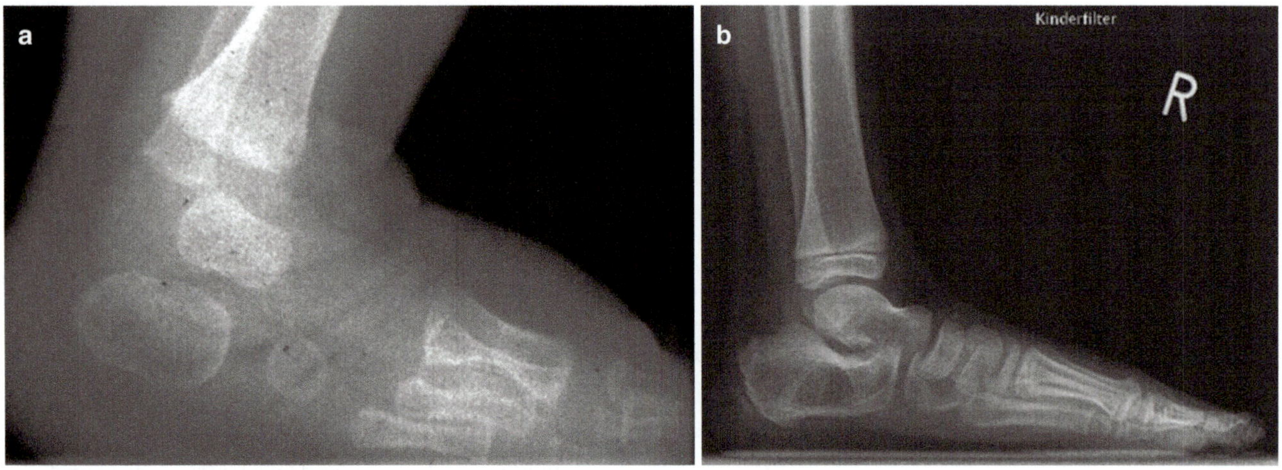

Fig. 1.51 Clubfoot before peritalar release including lengthening of Achilles tendon and flexor tendons at 6 months (**a**), clinical and radiological result at 13 years (**b**) very good, slight hindfoot valgus

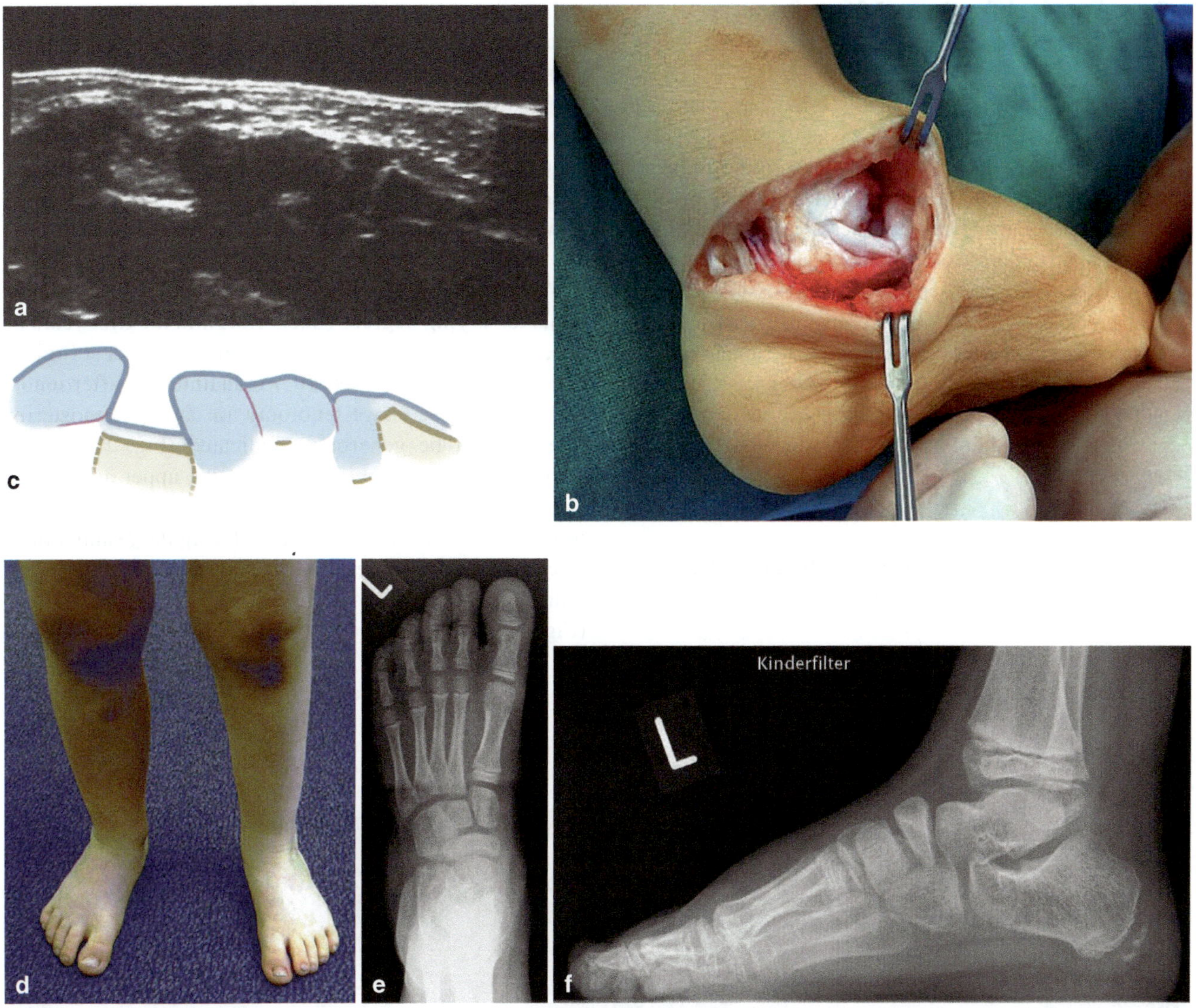

Fig. 1.52 Clubfoot patient with treatment takeover at the age of 4 months, plaster redression and tenotomy at the age of 5 months, followed by retention in the long-leg-splint with clinically clear improvement of findings. Sonographically hardly corrected at 12 months (**a** and **c**), limited dorsomedial peritalar release at 14 months (**b**), clinical result at 4 years (**d**) and radiological result at 10 years (**e** and **f**) very satisfactory. The close spatial proximity of the medial navicular pole and the medial malleolus as shown by sonography (**a** and **c**) was confirmed intraoperatively (**b**). Probably a longer period of plaster redression initially would have been superior

Typical Complications After Peritalar Release

- Wound edge necroses.
- Stiffening by scarring around the talocalcaneal-navicular complex.
- Muscular insufficiencies due to scarring around the tendons.
- Skeletal misalignments.
- Talar necrosis leading to flat top talus.
- Recurrence (especially in case of insufficient follow-up treatment).
- Overcorrection (may still develop after years).

1.6 Surgical Treatment After Primary Correction

The indication for surgical secondary corrections is very individual (Tarraf and Carroll 1992; Raab and Krauspe 1999). In addition to the components of deformity requiring correction, the age of the child in particular determines whether predominantly soft tissue procedures ("toddler" age) or more or additional bony procedures (older children and adolescents) are applied. However, a strict separation is not possible; therefore typical procedures for these age groups are presented. The recurrence problem after Ponseti primary treatment is different from earlier primary surgical concepts. Radler and Mindler (2016) provide an instructive overview of how to deal with a relapse after Ponseti primary therapy.

1.6.1 Recurrence Treatment in Infancy: Soft Tissue Interventions

A clubfoot recurrence during Ponseti primary treatment can develop during the retention phase (foot abduction orthosis), but more frequently afterwards. This can be a "real" relapse or a consequence of primarily incomplete corrected deformities. In many cases, relapse development begins with the decrease in dorsal extension, which should therefore be precisely measured and documented during follow-up. Many factors can favor a relapse: severe initial condition, insufficient primary correction, problems with retention splinting, overactivity of the anterior tibial muscle, etc.

A relapse may affect any of the five clinical components to varying degrees (Sect. 1.3.1). In the first years of life, it is particularly important to ensure that a sufficient dorsal extension (at least 10°) is maintained after tenotomy. Otherwise, a re-tenotomy or an open posterior release must be generously indicated (Fig. 1.53). The decrease in the dorsal extension of the upper ankle joint can be compensated by hypermobility of the Chopart joint line and thus be overlooked during the examination. In case of doubt, a lateral X-ray should be taken in maximum dorsal extension or in a weight-bearing position (Fig. 1.53a, b). Mitchell et al. (2018) found changes in the talar contour with reduced anterior offset as a possible cause in MRI examinations of patients in infancy

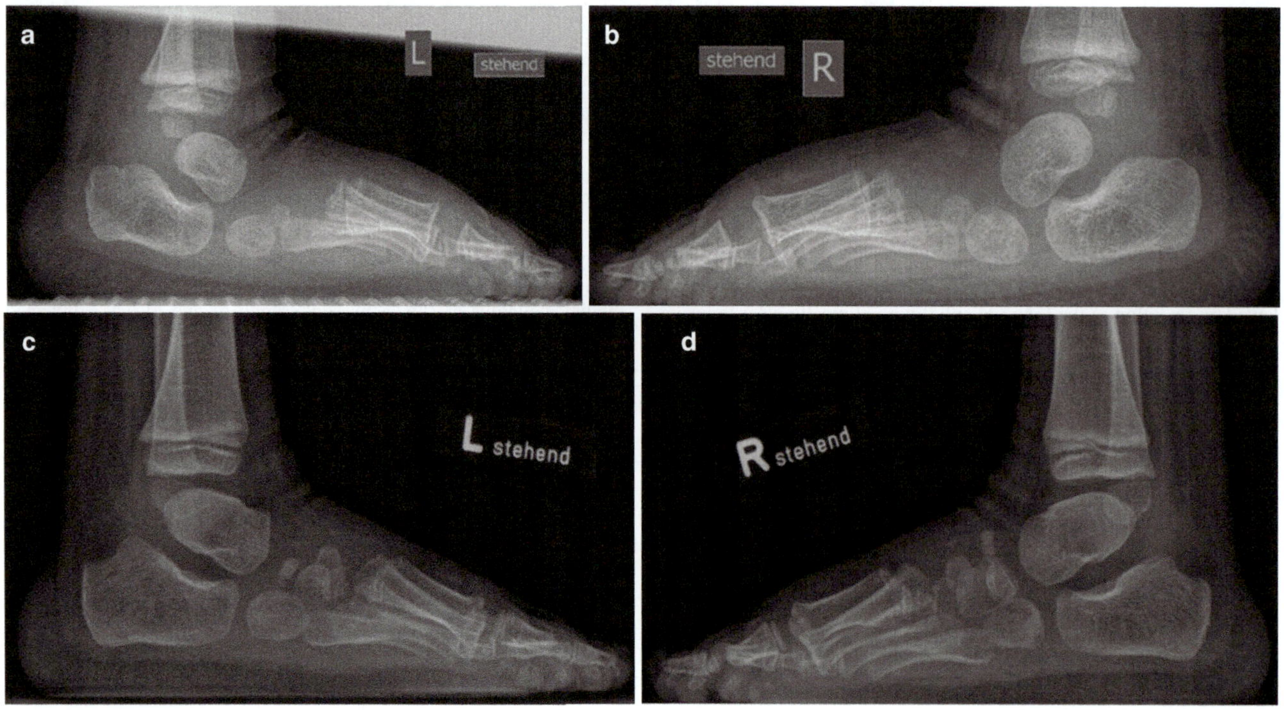

Fig. 1.53 2.5-year-old child with condition after Ponseti primary therapy and good compliance with retention treatment in the foot abduction splint. Significant decrease of the primary clinically sufficient dorsal extension of the ankle joint on both sides (**a** and **b**), indicating an open dorsal release. 32 months postoperatively, improvement of the calcaneus position, but still significantly reduced calcaneal pitch angle (**c** and **d**)

with insufficient dorsal extension despite posterior release.

In pre-school age, the primarily not completely eliminated inversion of the peritalar complex (Fig. 1.54) in combination with a contracture of the posterior soft tissues (equinus component) is the most common situation favoring relapse (Fig. 1.58), but also the middle forefoot adduction (Fig. 1.59) or the cavus component (Fig. 1.67) can be predominant.

1.6.1.1 Repeated Casting

The first measure in the case of an imminent or already manifest recurrence of clubfoot deformity during or after the retention phase is the initiation of a new long-leg redressive plaster treatment. In younger children, the retention is then continued in the abduction orthosis. As a rule, re-entry using the foot abduction orthosis is only possible if the child is still used to it. In most cases, the recurrence is based on an inconsistent splint treatment, which can often hardly be reversed. As a rule, the repeated redressive plaster treatment will be successful in infancy, but the probability of a further relapse is not low, depending also on the possibilities of further retention. Therefore, in many cases a surgical measure should be considered once the hindfoot correction has been achieved. Ponseti recommends this after the first or second relapse (Ponseti 1997).

1.6.1.2 Surgical Relapse Correction in Infancy and Pre-school Age

The majority of correction procedures to be used here are pure soft tissue components, but it may also be necessary to use bony procedures, as explained in more detail in Sect. 1.6.2. The following procedures are usually considered:

Typical Procedures for Clubfoot Recurrence in Toddler Age

- Posterior release with Z-shaped Achilles tendon lengthening and posterior capsulolysis of the ankle joint, if dorsal extension is not sufficient (see Sect. 1.5.8.1).
- Medial talonavicular release (see text).
- Percutaneous release of the long flexor tendons at MTP joint level (Mosca 2014).
- Anterior tibial tendon transfer to the lateral cuneiform to prevent relapse (Sect. 1.6.1.3).
- If necessary, shortening of the lateral foot column by cuboid osteotomy or resection arthroplasty of the calcaneocuboid joint (Sect. 1.6.2.1).

The lateral patient position with support in the thoracic region has proven to be useful for interventions requiring posterior access to the ankle joints, when anteromedial

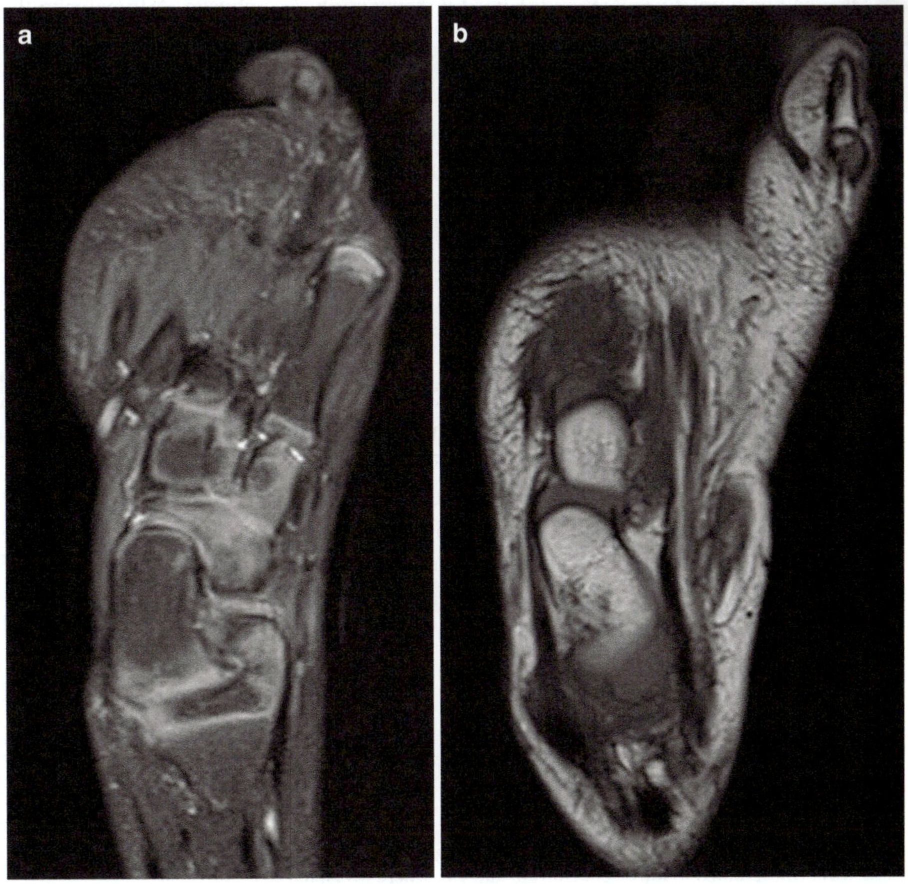

Fig. 1.54 Magnetic resonance tomographic transverse sections of a 4.5-year-old patient with arthrogrypotic clubfoot and tarsal inversion not sufficiently corrected primarily (no Ponseti primary therapy). The pronounced talonavicular malposition and deformation of the still cartilaginous navicular (**a**) as well as the calcaneocuboid deformity (**b**) are clearly visible

access to the foot is also required. The posterior release is performed as described in Sect. 1.5.8.1. If a moderate inversion contracture of the talocalcaneal-navicular complex exists, an additional medial release around the talonavicular joint can be added. Via a longitudinal incision above the posterior tibial tendon, the talonavicular joint is incised semicircularly, contracted parts of tibionavicular ligament connections are severed, and the posterior tibial tendon in the inframalleolar region is lengthened in a Z-shaped form. This allows a limited lateral repositioning of the os naviculare on the talar head. This effect can be enhanced by shortening osteotomies on the lateral column (Fig. 1.63). If the inversion contracture of the talocalcaneal-navicular complex is pronounced, a peritalar release (Sect. 1.5.8.2) should be considered alternatively in the younger child.

If a severe toe flexion contracture is recognizable after soft tissue release, this can be corrected by a percutaneous release of the long flexor tendons at the MTP joint level (Mosca 2014).

Technique

An Nr. 11 knife is inserted at the flexion crease of the MTP joint by stab incision and the long flexor tendon is severed. A clear loss of resistance of the toe is noticeable. A clinically significant weakness of the active toe flexion was not observed after such tenotomies. It should be emphasized that the release of long toe flexors also has a positive effect on the peritalar inversion contracture.

1.6.1.3 Anterior Tibial Tendon Transfer (TAT)

The lateral transfer of the anterior tibial tendon attachment (Fig. 1.55) has been a proven procedure in relapse surgery for decades (overview in Lampasi et al. 2009). The often persistent muscular disbalance in idiopathic clubfoot (Sect. 1.2.4) with weakness of the peroneal musculature (especially the long peroneal muscle) and the resulting relative predominance of the inverting musculature (especially the anterior tibial muscle) can thus be effectively treated (Kuo et al. 1994). The indication is given when a peroneal muscle weakness exists, when the medial foot ray is lifted much more pronounced than the lateral forefoot during active foot lifting (Fig. 1.56), and when a gait pattern is observed where the heel is initially contacting the ground in varus position. This can be observed particularly in clinical gait analysis, preferably by filming and viewing in slow motion. The inward rotation gait is also improved to a certain extent by the transfer. Very important is the fact that the anterior tibial tendon transfer is not a corrective measure and all contractures have to be treated by other procedures beforehand. In particular, a sufficient dorsal extension of the ankle joint is a prerequisite for the effectiveness of tendon transfer. The role of anterior tibial tendon transfer in relapse surgery is to improve function (cf. Fig. 1.57) and to provide prophylaxis against further relapse.

Depending on the insertion site, the effect of the tendon transfer can vary. As a rule, the os cuneiforme laterale, in some cases also the os cuneiforme intermedium should be chosen. A transfer to the peroneus brevis tendon attachment (Imhäuser 1984) leads to overcorrection and is not recommended. If tendon fixation is planned by means of a drill

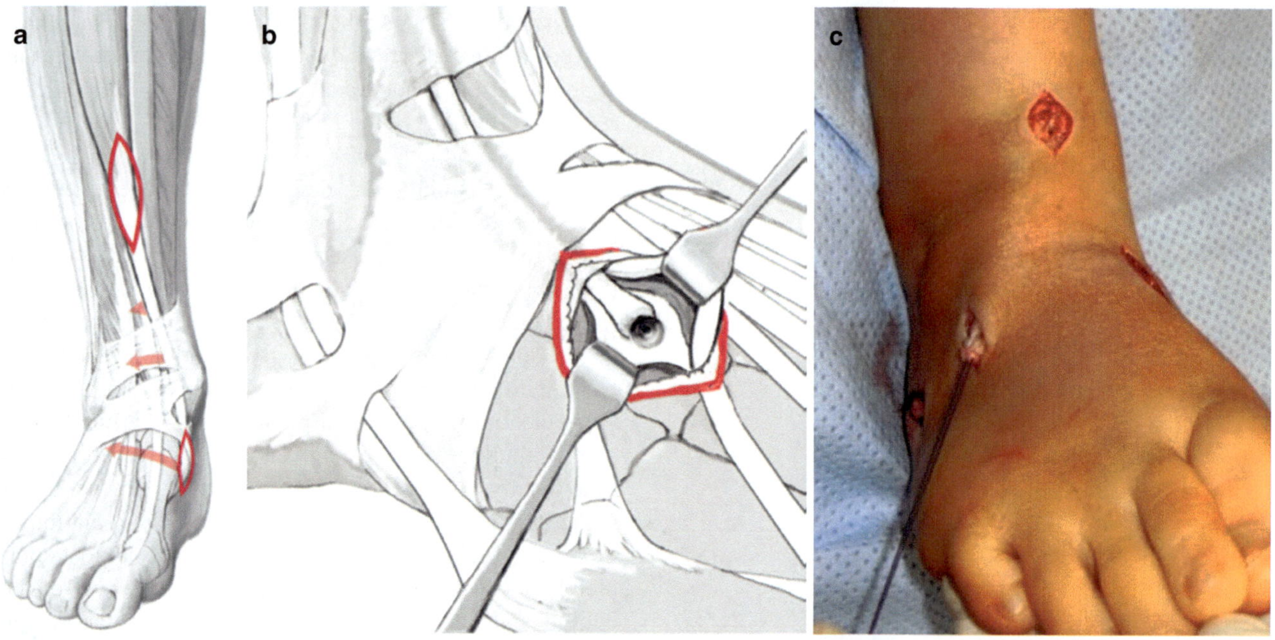

Fig. 1.55 Anterior tibial transfer to the os cuneiforme laterale via three incisions. The tendon is detached at its insertion, pulled out above the ankle level (**a**), rerouted to the os cuneiforme laterale, where it is fixed under tension (**b**). An intraoperative view of this three-incision technique is shown in (**c**)

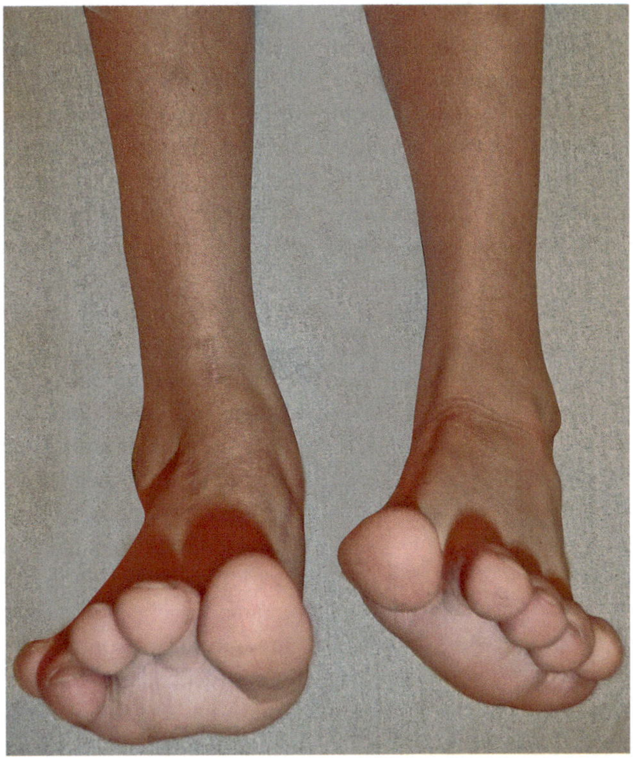

Fig. 1.56 6-year-old patient with bilateral clubfoot, 1.5 years after TAT at the right foot (more severely affected side), TAT on the left side is now planned due to clear muscular disbalance during active foot lifting

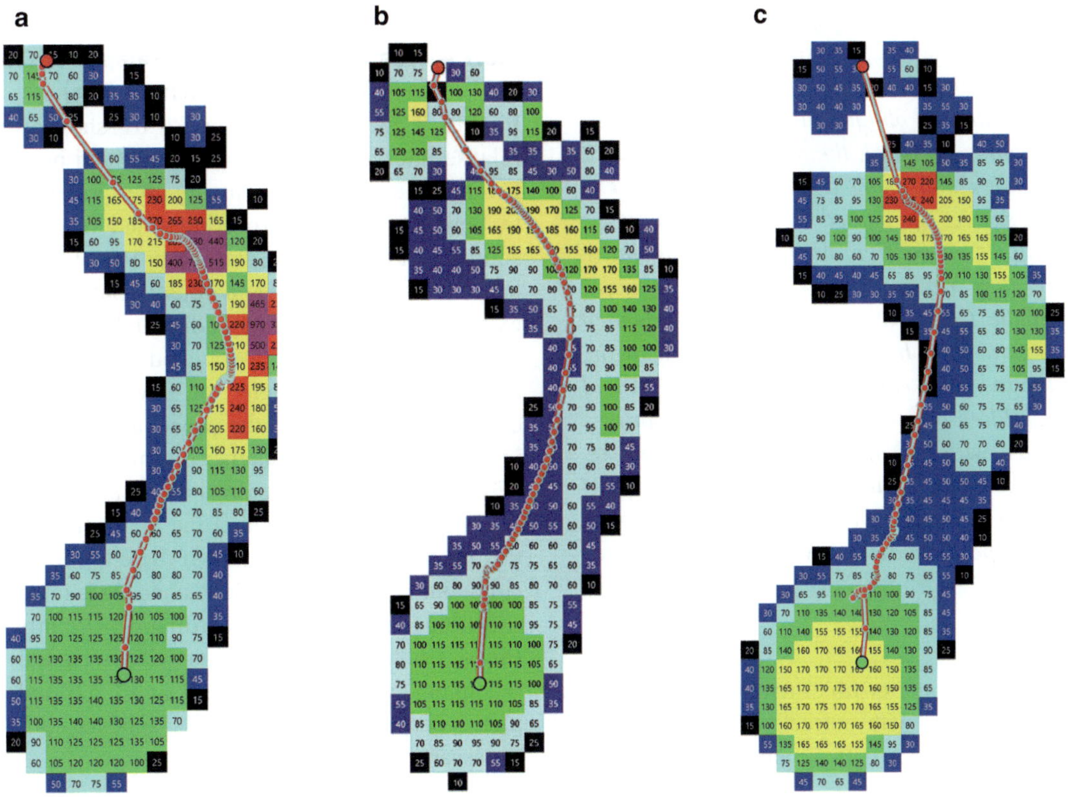

Fig. 1.57 6-year-old female patient, idiopathic clubfoot, pedographic peak pressure image before (**a**), 6 months (**b**) and 3.5 years after TAT (**c**), with clear normalization of load distribution in the metatarsal region. Due to the overactivity of the anterior tibial muscle with weakness of the long peroneal muscle at the same time, load transmission at the medial metatarsal ray is clearly reduced before the tendon transfer (**a**)

hole, the os cuneiforme should have reached a sufficient degree of ossification, which is usually the case from about 3 years of age. In order to avoid a disturbing protrusion of the transferred tendon, the course below the retinaculum should be chosen. The two-incision technique without supramalleolar access is commonly used, as is the three-incision technique, which has a more pronounced effect (Knutsen et al. 2015) and is preferred by the author and described here (Fig. 1.55):

Technique

A short medial longitudinal incision is made in the attachment area of the anterior tibial tendon at the first tarsometatarsal joint and the tendon is completely detached, trimmed, and neatly slung on with a Vicryl-0 suture. Adhesions of the tendon are released proximally as far as possible. The tendon is pulled out via a supramalleolar second incision slightly lateral of the palpable tibial bony edge and placed on a moistened compress. The os cuneiforme laterale is marked with a K-wire, localized in the image intensifier, and a third access is made in this area. In this access, the extensor-digitorum-longus tendons are displayed, and a slender tunneling clamp in the tendon sheath of these tendons is inserted proximally into the supramalleolar incision. The sutures of the anterior tibial tendon are grasped, and the tendon is transferred to its new insertion site. Via a 4.5 mm drill hole central in the bone core of the os cuneiforme laterale in a slightly oblique direction from dorsal-distal to plantar-proximal, the tendon can be pulled into the bone canal using a blunt loop wire. The attachment sutures are passed through the skin via a small plantar stab incision. At the end of the entire procedure, they are knotted over a compress under tension of the tendon in a slightly dorsal-extended position of the foot. In addition, the fixation in the area of the insertion can be secured with periosteal sutures. Children below the age of 7–8 are kept in a long-leg cast with 90° of knee flexion for 3 weeks. After removal of the sutures a short leg walking cast is applied for another 3 weeks. Only in case of pronounced preoperative deformity further night splinting is advisable.

The effect of the anterior tibial tendon transfer is usually clearly noticeable with correct execution and good tendon tensioning (Fig. 1.56). Function and loading behavior of the foot normalizes impressively (Fig. 1.57), as could also be shown in the pedographic study by Wallace et al. (2016). A disturbing "dropping" of the medial foot ray in the swing phase of gait due to overactivity of the antagonistic peroneal longus muscle is hardly observed in idiopathic clubfoot, probably because of the persistent weakness of this muscle. By eliminating the antagonistic effect of the anterior tibial muscle, however, the plantarizing effect of the peroneal longus muscle on the first ray can be improved, as well as the loading of the medial metatarsal ray (Fig. 1.57).

When carrying out this tendon transfer, one should always be aware that any secondary correction, e.g., "retensioning" or a repeated relocation as with any tendon transfer, is rather problematic, and the transfer thus has the character of a definitive, almost irreversible measure. If, for example, it is carried out without prior restoration of the dorsal extension by sufficient posterior release, it remains largely ineffective, and thus an important procedure of relapse prophylaxis is lost. The effect of the transfer also depends on whether there is a complete correction in the transversal plane of the foot, a prerequisite for the new insertion site actually assuming a more favorable position in relation to the subtalar axis of motion (cf. Fig. 1.10). Overcorrection of anterior tibial tendon transfer as well as clubfoot relapse despite of transfer has been observed but is not common.

1.6.1.4 Treatment Examples (Relapse of Clubfoot in Infancy and Pre-school Age)

Figures 1.58, 1.59, 1.60 and 1.61 show examples of relapse interventions in late infancy and pre-school age. It is not uncommon for scarring after previous operations to limit the surgical procedures and force compromise solutions. For example, the repetition of an earlier peritalar release is difficult and not without danger due to the existing scarring. For each individual measure, it must be estimated whether the associated disadvantage of scarring processes outweighs the advantages of deformity correction. Frequently, the procedure can be carried out in a purely soft tissue manner during the first years of age (Fig. 1.58). Bony shortenings of the lateral tarsal column are applied in the cuboid, if the malposition is localized tarsometatarsally (Fig. 1.59); if there is still a clear inversion contracture of the talocalcaneal-navicular complex, resection arthroplasty according to Lichtblau (1973) (Sect. 1.6.2.1) in conjunction with a medial release is recommended (Figs. 1.60, 1.61 and 1.62), unless a complete peritalar release still appears possible and necessary.

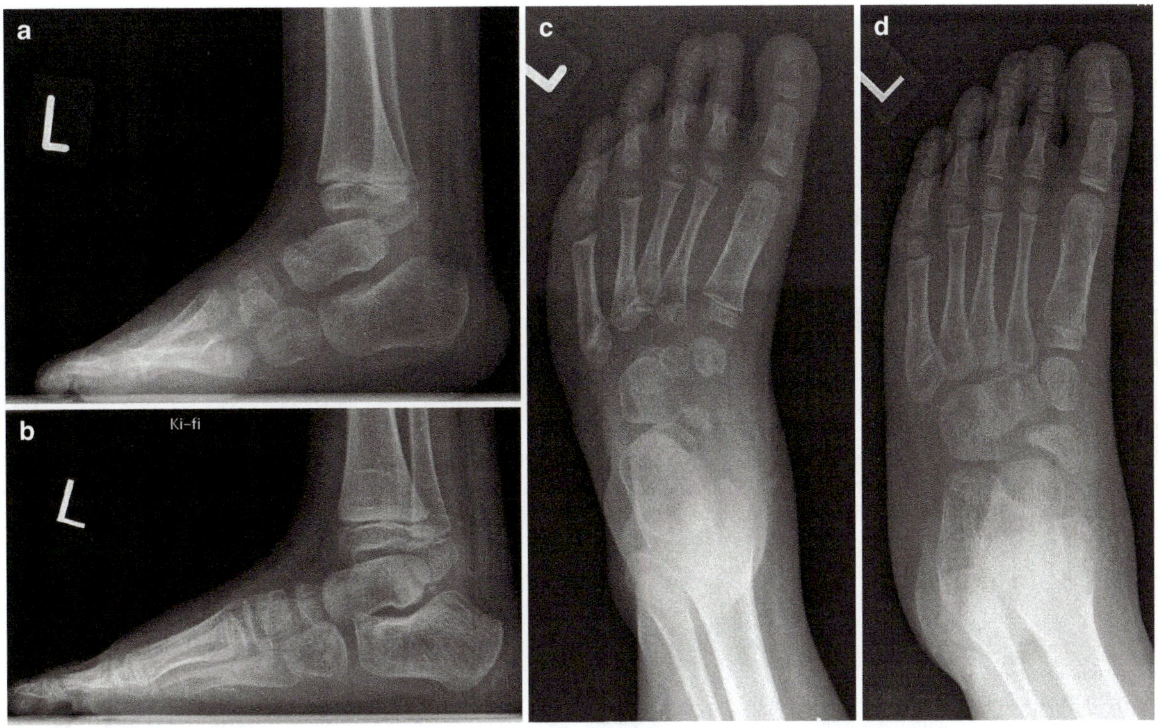

Fig. 1.58 4.5-year-old female patient with a pronounced clubfoot relapse and persisting severe peritalar inversion contracture after external pre-treatment with dorsal release (**a** and **c**). Still about 7° equinus deformity contracture after four preoperative redressive plaster dressings. After lengthening of the Achilles tendon and posterior ankle joint and subtalar capsular release, dorsal extension improved to almost 15°, additionally anterior tibial tendon transfer to the midline of the foot. The talocalcaneal-navicular complex could only partially corrected thereby (**d**), possibly a lateral column shortening measure in conjunction with a medial release would have been advisable. However, the further development was favorable, the postoperative images were taken approx. 1.5 years after the procedure (**b** and **d**)

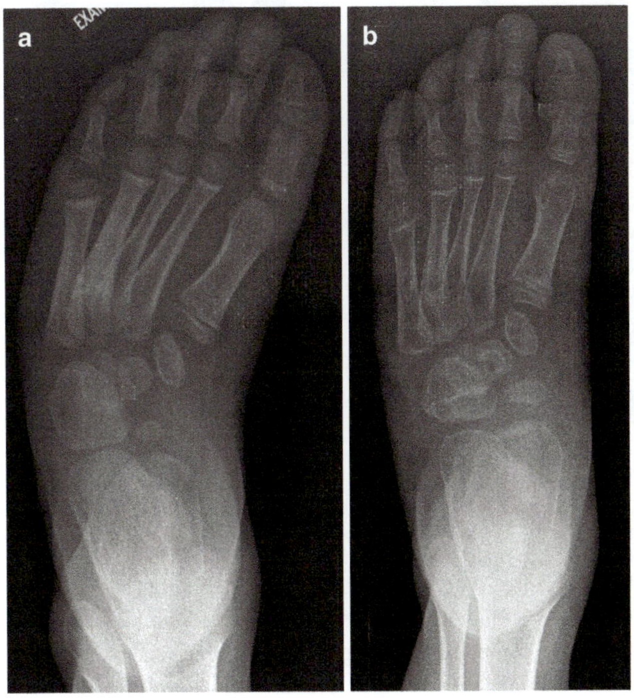

Fig. 1.59 5-year-old female patient with idiopathic clubfoot with residual deformity, especially in the sense of a mid-forefoot adduction contracture, before (**a**) and 8 months after TAT and cuboid osteotomy (**b**). Since in this case the adduction was rather tarsometatarsally localized, a cuboid osteotomy seemed adequate. The drill hole for anchoring the anterior tibial tendon in this case in the os cuneiforme intermedium is clearly visible

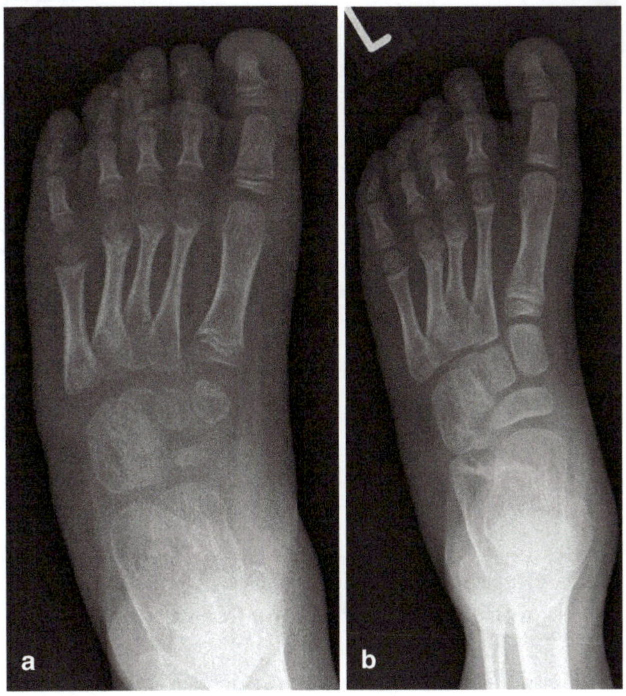

Fig. 1.60 4.3-year-old female patient with status after peritalar release in the first year of life and relapse (**a**) with still moderate inversion contracture in the talocalcaneal-navicular complex. 66 years after medial talonavicular release, resection of the anterior calcaneal portion and anterior tibial tendon transfer, favorable development of alignment (**b**)

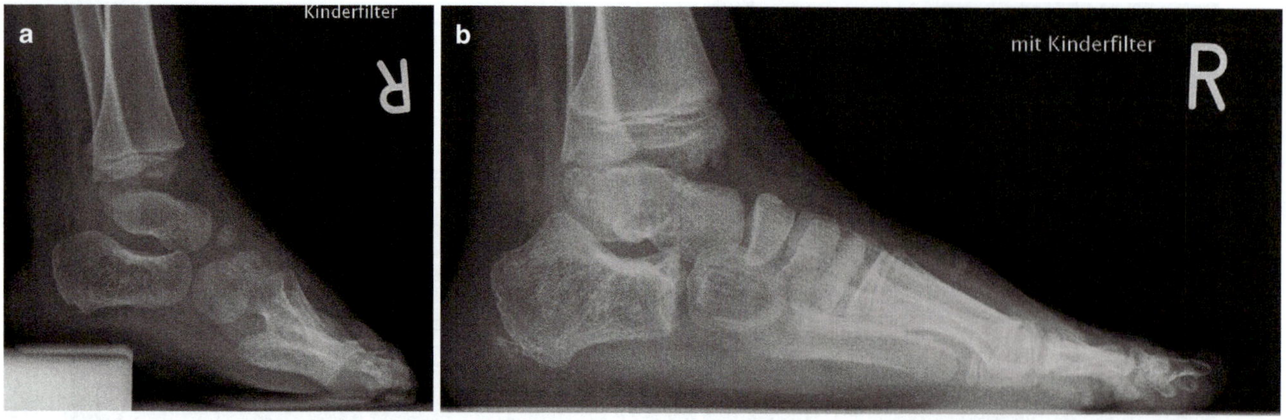

Fig. 1.61 3.5-year-old patient with status after external peritalar release in the first year of life and severe relapse (**a**). After six redression plaster dressings, posterior release, anterior tibial tendon transfer, and resection arthroplasty according to Lichtblau at the calcaneocuboid joint, to shorten the lateral foot ray. 5 years postoperatively (**b**) relapse-free with ankle range of motion of 10°–0°–25°

Fig. 1.62 Pedographic image of peak pressure distribution in an 11-year-old patient with clubfoot relapse before (**a**) and after 4-week preoperative treatment with the lower leg redressive walking cast (**b**) showing clear functional improvement with increased and prolonged heel loading, recognizable by the center of pressure line

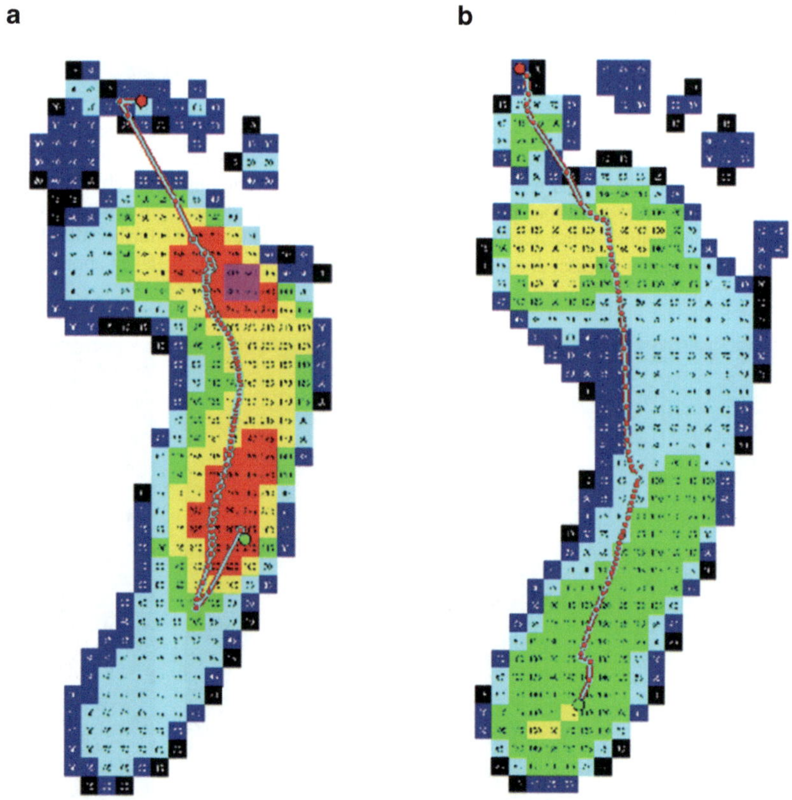

1.6.2 Relapse Treatment in Schoolchildren and Adolescents: Bony Corrections

Also in the older clubfoot child a relapse or also a not pre-treated "overlooked" clubfoot (see also Sect. 1.7) is first treated by redression casts. In this case, the much less invasive treatment with lower leg "hybrid" walking cast dressings has proved very effective with very precise casting techniques: With only minimal padding and the use of white plaster in the ankle joint region with precise counter pressure at the lateral talar head in the Ponseti technique, the deformity is first corrected, and then the necessary stability is achieved with a second layer of synthetic hard cast. A reduction of the dorsal extension under about 10° can often be significantly improved by a few treatment weeks with such weekly changed redressive casts. The progress can also be well checked pedographically (Fig. 1.62). In minor cases, a dynamic lower leg night splint with condylar socket and continuous dorsal-extending pressure can then secure the achieved correction in the longer term (Fig. 1.41).

More pronounced and not completely redressable recurrent malpositions or late primary corrections require surgical interventions after a redressive period with serial plaster dressings as described above. Surgery is performed, when a plateau phase is reached with no further improvement. Such procedures usually begin with a soft tissue release but usually require additional bony corrections in the older child, if possible without joint fusion. The older the patient and the more contracted the foot, the more bony corrective measures will be applied in addition to the soft tissue interventions described in Sect. 1.6.1, and the sooner a pure soft tissue release may be refrained from. In some cases, (partial) fusion of the tarsal skeleton cannot be avoided in order to achieve full and long-lasting correction. The aim always will be to adjust the upper ankle joint as the most important joint to a favorable range of motion (see Sect. 1.8). Typical surgical procedures for this age group in addition to the soft tissue release measures described in Sect. 1.6.1 are:

Typical Procedures for Clubfoot Relapse in Schoolchildren and Adolescents

- Medial release of the talonavicular joint with shortening of the lateral tarsal column by Lichtblau resection arthroplasty (Fig. 1.63) or calcaneocuboid resection arthrodesis.
- Lesser tarsal osteotomies for pes adductus deformity (Fig. 1.66).
- Naviculo-cuneiforme correction arthrodesis for cavus deformity (Fig. 1.68).
- Sliding osteotomy of the calcaneus to correct hindfoot varus (Fig. 1.69).
- Supramalleolar extension osteotomy or epiphysiodesis and notch plasty of the talus (Fig. 1.71).
- Supramalleolar varization by osteotomy or medial hemiepiphysiodesis in case of supramalleolar valgus (Fig. 1.70).
- In cases of pronounced tarsal malposition, Chopart or triple corrective fusion (Fig. 1.76).

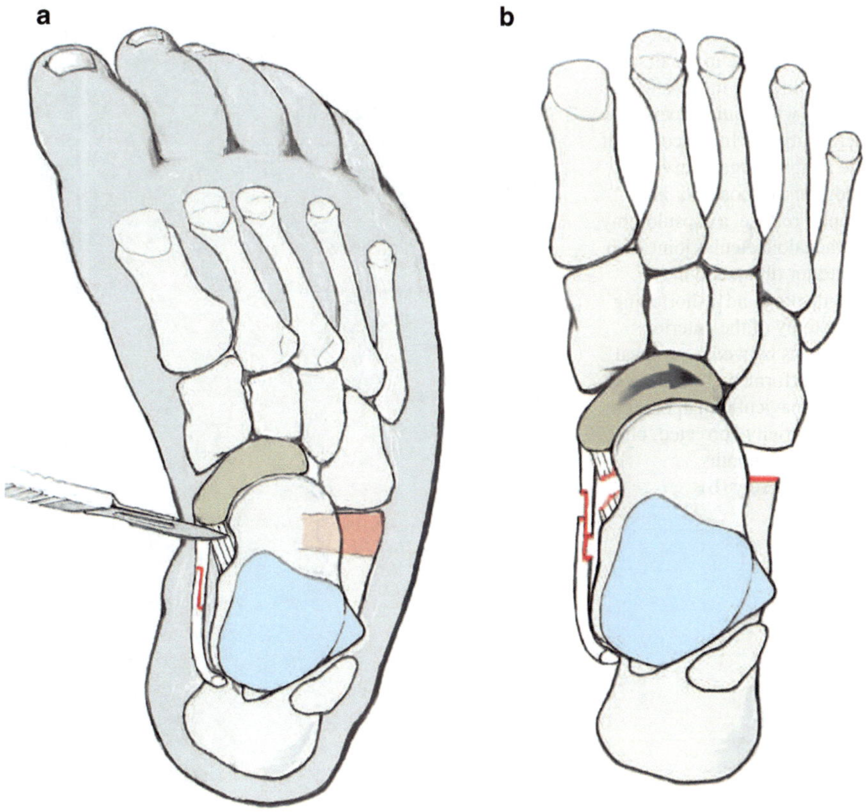

Fig. 1.63 Correction of a (moderate) inversion contracture of the talocalcaneal-navicular complex (**a**) by medial soft tissue release with shortening of the lateral tarsal column according to Lichtblau (1973) (**b**)

1.6.2.1 Medial Talonavicular Joint Release with Shortening of the Lateral Tarsal Column

A peritalar inversion still existing in schoolchildren or adolescents can no longer be completely corrected by a peritalar release. In some cases however, the combination of a capsular release of the talonavicular joint with inframalleolar lengthening of the posterior tibial tendon and release of the adductor hallucis muscle in conjunction with a shortening of the lateral column in the area of the anterior calcaneus is sufficiently effective (Fig. 1.63).

Options to Shorten the Lateral Tarsal Column

- Calcaneus shortening osteotomy (lateral base wedge removal).
- Resection arthroplasty according to Lichtblau (1973).
- Calcaneocuboid resection arthrodesis according to Evans (1961).
- Cuboid osteotomy (no effect on the peritalar complex).

The resection arthroplasty according to Lichtblau (1973) is a very valuable method for this age group which, in contrast to cuboid wedge resection (Fig. 1.66a), not only shortens the lateral tarsometatarsal ray but also allows (limited) correction of the talocalcaneal-navicular complex (Lichtblau 1973; Mehrafshan et al. 2009). The os naviculare can be shifted laterally to a limited extent with additional medial release of the talonavicular joint. The resection arthroplasty of the calcaneocuboid joint even results in some improvement of the dorsal extension. It is important that the cartilage of the os cuboideum remains completely intact during the resection of the anterior portion and joint surface of the calcaneus so that a nearthros can form subsequently (Fig. 1.65). In principle, a similar, but considerably smaller effect can also be achieved with a wedge resection at the anterior calcaneal region. Also a resection of the complete calcaneocuboid joint with fusion is possible (Lehman et al. 1999) but may result in overcorrection if performed in an early age. Figures 1.64 and 1.65 show treatment examples from this age group; further examples from the infant period can be found in Sect. 1.6.1.4.

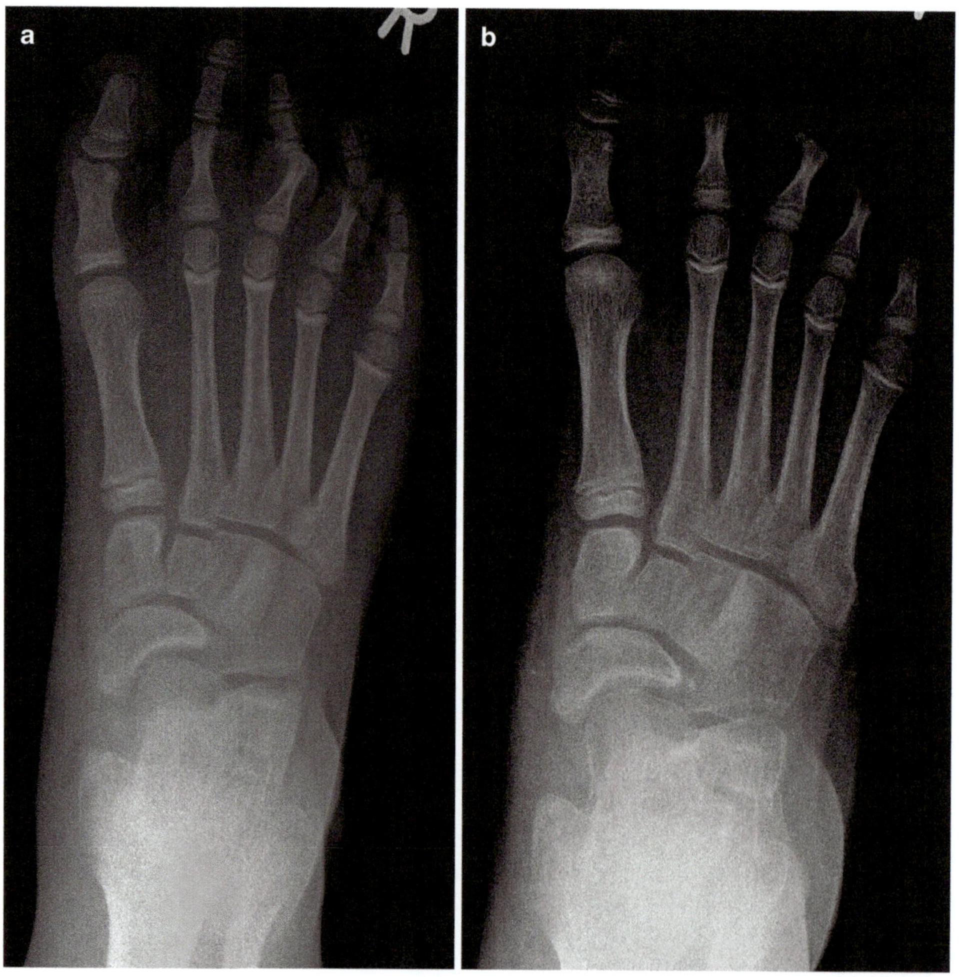

Fig. 1.64 9-year-old boy with status after external peritalar release in the first year of life and moderate relapse with equinocavus foot deformity (**a**). In the course of the relapse surgery, in addition to a posterior and plantar release, a capsulotomy of the talonavicular joint with posterior tibial tendon lengthening and a shortening osteotomy of the anterior calcaneus by wedge removal were performed. This allowed the talonavicular malposition to be partially corrected, on the right, 5 months postoperatively (**b**)

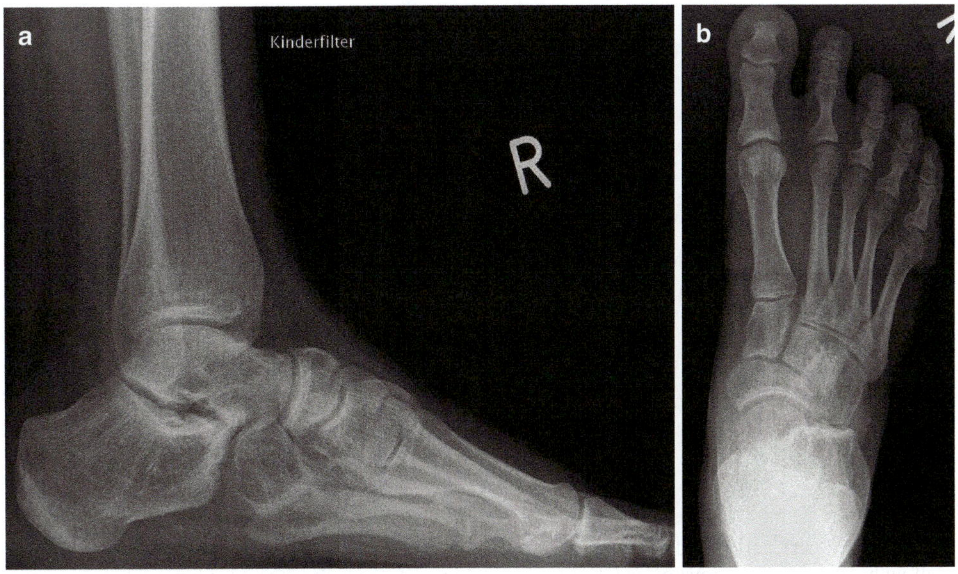

Fig. 1.65 9.5 years after clubfoot relapse correction at the age of about 5.5 years, including Lichtblau resection arthroplasty (**a** and **b**). A painless nearthros has formed with good deformity correction

Technique (Lichtblau Procedure)

The skin incision is made over the anterior aspect of the calcaneus in the course of the peroneus brevis tendon. The sural nerve must be carefully protected. The calcaneus is exposed epiperiostally and osteotomized about 10–12 mm proximal to the calcaneocuboid joint. This can be started with a scalpel in smaller children; otherwise an oscillating saw is used. The osteotomy is finished with a chisel. During the resection of the distal calcaneal portion, the cartilaginous joint surface of the os cuboideum is carefully protected after the opening of the calcaneocuboid joint. After the resection, it is checked whether an increased amount of eversion is possible. The procedure is usually combined with a medial soft tissue release (Sect. 1.6.1.2, Fig. 1.63).

1.6.2.2 Osteotomies of the Lesser Tarsus

If there is a distinct residual adduction and this is mainly located at the level of the anterior tarsus, a lesser tarsal osteotomy (Fig. 1.66) with complete joint preservation and without any capsular release can bring about a clear correction (McHale and Lenhart 1991; Schäfer and Hefti 2000). If, on the other hand, there is still an inversion of the hindfoot complex (Fig. 1.63a) or if the deformity is located at the level of the metatarsal bases, as is typically the case the in scewfoot (see Chap. 2), the correction must be carried out directly at these different locations of the deformity. The author was able to prove by cadaver investigations that the "Center of Rotation of Angulation (CORA)" (Paley 2002) of the correction is located centrally in the anterior tarsus in the double osteotomy of the lesser tarsus, whereas it is located far proximally in the case of cuboid wedge removal alone (Fig. 1.66c). Figure 1.67 shows an example of cuboid/cuneiforme double osteotomy.

Technique (Cuboid/Cuneiforme Osteotomy)

The cuboid wedge removal is carried out after marking and under protection of the calcaneocuboid and the lateral tarsometatarsal joint. A thin K-wire should be inserted into the bone at the site of the planned wedge for better manipulation of the bone graft. The wedge of bone should not be too small and is cut out with a small oscillating saw. Even if the osteotomy cannot be closed completely later, it will always heal safely. The planned osteotomy on the medial cuneiform should be marked intraoperatively with the image intensifier. The osteotomy can be opened with two strong K-wires proximally and distal to the osteotomy using an osteotomy spreader. When placing the cuboid wedge, it is very helpful, if it is reinforced with a thin K-wire (see above)—similar to a shashlik skewer—for better manipulation.

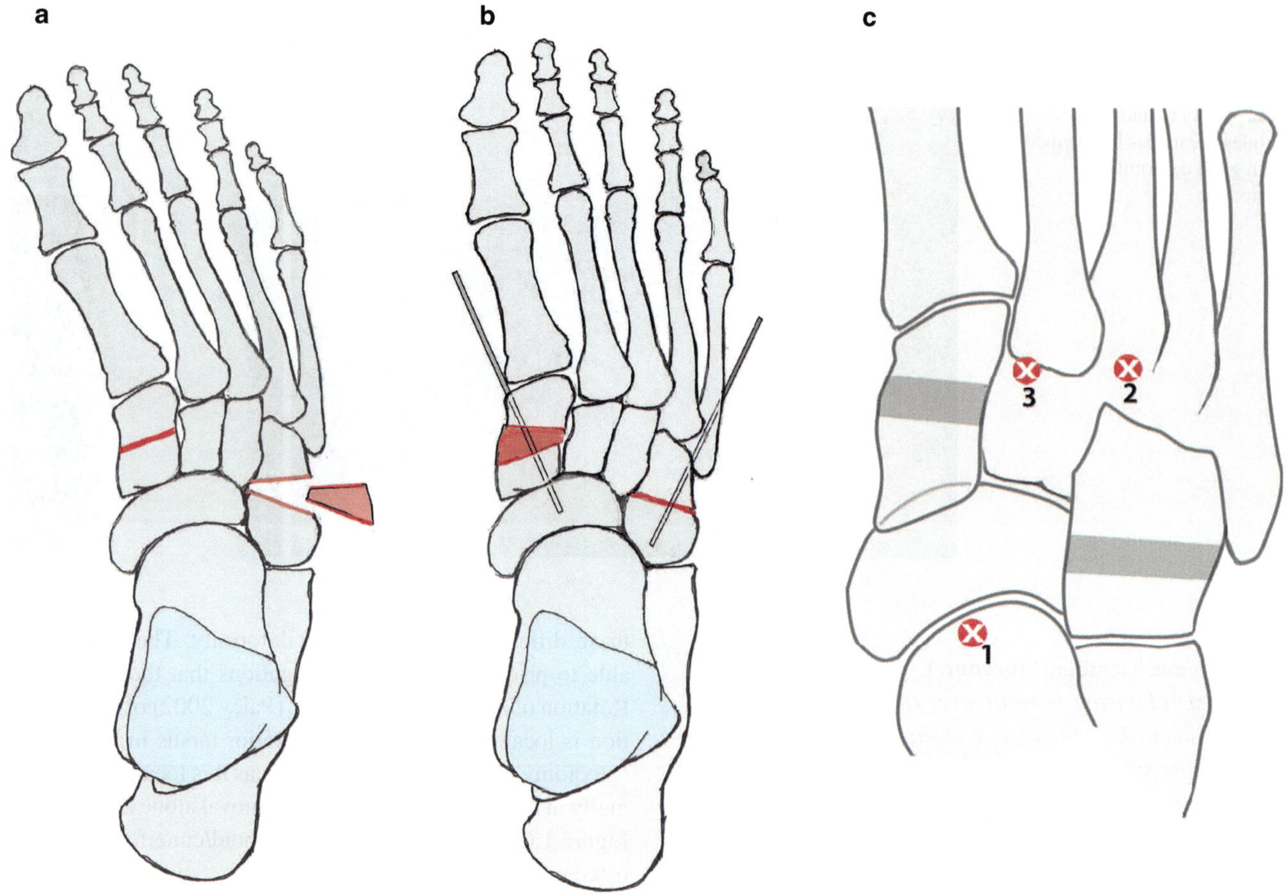

Fig. 1.66 Lesser tarsal cuboid/cuneiforme double osteotomy with wedge removal from the os cuboideum (**a**) and open-wedge osteotomy of the os cuneiforme mediale (**b**). The resulting CORA of the cuboid wedge removal (1), the isolated cuneiform osteotomy (2), and the combination of both osteotomies (3) from cadaver examinations on adult foot specimen are marked in (**c**)

1.6.2.3 Cavus Correction at the Lesser Tarsus

If marked cavus deformity is observed in the older child beyond 8–10 years of age and simple plantar fascial release with subsequent stretching does not seem to be sufficient, wedge resection at the lesser tarsus or the naviculo-cuneiforme joint line may be considered. This procedure was described by Cole (1940) (American literature) and Meary (French literature) and is described in Chap. 7. An example is presented in Fig. 1.68. As a positive side effect, the talus is slightly plantar-flexed by cavus correction, improving the capacity of the tibiotalar joint for dorsal extension. However, especially in idiopathic clubfoot, any fusion should be avoided if possible.

1.6.2.4 Osteotomies of the Tuber Calcanei for Varus Correction

To correct a hindfoot varus that remains despite soft tissue correction, a Dwyer osteotomy (lateral closing wedge resection at the tuber calcanei), a sliding osteotomy or a calcaneus scarf osteotomy (see Chap. 7) can be performed. The latter two forms of osteotomy may be associated with compression of the tibial nerve due to impingement by the laciniate ligament, so that a prophylactic splitting of the tarsal tunnel should be considered depending on the amount of displacement. Figure 1.69 shows an example of a sliding osteotomy (in combination with other tarsal osteotomies).

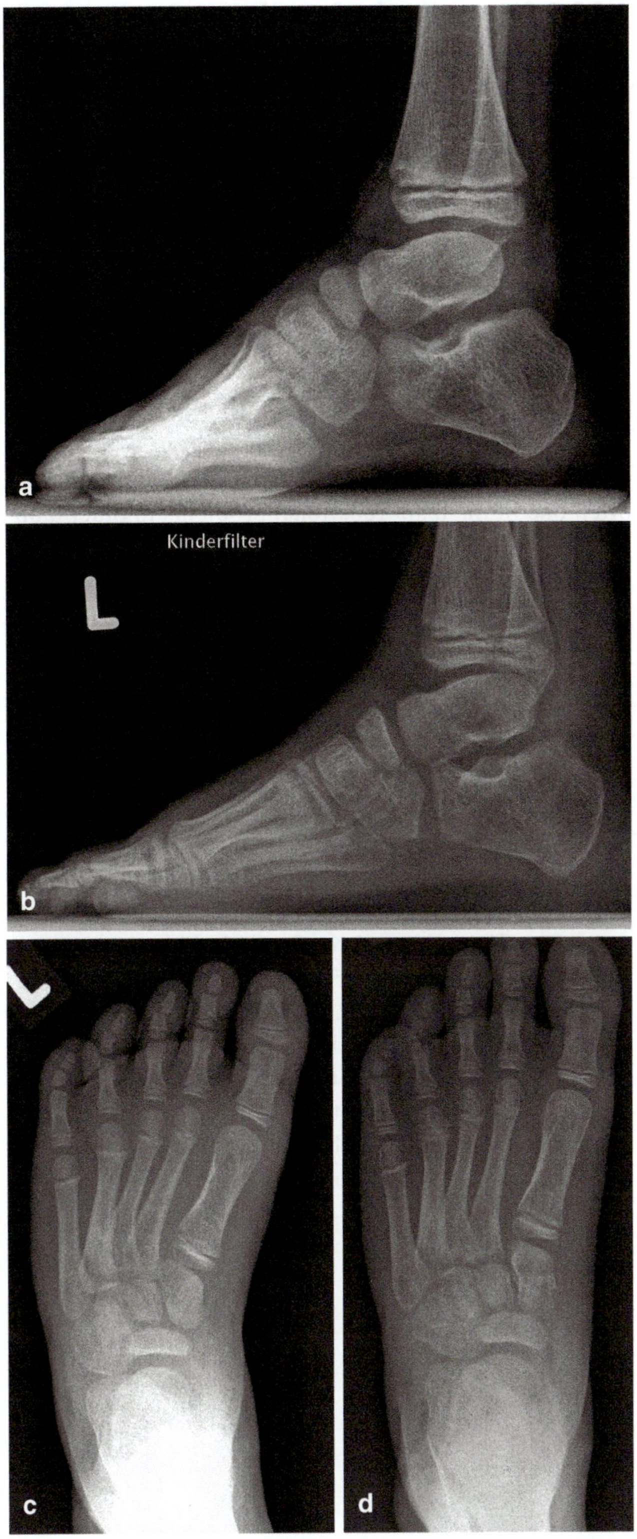

Fig. 1.67 7-year-old boy with external pretreatment according to the Ponseti concept with first percutaneous tenotomy, later open Achilles tendon lengthening and clubfoot relapse with distinct cavus and adductus components (**a** and **c**). Relapse surgery was performed with posterior and plantar release, cuboid/cuneiforme osteotomy, and anterior tibial tendon transfer. 3 years postoperatively significantly improved tarsal alignment, however with persistent moderate flattening of the trochlea tali (**b** and **d**)

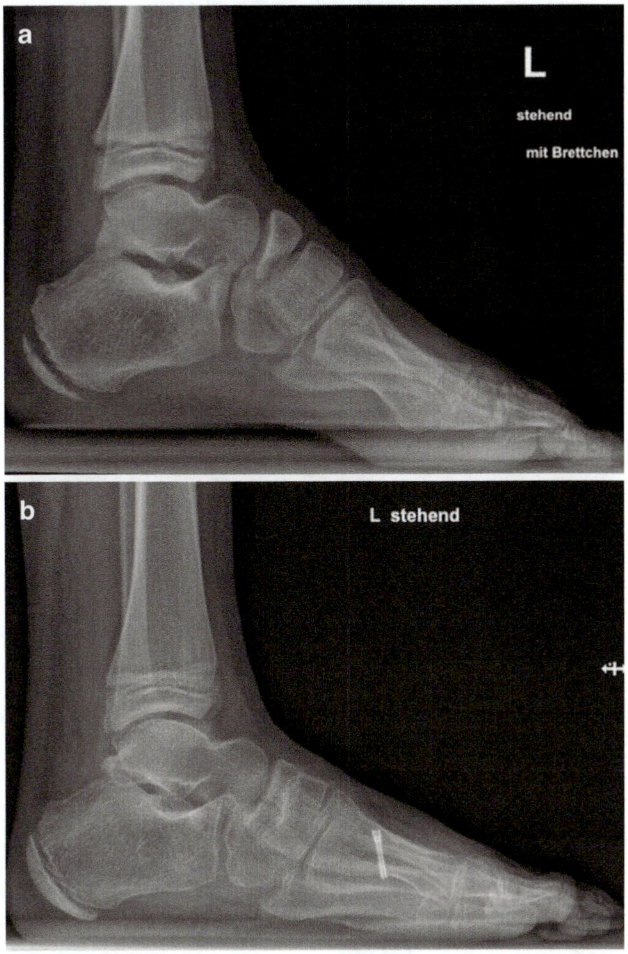

Fig. 1.68 10-year-old boy with idiopathic clubfoot after uneventful Ponseti treatment, who developed cavus relapse (**a**). The hindfoot-centered lateral projection with Coleman blocktest shows the talometatarsal angle markedly increased. 6 months after Cole procedure, elevating osteotomy of the first metatarsal bone and transfer of the long peroneal muscle improved tarsometatarsal alignment (**b**)

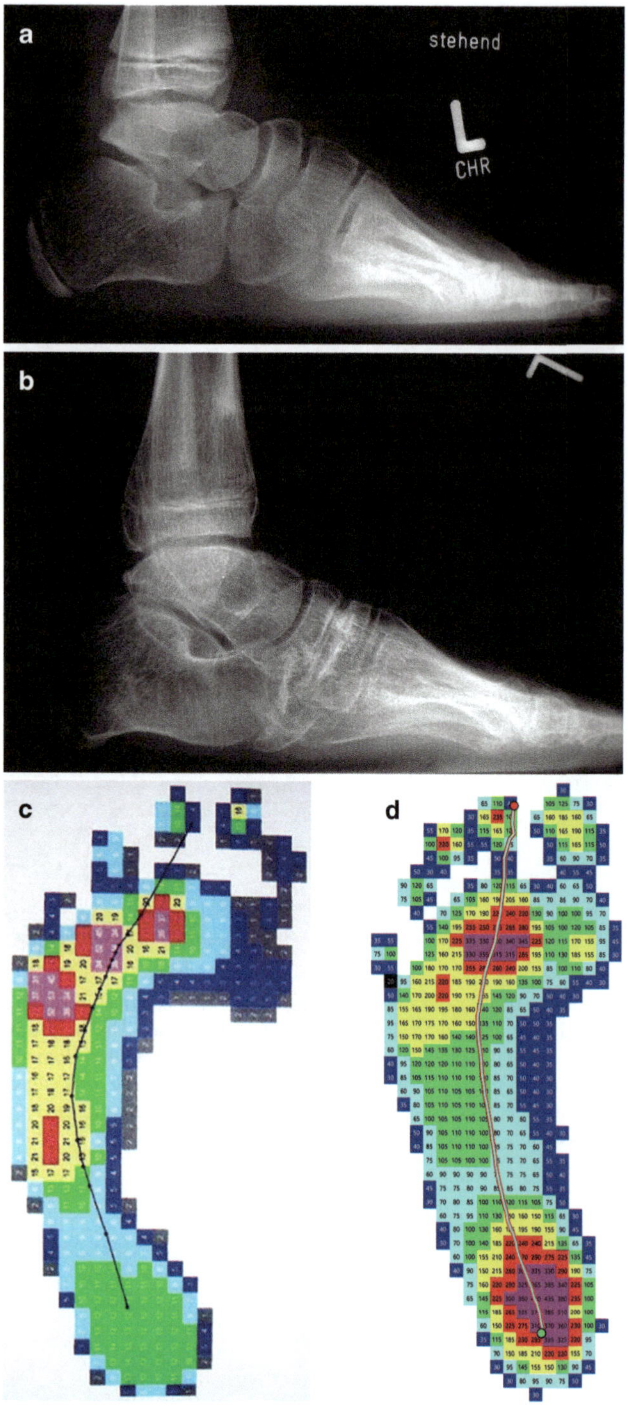

Fig. 1.69 13-year-old patient with condition after external posterior release and clear relapse (**a**). More impressive than the X-ray image is the pedographic peak pressure representation with reduced load on the heel and marked overload at the lateral metatarsus (**c**). 1.5 years after relapse correction including multiple tarsal osteotomies (among those a lateralizing osteotomy of the tuber calcanei) and anterior tibial tendon transfer (**b**), pedographically documented significant functional improvement (**d**)

1.6.2.5 Supramalleolar Procedures and Arthroplasty of the Talus

Growth of the supramalleolar region in the frontal plane should be controlled in idiopathic clubfoot. Valgus deformity is observed quite frequently (Stevens and Otis 1999; Burghardt et al. 2016), especially in overcorrection conditions (Sect. 1.6.3) but also in relapses (Fig. 1.70). The pathogenesis of this growth disturbance remains unclear; probably deloading of the medial metatarsal ray plays a role. Napiontek (2003) found fibular shortening connected with weakness of plantarflexors. Here, medial epiphysiodesis with a small fragment screw or eight-plate can be used at a suitable age (Stevens et al. 2011; Rupprecht et al. 2015).

The deficient dorsal extension of the ankle joint is often one of the main functional problems in older clubfoot patients (Fig. 1.111). The dorsal extension capacity of the tibiotalar joint can be enhanced by supramalleolar removal of an anterior-based wedge, reducing plantar flexion at the same amount (Coleman 1983). This is particularly indicated when the natural slope of the distal tibial joint surface is absent or even negative. In addition to the loss of correction due to remodeling in cases with still open physis, one additional disadvantage is that the center of rotation of the talus is moved anteriorly (Fig. 1.71). The same effect over time is achieved by an anterior epiphysiodesis of the distal tibial physis in case of sufficient residual growth to be expected (Figs. 1.72 and 1.79). The published results with this procedure are partly encouraging (Flöter et al. 2015), partly not convincing (Al-Aubaidi et al. 2011). In suitable cases, an arthroplastic reduction at the talar neck can also be considered ("notch plasty") to improve dorsal extension (Fig. 1.73b), although limited experience exists with this and only minor effect can be expected.

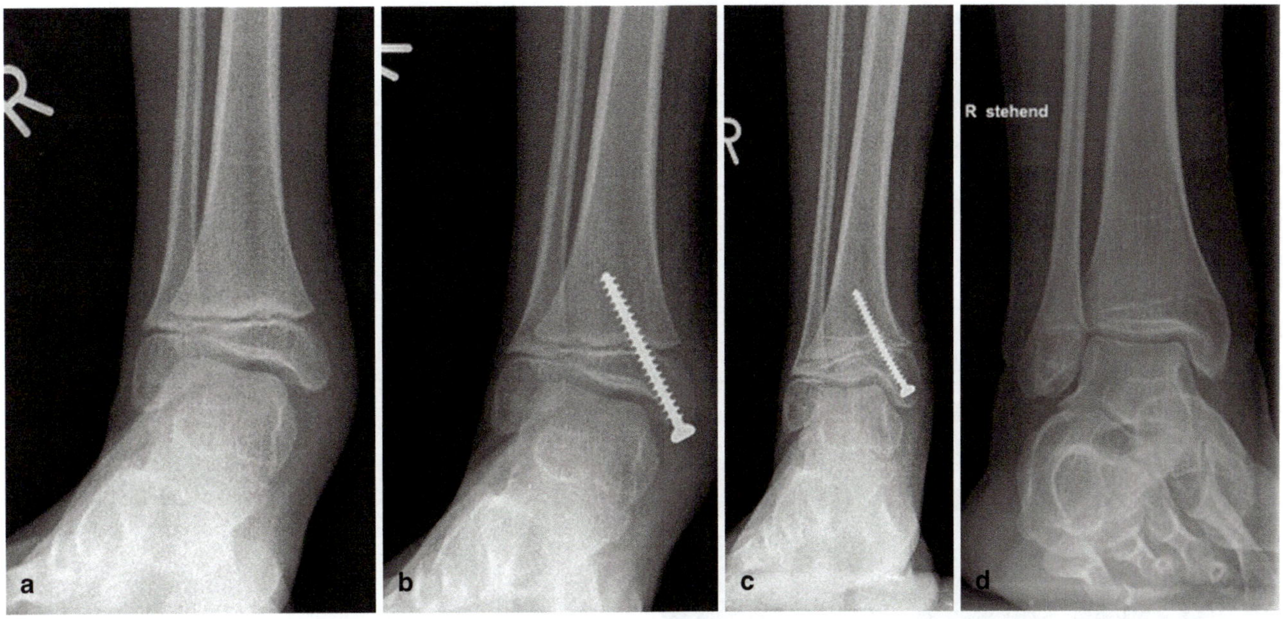

Fig. 1.70 8-year-old girl with multiple clubfoot correction because of relapse, now supramalleolar valgus malformation (**a**). Temporary hemiepiphysiodesis (**b**) resulted in slight overcorrection within 20 months (**c**). At the end of growth orthograde tibiotalar angle could be observed with 13 years of age (**d**)

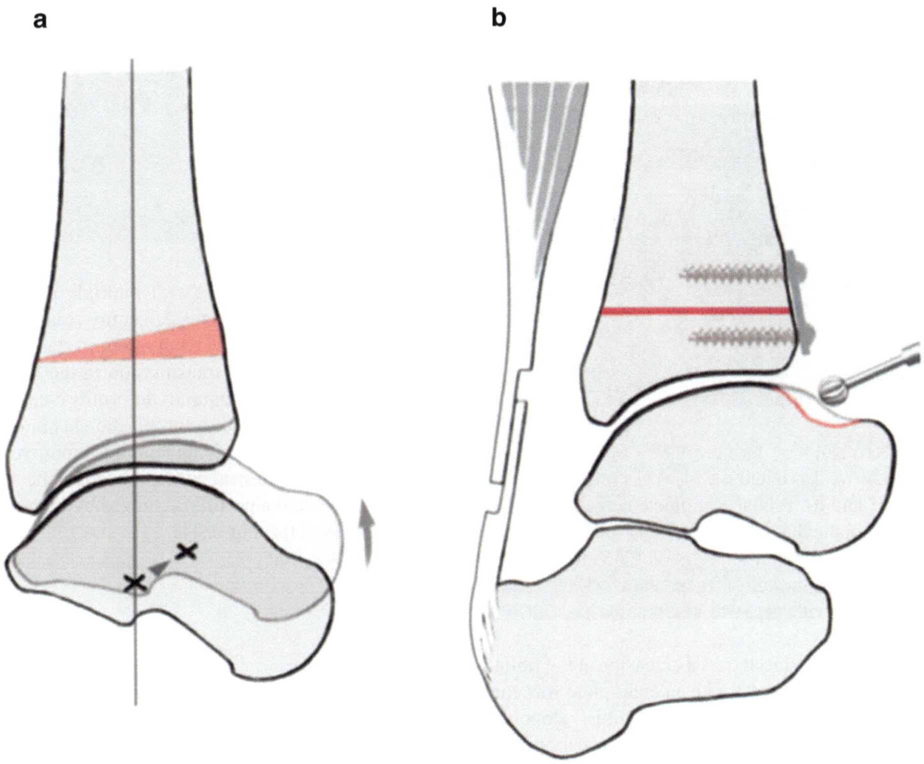

Fig. 1.71 Improvement of the dorsal extension of the upper ankle joint by supramalleolar osteotomy (or epiphysiodesis). This, however, results in a shift of the center of talar rotation (**a**) and a reduction of the anterior stability of the tibiotalar joint. In individual cases, arthroplastic shaping of the talar neck for improvement of the dorsal extension may be useful ("Notch plasty") (**b**). All such measures are only justified after soft tissue contracture treatment has been exhausted (e.g., lengthening of Achilles tendon and capsular release)

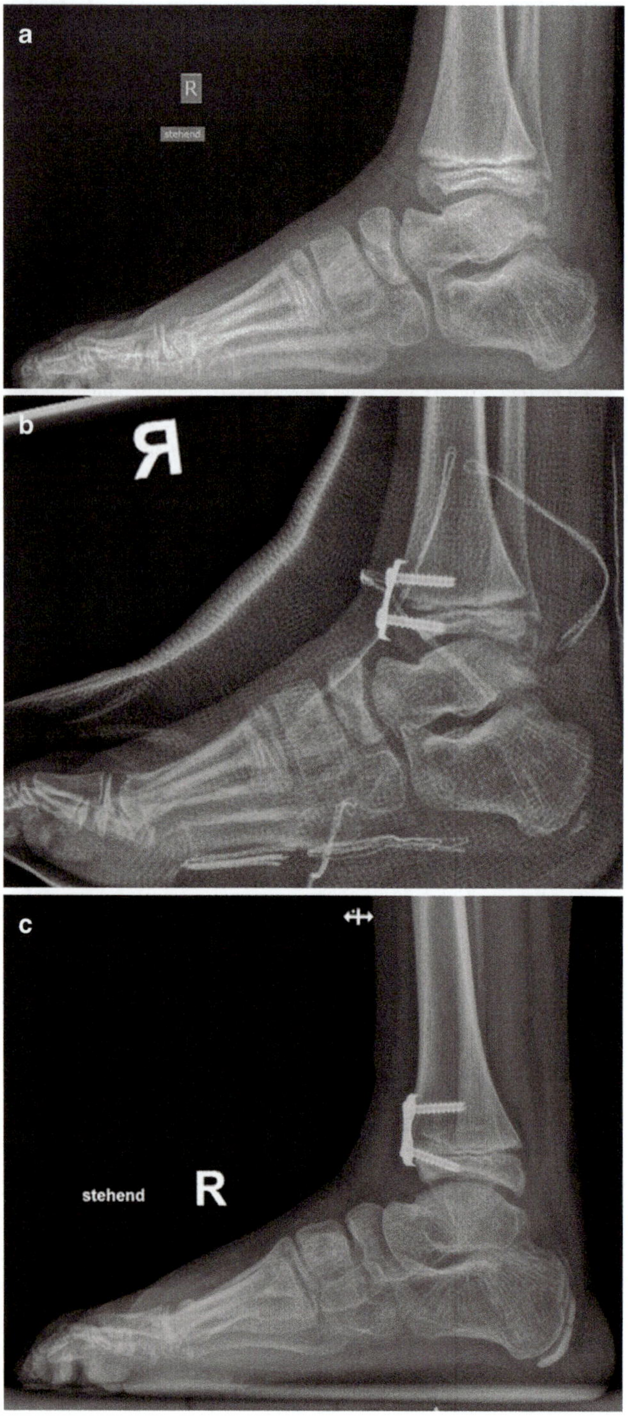

Fig. 1.72 10-year-old boy with reduced dorsal extension at the tibiotalar joint (**a**). Anterior hemiepiphysiodeses with an eight-plate was combined with posterior release (**b**). After 1.5 years tibial slope had improved to a normal range (**c**). The effect of the temporarily physeal closure can be evaluated by the increased angle of the inserted screws

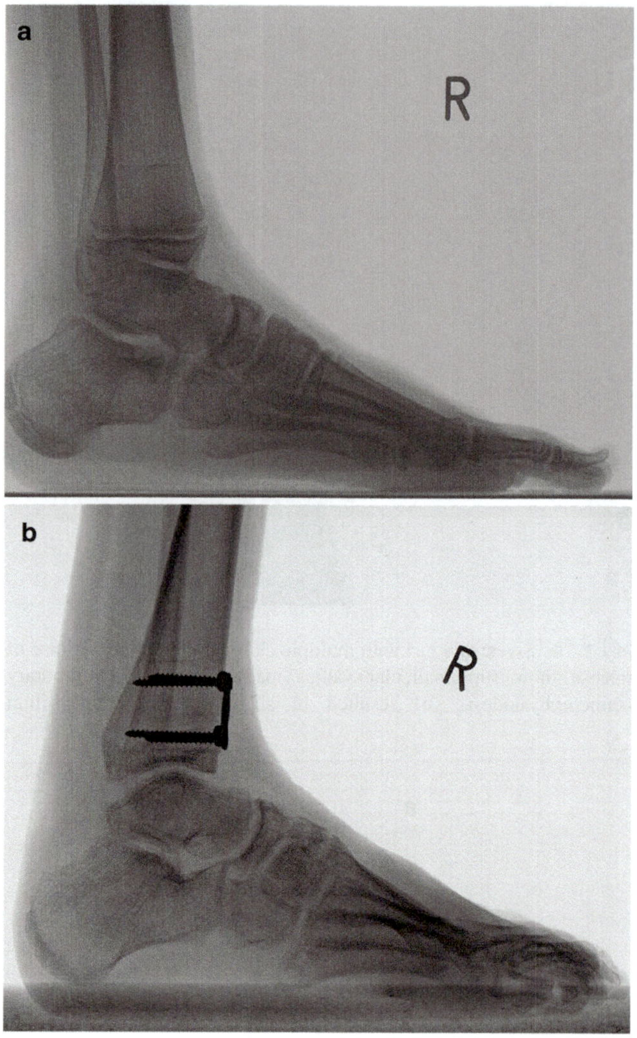

Fig. 1.73 13-year-old boy with multiple previous surgeries for the treatment of recurrent equinus deformity contracture (**a**). With 16 years clinically pronounced knee recurvatum in standing position and nearly completely missing load transmission in the heel region in pedogram with clinically about 15° equinus deformity contracture. Supramalleolar extension osteotomy with arthroplastic shaping of the talar neck and repeated Achilles tendon lengthening to improve dorsal extension (**b**). Postoperatively, 5° dorsal extension could be maintained, a further improvement could have been achieved by cavus correction in the anterior tarsal region (cf. Fig. 1.74)

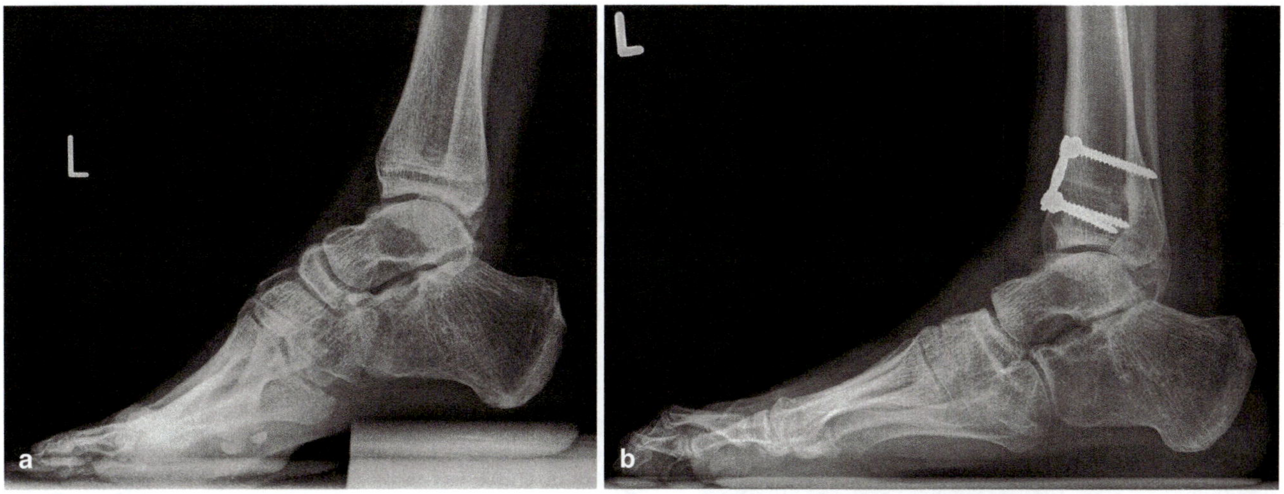

Fig. 1.74 15-year-old patient with severe recurrence of an equinocavus foot deformity after several previous surgeries including an anterior tibial tendon transfer without major tarsal malalignment and still partially mobile peritalar joint complex (**a**). Supramalleolar extension osteotomy and naviculo-cuneiforme correction arthrodesis with cuboid osteotomy (Cole procedure) resulted in a plantigrade foot position (**b**). Alternatively, a Lambrinudi correction arthrodesis would also have been possible, but seemed less recommendable from a functional point of view with a partially mobile hindfoot

1.6.2.6 Supramalleolar Rotational Osteotomy

Intoeing gait has been one of the most frequently observed sequelae of idiopathic clubfoot in former times. It seems to be less frequent in patients treated according to the Ponseti concept (Mindler et al. 2014), probably due to the effect of the foot abduction brace. In rare exceptional cases, an outward rotating supramalleolar rotational osteotomy of the tibia may be useful. This should only be performed if more proximal located common causes of the inward rotation gait (e.g., Coxa antetorta) are excluded and all other inframalleolar malposition causes have been addressed beforehand. Figure 1.75 shows the clinical examination to check the rotational profile of the lower leg.

Surgical Options for Correction of the Persistent Intoeing Gait

- Elimination of inversion contracture (peritalar complex).
- Removal of a remaining adductus deformity.
- Posterior tibial tendon lengthening.
- Anterior tibial tendon transfer (particularly effective with full correction of the peritalar joint complex).
- Supramalleolar rotation osteotomy (very rarely indicated, as the intermalleolar axis often tends to outward rotation per se in clubfoot).

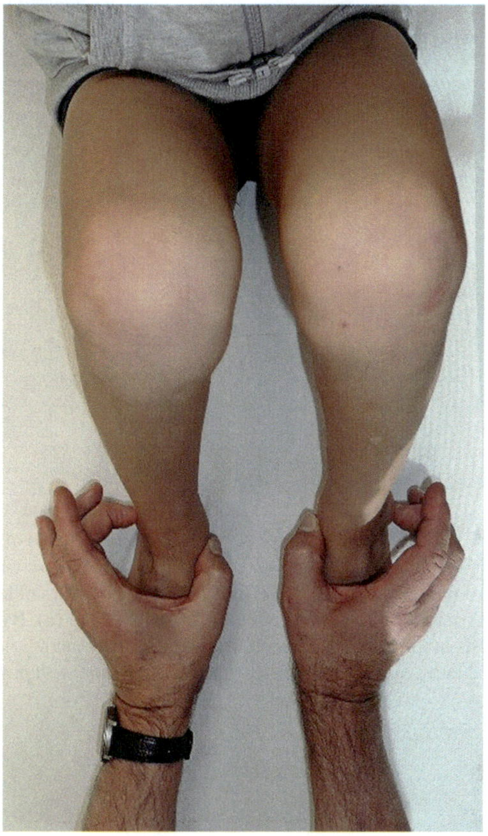

Fig. 1.75 6-year-old boy with complete correction for idiopathic clubfoot on both sides. In addition, there is a lower leg inward rotational component which has already been corrected on the right leg by supramalleolar outward rotation osteotomy. On the left lower leg, the knee joint flexion axis and the intermalleolar axis (marked by the palpating examiners fingers) are still almost parallel and lack the physiological outward rotation of about 25° (right leg). Clinically there is a pronounced intoeing gait

1.6.2.7 Realigning Peritalar Fusions

Corrective procedures that sacrifice tarsal joints should generally better be avoided in idiopathic clubfoot, since all joints of the tarsometatarsal region including the ankle joint are less flexible and more or less non-anatomically shaped, and therefore the compensation mechanisms of the neighboring joints are less effective than in other underlying diseases. Nevertheless, there are indications for tarsal fusions already in late childhood and adolescence, if a functionally better adjustment of adjacent joints—especially the ankle joint—can thus be achieved. A persisting cavus component can be corrected by naviculo-cuneiforme corrective arthrodesis with dorsal wedge removal, which runs out laterally into the os cuboideum (Cole 1940) (Figs. 1.68 and 1.74). With pronounced, contracted inversion malpositions of the tarsus, a Chopart fusion, or a triple arthrodesis can be advisable, for example, in the technique according to Lambrinudi (1927) (cf. section "(Extreme) Lambrinudi"), in particular in order to adjust the upper ankle joint to a more favorable working range (Fig. 1.76).

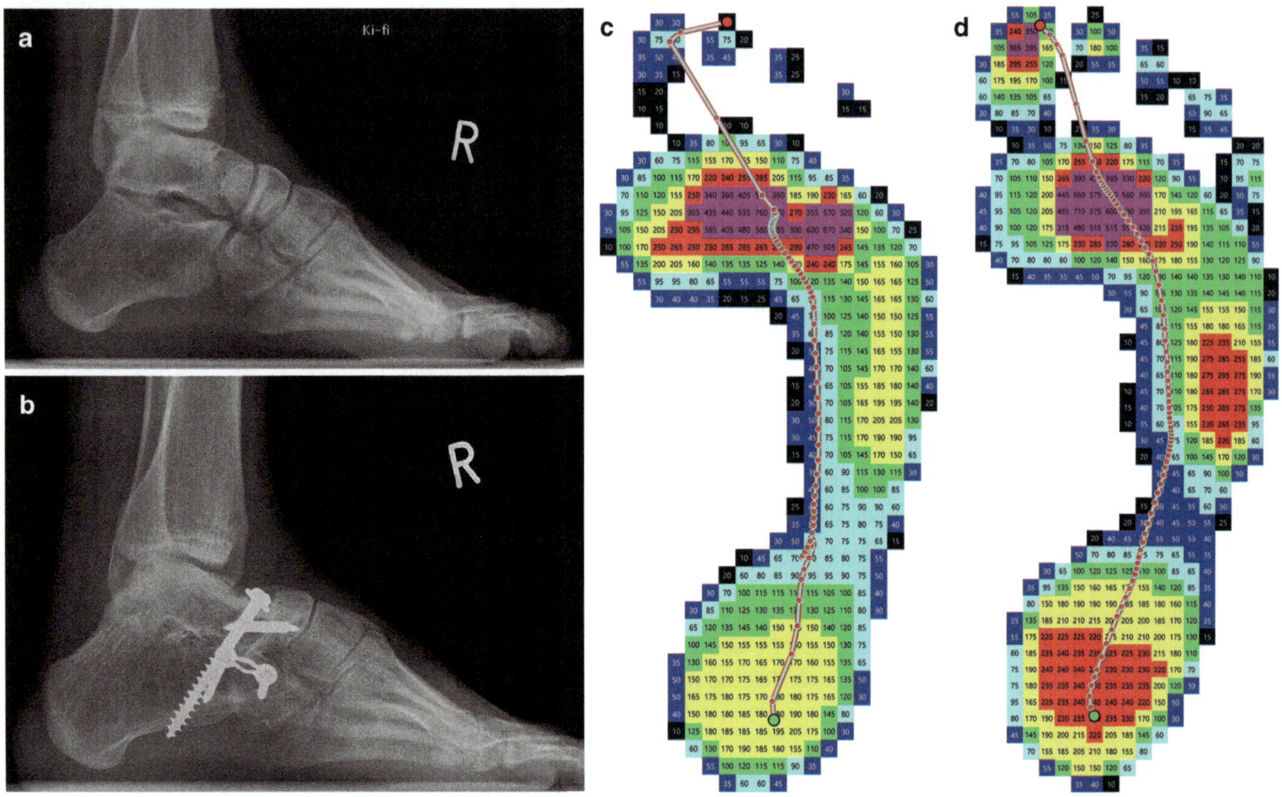

Fig. 1.76 15.5-year-old male adolescent patient with status after peritalar release in the first year of life. Clinically distinct relapse with overloading of the lateral border of the foot and a tendency for ankle sprain, as well as anterior impingement of the upper ankle joint (**a**). By a triple arthrodesis in the Lambrinudi modification, the upper ankle joint could be moved into a significantly better functional position with now 10° of dorsal extension (**b**). Pedographically, 15 months postoperatively (**d**), a normalized early stance phase is observed with temporally extended heel loading after the initial contact compared to preoperative status (**c**). However, a non-physiological loading of the metatarsal V base persists and could have been avoided by even more increased pronation of the middle forefoot segment

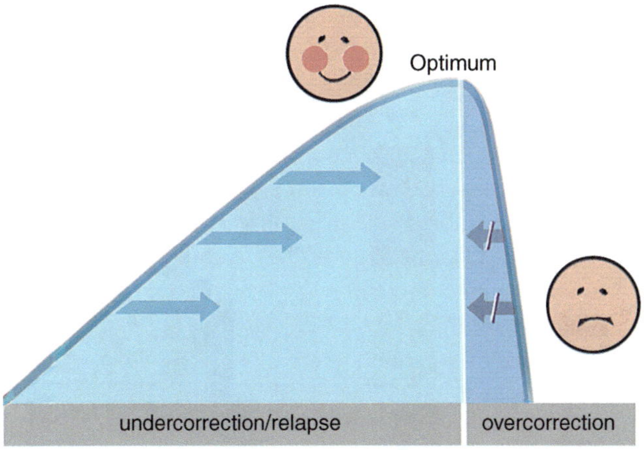

Fig. 1.77 While undercorrections (to the left of the "optimum") can be controlled secondarily, optimal results and overcorrection (to the right of the "optimum") are close together, and the latter pose considerable therapeutic problems

1.6.3 Clubfoot Overcorrection

When correcting an idiopathic clubfoot, the aim is to achieve a full correction as the optimum possible result (curve summit in Fig. 1.77). This can lead to undercorrections or recurrences, as can often be observed at previous treatment concepts with purely posterior release, or with the Ponseti concept and early discontinuation of the retention splint. However, overcorrections can also occur, which most frequently appeared after previous extensive surgical release. Overcorrection phenomena were observed after Ponseti primary treatment as well: Hayes et al. (2018) described 12% of hindfoot valgus alignment. Severe complex overcorrections, however, seem to be less frequent after this primarily conservative treatment concept and were not observed by the author up to now. While undercorrections and recurrences are generally well treatable, overcorrections are hardly reversible dysfunctions, which require complex surgical measures.

1.6.3.1 Pathomorphology and Dysfunction

Each of the five malalignment components of clubfoot deformity (see Sect. 1.3.1) can be iatrogenically overcorrected (Haslam et al. 2006; Hamel 2011). This danger exists especially after extensive release procedures on joint capsules of the peritalar complex and tendons, as they were common before the "Ponseti era." Mosca (2014) and previously Simons (1993) distinguish a subtalar malrotation ("rotatory valgus," especially with persistent calcaneocuboid deformity) from an excessive subtalar translation ("translatory valgus" with talocalcaneal ad-latim malalignment). Eberhardt et al. (2018) recommended triple fusion for these cases with translatory valgus deformity. After treatment with the Ponseti concept, overcorrection phenomena are observed much less frequently, so that a reduction of cases of this kind as shown below can be expected in the future. From a functional and therapeutic point of view, overcorrections are generally less favorable than recurrences and tend to worsen continuously (Fig. 1.77). In particular, with increasing age and body weight, the affected patients are no longer able to transfer sufficient strain on their forefoot (calcaneus gait) and thus dynamic walking is no longer possible. The following components are often observed in combination:

Components of Clubfoot Overcorrection
- Calcaneus foot deformity with insufficiency of the calf muscles and compensatory overactivity of the long toe flexors (cf. Sect. 6.1).
- Excessive peritalar eversion with insufficiency of the tibialis posterior muscle, in severe cases fibulocalcaneal impingement.
- Supramalleolar valgus malgrowth with malformation of the medial upper ankle compartment.
- Middle forefoot supination.
- Dorsal-bunion problem with elevation and destabilization of the medial ray and flexion contracture of the metatarsophalangeal joint (section "Correction of the Dorsal Bunion").
- Peroneal tendon dislocation.

Radiologically, the characteristics of excessive hindfoot eversion can be seen in the lateral and dorsoplantar X-ray image or—better—in the (weight-bearing) DVT. Frequently a supramalleolar valgus deformity adds to the hindfoot deformity and can be observed in the ankle ap projection. Elevation of the medial metatarsal ray or supination of the whole mid-forefoot is shown in the lateral projection. The development of the often detrimental functional consequences of overcorrection can best be documented pedographically (Hamel 2011) (Fig. 1.78). The cause of the frequently observed supramalleolar valgus malgrowth (Stevens and Otis 1999) could be the fact that in the case of clubfoot sequelae—and in particular in the case of overcorrection—a normal load on the medial foot ray can rarely be observed and this might result in altered force ratios at the growing supramalleolar structures.

Pedographic Signs of Clubfoot Overcorrection
- Missing indentation of the pedographic footprint in the midfoot area.
- Reduction of pressure and force in the forefoot area.
- Overloading of the anterior tarsal region with reduced heel loading.
- Missing load transfer at the metatarsal I (in contrast to flexible flatfoot).
- High load transfer at the big toe (compensation).

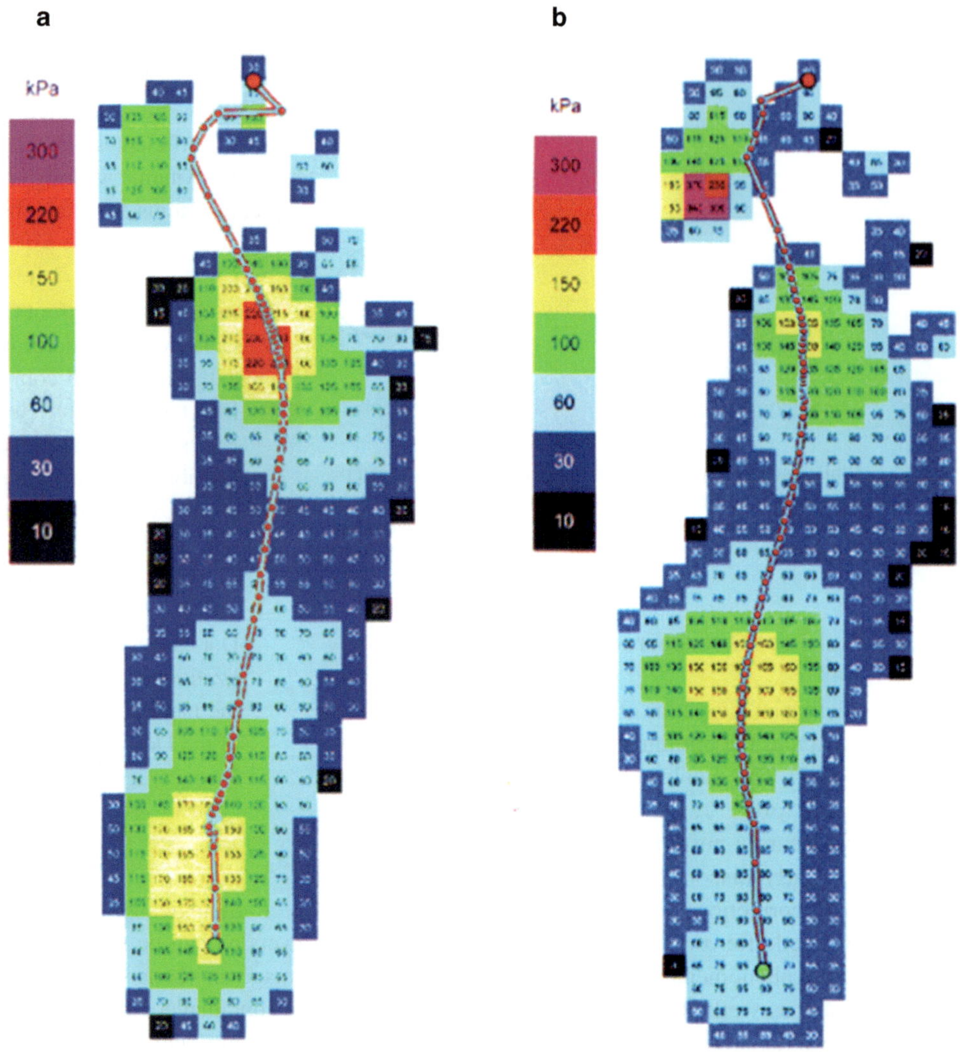

Fig. 1.78 Clubfoot patient with condition after externally performed peritalar release in the first year of life. The pedographies (peak pressure pictures) with 9 (**a**) and 12 years (**b**) show the serious and progressive increase of the dysfunction with complete missing of load transfer at the medial ray

1.6.3.2 Principles of Surgical Treatment

Surgical corrections of clubfoot overcorrection should not be delayed and are recommended already in growth age in the case of manifest functional impairment. Surgery can significantly improve function in the long term or prevent the otherwise threatening deterioration (O'Brien et al. 2004; Hamel 2011). Simple solutions such as isolated arthroereisis are to be evaluated critically (Fig. 4.33). Typical operative measures are:

- Strengthening of the calf muscles and the posterior tibial muscle by tendon transfer and Achilles tendon shortening (limited effect).
- Stabilization of the talocalcaneal-navicular complex by osteotomies or arthrodesis (calcaneal osteotomy, calcaneocuboid interposition arthrodesis, Grice procedure, arthroereisis in less rigid conditions, Chopart, or triple arthrodesis), thereby increasing the efficiency of calf muscles function.
- Supramalleolar valgus corrections by osteotomies or guided growth.
- Plantarization or stabilization of the medial foot ray by osteotomy, or arthrodesis (e.g., naviculo-cuneiforme fusion), flexor hallucis longus transfer to the metatarsal I, and the anterior tibial tendon to the second ray (see section "Correction of the Dorsal Bunion").

1.6.3.3 Treatment Examples

Since the indication for the combination of procedures is very individual, the treatment concept will be described case based. For example, in individual cases and depending on age, it must be considered, whether a Chopart joint line with excessive compensatory mobility should be fused to stabilize the foot (Fig. 1.81) or rather left hypermobile (Fig. 1.80) in order to further compensate for the reduced mobility of the upper ankle joint. The reversed Coleman block test can be helpful to estimate the stability of the joints of the medial ray (Fig. 1.89). If the ankle joint is anatomically developed close to normal, triple fusion is the standard procedure in adolescents for three-dimensional realignment of the hindfoot with special regard to sufficient medial forefoot pronation.

Complex Interventions for Overcorrection Conditions

The surgical treatment of clubfoot overcorrection usually requires multiple measures in the hindfoot and midfoot area

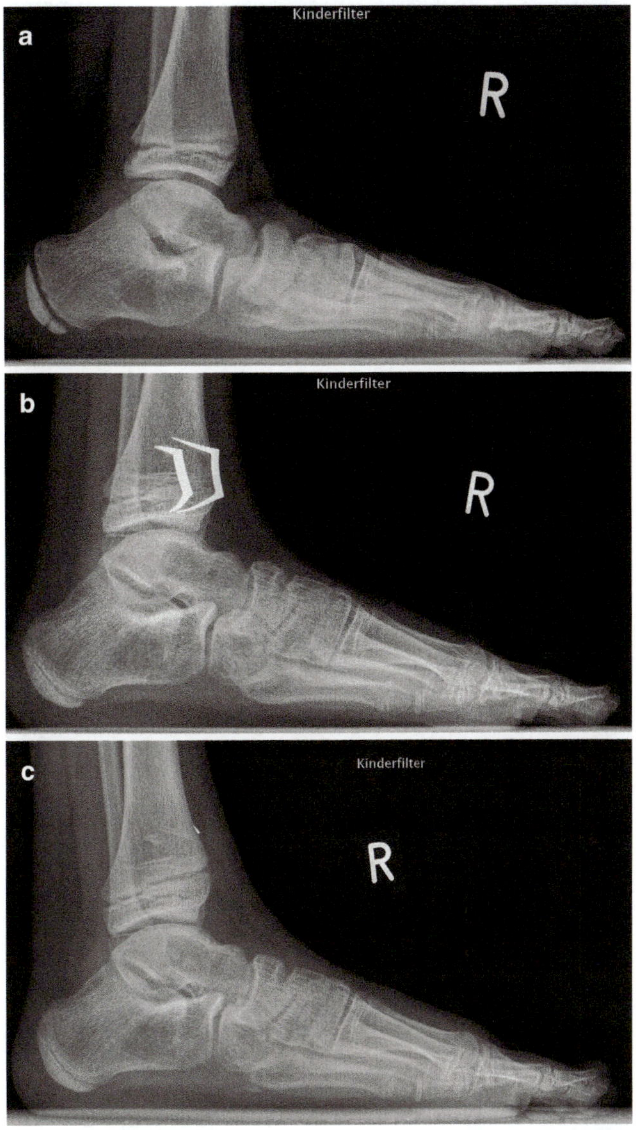

Fig. 1.79 11-year-old patient, idiopathic clubfoot, externally treated purely conservatively, clinically marked overcorrection (**a**). After Achilles tendon lengthening, calcaneus double osteotomy, and temporary anteromedial epiphyseodesis of the distal tibial physis, distinct effect on supramalleolar correction after 15 months (**b**). After removal of the staples 27 months postoperatively (**c**) clinically marked improvement of function

as well as sometimes the supramalleolar region. In minor cases, the tarsal joints can be preserved (Fig. 1.79). If stabilization of the hindfoot by arthrodesis appears necessary, the talocalcaneal joint and the naviculo-cuneiforme joint line should be considered first (Fig. 1.80) and only in more pronounced cases the functionally particularly important Chopart line (Fig. 1.81). In addition to hindfoot stabilization, the simultaneous correction of a middle forefoot supination is always essential (Fig. 1.82). Marked supramalleolar valgus deformity requires bony correction (Figs. 1.83 and 1.84). Complete tarsal collapse should be corrected by bony interpositional fusions (Fig. 1.85).

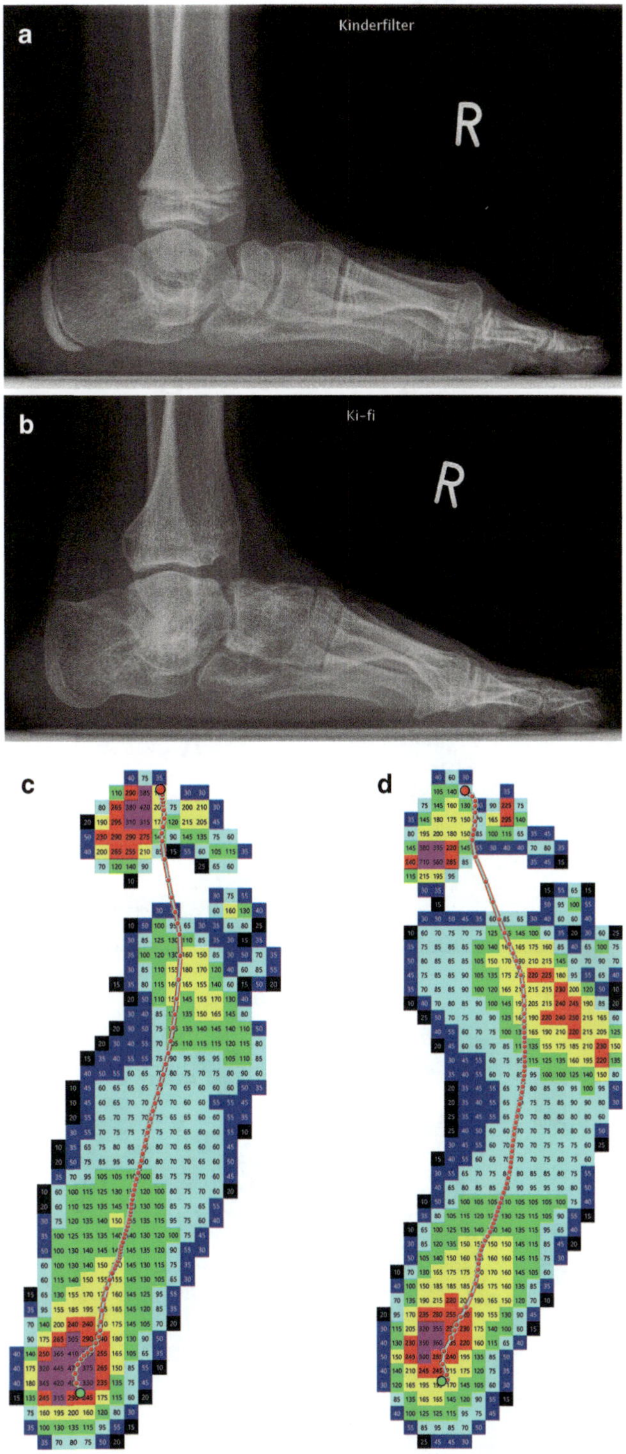

Fig. 1.80 13-year-old patient, status after peritalar release in idiopathic clubfoot (**a** and **c**). Tarsal stabilization by Grice extra-articular fusion and calcaneus sliding osteotomy, as well as stabilization of the medial ray by naviculo-cuneiforme arthrodesis. The dorsal-bunion deformity was corrected by FHL rerouting and proximal closing wedge osteotomy of the first metatarsal. The compensatory hypermobile Chopart line was left untouched, because of the limited mobility of the tibiotalar joint, due to flat top talus. 2.5 years postoperatively (**b** and **d**) clinically clearly improved function with still distinctly lateral forefoot loading

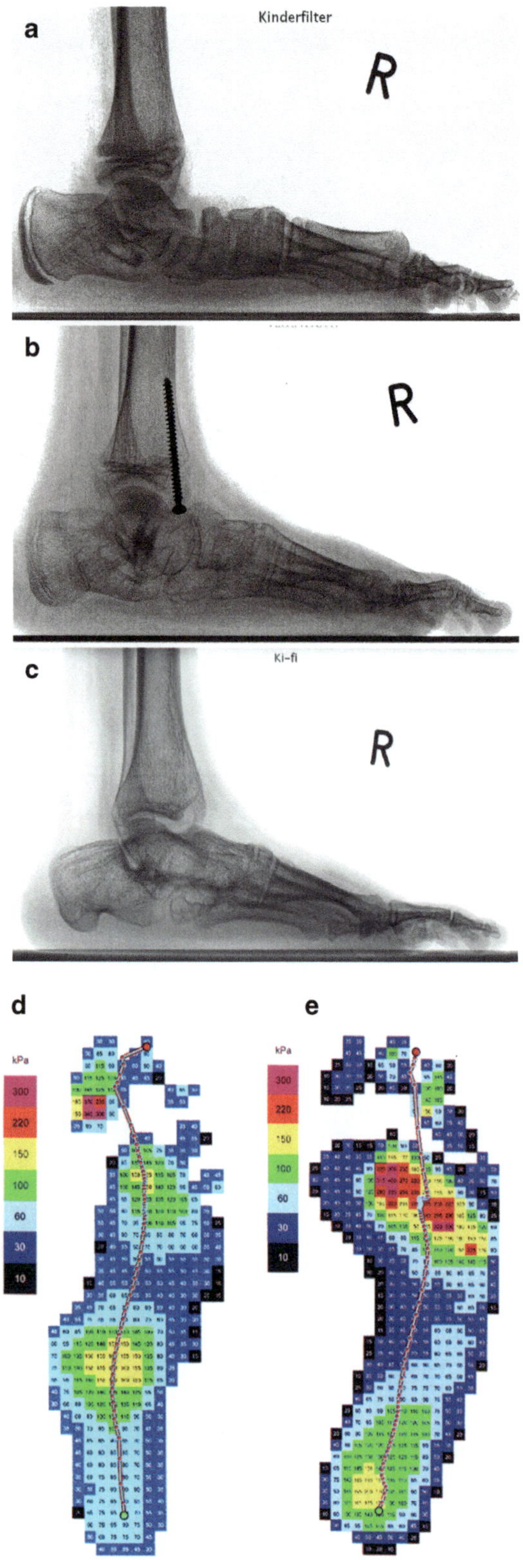

Fig. 1.81 12-year-old boy, status after peritalar release externally in the first year of life, clinically most severe overcorrection (**a** and **d**). After extensive bone and soft tissue stabilization, leaving the Chopart line (**b**) unchanged, an inadequate overall correction was observed due to the highly unstable talonavicular joint (underestimated during the first intervention), which had to be fused in a second procedure (**c**). Only 1 year after this second intervention, at the age of 14, major improvement of function could be observed (**e**)

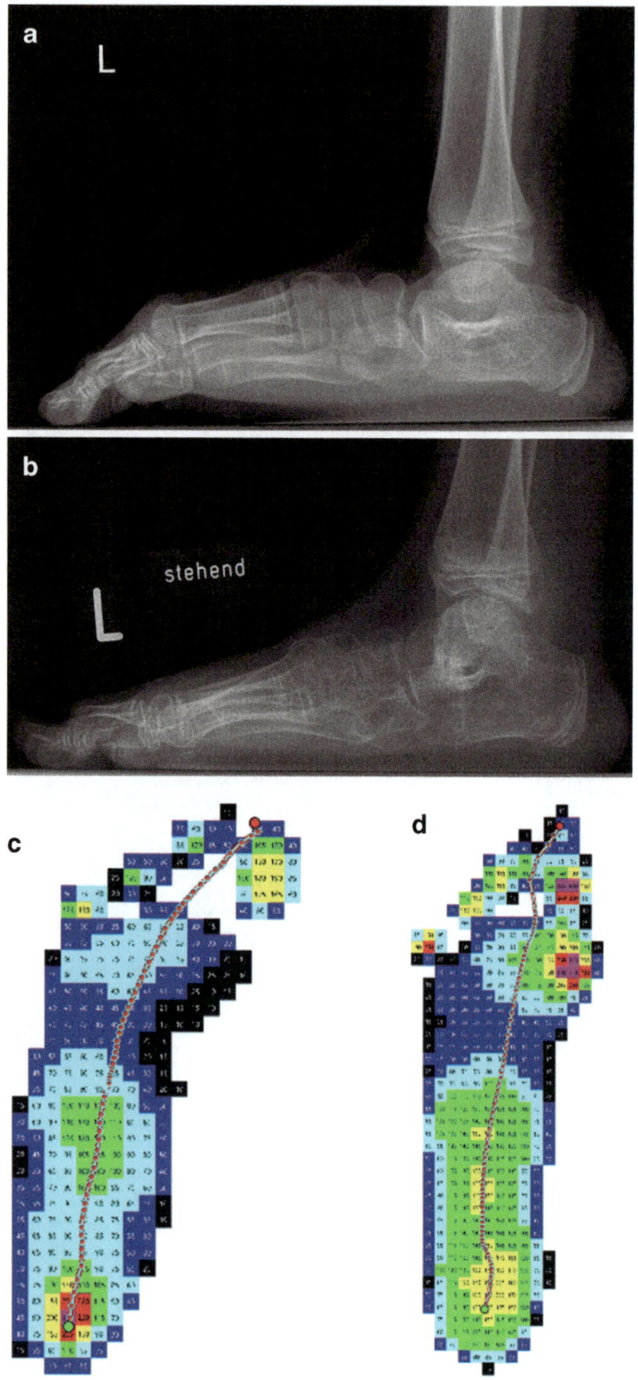

Fig. 1.82 9-year-old girl with status after peritalar release in the first year of life and severe overcorrection with supination of the mid-forefoot complex and dorsal bunion symptoms (**a** and **c**). Talocalcaneal stabilization with Grice procedure and correction of the dorsal bunion with plantarizing cuneiform medial osteotomy, rerouting of the flexor hallucis longus tendon back to the metatarsal I and transfer of the anterior tibial tendon to the second ray (**b**). Almost 2 years postoperatively (**b** and **d**), the load distribution at the forefoot is clearly normalized

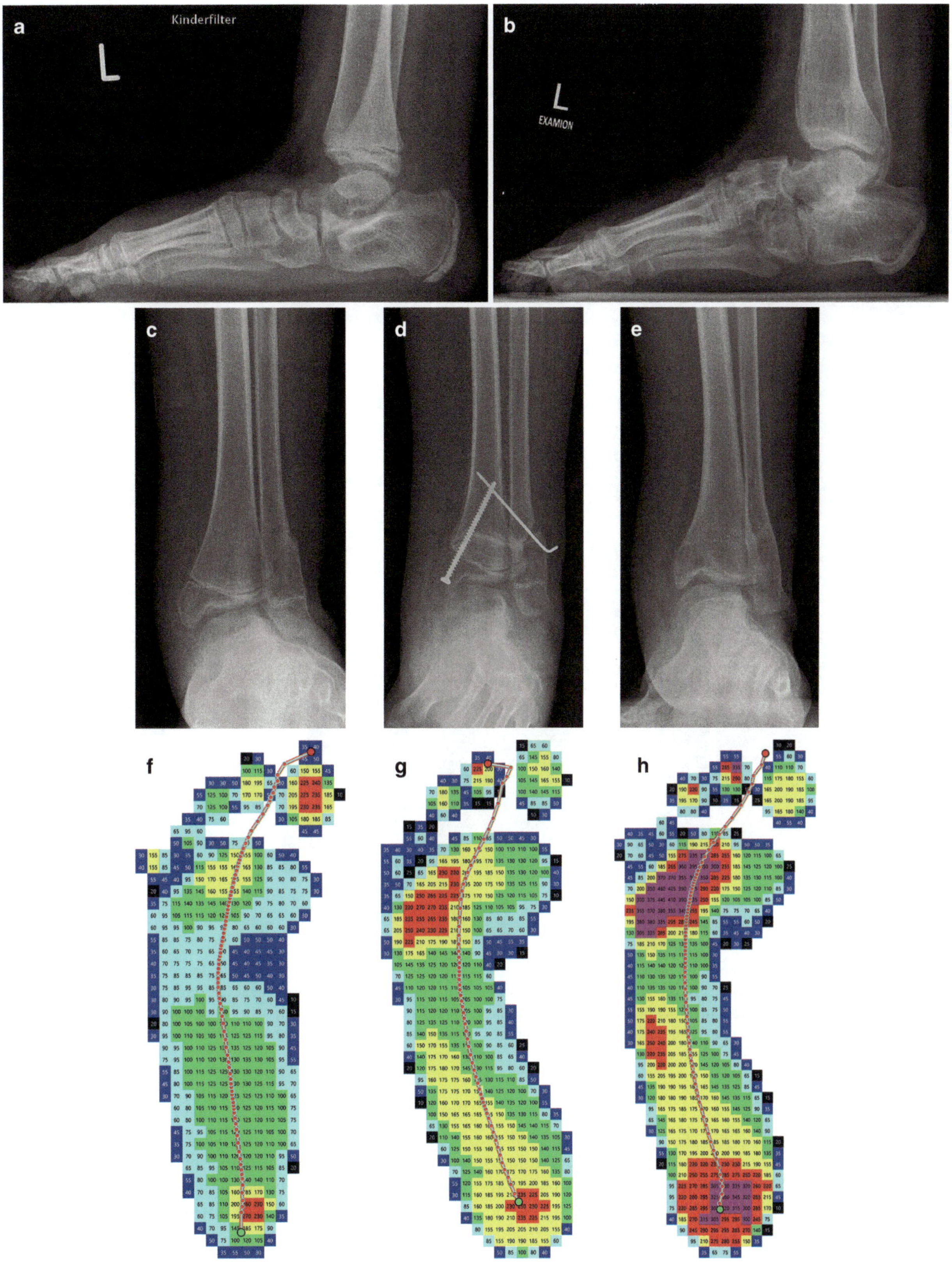

Fig. 1.83 9-year-old girl after external peritalar release in the first year of life with severe overcorrection and ad-latim talocalcaneal translocation (translational hindfoot valgus) as well as supramalleolar valgus malformation (**a** and **c**). Pedographically signs of significant weakness during late stance phase, tiptoe gait hardly possible (**f**). Talocalcaneal stabilization by extra-articular Grice arthrodesis as well as pronating rotational osteotomy of the anterior tarsus with corrective fusion of the naviculo-cuneiforme joint line for stabilization of the medial ray, Achilles tendon lengthening, additionally supramalleolar varus osteotomy with temporary epiphysiodesis tibial medial (**b**, **d**, and **e**). Clinically 1 year (**g**) and 2.5 years p.o. (**h**) still unphysiological pressure distribution, but functionally improved, tiptoe gait possible

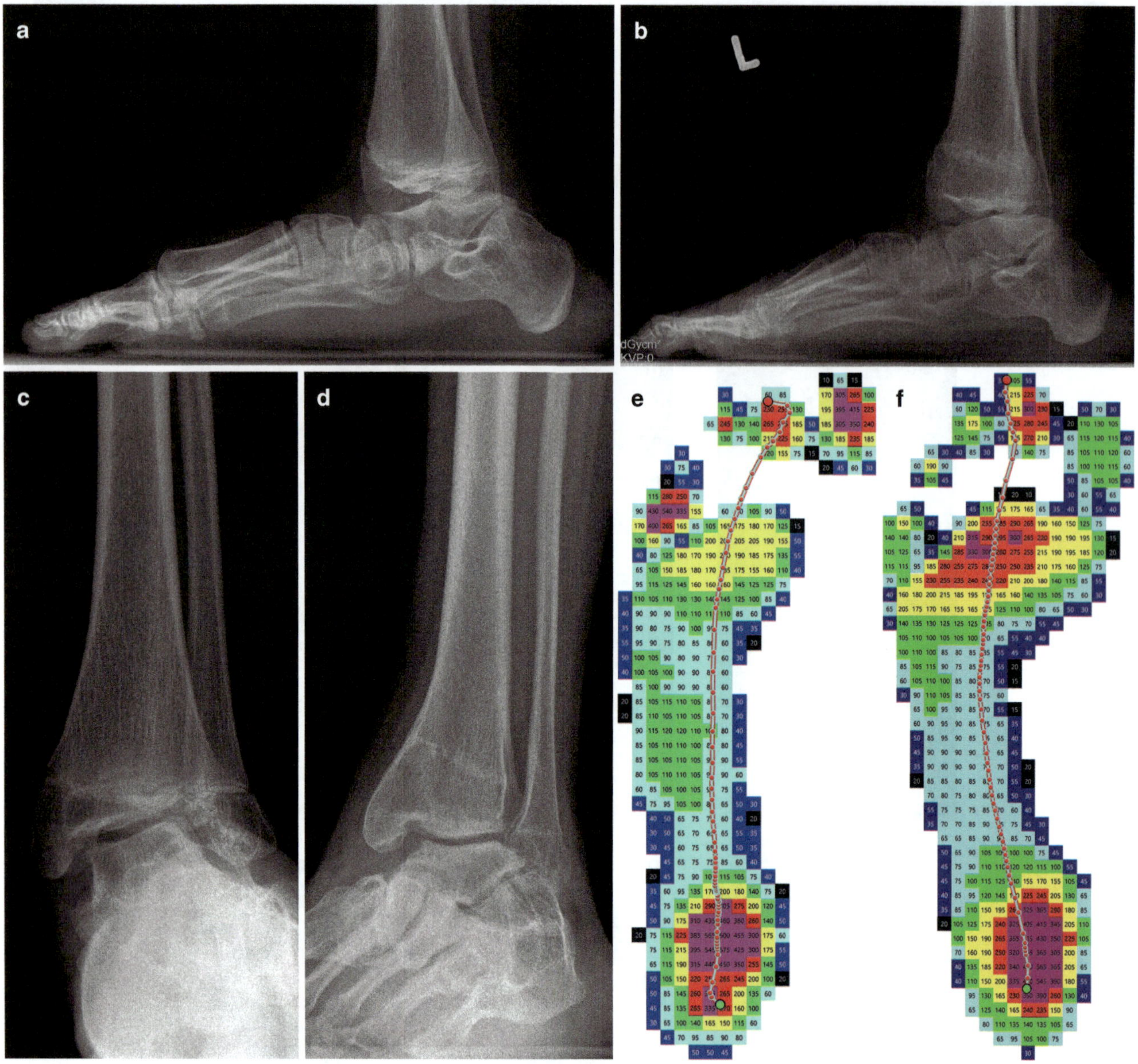

Fig. 1.84 12-year-old girl with status after peritalar release in the second year of life externally, now clinically severe overcorrection problem with inability of the tiptoe gait (**e**). Radiologically distinct talar deformity, supramalleolar malformation, and dorsal bunion (**a** and **c**). After supramalleolar osteotomy with dorsal bunion correction (anterior tibial tendon transfer), metatarsal I base osteotomy and flexor-hallucis longus rerouting, (**b** and **d**) significant functional improvement pedographically recognizable by an increased forefoot load (**f**)

Correction of the Dorsal Bunion

Dorsal bunion correction often is part of a combined hindfoot-forefoot procedure (section "Complex Interventions for Overcorrection Conditions") but in some cases can also be treated in isolation (McKay 1983a, b; Yong et al. 2007). Pathogenetically, the dorsal bunion is the consequence of reduced power of the calf musles due to weakening and inability of the hindfoot complex to sufficiently stabilize the foot for rigid lever function in late stance phase with compensatory overactivity of the toe flexors, especially the flexor hallucis longus muscle. Also disbalance of the tibialis anterior-peroneus longus antagonism contributes to elevation of the medial metatarsal ray. The overactivity of the flexor hallucis longus muscle thus represents an (effective) compensation attempt, however with the consequence of a non-physiological load distribution of the first ray (deloading of the metatarsal I and high impact of the big toe, cf. Fig. 1.84e) (Hamel and Nell 2016). In some cases this only affects the medial foot ray, in others, in particular the activity of the anterior tibial muscle in combination with weak peroneal longus muscle, leading to a supination of the entire middle forefoot complex (e.g., in Fig. 1.82). In the long term, this results in a shoe conflict above the metatarsal I head and in flexion contracture and degeneration of the first metatarsophalangeal joint, often accompanied by secondary deformities of the lesser toes. This can be prevented by early

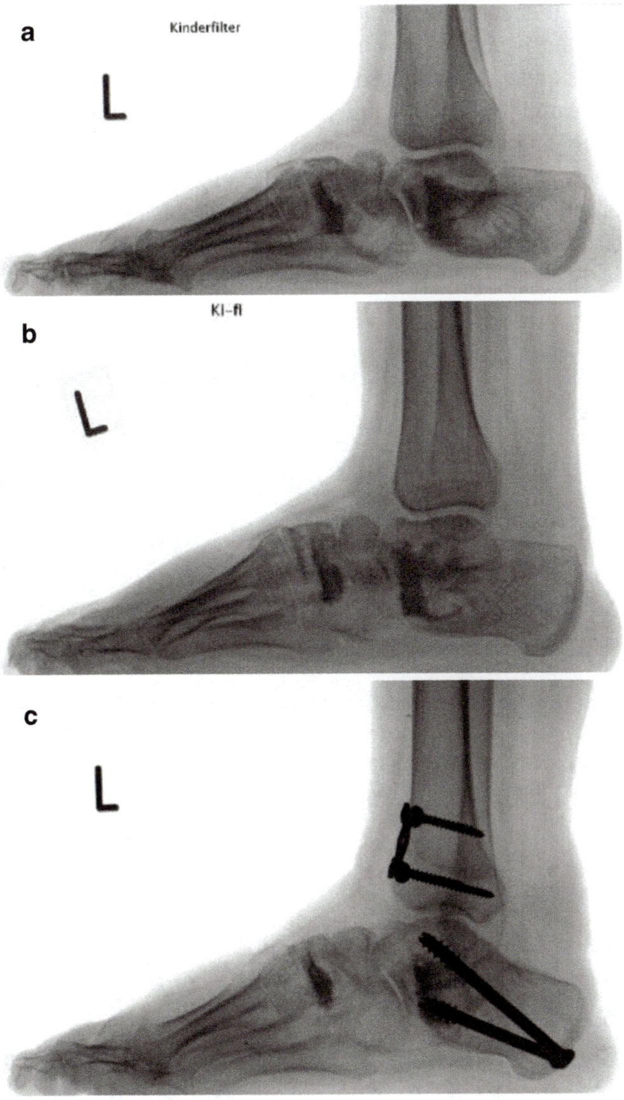

Fig. 1.85 14-year-old female patient with severe overcorrection and painful fibulocalcaneal impingement after peritalar release in the first year of life (**a**). After talocalcaneal Grice arthrodesis and plantarization of the medial ray, improved hindfoot position, but increasing discomfort in the sense of an anterior upper ankle impingement due to increased horizontal position of the talus (**b**). A talocalcaneal interpositional fusion with supramalleolar extension osteotomy was able to bring the upper ankle joint into an improved functional position (**c**)

correction intervening in this pathogenetic process (Kuo 1993). Figure 1.86 shows the typical combination of procedures to correct dorsal bunion deformity.

Corrective Procedures for Dorsal Bunion Deformity (Fig. 1.86)

- Plantarization and stabilization of the medial ray.
- Rerouting of the flexor hallucis longus tendon.
- Anterior tibial tendon transfer to second ray.
- Periarticular osteotomies of the first metatarsophalangeal joint as required.

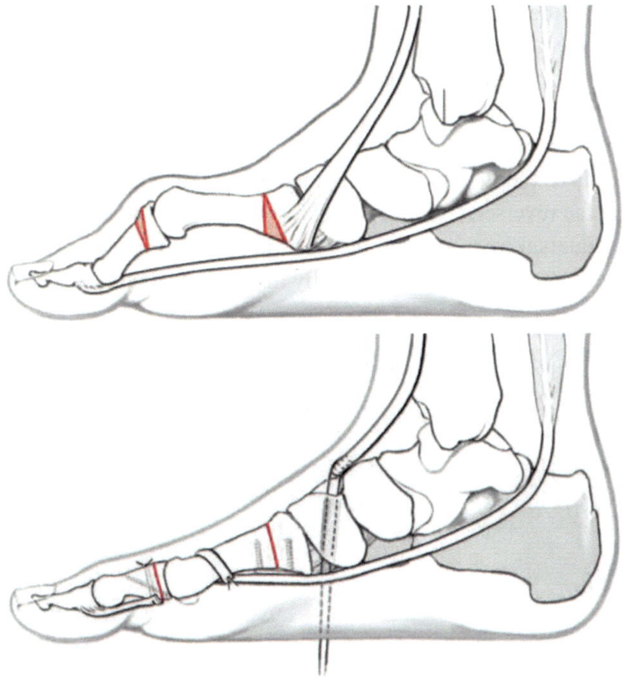

Fig. 1.86 Correction principle for dorsal bunion. In addition to the bony corrections on the medial ray, the FHL tendon is transferred to the distal metatarsal I and the anterior tibial tendon to the second ray, to eliminate its effect on the first ray

Technique

The flexor hallucis longus tendon is sectioned approximately at the base of the proximal phalanx via a medial longitudinal incision at the medial rim of the foot. The distal stump is fixed as a tenodesis with sutures at the base of the proximal phalanx to prevent hyperextension of the interphalangeal joint; the proximal stump is anchored in the distal metaphysis of metatarsal I via a drill hole. Depending on the malposition and instability, the medial tarsometatarsal ray is stabilized and plantarized. In addition, the anterior tibial tendon is transferred to the second ray (cuneiforme intermedium or base of metatarsal II) to eliminate the elevating effect of this muscle on the medial ray. Periarticular osteotomies in the retrocapital area of the metatarsal I and the base of the proximal phalanx restore the dorsal extension of the metatarsophalangeal joint while reducing the usually excessive plantar flexion.

As the cases in Figs. 1.87 and 1.88 show, plantarization of the elevated medial ray can be achieved either by osteotomies at the cuneiformia and/or metatarsal I base or also by corrective arthrodesis of the naviculo-cuneiforme joint line in case of significant hypermobility. A diagnostic tool to localize the instability at the medial tarsometatarsal ray can be the reversed Coleman blocktest with elevation of the first metatarsal by a wooden block (Fig. 1.89). In a group of 11 children (13 feet) with surgically treated dorsal bunion deformity after surgically treated clubfoot, it could be shown that after an average of 24.4 months, the proportion of maximum force under the metatarsal I in relation to the entire forefoot increased from 7.9% preoperatively to 23.1% postoperatively and the maximum force under the big toe postoperatively still amounted to 82.6% of the initial value, despite the rerouting of the tendon of the flexor hallucis longus muscle (Hamel and Nell 2016).

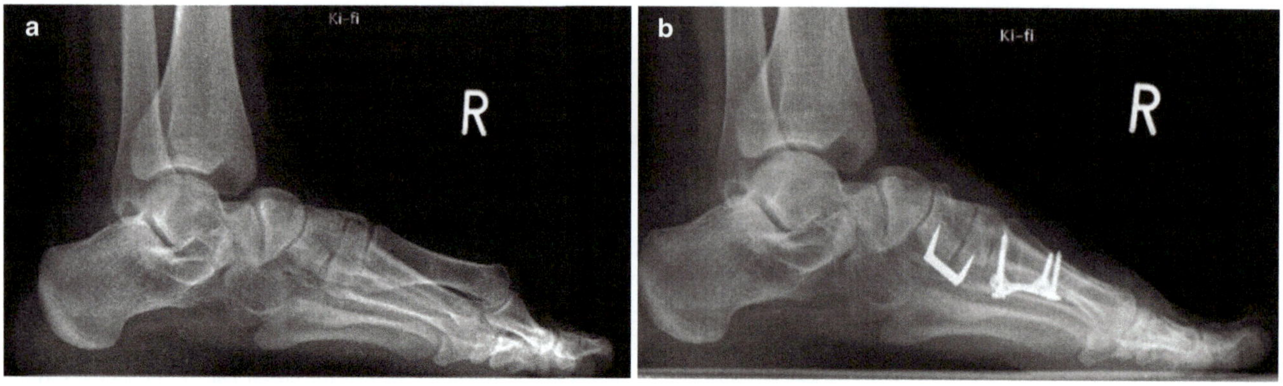

Fig. 1.87 16-year-old female patient, idiopathic clubfoot, status after peritalar release, largely free of pain, but severe forefoot deformity with dorsal bunion (**a**) and varus toes 2–5. Plantarization of the medial ray at the level of the cuneiformia and MT-I base, periarticular osteotomies of the metatarsophalangeal joint of the big toe, tendon transfers of flexor hallucis longus and anterior tibial tendon, tenotomy of the flexor tendons 2–5. 5 months postop. (**b**), very satisfied

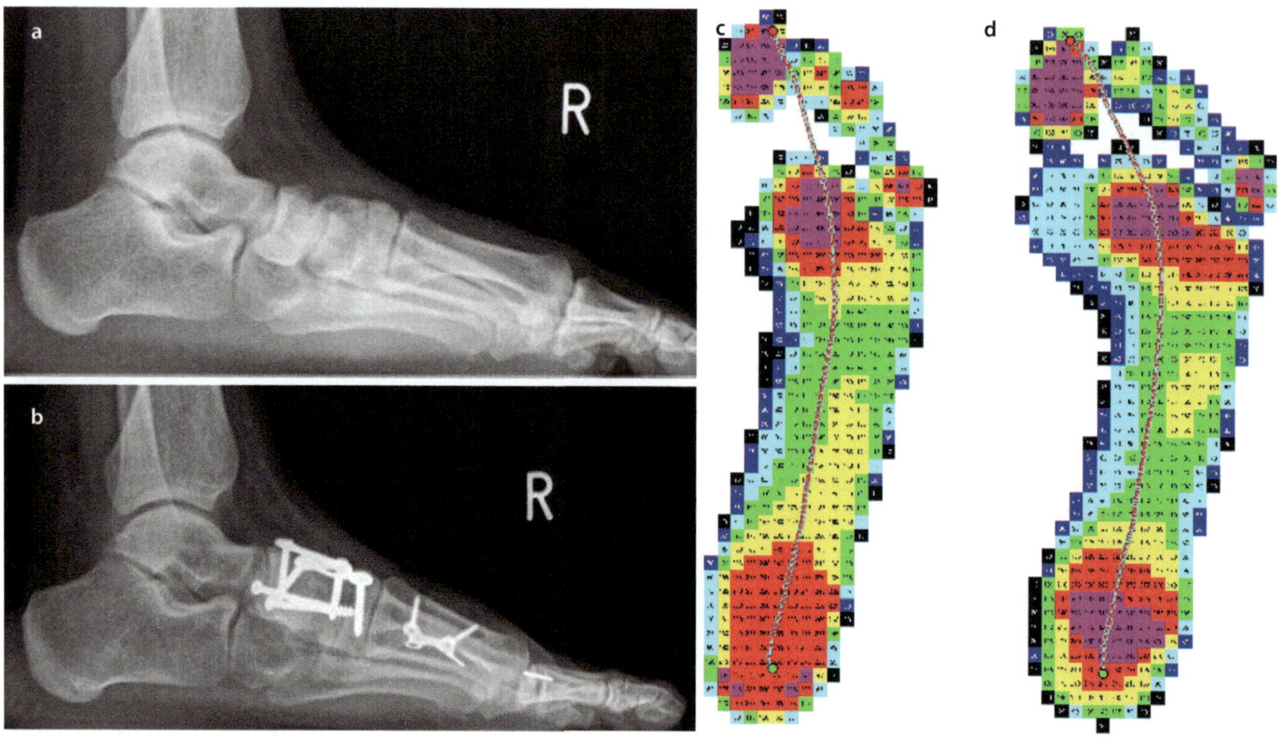

Fig. 1.88 20-year old patient with dorsal bunion in idiopathic clubfoot (**a** and **c**). Stabilization of the naviculo-cuneiforme hypermobility by arthrodesis, additionally metatarsal I base and proximal phalanx osteotomy as well as transfer of flexor hallucis longus tendon (**b**). The load distribution in the midfoot area was improved 15 months after the procedure, but the pressure in the big toe was still high due to limited dorsal extension of the metatarsophalangeal joint (**d**). In the case of surgical correction at an earlier age (cf. Fig. 1.82), significantly better results can be expected

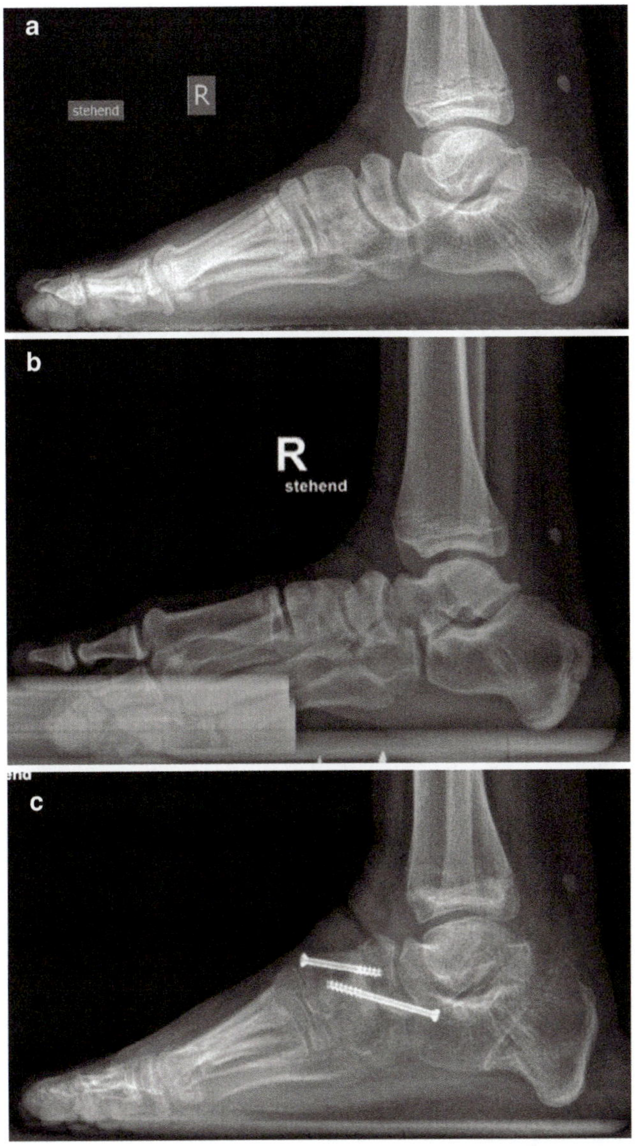

Fig. 1.89 Overcorrected clubfoot (**a**) with instability of the medial tarsometatarsal ray. The hypermobility of the naviculo-cuneiforme joint line is not apparent in the lateral X-ray projection (**a**) but could be localized by the reversed Coleman-blocktest (**b**) and was treated by interpositional fusion in combination with calcaneal slide osteotomy (**c**)

1.7 Clubfoot Treatment in Developing Countries

Through several terms with the "Feuerkinder-Team" in Northern Tanzania, the author has gained experience with clubfoot treatment under the conditions in developing countries. The frequency of idiopathic clubfoot is significantly higher here than in Central Europe. The therapeutical approach described here does not claim to be valid in other regions as well. However, much is also applicable in more developed health systems and appears also of general interest in our globalized world with increasing migration (Fig. 1.90).

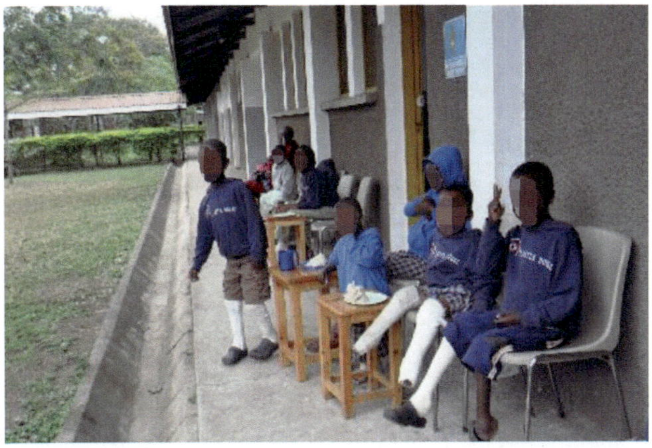

Fig. 1.90 Outpatient clubfoot clinic consultation in Usa River, Northern Tanzania with presentation of children with untreated or relapsed clubfeet in different age

1.7.1 Primary Treatment

The primary therapy of idiopathic clubfoot is the Ponseti concept, which is widespread all over the world today and which seems especially practicable and adequate in regions of less developed health systems. However, structures must be provided which guarantee sufficient knowledge of the redression technique, tenotomy, and the manufacture and application of abduction orthoses. Some experiences of the "Usa River Clubfoot Clinic" (Figs. 1.91, 1.92 and 1.93) will be presented here as an example for the establishment of such structures. The Ponseti treatment itself is described in detail in Sect. 1.5.2. Cooperation in networks and, for example, within the framework of MiracleFeet (NGO for the worldwide propagation of the Ponseti method) is helpful.

The treatment with redression plaster dressings can in principle be learned by doctors, medical officers, physiotherapists, and possibly also by non-medical personnel. Careful training and continuous interest on the part of the trainee are crucial. The quality of the plaster material available does not always meet higher demands. Continuous monitoring with the Pirani score is very helpful (Fig. 1.94).

The tenotomy is a limiting factor, as it is an essential part of the Ponseti concept, but experience has shown that training of non-surgical medical staff causes difficulties. Thus, one is dependent on cooperation with a surgeon or medical officer whose interest in clubfoot treatment has to be aroused.

The abduction orthoses can be manufactured in local orthopedic technical units by simple means (Steenbeek 2002). MiracleFeet provides alternatively prefabricated splints. The quality of the splints and the experience in handling them are of decisive importance for compliance.

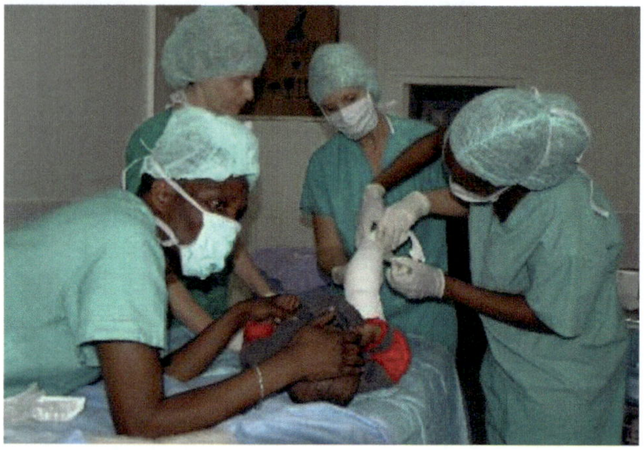

Fig. 1.91 Training situation with the Ponseti cast technique

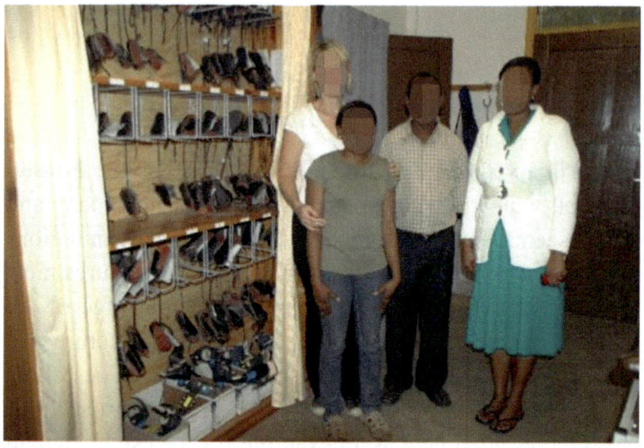

Fig. 1.92 The clubfoot team in Usa River and the Steenbeek abduction orthoses manufactured in the company's own workshop

1.7.2 Late Primary Correction ("Neglected Clubfoot") and Relapses

Every clubfoot treatment can be divided into the phases of redression, (surgical) release, and retention. The treatment objective for older, non-pretreated, or recurrent clubfeet after insufficient pretreatment is in principle a foot as similar as possible to the normal condition in terms of form and function. Since this is usually unattainable regarding the severity of initial conditions encountered here (Fig. 1.93), the realistic treatment objective can approximately be formulated as follows:

Treatment Goal for Late Correction

- Plantigrade foot with full ability for weight-bearing.
- Possible to be supplied with regular shoes.
- Absence of pain.
- Functionally usable residual mobility at least of the upper ankle joint.

Since possibilities for the retention phase under the conditions of limited resources are restricted and sometimes not feasible at all, the prophylaxis of repeated recurrence by arthrodesis and/or tendon transfer is one of the most important treatment goals of surgical clubfoot treatment. Penny (2005) has summarized his several years of experience with clubfoot treatment in Uganda, including a good literature review, which was of great help to the author. In the more recent literature, there is an increasing body of work that reports good results with Ponseti primary therapy, even in older children, so that it can always be used initially. Success will depend on very careful follow-up, which unfortunately is usually not always given. The presentation of the alternatively possible gradual correction using external fixators is omitted here, and reference is made to the corresponding literature.

1.7.2.1 Redression

The correction of older children with non-pretreated clubfoot (neglected clubfoot) or severe recurrences after previous surgery should always begin with pretreatment according to the Ponseti principles ("pre-casting"). This requires long-leg redressive plaster dressings with a cast change every 1–2 weeks, which do not allow weight-bearing, if applied in the usual manner. This, however, is possible with very short thigh casts in only 30°–40° knee flexion with pure forefoot loading, which significantly increases practicability ("walking cast"). For older children and adolescents—at least if the deformity has already been partially corrected—a lower leg walking cast can also be applied using a very precise plaster technique (see Sect. 1.6.2). The redressive phase should ideally be carried out until a "plateau" is reached, i.e., no more or only insignificant further progress in further correction (Pirani score) is achieved (Fig. 1.94). The effect is most obvious with the first redressive plaster treatments, so that at least this phase should not be omitted as pretreatment for pre-stretching soft tissues and skin prior to surgery (Fig. 1.95).

Limited corrective effects can also be expected postoperatively through redressive cast dressings ("post-casting"), therefore it should be considered intraoperatively, whether slight residual deformities can be left depending on the flexibility of the foot and the age of the patient, provided that the possibility of a post-redression phase is given. However, this procedure should not be exaggerated as otherwise a relapse will be more likely to occur.

1.7.2.2 (Surgical) Correction

The surgical procedure must be chosen individually but can be structured and divided into four complexes. The release of soft tissue contractures is always the first part of the procedure. In early infancy, this alone can be sufficient.

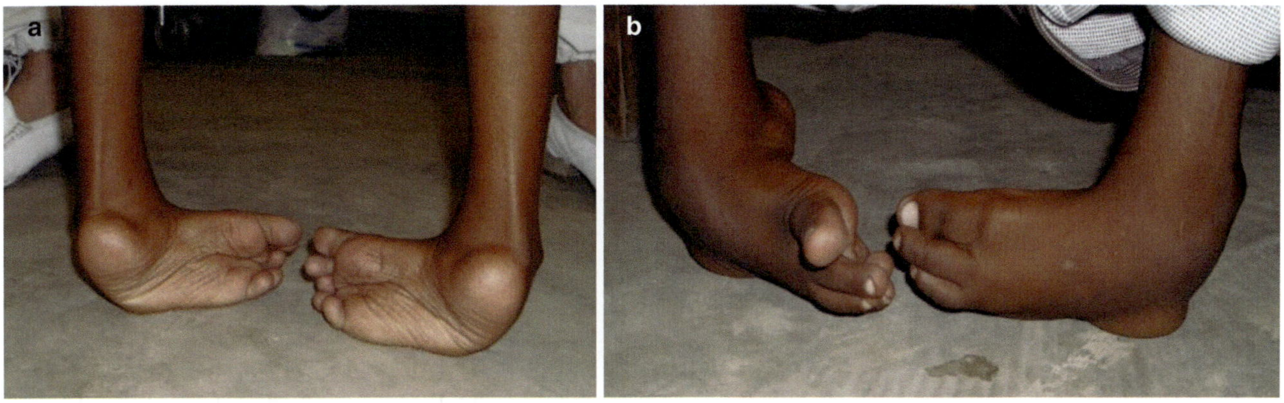

Fig. 1.93 6-year-old boy with untreated idiopathic bilateral clubfoot before the redression phase (**a** and **b**)

	Start of treatment 09.04.14		Mid-treatment 17.07.14		Pre-surgery 11.09.14		Post-surgery 14.11.14	
Foot	Right	Left	Right	Left	Right	Left	Right	Left
Curvature Lat.Border	1	1	1	1	0.5	0.5	0	0
Medial crease	1	1	0	0	0	0	0	0
Lateral Head of Talus	1	1	0.5	1	0.5	0.5	0	0
Posterial crease	1	1	0	0	0	0	0	0
Empty Heel	1	1	0	0	0	0	0	0
Rigidity Equinus	1	1	0.75	1	1	1	0	0
Total Score	**6**	**6**	**2.25**	**3**	**2**	**2**	**0**	**0**

Fig. 1.94 Example of a course of treatment with documentation of the Pirani score in the case of bilateral untreated clubfoot at the age of 6 years (same patient as in Fig. 1.93). In this case of a very severe initial deformity (score 6), the plateau phase was only reached after about 5 months (score 2), so that the surgical correction was postponed until then

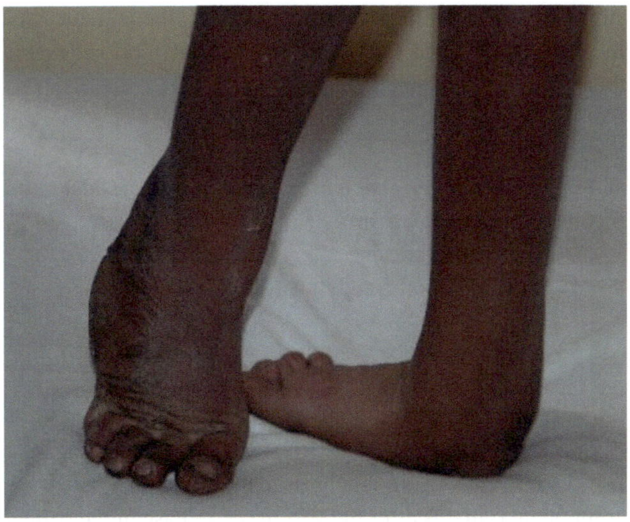

Fig. 1.95 9-year-old patient with bilateral idiopathic clubfoot. The patient's right foot was already prepared for surgical correction by pre-casting

If, on the other hand, it is not possible in severe cases in schoolchildren and adolescents to bring the hindfoot into a sufficiently plantigrade position, a remaining equinus, varus, or cavus component must be additionally adjusted by bony correction. As early as around the age of 4–5 years, a middle forefoot adduction component often cannot be realigned by soft tissue procedures alone and requires a measure to shorten the lateral ray of the foot. Finally, a relocation of the anterior tibial tendon to improve dynamics and thus to prevent recurrence should be considered in most cases. In the following, some aspects of individual procedures that concern late primary correction (neglected clubfoot) will be addressed.

Sequence of Surgical Measures for Clubfoot Correction

1. Soft tissue release (always required).
2. Bony hindfoot correction (from approx. about 8–9 years of age).
3. Shortening of the lateral ray of the foot (from approx. 4–5 years of age).
4. Anterior tibial tendon transfer (from approx. 3 years of age).

Soft Tissue Release

Before the soft tissue release, it is necessary to consider, which goal should and can be achieved by the release. However, this can often not be exactly estimated preoperatively. In any case, the dorsal structures must be released in order to correct the equinus component as far as possible. At a younger age, the contracture of the talocalcaneal-navicular complex must also be corrected by capsulotomies of the talocalcaneal and talonavicular joints. At the latest from the age of schoolchildren, this is less promising as a sole corrective measure. Optionally, a plantar and medial release can be performed. In older patients, part of the overall correction is more likely to be achieved by bony procedures. With all release measures, it should be kept in mind that the inevitable postoperative scarring and adhesions have to be accepted as negative consequences. In the course of further growth, they can give rise to new malpositions.

The well-known peritalar release via a Cincinnati incision (Sect. 1.5.8.2) with complete capsulolysis of the peritalar joints in the patient's prone position in general is not advisable for settings with limited anesthesiological possibilities and can also only be considered up to the age of about 4 or 5 years. Therefore, a generous dorsomedial soft tissue release is usually the main soft tissue component of the procedure (Figs. 1.96 and 1.97).

Technique

The procedure usually begins with a slightly curved incision posteromedially with careful preparation of the neurovascular bundle until it enters the adductor hallucis muscle (Fig. 1.96). The Achilles tendon is severed in a long Z-shape leaving the lateral calcaneal attachment intact for later suturing with controlled lengthening under slight tension. The posterior capsule of the upper ankle joint is opened by an exploratory longitudinal incision and completely split medially up to the posterior parts of the deltoid ligament and laterally up to the peroneal tendons. The peroneal tendon sheaths are opened lengthwise and, after identification of both tendons, are completely cut transversely. This often results in a noticeable increase in dorsal extension. As far as possible from this approach, the fibulocalcaneal ligament is relaxed at its calcaneal attachment. At the long toe flexors, far proximal intramuscular releases can be performed or—also at the posterior tibial tendon—Z-shaped lengthening. Alternatively, a percutaneous tenotomy at the level of the metatarsophalangeal joints is also very effective (Mosca 2014). If a visualization of the medial talonavicular region by further elongation of the skin incision or through an additional incision is planned, the posterior tibial tendon can be lengthened better in an inframalleolar Z-shaped form and enables identification of the talonavicular joint.

With a clear cavus component and palpably tensed plantar fascia, a percutaneous or open release is performed, preferably before the posterior release. The adductor hallucis muscle can be relaxed by detachment of its origin or also intramuscularly open or percutaneous.

Bony Tarsal Correction

In severe untreated cases from school age or older, it will often not be possible or even reasonable to achieve the correction solely by soft tissue release. For the correction required in this case, special attention should always be paid to the adjustment and range of motion of the upper ankle joint. In many cases it will be possible to avoid talectomy as the ultimate ratio and to use it only for arthrogrypotic forms of the clubfoot. A useful residual mobility of the upper ankle joint can be achieved by bony correction of the cavus component at the level of the Chopart line or further distally—but especially with the Lambrinudi modification of the triple arthrodesis. Surgical technique has to be adjusted to the local facilities. If no image intensifier is available this will have strong impact on the usage of osteosynthetic materials: K-wires, staples and clawplates seem to be more advisable than screws and plates.

Bony Hindfoot Correction in Severe Clubfoot of Older Children and Adolescents

- Chopart arthrodesis
- (Extreme) Lambrinudi arthrodesis
- Talectomy
- Pantalar fusion

Chopart Arthrodesis

If a distinct cavus component or a slight equinus deformity component remains after the soft tissue release in the patient

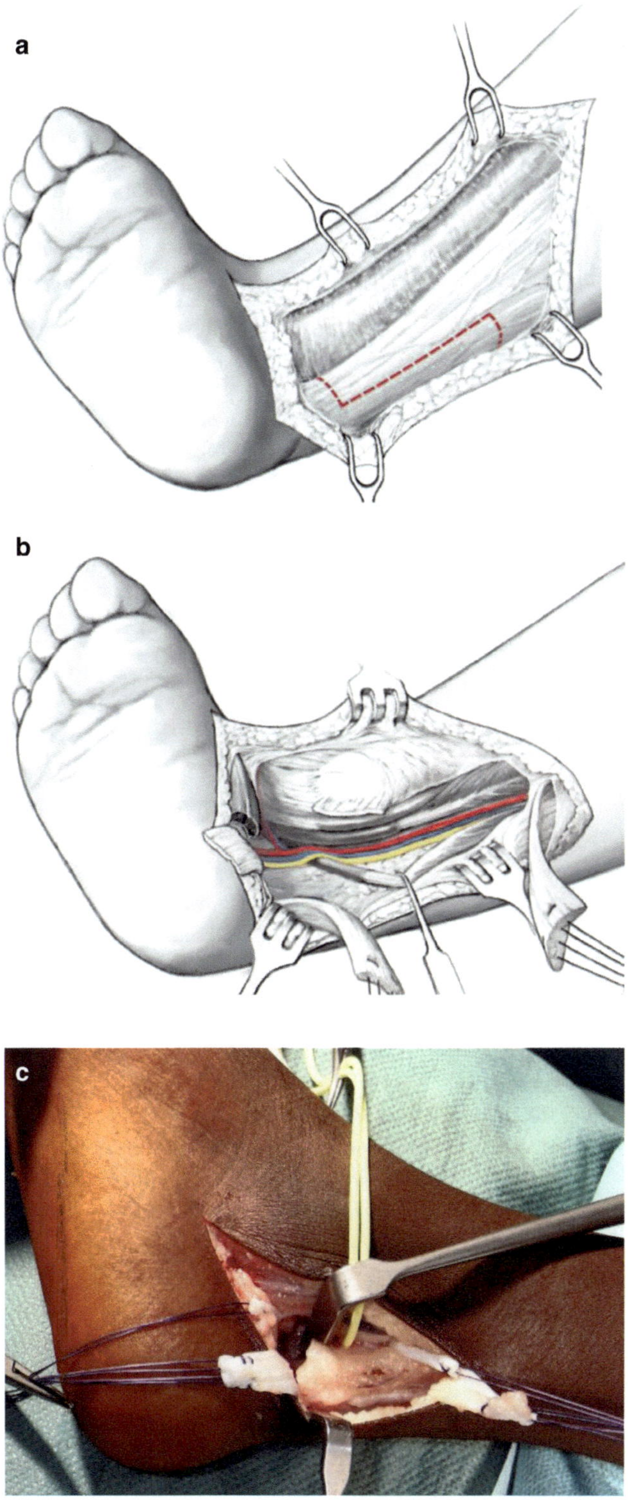

Fig. 1.96 Dorsomedial access for extensive soft tissue release of the flexor tendons and joint capsules with Z-shaped severance of the Achilles tendon (**a**) and further soft tissue release as required (**b**); in **c**, the Achilles tendon and the flexor hallucis longus tendon are severed in Z-shape, the neurovascular bundle is slung on, and the pre-ancillary fat was distally mobilized

Dorsomedial Release
- Achilles tendon (Z-shaped)
- Posterior tibial tendon
- Toe flexors
- Peroneal tendon sheaths
- Dorsal upper ankle joint capsule (with lig. fib. calc.)
- (Subtalar joint capsule)

Optional
- Plantar fascia
- M. adductor hallucis
- Toe flexors at the MTP joint level

from around the age of 8 years, this can be corrected in the Chopart line. The often existing adductus component can also be addressed thereby. The hindfoot varus deformity usually corrects itself sufficiently as well. If, however, the dorsal base wedge removal is carried out in excess, an undesirable rocker bottom foot adjustment occurs, and a Lambrinudi intervention would be preferable. Access is best chosen via two incisions, one medial to the talonavicular joint and a second curved incision laterally with temporary L-shaped detachment of the extensor digitorum longus origin to the calcaneocuboid joint (Hamel and Becker 1997). For the osteosynthesis, K-wires, bone staples or claw plates have proven effective, if screws do not seem appropriate when an image intensifier is not available (Fig. 6.7).

(Extreme) Lambrinudi

If a distinct equinocavus deformity component remains after the posterior soft tissue release, an anterior base wedge removal from the subtalar joint with dorsal relocation of the navicular and cuboid from about the age of 8–10 years represents a very good option (Lambrinudi 1927; Penny 2005) (Fig. 1.98). By abandoning the subtalar mobility (which is often low anyway), a high correction potential in the sagittal plane, but also in the frontal plane (hindfoot varus), is given with preservation of a functionally important residual mobility of the upper ankle joint and its stability. Since the blood circulation of the residual talus via the lateral tarsi sinus is almost completely destroyed, the medial structures in the area of the deltoid ligament and the medial talonavicular region should be kept untouched to prevent talar necrosis. In extreme cases, the "extended Lambrinudi modification" with resection of the navicular bone might be superior (Fig. 1.99c, d).

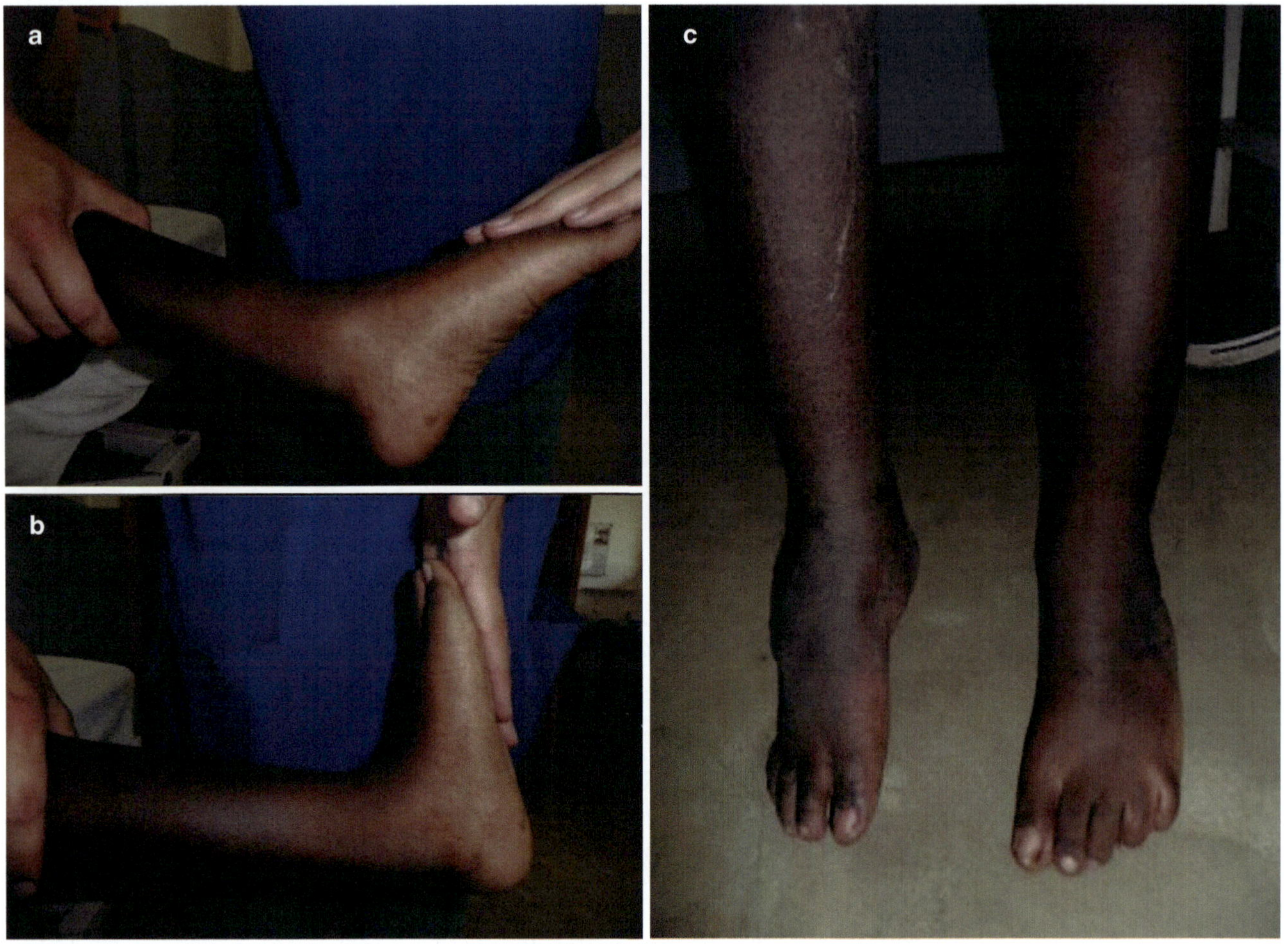

Fig. 1.97 8-year-old patient, 1 year after dorsomedial soft tissue release, cuboid osteotomy, and TAT on the left with good mobility of the upper ankle (**a** and **b**), now prepared for correction on the right with redressive plaster casts (**c**)

Technique

Via an S-shaped incision at the lateral side of the tarsus (Fig. 7.25), the extensor digitorum brevis origin is first generously detached in an L-shaped manner, and the sinus tarsi and the joints of the Chopart line are exposed. The calcaneocuboid joint is resected with a slightly dorsal based bone resection on the calcaneal side. The navicular side of the talonavicular joint is resected sparingly. An anterior based wedge is removed from the talocalcaneal joint, the extent of which corresponds to the existing equinovarus contracture (after posterior soft tissue release already performed) (Figs. 1.98 and Fig. 7.24). When positioning the arthrodesis, care must be taken to adjust the os naviculare clearly dorsally in relation to the talar head (Fig. 1.98c). Major corrections are possible by the Lambrinudi procedure (Figs. 1.99 and 1.100). Osteosynthesis is performed with a talocalcaneal compression screw in older patients and a claw plate or a staple talocuboidal (Figs. 1.101 and Fig. 7.26); additionally, K-wires at the talonavicular joint can be used and inserted percutaneously. Especially simple bone staples or adjusted claw plates talocuboidal have proved to be effective. This provides sufficient stability for follow-up treatment in the hard cast.

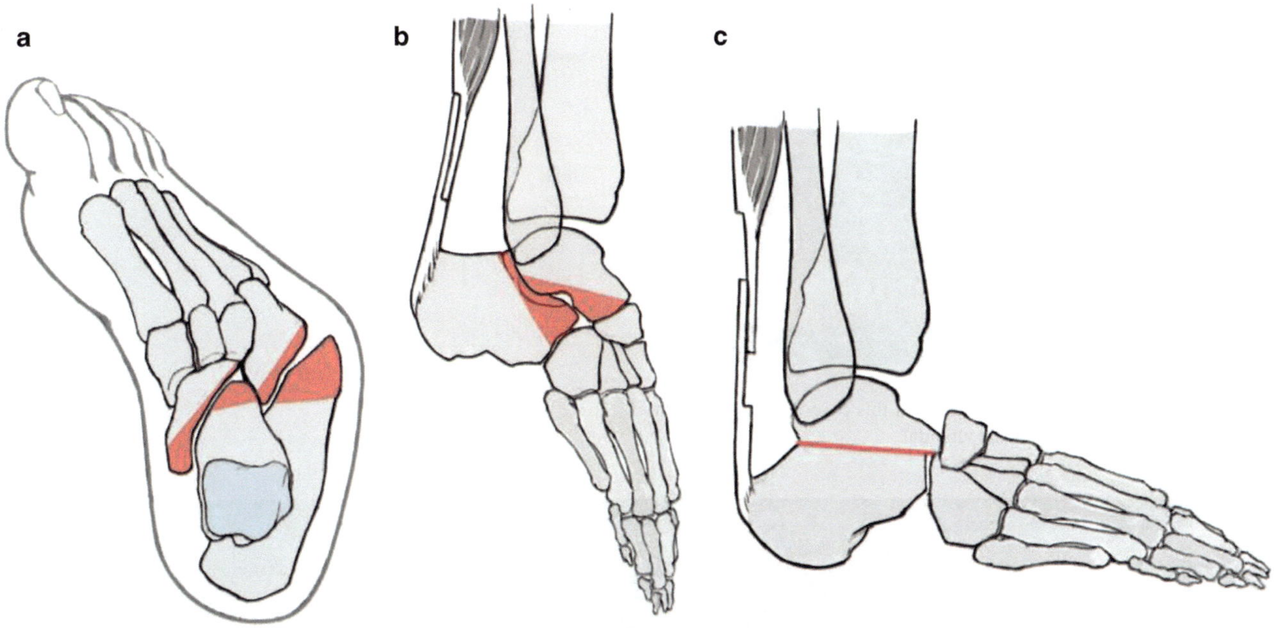

Fig. 1.98 Hindfoot correction by extreme Lambrinudi arthrodesis. This allows, under abandonment of the talocalcaneo-navicular complex, a correction in all planes (**a** and **b**) and adjustment of the upper ankle joint to an optimal range of motion (**c**)

Fig. 1.99 Pre- and postoperative X-ray of an older patient with severe neglected clubfoot with marked equinocavus deformity (**a**). Correction was performed by extreme Lambrinudi fusion (**b**). In such extreme deformities also resection of the os naviculare ("extended Lambrinudi procedure") could have been considered (**c** and **d**). The main objective of tarsal correction is to transfer the available tibiotalar motion in a functionally usable position

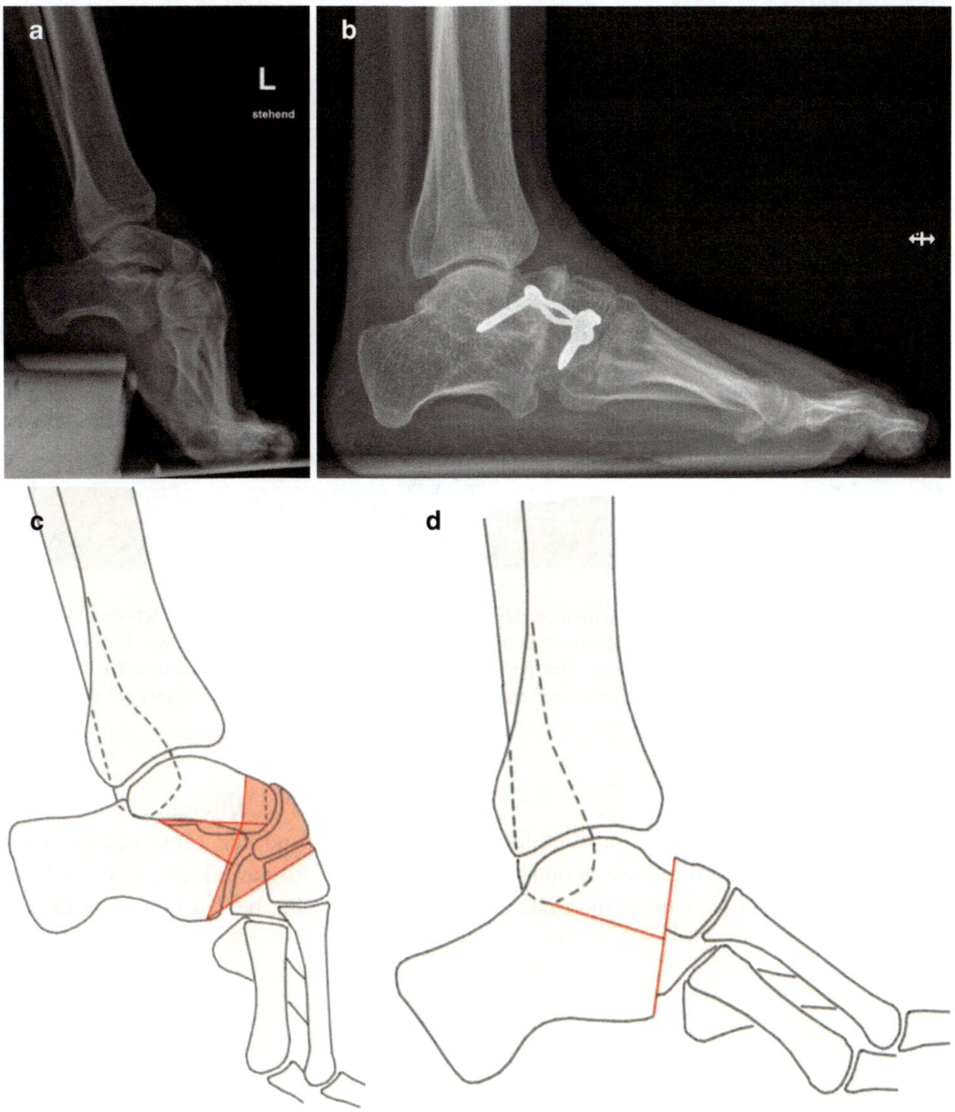

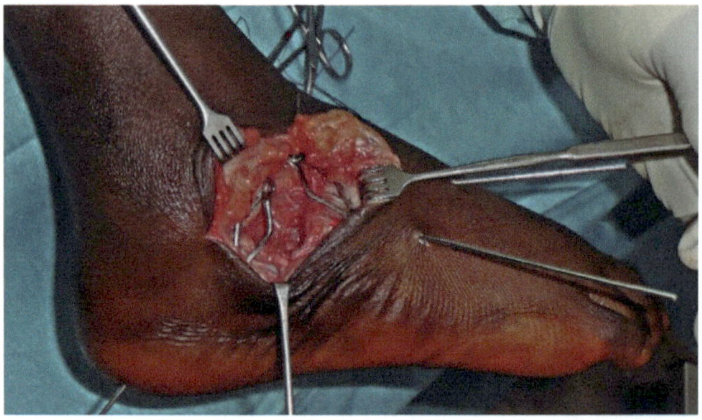

Fig. 1.100 The Lambrinudi arthrodesis in this case is fixed with two claw plates, talocalcaneal and talocuboidal

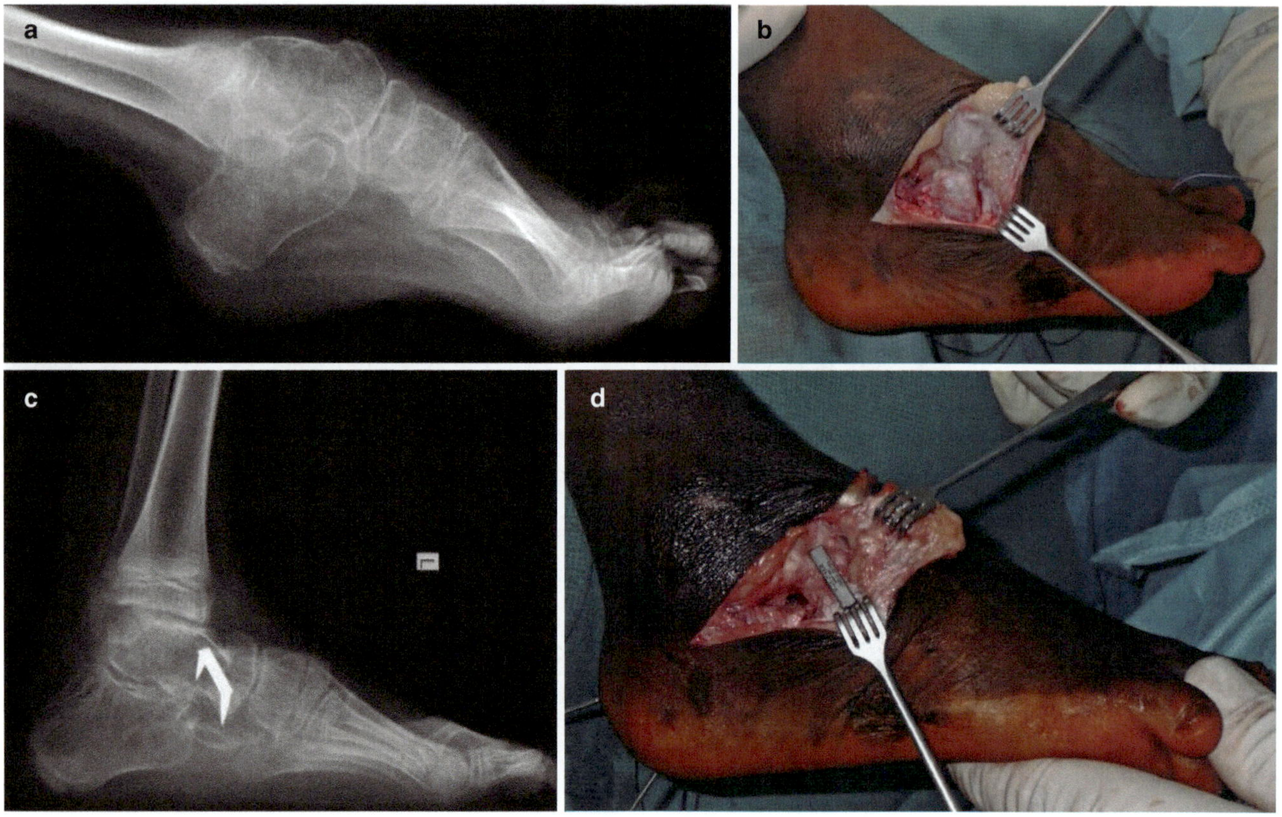

Fig. 1.101 (**a–d**) 10-year-old patient with most severe untreated clubfoot (**a**). The dorsomedial release (same patient as in Fig. 1.96c) significantly reduced the equinus component. The peritalar complex was visualized anterolaterally (**b**). After Lambrinudi arthrodesis a complete correction was achieved, the image was taken 1 year postoperatively (**c**). In this case, a talocuboidal staple was sufficient for fixation. Anterior tibial transfer was additionally performed for muscular rebalancing and recurrence prophylaxis

Talectomy

Only in extreme cases should the complete removal of the talus be used if none of the above options appear suitable to achieve full correction with plantigrade foot adjustment. The differential indication between extreme Lambrinudi and talectomy occurs after the generous dorsomedial soft tissue release. If partial mobility of the upper ankle joint has been achieved by this, preference should be given to the

Lambrinudi procedure; if complete rigidity persists, only the talectomy remains as an option. This is a resection arthroplasty with abandonment of the upper ankle, subtalar and talonavicular joints. Often the calcaneocuboid joint also has to be sacrificed by a corrective arthrodesis or arthroplasty. Problems are the resulting instability with the danger of secondary malpositioning (Legaspi et al. 2001) (Fig. 1.102), the progressive reduction of mobility, which is often still present at the beginning, and in the long run the danger of developing painful arthrosis. The best results of a talectomy can be expected at the age of about 7–10 years, since adaptive growth processes can still be observed. Coleman (1983) limits this—rarely indicated—intervention to the age of 4–8 years. In extreme cases, a talectomy with tibio-calcaneal fusion can also be considered with fixation of the os naviculare to the anterior tibial portion (Fig. 1.103).

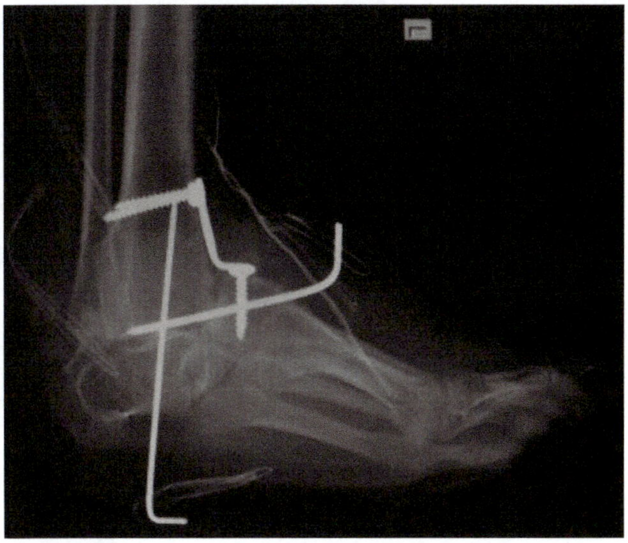

Fig. 1.102 Talectomy with pantalar fusion in a most severe clubfoot of an upgrown patient. A plantigrade position of the foot is achieved thereby; however tarsal mobility is sacrificed completely, and this patient will need special shoes

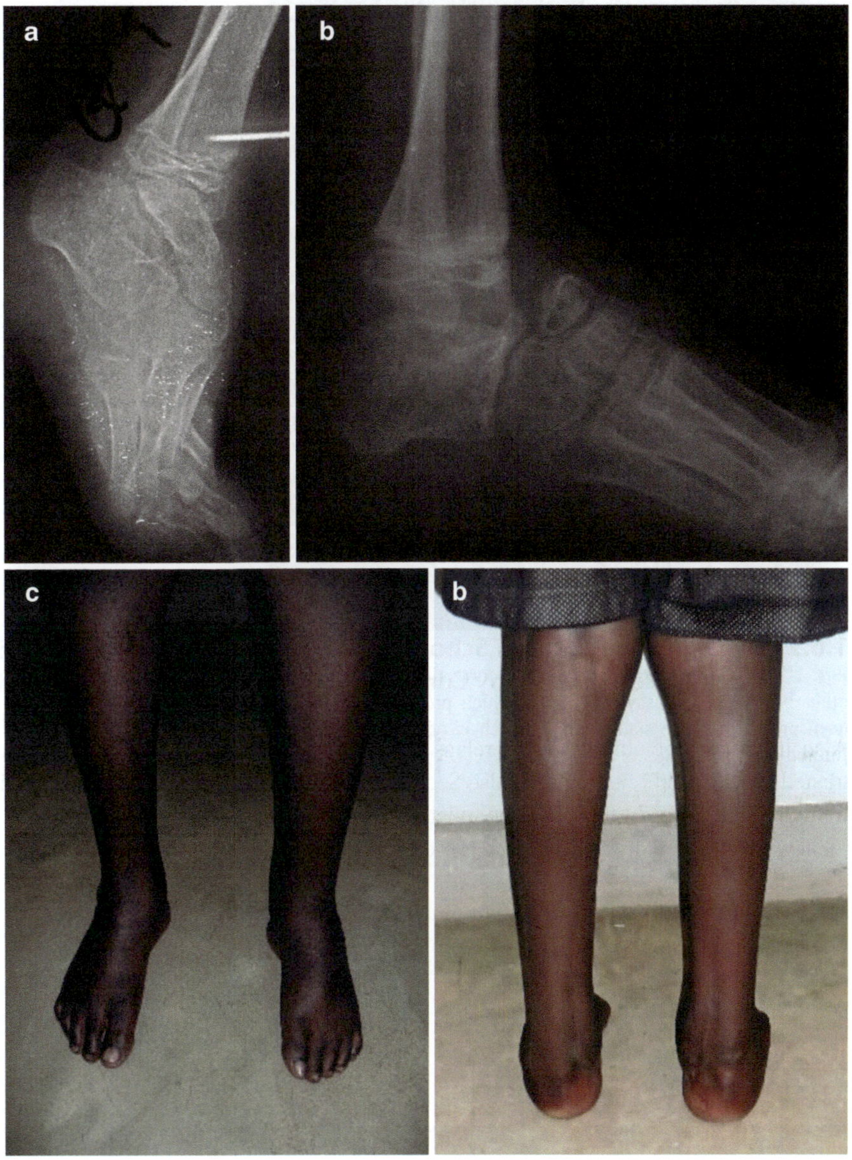

Fig. 1.103 12-year-old boy with untreated club feet on both sides (**a**), status after dorsomedial release, talectomy, and Lichtblau resection arthroplasty 2 and 3 years ago (**c** and **d**) (preoperative findings; see Fig. 1.95), slight residual deformity on the left. Radiologically favorable finding with os naviculare positioned clearly dorsal in front of the distal tibial region (**b**)

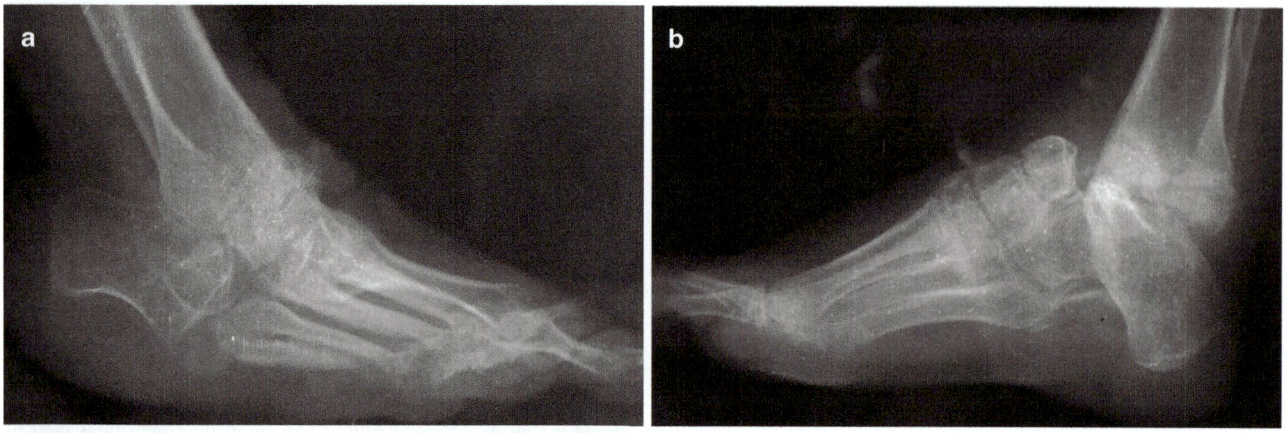

Fig. 1.104 Two postoperative findings clearly showing the problems of the talectomy. The calcaneus has adjusted postoperatively to equinus position (**a**) and calcaneus position (**b**) respectively. This is probably due in part to inadequate retention in the months following the operation, as unfortunately is a common problem in developing countries

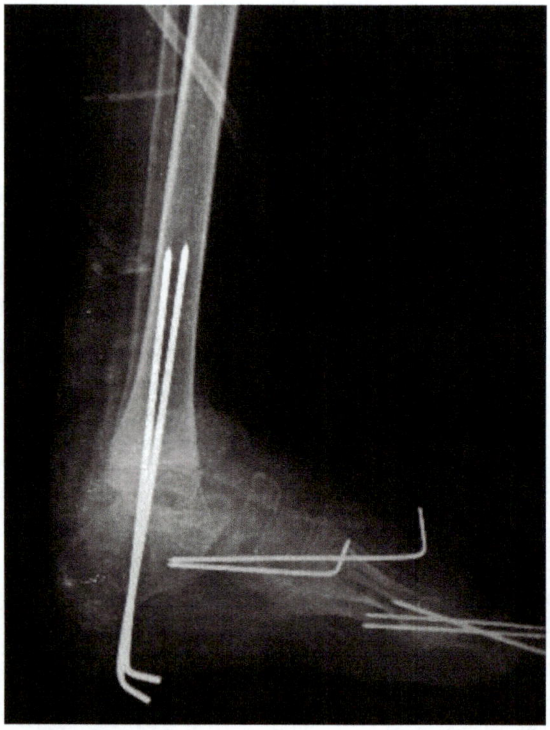

Fig. 1.105 Stabilization of a clubfoot correction with talectomy and other bony procedures with K-wires. Such procedures require long-term precise orthotic stabilization, which is often only possible to a limited extent

Technique

The procedure can be performed from an anterolateral incision that also allows access to the calcaneocuboid joint. It is important to completely remove the talus, which is usually only possible in portions, as any remaining parts can cause new malpositions due to growth-induced increase in size. It must be ensured intraoperatively that the os naviculare is positioned anterior to the tibial portion and that the desired correction actually occurs (Fig. 1.104b). A shortening measure at the lateral column of the foot is usually additionally necessary. Postoperatively, K-wires (Fig. 1.105) and plaster fixation must be used for several weeks to stabilize the foot, later with a lower leg orthosis, until sufficient stability has been achieved through scar tissue formation.

Shortening of the Lateral Foot Column (See Sect. 1.6.2)

The wedge removal from the cuboid is a joint-preserving correction with limited effect, which, however, unfolds its effect outside the peritalar complex. The main indications are minor to moderate residual adductus malpositions in younger children without significant calcaneocuboid malposition.

Resection of the anterior portion of the calcaneus (Lichtblau procedure) is a very proven measure, especially in addition to a medial-sided talonavicular joint release (Sect. 1.6.2.1), with a correction effect also on the entire peritalar complex at the age of about 5–10 years. By maintaining the joint cartilage on the cuboid side, arthrodesis generally does not occur, and a neo-joint is formed with a certain residual function and a rather low risk of arthrosis (Fig. 1.65). If the equinus component in the smaller child cannot be sufficiently reduced by soft tissue release, resection of the os naviculare in conjunction with a Lichtblau surgery may be considered. The talar head then articulates with the cuneiformia row.

The effect of the resection and fusion of the calcaneocuboid joint corresponds approximately to that described for the Lichtblau procedure (Lehman et al. 1999). Particularly after previous operations in the medial tarsal skeleton, stabilization by calcaneocuboid arthrodesis may be desirable. The correction potential is limited by the flexibility of the medial column. If too much bone is resected, the arthrodesis can no longer be closed. The procedure should not be used before approximately the age of 6, as this can lead to later growth-related overcorrection.

Anterior Tibial Tendon Transfer (TAT)

The transfer of the anterior tibial tendon slightly lateral to the middle of the foot (Sect. 1.6.1.3) is an indicated measure in most cases of untreated or recurrent clubfeet from about the late third to the fourth year of life to improve the dynamics and to prevent recurrence, especially in cases of limited possibilities of postoperative retention measures. The effect of the tibial muscle on the dorsal extension of the foot should be examined preoperatively, and in many cases a deformity enhancing effect will be observed. The effect of the anterior tibial transfer can be dosed by selecting the insertion site in relation to the center of the foot. The transfer can only be omitted if major hindfoot fusion is performed, but even then it often represents a significant improvement in the overall result. De facto anterior tibial tendon transfer should be included in the majority of surgical corrections under the conditions in developing countries.

Dealing with Skin Restrictions

A basic problem in the surgical treatment of severe clubfoot deformities is the dorsomedial skin closure after correction. The following measures have proven successful:

Measures in Dealing with the Dorsomedial Skin Deficit

- Pre-stretching by pre-casting.
- Pricking of the skin close to the wound edges.
- (Multiple) Z-plastics
- Rotational soft tissue flaps.
- (Open wound treatment with secondary skin coverage).

An important effect of pre-casting is the stretching of the dorsomedial contracted soft tissues including the skin. Multiple prickings of the skin close to the wound edge at a distance of up to about 2–3 cm from the wound result in significant relaxation of the skin suture (Fig. 1.106a). Multiple

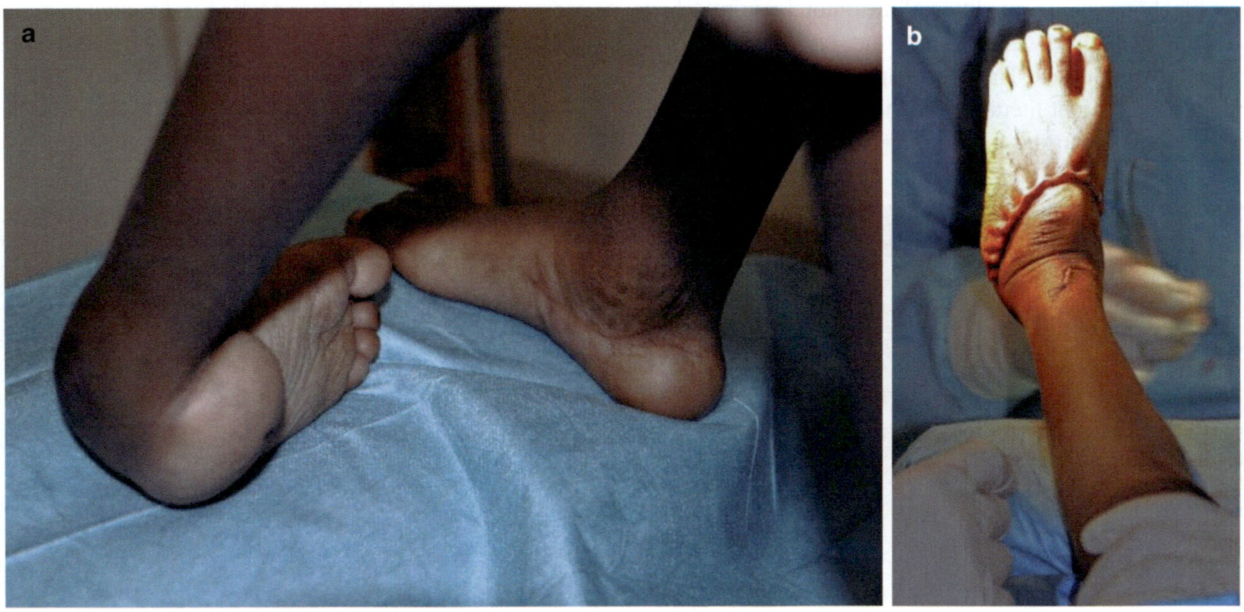

Fig. 1.106 Condition after correction right with pricking of the skin close to the wound margin (**a**) and before (**a**) and after correction on the left side with rotational soft tissue flap (**b**)

Z-plasties, which should not be designed too small, can also be used to enable dorsomedial skin closure. A very effective solution is the rotation soft tissue flap (Reize and Exner 2007), in which the skin and subcutaneous tissue, which is present in excess laterally after correction, is shifted medially over the dorsal aspect of the foot (Fig. 1.106b).

1.7.2.3 Retention

Orthopedic devices such as well-molded ankle foot orthosis for older children are not available in all regions. Long distances to the therapist, communication, and comprehension problems and lack of financial means are only some of the frequently encountered obstacles to continuous splinting. Often redressive plaster phases are required for mild recurrences. An effective retention measure after surgical correction is the use of long-leg hard cast splints, which are manufactured without an orthopedic workshop and can sometimes be used for months.

For the surgeon, the uncertainties of an optimal follow-up treatment should result in as complete a correction as possible and, for example, the generous use of the anterior tibial tendon transfer to prevent a relapse as well as possible. If there is a complete lack of long-term follow-up care however, the benefit of surgical clubfoot treatment overall seems questionable.

1.8 Importance of the Tibiotalar Joint for Long-Term Prognosis

The talocalcaneal-navicular joint complex is the center of clubfoot deformity. For long-term overall foot function in later life, however, the condition of the tibiotalar joint, which is functionally closely connected to the subtalar complex, is particularly important. This aspect appears clearly underrepresented in clubfoot literature (Hamel 2015). Adult patients that are referred to the foot and ankle surgeon today with clubfoot sequelae usually had some form of primary surgical therapy in infancy and may present a wide range of disorders around the ankle (Alkar et al. 2017; Kolb et al. 2017), either primarily clubfoot-associated or of iatrogenic nature. While for persistent subtalar malpositions and degenerative changes there are usually good therapeutic options, this is often not the case for the tibiotalar joint, so that in many cases this joint is decisive for the overall function in adulthood.

Problems of the Upper Ankle Joint in Clubfoot

1. Developmental malformation of the trochlea tali (Figs. 1.107 and 1.108).
2. Sequelae of talar (partial) necrosis (Fig. 1.109).
3. Range of motion and impingement phenomena (Figs. 1.110, 1.111 and 1.112).
4. Fibulocalcaneal impingement (Fig. 1.113).
5. Supramalleolar valgus deformity (see Sect. 1.6.3).
6. Malshaping of the medial compartment (Fig. 1.114).

The following problem areas will be addressed using examples of surgically treated clubfeet in comparison to what we might expect after uncomplicated Ponseti primary treatment. Twenty-two of the group of 25 severe clubfeet described in Sect. 1.5.6.2 were followed by the author radiologically up to the age of 10–14 years and compared to a normal patient group of the same age (Hamel et al. 2020, publication prepared).

1. The primarily dysplastic talar shape that is associated with idiopathic clubfoot (Sect. 1.2.1) often does not recover completely. Reduced talar height and length may persist to a certain degree (Fig. 1.107) as well as an enlarged radius of the trochlea tali (in severe cases a flat top talus) or a "small dome talus" (Fig. 1.113a). However, as we know already from sonographic evaluation of the

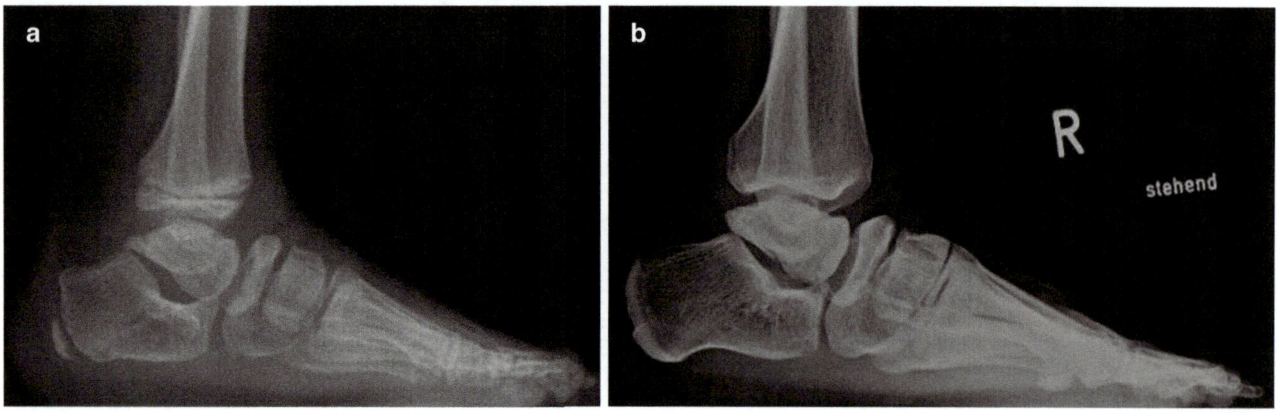

Fig. 1.107 Lateral X-ray of a clubfoot patient at the age of 10 years (**a**) and 17 years (**b**) treated with peritalar release in infancy. The strongly dysplastic talus with a large radius of the trochlea tali persists into adulthood without significant longitudinal growth

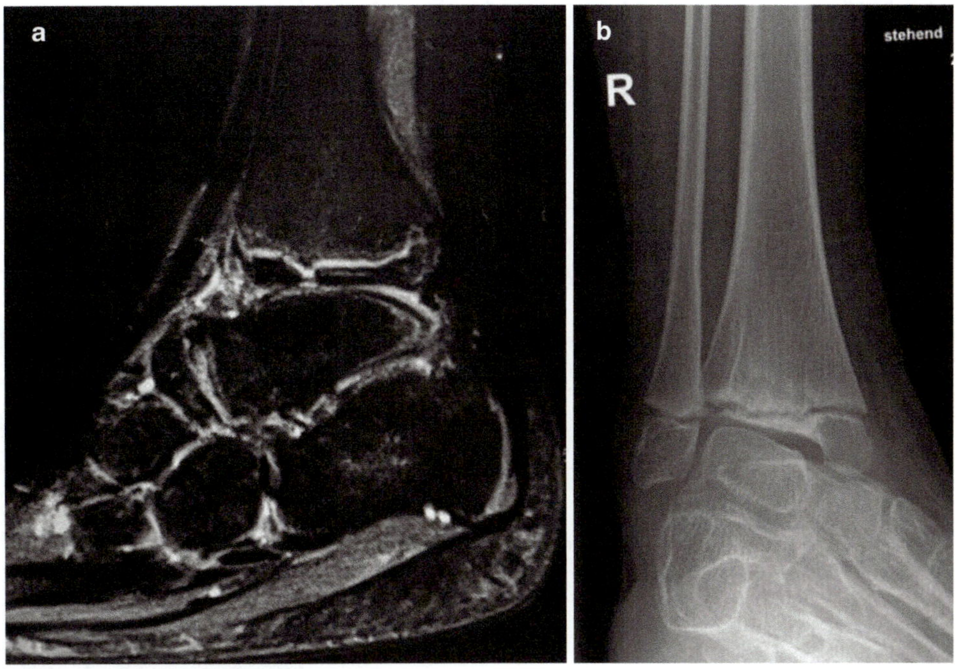

Fig. 1.108 Magnetic resonance tomography of a 7-year-old clubfoot patient with severe initial findings and equinus component persisting into the second year of life due to an accessory soleus muscle (same patient as in Fig. 1.47). The considerable flattening of the trochlea tali, an ossification disorder of the distal tibial epiphysis (**a**), and supramalleolar valgus (**b**) are visible

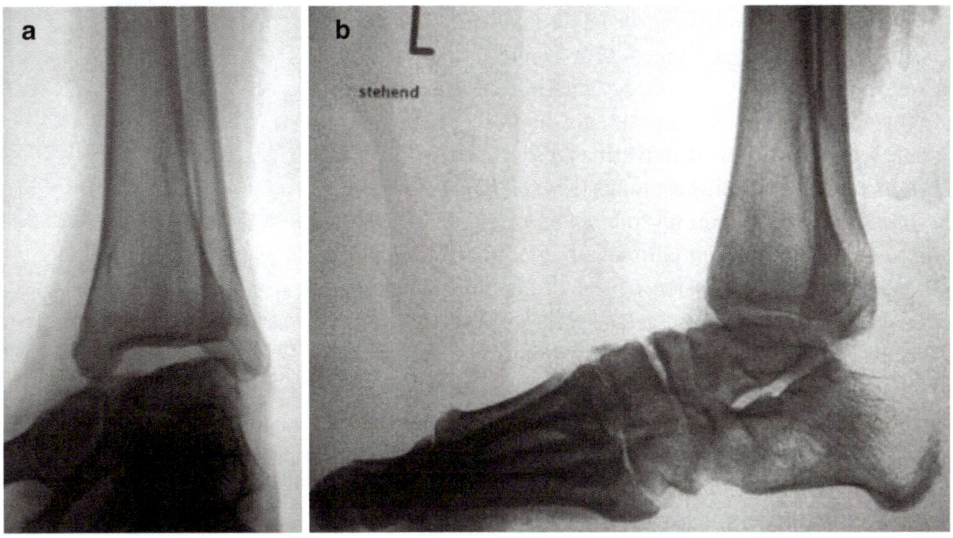

Fig. 1.109 22-year-old female patient with bilateral clubfoot (**a** and **b**), treated on both sides in the first year of life with an extended peritalar release. Apparently iatrogenic talus necrosis (on both sides) has occurred with severe talus malformation and joint incongruence. The patient is almost unable to walk due to pain in both upper ankle joints and appears in a wheelchair

talonavicular region (Sect. 1.5.6.2), remodeling can occur to a certain extent. After Ponseti treatment, talar length reached 95.5% of the normal group, and there was only slight difference in radius-length ratio [unpublished data]. These results seemed much better than what is known from primary surgically treated patients (Alkar et al. 2017; Kolb et al. 2017). It can be assumed that the trochlea tali can develop in a more physiological way under favorable conditions even in severe clubfeet. These favorable conditions include in particular free mobility as early as possible, since joint formation is strongly dependant on function. The earlier the equinus deformity contracture is overcome during primary therapy, the better the joint surfaces will be able to form. Therefore, the early time of tenotomy within the Ponseti primary therapy concept at already about 6–10 weeks of life seem to be a big advantage compared to former concepts where equinus correction was achieved only at about 4–12 months. If, on the other hand, a free dorsal extension occurs late, the trochlea tali will form less anatomically contoured (Fig. 1.108).

2. High iatrogenic compression forces and damage to the talar blood circulation during extensive release procedures have an unfavourable effect on the development of the talus. Necroses of the corpus tali are always of iatrogenic origin and considerably impair the function in the long term (Fig. 1.109). This complication was not yet observed after uncomplicated Ponseti treatment.

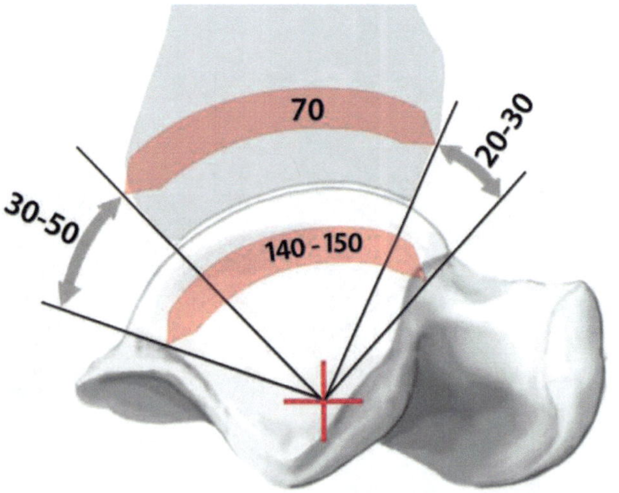

Fig. 1.110 The radius of curvature of the trochlea tali and the "off-set" of the talus determine—among other factors—the segment of motion of the upper ankle joint. In clubfeet especially the Anterior Talar Motion Segment is limited. In clubfoot especially the Anterior Talar Motion Segment is limited (see Fig. 1.23)

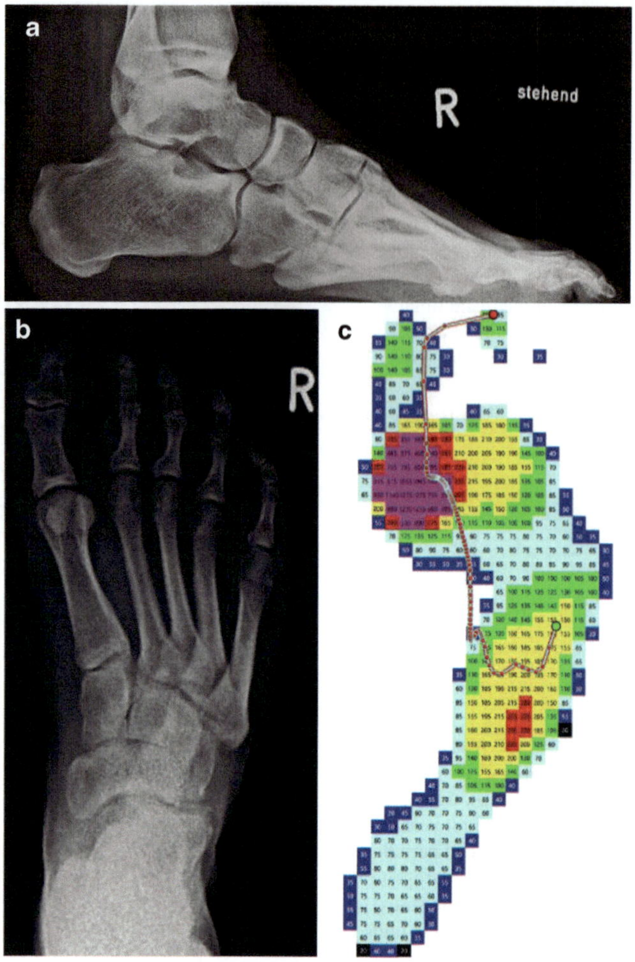

Fig. 1.111 27-year-old patient with status after posterior release in childhood. Radiologically moderate inversion of the hindfoot complex (**a** and **b**) and clinically complete lack of dorsal extension at about −5°. The already beginning painful anterior impingement of the upper ankle joint has by then formed a talar osteophyte (**a**). The pedography shows the extent of the gait disorder with inverse forefoot-hindfoot loading, almost completely unloaded heel region, overloading of the lateral foot region and the medial metatarsal ray (**c**). This can probably be improved surgically only by sacrificing important subtalar joints

3. Functionally of particular importance is the available motion segment of the upper ankle joint (Fig. 1.110). If dorsal extension is limited (Fig. 1.111), this leads to impingement problems in the anterior ankle section, to considerable functional problems (Fig. 1.111c), and in the long term to degenerative changes or to compensatory hypermobility of adjacent joints (Fig. 1.112). Ankle range of motion depends on several factors, some of which are radius of the trochlea tali (see above), talar inclination, anteroposterior extension of the distal tibia, and especially the contour of the talar neck ("off-set"). Mitchell et al. (2018) found by MRI evaluation missing talar offset, that means missing indentation of the dorsal talar neck region, to be the main reason for restricted dorsal extension after posterior soft tissue release in infants. In the quantitative analysis of the group of 22 clubfeet after Ponseti treatment, the markedly reduced ATM-segment (Sect. 1.4.1) was one of the main features in comparison to normal feet (Fig. 1.23). If dorsal extension is limited by the posterior soft tissues, hypermobility of tarsal joints might develop (Fig. 1.112).
4. In case of dysplastic formation of the talus with reduced talar height or "small dome talus," a fibulocalcaneal impingement may result due to the reduced height of the corpus tali (Fig. 1.113). This problem can only be solved with a build-up of height by interpositional talocalcaneal arthrodesis and was not observed after Ponseti treatment.
5. Supramalleolar valgus malgrowth is most frequently observed in the context of overcorrection symptoms but can also be observed in other cases and is pathogenetically probably associated with reduced loading of the medial foot ray. Napiontek (2003) determined a connection between supramalleolar valgus malgrowth and a reduction in the strength of the plantar flexors. If a hindfoot valgus position is observed in children with clubfoot during growth, an upper ankle ap X-ray should be taken. Through hemiepiphysiodesis and stabilization of the medial foot ray, effective growth control can be achieved (Fig. 1.114 and Chap. 8) later through supramalleolar osteotomy (Figs. 1.83 and 1.84). In the group of 22 clubfeet treated by the Ponseti concept, severe valgus only was observed in one child with bilateral clubfoot and accessory soleus muscle, which was resected by open posterior release in the second year of life (Fig. 1.108b).
6. In the context of valgus malgrowth, the medial compartment may be malshaped, and the medial talus shoulder rounded off (Fig. 1.114) similar to a ball and socket ankle joint. This leads to medial instability with tilting of the talus and requires complete realignment of the valgus component and sufficient stabilization of the medial ray.

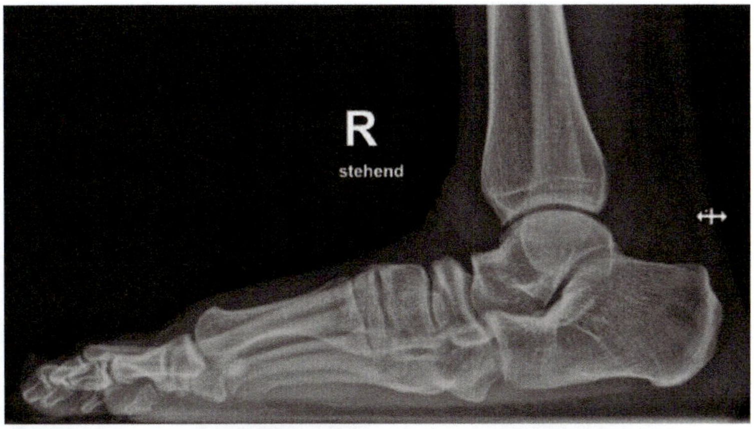

Fig. 1.112 In this case, repeatedly advised posterior release measures were not performed after an Achilles lengthening procedure in the infant period. Due to the hindfoot equinus component, a (compensatory) hypermobility of the Chopart line with destabilization of the medial column developed, which was already painful at a young adult age—a therapeutically difficult situation

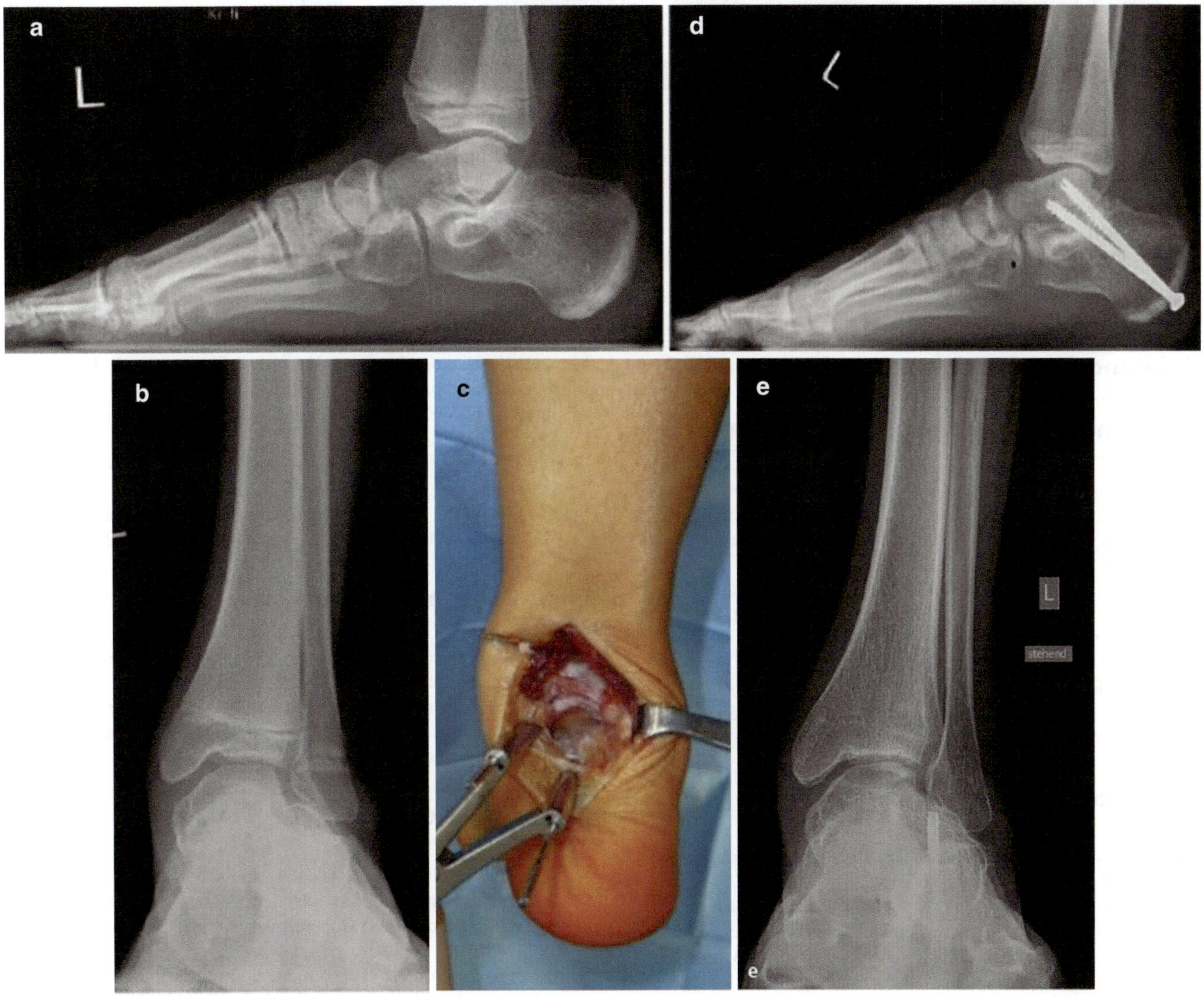

Fig. 1.113 14-year-old patient with status after surgical clubfoot treatment. Clinically, with only a slight hindfoot valgus, there is a painful fibulocalcaneal impingement, caused by the reduced height of the dysplastic corpus tali and a slightly spherical trochlea tali with rounding of the medial talus edge (**a** and **b**). With a talocalcaneal interposition arthrodesis from a posterior access (**c**), the fibulocalcaneal impingement could be removed (**d** and **e**)

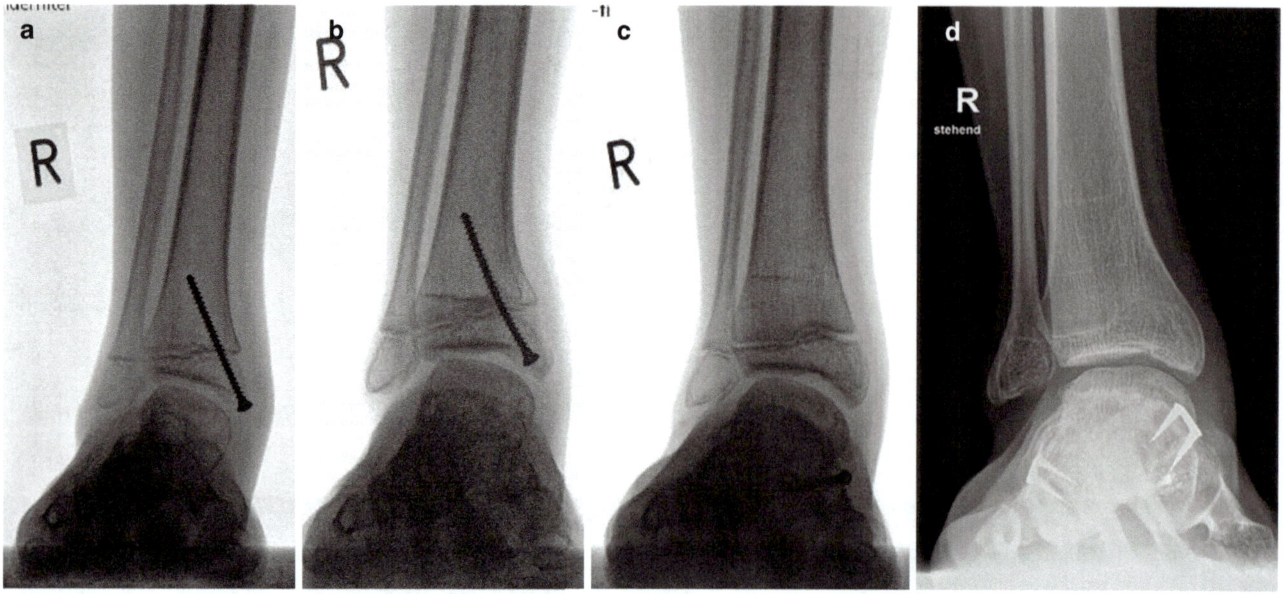

Fig. 1.114 Supramalleolar valgus with reshaping of the medial ankle joint compartment, resulting in significant medial instability in the context of an overcorrected clubfoot (**a**). By medial hemiepiphysiodesis for 16 months, the supramalleolar axial misalignment could be corrected (**b**), but not the rounding off of the medial compartment with the instability, in (**c**) 21 months later. In this case, the problem of hemiepiphysiodesis becomes particularly clear: Due to the persistent fibula shortening, the lateral counter support for the talus is not given, so that the talus is tilting in valgus again. Medial column stabilization was helpful to realign the hindfoot. At the end of growth, a situation similar to a ball and socket joint with orthograde hindfoot could be observed (**d**)

References and Recommended Literature

Recommended Monographs and Manuals

Döderlein L, Wenz W, Schneider U (1999) Der Klumpfuß. Springer, Berlin

Krauspe R, Westhoff B, Wild A (2006) Der Klumpfuß. Thieme, Stuttgart

Mosca VS (2014) Principles and management of pediatric foot and ankle deformities and malformations. Wolters Kluwer, Philadelphia

Ponseti IV (1996) Congenital clubfoot—fundamentals of treatment. Oxford University Press, Oxford

Ricco AI, Richards BS, Herring JA (2014) Disorders of the foot (Chapter 23). In: Tachdjian's pediatric orthopaedics. Elsevier Saunders, Philadelphia

Pathomorphology/Pathophysiology

Farsetti P, Dragoni M, Ippolito E (2012) Tibiofibular torsion in congenital clubfoot. J Pediatr Orthop B 21:47–51

Gelfer Y, Dunkley M, Jackson D et al (2014) Evertor muscle activity as a predictor of the mid-term outcome following treatment of the idiopathic and non-idiopathic clubfoot. Bone Joint J 96-B:1264–1268

Ippolito E (1995) Update on pathologic anatomy of clubfoot. J Pediatr Orthop 4-B:17–24

Ippolito E, Ponseti IV (1980) Congenital clubfoot in the human fetus: a histological study. J Bone Joint Surg 62-A:8–22

Kolb A, Willegger M, Schuh R, Kaider A, Chiari C, Windhager R (2017) The impact of different types of talus deformation after treatment of clubfeet. Int Orthop 41:93–99

McKay DW (1982) New concept of and approach to club-foot treatment: Section I—Principles and morbid anatomy. J Pediatr Orthop 2:347–356

Mitchell J, Bishop A, Feng Y, Farley D, Hetzel S, Ploeg HL, Nguyen J, Noonan KJ (2018) Residual equinus after the Ponseti method: an MRI-based 3-dimensional analysis. J Pediatr Orthop 38:e271–e277

Shapiro F, Glimcher M (1979) Gross and histological abnormalities of the talus in congenital club foot. J Bone Joint Surg 61-A:522–530

Simons GW (1993) Calcaneocuboid joint deformity in talipes equinovarus: an overview and update. J Pediatr Orthop B 4:25–35

Clinical Diagnostics and Classification

Dimeglio A, Bensahel H, Soutchet P, Mazeau P, Bonnet F (1995) Classification of clubfoot. J Pediatr Orthop B 4:129–136

Pirani S (2004) A reliable and valid method of assessing the amount of deformity in the congenital clubfoot. Presented at the Pediatric Orthopaedic Society of North America, St. Louis

Imaging and Gait Analysis

Aurell Y, Andriesse H, Johannson A, Jonsson K (2005) Ultrasound assessment of early clubfoot treatment. A comparison of the Ponseti method and a modified Copenhagen method. J Pediatr Orthop B 14:347–357

Beatson TR, Pearson JR (1966) A method of assessing correction of clubfoot. J Bone Joint Surg 48-B:40–50

Desai S, Aroojis A, Mehta R (2008) Ultrasound evaluation of clubfoot correction during Ponseti treatment. J Pediatr Orthop 28:53–59

Grayhack JJ, Zwavin JK, Shore RM et al (1995) Assessment of calcaneocuboid joint deformity by magnetic resonance imaging in talipes equinovarus. J Pediatr Orthop B 4:36–38

Hamel J (2012) Klumpfuß-Primärbehandlung nach dem Ponseti-Konzept – sonographische Verlaufsbeobachtungen bis zum 4. bis 7. Lebensjahr. FussSprunggel 10:166–174

Hamel J, Becker W (1993) Sonographische Diagnostik bei idiopathischem Klumpfuß im Kindesalter. Ultraschall Klin Prax 8:78–82
Hamel J, Becker W (1996) Sonographic assessment of clubfoot deformity in young children. J Pediatr Orthop B 5:279–286
Huber H, Dutoit M (2004) Dynamic foot-pressure measurement in the assessment of operatively treated clubfeet. J Bone Joint Surg 86-A:1203–1210
Kang S, Park SS (2015) Lateral tibiocalcaneal angle as a determinant for percutaneous Achilles tenotomy for idiopathic clubfeet. J Bone Joint Surg 97-A:1246–1254
Kelly AJ, Erdman AL, Karol LA (2017) Plantar pressures after nonoperative treatment for clubfoot: intermediate follow-up at age 5 years. J Pediatr Orthop 37:53–57
Lampe R, Mitternacht J, von Pfister L et al (2017) Development of congenital clubfoot during growth: a long-term study on the basis of pedobarography, biomechanics, and magnetic resonance imaging measurements of muscle volumes. J Pediatr Orthop B 26:122–132
Moon DK, Gurnett CA, Aferol H, Siegel MJ, Commean PK, Dobbs MB (2014) Soft-tissue abnormalities associated with treatment-resistant and treatment-responsive clubfoot: findings of MRI-analysis. J Bone Joint Surg 96-A:1249–1256
Pirani S, Zeznik L, Hodges D (2001) Magnetic resonance imaging study of the congenital clubfoot treated with the Ponseti method. J Pediatr Orthop 21:719–726
Ponseti IV, El-Khoury GY, Ippolito E, Weinstein SL (1981) A radiographic study of skeletal deformities in treated clubfeet. Clin Orthop 160:30–42
Pullinger M, Southorn D, Easton V et al (2014) An evaluation of prenatal ultrasound screening for CTEV. J Bone Joint Surg 96-B:984–988
Radler C, Manner HM, Suda R et al (2007) Radiographic evaluation of idiopathic clubfeet undergoing Ponseti treatment. J Bone Joint Surg 89-A:1177–1183
Simons GW (1978) A standardized method for the radiographic evaluation of clubfeet. Clin Orthop 135:107–118
Sinclair MF, Bosch K, Rosenbaum D, Böhm S (2009) Pedobarographic analysis following Ponseti treatment for congenital clubfoot. Clin Orthop Relat Res 469:1223–1230
Suda R, Suda AJ, Grill F (2006) Sonographic classification of idiopathic clubfoot according to severity. J Pediatr Orthop B 15:134–140
Wallace J, White H, Xi J et al (2016) Pedobarographic changes in Ponseti-treated clubfeet with and without anterior tibialis tendon transfer: changes during growth and surgical intervention. J Pediatr Orthop 25-B:89–95

Primary Treatment and Results

Alkar F, Louahem D, Bonnet F et al (2017) Long-term results after extensive soft tissue release in very severe congenital clubfeet. J Pediatr Orthop 37:500–503
Cooper DM, Dietz SR (1995) Treatment of idiopathic clubfoot. Thirty-year follow-up. J Bone Joint Surg 77-A:1477–1498
Crawford AH, Marxen JL, Osterfeld DL (1982) The Cincinnati incision: a comprehensive approach for surgical procedures of the foot and ankle in childhood. J Bone Joint Surg 64-A:1355–1358
Dobbs MB, Nunley R, Schoenecker PL (2006) Long-term follow-up of patients with clubfeet treated with extensive soft-tissue release. J Bone Joint Surg 88-A:986–996
George HL, Unnikrishnan PN, Garg NK, Sampath J, Bruce CE (2011) Unilateral foot abduction orthosis: is it a substitute for Denis Browne boots following Ponseti technique? J Pediatr Orthop 20-B:22–25
Hosseinzadeh P, Steiner RB, Hayes CB et al (2015) Initial correction predicts the need for secondary Achilles tendon procedures in patients with idiopathic clubfoot treated with Ponseti casting. J Pediatr Orthop 36:80–83
Imhäuser G (1984) Die Behandlung des idiopathischen Klumpfußes. Ferdinand Enke Verlag, Stuttgart
Ippolito E, Farsetti P, Caterini R, Tudisco C (2003) Long-term comparative results in patients with congenital clubfoot treated with two different protocols. J Bone Joint Surg 85-A:1286–1294
Jauregui JJ, Zamani S, Abawi HH, Herzenberg JE (2017) Ankle range of motion after posterior subtalar and ankle capsulotomy for relapsed equinus in idiopathic clubfoot. J Pediatr Orthop 37:199–203
Krauspe R, Parsch K (1995) Die peritalare Arthrolyse zur Klumpfußkorrektur über den sogenannten Cincinnati-Zugang. Oper Orthop Traumatol 7:125–140
Laaveg SJ, Ponseti IV (1980) Long-term results of treatment of congenital club foot. J Bone Joint Surg 62-A:23–31
McKay DW (1983a) New concept of and approach to clubfoot treatment: Section II—Correction of the clubfoot. J Pediatr Orthop 3:10–21
Mindler GT, Kranzl A, Lipkowski CAM et al (2014) Results of gait analysis including the Oxford foot model in children with clubfoot treated with the Ponseti method. J Bone Joint Surg 96-A:1593–1599
Napiontek M (2003) Fibular shortening in clubfeet. J Pediatr Orthop B 12:56–58
Ponseti IV (1992) Treatment of congenital club foot – current concepts review. J Bone Joint Surg 74-A:448–454
Ponseti IV (1997) Common errors in the treatment of congenital club foot. Int Orthop 21:137–141
Richards BS, Faulks S, Rathjen KE et al (2008) A comparison of two nonoperative methods of idiopathic clubfoot correction: the Ponseti method and the French functional physiotherapy method. J Bone Joint Surg Am 90-A:2313–2321
Simons GW (1985) Complete subtalar release in club feet: Part I. A preliminary report. J Bone Joint Surg 67-A:1044–1055
Smith PA, Kuo KN, Graf AN et al (2014) Long-term results of comprehensive clubfoot release versus the Ponseti method: which is better? Clin Orthop Relat Res 472:1281–1290
Zionts LE, Sangiorgio SN, Ebramzadeh E et al (2012) The current management of idiopathic clubfoot revisited: results of a survey of the POSNA membership. J Pediatr Orthop 32:515–520

Atypical Clubfoot

Boehm S, Limpaphayoum N, Alaee F, Sinclair MF, Dobbs MB (2008) Early results of the Ponseti method for the treatment of clubfoot in distal arthrogryposis. J Bone Joint Surg 90-A:1501–1507
Eberhardt O, Peterlein CD, Fernandez F et al (2012) Die Behandlung komplexer atypischer Klumpfüße mit der modifizierten Ponseti-Redression. Dt Ärzte Verlag, Köln, pp 212–217
Gerlach DJ, Gurnett CA, Limpaphayom N et al (2009) Early results of the Ponseti method for the treatment of clubfoot associated with myelomeningocele. J Bone Joint Surg 91-A:1350–1359

Surgical Treatment After Infancy, Clubfoot relapse

Al-Aubaidi Z, Lundgaard B, Pedersen NW (2011) Anterior distal tibial epiphysiodesis for the treatment of recurrent equinus deformity after surgical treatment of clubfeet. J Pediatr Orthop 31:716–720
Cole WH (1940) The treatment of claw-foot. J Bone Joint Surg 22-A:895–908
Evans D (1961) Relapsed clubfoot. J Bone Joint Surg 43-B:722
Flöter N, Stücker R, Rupprecht M (2015) Wachstumslenkung am distalen Unterschenkel und Fuß. Orthop Unfallchir Praxis 4:370–375
Hamel J (2015) Knöcherne Deformitäten des Oberen Sprunggelenkes beim operativ behandelten idiopathischen Klumpfuß. Orthop Unfallchir Praxis 4:349–355
Hamel J, Becker W (1997) Die Korrekturarthrodese des Chopart-Gelenkes bei neurogenen Fußdeformitäten. Oper Orthop Traumatol 9:109–119

Knutsen AR, Avoian T, Sangiorgio SN et al (2015) How do different anterior tibial tendon transfer techniques influence forefoot and hindfoot motion. Clin Orthop Relat Res 473:1737–1743

Kuo KN, Hennigan SP, Hastings ME (1994) Anterior tibial tendon transfer in residual dynamic clubfoot deformity. J Pediatr Orthop 21:35–41

Lampasi M, Bettuzzi C, Palmonari M, Donzelli O (2009) Transfer of the tendon of tibialis anterior in relapsed congenital clubfoot. J Bone Joint Surg 92-B:277–283

Lehman WB, Atar D, Bash J et al (1999) Results of complete soft tissue clubfoot release combined with calcaneocuboid fusion in the 4-year to 8-year age group following failed clubfoot release. J Pediatr Orthop B 8:181–186

Lichtblau S (1973) A medial and lateral release operation for clubfoot. J Bone Joint Surg 55-A:1377–1384

McHale KA, Lenhart MK (1991) Treatment of residual clubfoot deformity – the "bean-shaped" foot – by opening wedge medial cuneiform osteotomy and closing wedge cuboid osteotomy. Clinical review and cadaver correlations. J Pediatr Orthop 11:374–381

Mehrafshan M, Rampal V, Seringe R et al (2009) Recurrent club-foot deformity following previous soft-tissue release. J Bone Joint Surg 91-B:949–954

Paley D (2002) Principles of deformity correction. Springer, Berlin

Raab P, Krauspe R (1999) Das Klumpfußrezidiv. Orthopade 28:110–116

Radler C, Mindler GT (2016) Kindlicher Klumpfuß – Rezidivbehandlung. Orthopade 45:909–924

Schäfer D, Hefti F (2000) Combined cuboid/cuneiform osteotomy for correction of residual adductus deformity in idiopathic and secondary club feet. J Bone Joint Surg 82-B:881–884

Tarraf YN, Carroll NC (1992) Analysis of the components of residual deformity in clubfeet presenting for reoperation. J Pediatr Orthop 12:207–216

Overcorrection, Dorsal Bunion and Supramalleolar Valgus

Burghardt RD, Tettenborn LP, Stücker R (2016) Growth disturbance of the distal tibia in patients with idiopathic clubfeet: ankle valgus and anteflexion of the distal tibia. J Pediatr Orthop 36:343–348

Eberhardt O, Wachowsky M, Wirth T, Fernandez FF (2018) Limitation of flatfoot surgery in overcorrected clubfeet after extensive surgery. Arch Orthop Trauma Surg 138:1037–1043

Hamel J (2011) Die Überkorrektur-Problematik beim idiopathischen Klumpfuß – Übersicht, Einteilung und Behandlungsbeispiele. FussSprunggel 9:61–71

Hamel J, Nell M (2016) Pedobarographie zur Diagnostik und Therapiekontrolle am Beispiel der Dorsal-Bunion-Deformität. Orthopädie-Technik 8(16):20–23

Haslam PG, Goddard M, Flowers MJ, Fernandes JA (2006) Overcorrection and generalized joint laxity in surgically treated congenital talipes equino-varus. J Pediatr Orthop B 15:273–277

Hayes CB, Murr KA, Muchow RD et al (2018) Pain and overcorrection in clubfeet treated by Ponseti method. J Pediatr Orthop 27-B:52–55

Kuo KN (1993) "Reverse Jones" procedure for dorsal bunion following clubfoot surgery. In: Simons GW (ed) The clubfoot, the present and a view of the future. Springer, New York

McKay DW (1983b) Dorsal bunions in children. J Bone Joint Surg 65-A:975–980

O'Brien SE, Karol LA, Johnston CE (2004) Calcaneus gait following treatment for clubfoot: preliminary results of surgical correction. J Pediatr Orthop 13-B:43–47

Rupprecht M, Spiro AS, Breyer S, Vettorazzi E, Ridderbusch K, Stücker R (2015) Growth modulation with a medial malleolar screw for ankle valgus deformity. Acta Orthop 5:1–5

Stevens PM, Otis S (1999) Ankle valgus and clubfeet. J Pediatr Orthop 19:515–518

Stevens PM, Kennedy JM, Hung M (2011) Guided growth for ankle valgus. J Pediatr Orthop 31:878–883

Yong SM, Smith PA, Kuo KN (2007) Dorsal bunion after clubfoot surgery. J Pediatr Orthop 27:814–820

Clubfoot Treatment in Developing Countries – Neglected Clubfoot

Coleman SS (1983) Complex foot deformities in children. Lea & Febiger, Philadelphia

Lambrinudi C (1927) New operation on drop-foot. Br J Surg 15:193

Legaspi J, Li YH, Chow W, Leong JCY (2001) Talectomy in patients with recurrent deformity in club foot. J Bone Joint Surg 83-B:384–387

Penny JN (2005) The neglected clubfoot. Tech Orthop 20:153–166

Reize C, Exner GU (2007) Acute correction of severe neglected club feet using a circumferential incision. J Pediatr Orthop B 16:213–215

Steenbeek M (2002) The Steenbeek foot abduction brace (SFAB). Presented at the Third International Clubfoot Congress, San Diego

Skew Foot/Serpentine Foot

2

Contents

2.1 Therapeutically Relevant Pathomorphology

The skew foot deformity is pathomorphologically characterized by an adduction contracture at the level of the Lisfranc joint line in the transverse plane of the foot. While there is typically a medial inclination of the distal articular surface of the medial cuneiform at the first ray, the CORA (Center of Rotation of Angulation) of the deformity is often localized at the level of the metatarsal bases at the second to fifth ray (Fig. 2.1). Often the deformity is associated with a certain cavus component of the medial ray or supinatory rotation of the midfoot.

The medial and sometimes also the plantar soft tissues of the foot show a shortening, especially of the adductor hallucis muscle, which additionally causes an abduction of the big toe. Typical is a medial skin crease formation, similar to the idiopathic clubfoot (Fig. 1.13c).

Often there is also a primary eversion of the talocalcaneonavicular complex (Fig. 2.2). If this is contracted and very pronounced, it is referred to as a serpentine foot. However, the hindfoot eversion can also be caused or intensified secondarily by iatrogenic influence, if therapeutic manipulations are imprecise or an unphysiological high force on the medial midfoot drives the talocalcaneo-navicular complex into eversion (Fig. 2.16). There is typically no shortening of the calf muscles, but often skew foot is associated with a lower leg internal rotation component. In the literature, the—harmless—metatarsus varus (skew foot) is sometimes sharply distinguished from the—more serious—metatarsus adductus (serpentine foot) (Coleman 1983). According to the author's experience, however, this distinction is somewhat artificial and the transitions can be fluent.

J. Hamel, *Foot and Ankle Surgery in Children and Adolescents*, https://doi.org/10.1007/978-3-030-58108-4_2

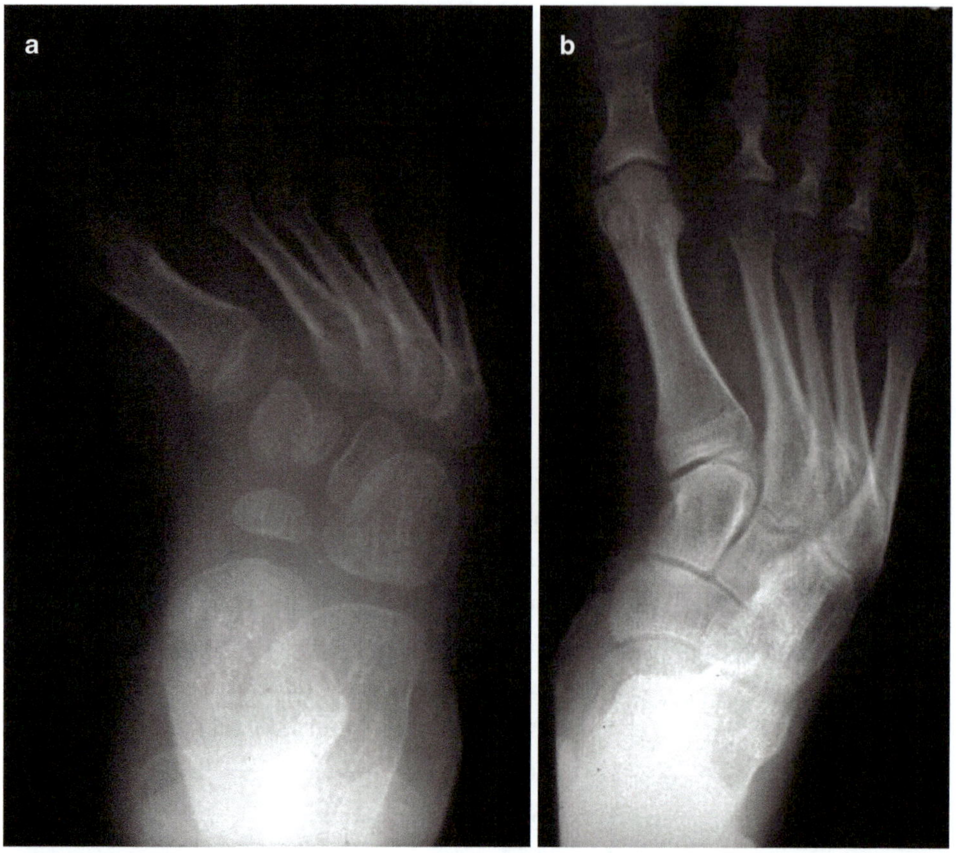

Fig. 2.1 Severe skew foot deformity of the same patient at infancy (**a**) and at the age of 15 years after insufficient purely soft tissue correction attempt (**b**). The inclination of the distal articular surface of the os cuneiforme mediale and the deformation of the metatarsal bases II–V are clearly visible (**b**)

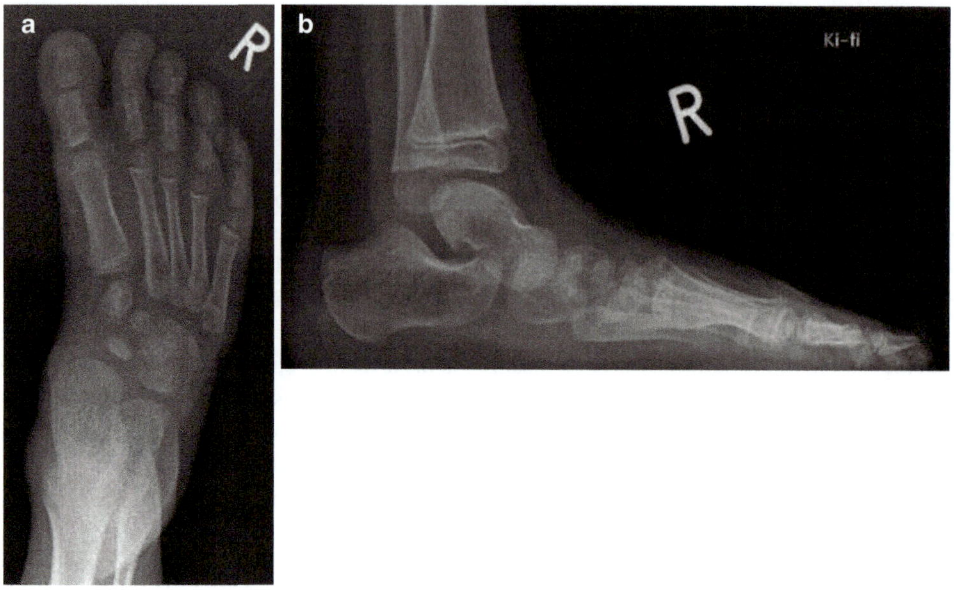

Fig. 2.2 Moderate serpentine foot deformity at the age of 5 years. The signs of hindfoot eversion are clearly visible in both planes (lateral positioning of the os navicular in (**b**) and plantar flexion of the talus in (**a**)). The calcaneus-metatarsal II angle in the ap-image is increased to almost 20°. In contrast, the TMT-I angle in the dorsoplantar projection is only slightly positive, since midfoot adduction and hindfoot eversion compensate each other. This angle therefore describes the deformity less conclusively

2.2 Clinical Diagnostic

The detection of the adduction contracture as the main component of the skew foot deformity is done by assessing the foot from plantar in spontaneous posture and with the greatest possible manual correction. In mild, less contracted cases, a correction up to the neutral position of the foot is almost completely possible, recognizable by the degree to which the lateral metatarsus has been straightened. In moderately severe cases, however, a deformity remains even after the correction attempt. A heel bisector can be formed, the extension of which in maximum correction meets the first or second interdigital space (Fig. 2.3). In severe cases, the banana shape of the foot

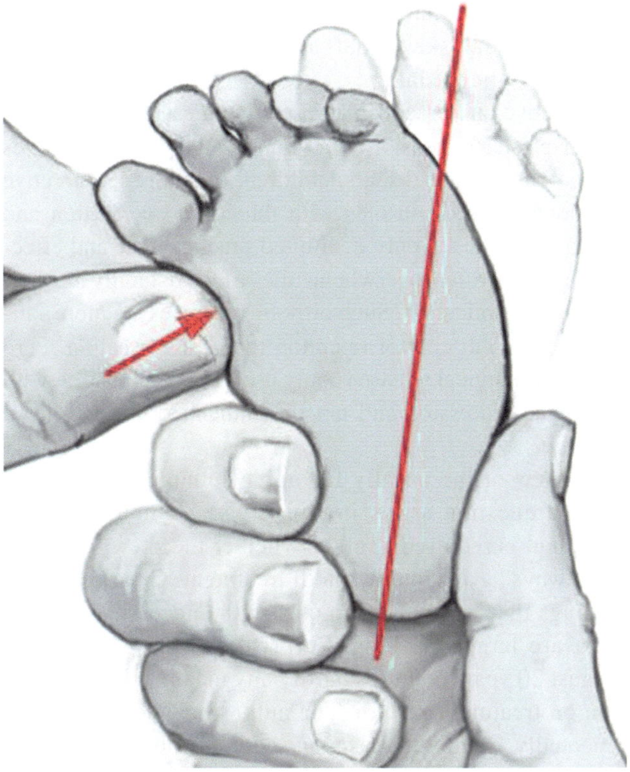

Fig. 2.3 In the clinical examination, it is assessed which interdigital space the heel bisector affects in spontaneous posture and in maximum correction position and to what extent the lateral foot rim can be straightened out

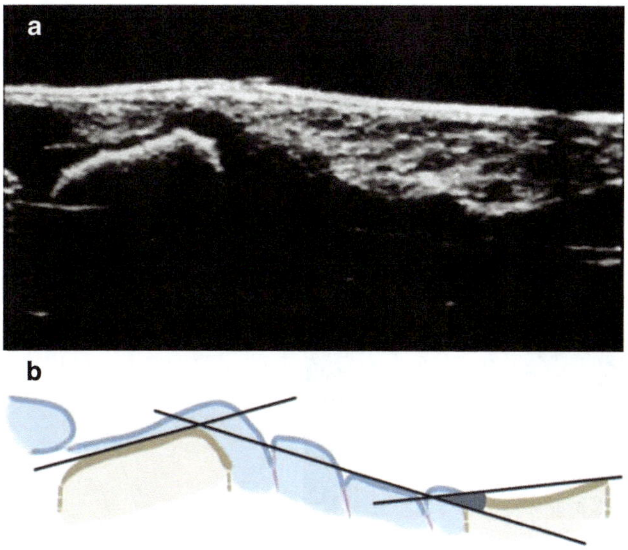

Fig. 2.4 Sonographic transversal section of the medial ray in a contracted skew foot at the age of four months (**a**) with explaining drawing (**b**); for the technique see Sect. 1.4.2. The plotted $TnCMT_E$-angle (**b**)—in this case about +20°—allows a quantification of the mid-forefoot adduction

is more pronounced, medial skin retraction is visible, and manual correction is incomplete.

2.3 Imaging

In the transverse plane, according to the pathomorphology (Sect. 2.1), there are essentially two phenomena that impress in imaging (see Fig. 2.2): adduction at the level of the Lisfranc joint line (skew foot) and often additionally an eversion of the hindfoot complex (serpentine foot). The transitions between the skew foot and the serpentine foot are fluent, meaning that a tendency towards hindfoot eversion can often also be seen in the "pure" skew foot.

Both phenomena can be quantitatively recorded in sonographic transverse section already in infancy: the hindfoot eversion based on the TnC_E angle (see Sect. 1.4.2) and adduction in the Lisfranc line based on the $TnCMT_E$ angle (**t**alus-**n**ucleus-**c**uneiform-**m**etatarsal-I angle in maximum **e**version), which is below 0° in the normal foot and reaches clearly positive values in the skew foot (Fig. 2.4). This angle is constructed from the tangents to the lesser tarsal skeletal elements (constructed similar as in clubfoot diagnostics) and the first metatarsal bone.

Corresponding to the sonographic imaging in infants, the skew/serpentine foot deformity in older children is assessed radiologically in the dorsoplantar projection (Fig. 2.5). For adduction in the Lisfranc joint line, numerous angular measures have been described. The calcaneus-metatarsal-II angle, which exclusively reflects the alignment of the subtalar footplate and is below approximately +10° at the normal foot, has proven particularly effective. In contrast, the TMT-I angle is not very informative, since both pathomorphological phenomena (see Sect. 2.1) change it in opposite directions and the deformity components therefore compensate each other (see Fig. 2.2). Another typical feature is the superposition of the metatarsal bases in the dorsoplantar X-ray projection (Fig. 2.1b).

The hindfoot eversion can be radiologically evaluated in the dorsoplantar projection using the TMT-I- base angle (see Sect. 4.4). Even more significant is the TMT index obtained from the dorsoplantar projection and the lateral projection (see Sect. 4.4). It should be taken into account that the ossification nucleus of the os naviculare in younger children is often located far laterally and this further reinforces the impression of an everted hindfoot position (Figs. 2.5, 2.6, and 2.19a).

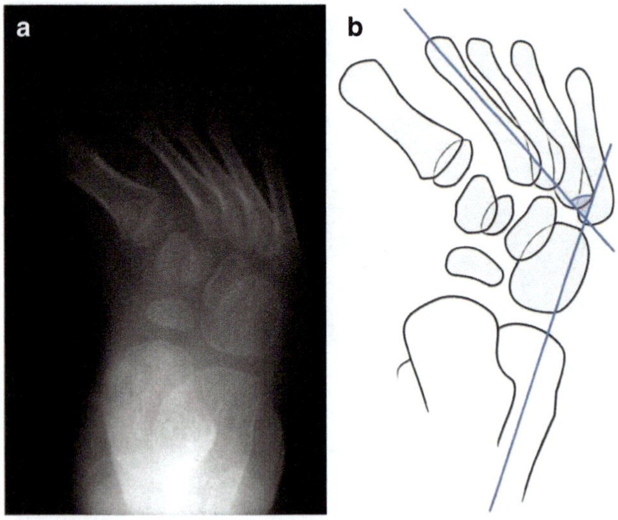

Fig. 2.5 The calcaneus-metatarsal-II angle quantifies the mid-forefoot adduction particularly conclusively. It is independent of the extent of a frequently additionally present hindfoot eversion and is therefore more suitable than the talus-metatarsal-I angle. In the presented case (**a**) it is about +60° (**b**)

Radiological Parameters of the Skew/Serpentine Foot in the Dorsoplantar Projection

Mid-forefoot-adduction	*Normal values*
– Calcaneal-metatarsal-II-angle	<10°
Hindfoot eversion	
– TMT-Index (including lateral projection)	Up to −35°
– TMT-I-base angle	Up to −20°

2.4 Natural Course and Treatment Indication

The congenital skew foot or the skew foot that becomes obvious in the first months of life in most of the cases has an absolutely favorable spontaneous prognosis in the milder forms (Farsetti et al. 1994). The long-term observation in Fig. 2.6 shows a continuous reduction of midfoot adduction component without any treatment. However, there are rare cases in which spontaneous correction is absent or incomplete or the adduction contracture of the Lisfranc joint line is compensated by increased eversion of the hindfoot complex ("compensated adductus deformity"). Cases are also observed in which a significant overload of the lateral metatarsus remains (Fig. 2.16). Therefore, the skew foot should on principle not be regarded to be trivial.

Effective and practicable corrective measures are in particular plaster redression at a younger age and osteotomies in small children and schoolchildren. In contrast, corrective positioning braces, insoles with three-point correction and antivarus shoes are only of limited practicability and effectiveness and often overwhelm the affected family in their consistent application. Such orthotic measures are more suitable for growth control retention than for correction. Pure soft tissue surgical release is only useful in combination with prolonged redression and not recommended as an isolated measure.

In view of the usually favorable spontaneous prognosis, the question arises in which cases a more invasive treatment is required at all or whether the skew foot does not always "grow out" without treatment. Clear scientific findings that would help to clarify the necessity of treatment are largely lacking. Surprisingly, the literature of the last 20 years contains hardly any meaningful information on treatment results. The author has, however, been repeatedly faced with cases in toddlers and early schoolchildren where, in retrospect, the skew foot was primarily underestimated and more complex treatment was then necessary (see Fig. 2.11). In severe cases, it has therefore proved to be effective in practice to initiate early redression with the application of long leg plaster of Paris casts in the first weeks of life, in moderately severe cases when no significant improvement is evident by about 3–4 months of life.

The indication for surgical treatment in young children and schoolchildren is derived from the degree of severity and, in particular, the monitoring of the course of the deformity (Fig. 2.6). Clear criteria can hardly be defined from the available literature. If left untreated, an internal rotation gait with overloading of the lateral metatarsus can persist (Fig. 2.16) and may cause stress fractures (Fig. 2.17). Real late adverse effects like hallux valgus or varus deformity are rarely observed or are difficult to prove completely conclusively (Figs. 2.7 and 2.8). Given the generally favorable results of surgical corrections, a surgical solution often appears to be advantageous over a lengthy and stressful attempt with purely orthotic measures.

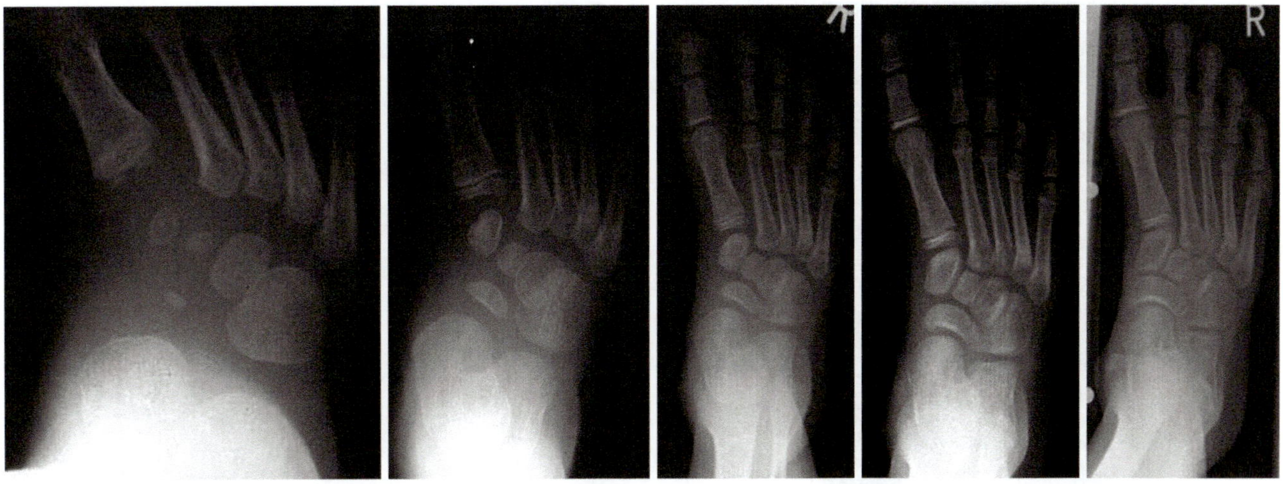

Fig. 2.6 Spontaneous course of a serpentine foot deformity without treatment at 21, 42, 68, 86, and 140 months of age. Continuous straightening can be observed with improvement of calcaneus-metatarsal-II angle from over 30° to below 20°, but a moderate hindfoot valgus component remains

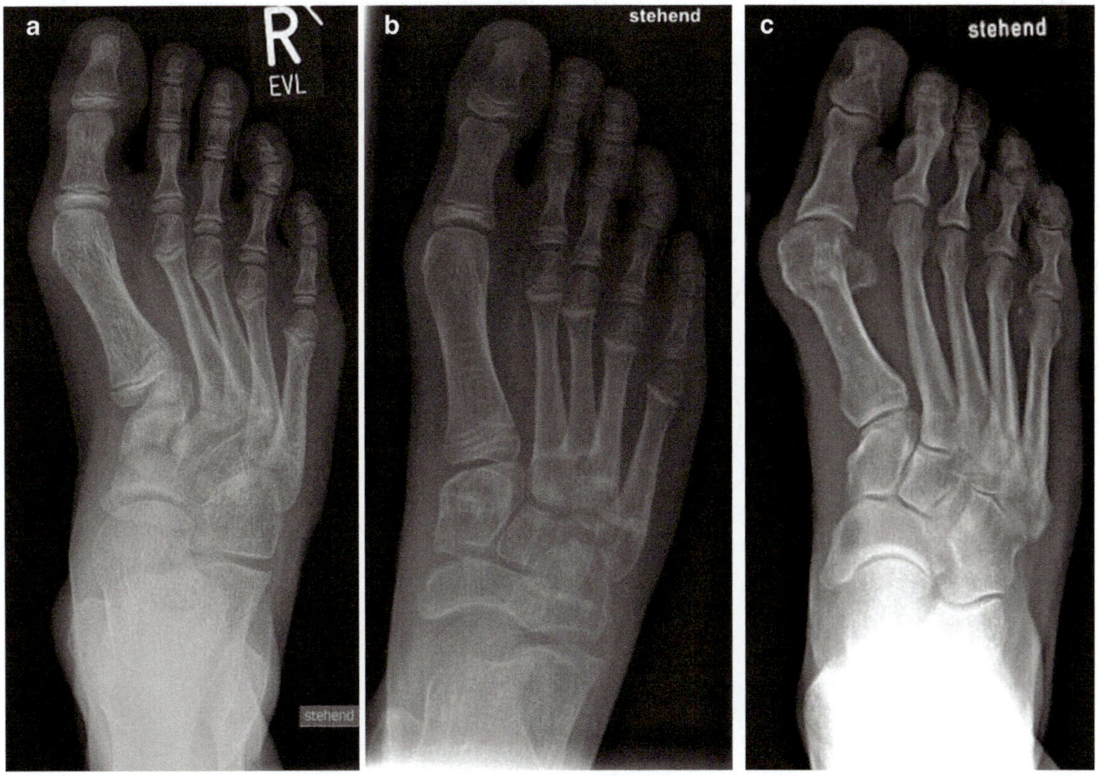

Fig. 2.7 Juvenile patient with skew foot deformity and additionally hallux valgus development (**a**). Skew foot correction could improve toe alignment, at least prevent further deterioration (**b**). The image given in (**c**) is taken from another patient with hallux valgus syndrome in adulthood and midfoot adduction. This latter patient was temporarily treated conservatively in early childhood because of a skew foot. To what extent the mid-forefoot adduction is a relic of the congenital deformity cannot be proven

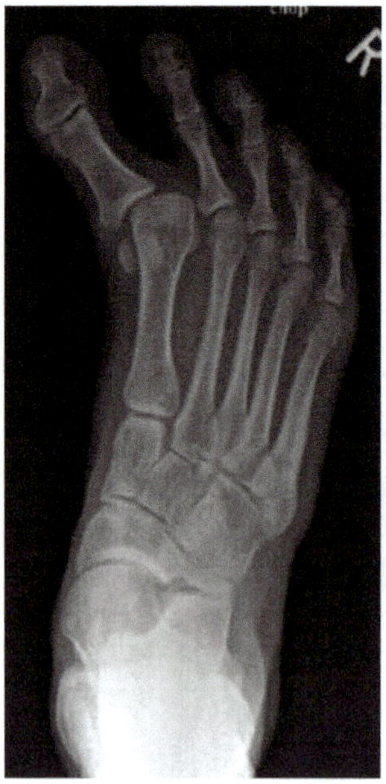

Fig. 2.8 Rare severe hallux-varus deformity with varus toe malpositioning also of the lesser toes in adulthood. In the infancy a skew foot deformity existed which was not treated

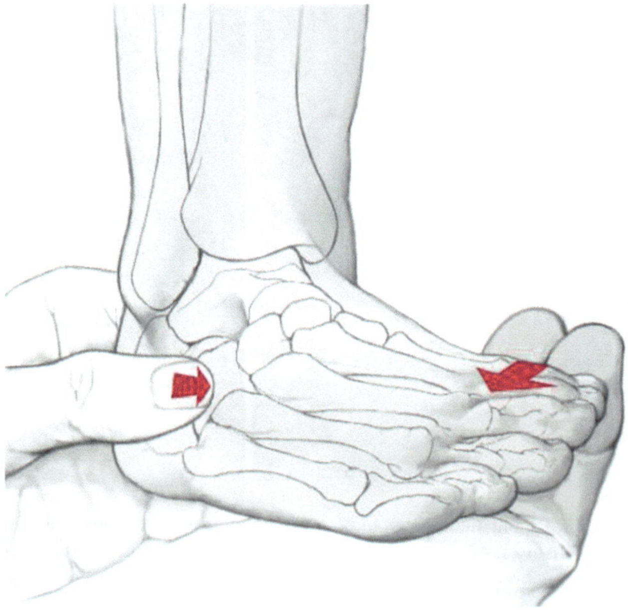

Fig. 2.10 Three-point redression grip on a right foot for correction of the skew foot deformity: The long fingers of the left hand of the therapist grasp the tuber calcanei from medial, and the thumb of the same hand holds precisely at the cuboid and provides counterpressure here (arrow), while the right hand of the therapist redresses the midfoot complex laterally (arrow). Without the counter support on the os cuboideum, this would increase the hindfoot eversion

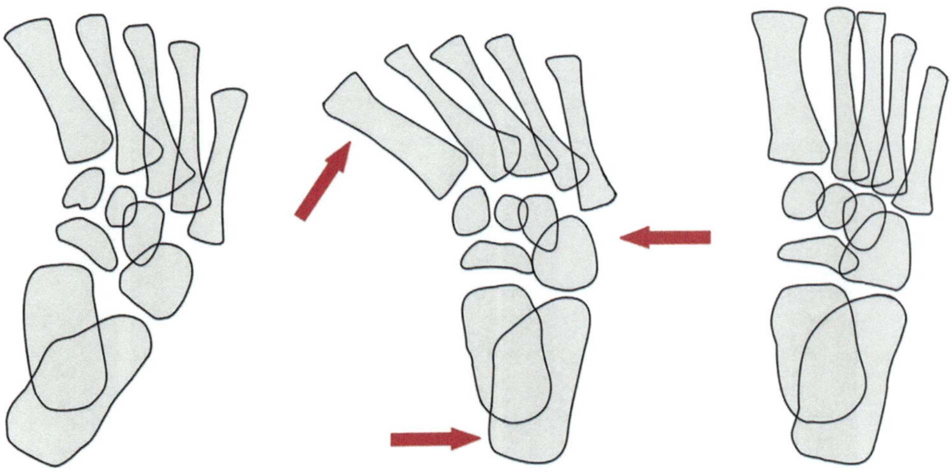

Fig. 2.9 Application of the correction forces in skew foot redression according to the three-point principle. It is important to provide exact counter support laterally on the os cuboideum to avoid iatrogenic reinforcement of the hindfoot eversion

2.5 Redression and Retention

The early treatment of severe and moderately severe cases in a long leg redression plaster of Paris cast with weekly cast changes is carried out—unlike with idiopathic clubfoot—according to the three-point correction principle (Fig. 2.9). It is extremely important to provide sufficient counter support on the cuboid (Fig. 2.10) to prevent iatrogenic serpentine foot development. This is only really possible with high precision in a plaster of Paris cast. All orthoses offered as alternatives do not achieve this precision sufficiently. In particular, the Denis Browne brace, which was originally developed for skew foot treatment, can also increase hindfoot eversion and therefore cannot be recommended.

The plaster treatment is continued until slight overcorrection to anticipate the high restoring forces (rebound phenomenon). Subsequently, braces are used—if at all necessary—only for retention after correction. Correction attempts with night braces and insoles with three-point correction (Fig. 2.11) can obviously develop a certain effect in the sense of growth guidance, but they are often associated with inconvenience and possible problems (e.g., difficult

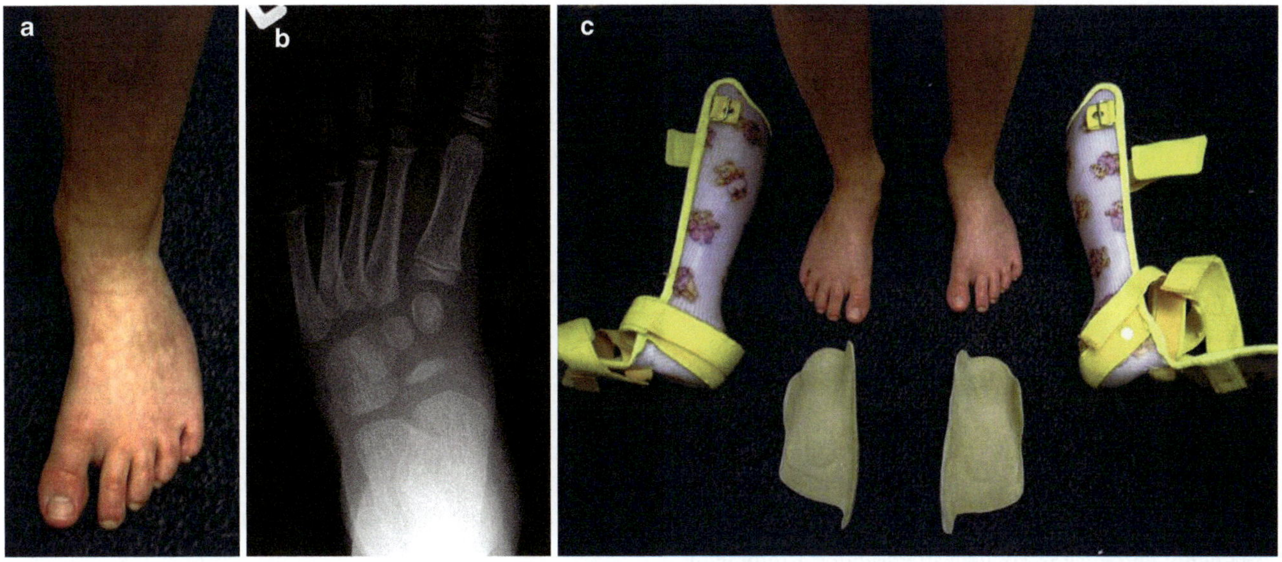

Fig. 2.11 5-Year-old girl with conservatively treated moderate skew foot (**a**, **b**). For years, she was treated with insoles according to the three-point correction principle and lower leg night braces (**c**) with considerable inconvenience for the child and the family

shoe fitting, pressure sore problems, imprecise correction effects, ineffectiveness due to rotation of the lower leg orthoses around the lower leg). It is therefore preferable to achieve correction by other means and leave the task of retention and growth guidance to the orthotic measures.

2.6 Soft Tissue Corrections: Medial Midfoot Release

In the literature, medial soft tissue surgery ("medial midfoot release") is indicated as an option for persistent skew feet at around 2–6 years of age (Asirvatham and Stevens 1997; Ghali et al. 1984; Thompson and Abaza 2010). The author has not been able to gain any experience with this but has instead subjected smaller children in exceptional cases to a redression plaster treatment with subsequent night bracing (at walking age, however, this is much more invasive for the child) but has usually waited for the spontaneous course of the deformity and, if necessary, planned later less invasive bony corrections (Sect. 2.7). However, since medial release can be useful at least in connection with osteotomies, it should be mentioned here.

Technique

A medial incision in the area of the tarsometatarsal junction is used to perform an intramuscular lengthening of the abductor hallucis muscle by cutting its tendinous part once or at several locations. The talonavicular joint is not exposed. The medial naviculo-cuneiform joint and the tarsometatarsal I joint are opened semicircularly on the medial side, so that the joint spaces are clearly gaping. In the tarsometatarsal I joint, the insertion of the anterior tibial tendon and the growth plate at the metatarsal I base must be carefully protected. If the attachment of the anterior tibial tendon is located far distally, it can be rerouted and reinserted proximal to the Lisfranc joint line if necessary, e.g., also by transposition of only the distal tendon insertion at the metatarsal I base with longitudinal splitting of the tendon close to the attachment (see Fig. 4.14). Postoperatively, the foot should be retained in clear abduction to ensure the desired adapting growth of the skeletal elements next to the joint and thus a permanent correction.

For several reasons, the previously recommended procedure according to Heyman and Herndon with capsulolysis of the central tarsometatarsal joints must be considered obsolete. It offers clear disadvantages compared to metatarsal base osteotomies (Sect. 2.7).

2.7 Osteotomies

In the literature there are suggestions for soft tissue surgical correction in the second and third year of life (see Sect. 2.6). In practice, however, the author has found it useful to wait for the further course of the condition and correct it by osteotomies at the site of the deformity from about the end of the third year of life if the spontaneous correction is insufficient (Cahuzac et al. 1993). The threshold of the indication for correction is set at approximately above +20° to +30°

calcaneus-metatarsal-II angle. It has been observed that, on the one hand, the spontaneous progression shows a continuous reduction of the angle (Fig. 2.6), therefore only more pronounced cases should be corrected surgically, if necessary also after radiological observation of the progression; on the other hand, the results after surgical correction are very convincing (Figs. 2.14, 2.15, and 2.16), so that in pronounced cases it is certainly advisable.

Technique

An oblique skin incision is made above the metatarsal II to V bases (Fig. 2.13). While carefully preserving neurovascular structures, the long extensor tendons, and the short foot muscles by means of longitudinal preparation, the metatarsal bases are exposed individually and each is circumvented subperiostally with small Hohmann hooks. A lateral wedge removal is performed close to the base with very small saw blades (Fig. 2.12), usually with complete dissection of the bone and, if necessary, also with intended slight loss of length. Via a separate skin incision medially above the medial cuneiform, an intramuscular lengthening of the M. abductor hallucis is initially performed. Subsequently, the medial cuneiform is visualized with the X-ray image intensifier, and a K-wire is inserted proximally and distally into the bone. The cuneiforme mediale is completely severed between the two wires and distracted with an osteotomy spreader placed on the K-wires. Depending on the age of the child, some bone material is placed in the osteotomy site. In smaller children this can be omitted; in older children and in cases with clearly inclined distal articular surface of the medial cuneiform, a corticospongious bone graft from the iliac crest may be used. Manual correction of the adductus deformity after osteotomy of all five rays is now possible. All five osteotomies are secured with thin K-wires. For this purpose, a dorsal entry hole with a thicker K-wire is first drilled in the distal osteotomy partner at the metatarsal II–V bases, which considerably eases the penetration of the thinner K-wire into the bone percutaneously from the distal side (Fig. 2.13). The only purpose of K-wire osteosynthesis is to precisely align the osteotomy partners one to the other and to prevent synostosis of adjacent metatarsals thereby. The maintenance of the correction position itself is carried out in the long leg hard cast with flexed knee joint. Secondary post-corrections with this semistable osteosynthesis are also still possible when changing the cast.

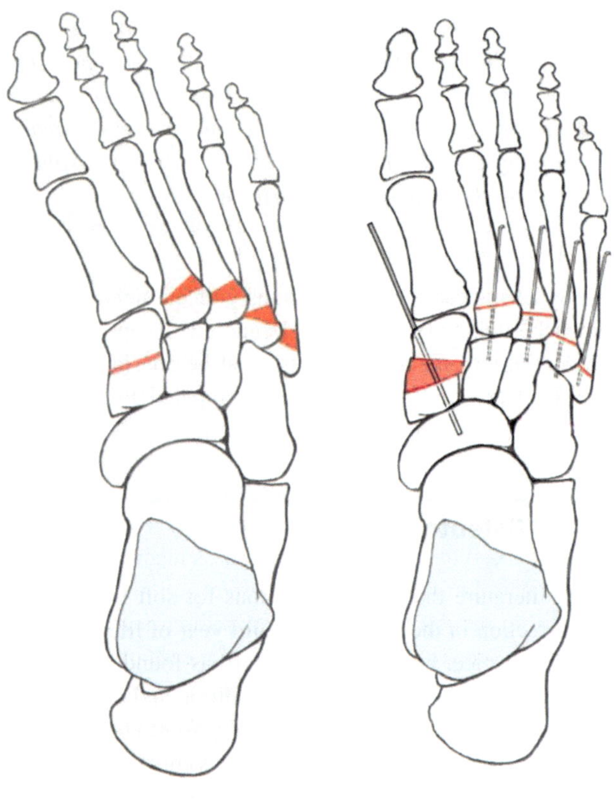

Fig. 2.12 Bony skew foot correction by multiple osteotomies of medial cuneiform bone and metatarsal bases II–V

Osteotomy of the medial cuneiform is performed as described by Mosca (2014). It has been shown that correction at the metatarsal II to V bases, that is, at the site of the deformity, is the most important corrective step in the treatment of skew foot deformity. Even without osteotomy of the medial cuneiform, correction of the articular surface can be achieved in milder cases through subsequent adaptive growth, as Fig. 2.14 shows and as a percutaneous surgical procedure without cuneiform osteotomy presented by Knörr et al. (2014) also confirmed. If the ossification state of the medial cuneiform is still insufficient, a metatarsal I base

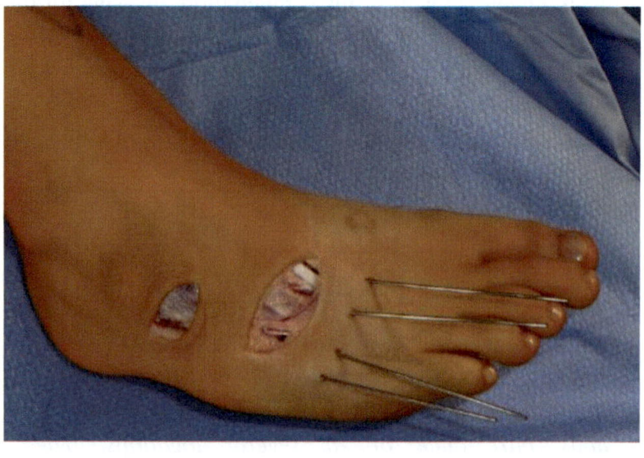

Fig. 2.13 Intraoperative image after preparation of the percutaneous K-wire osteosynthesis of metatarsal base osteotomies. In this case, an additional cuboid wedge removal was performed, and the bone wedge obtained here was inserted into the medial cuneiform

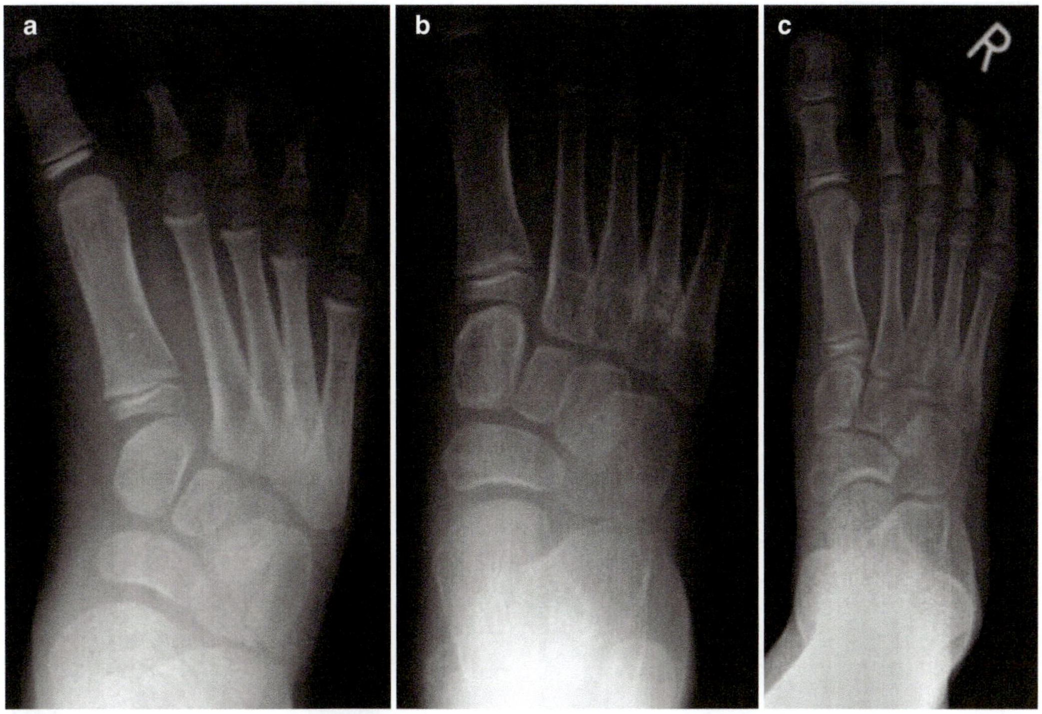

Fig. 2.14 5.5-Year-old female patient with distinct skew foot (**a**). 1 year (**b**) and 5 years (**c**) after metatarsal II–V base osteotomies and abductor hallucis release complete correction of the deformity. It is noteworthy that in this case the distal articular surface of the medial cuneiform has corrected itself completely even without an osteotomy

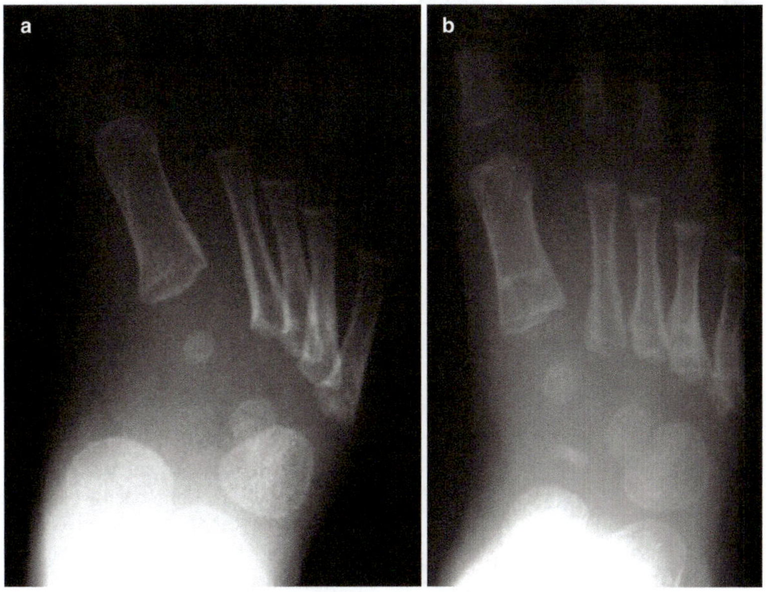

Fig. 2.15 2.8-Year-old boy with distinct skew foot and early ossification status of the medial cuneiform (**a**). 7 months after MT I–V osteotomy, abductor hallucis release, and TMT-I release, the foot shows good straightening (**b**)

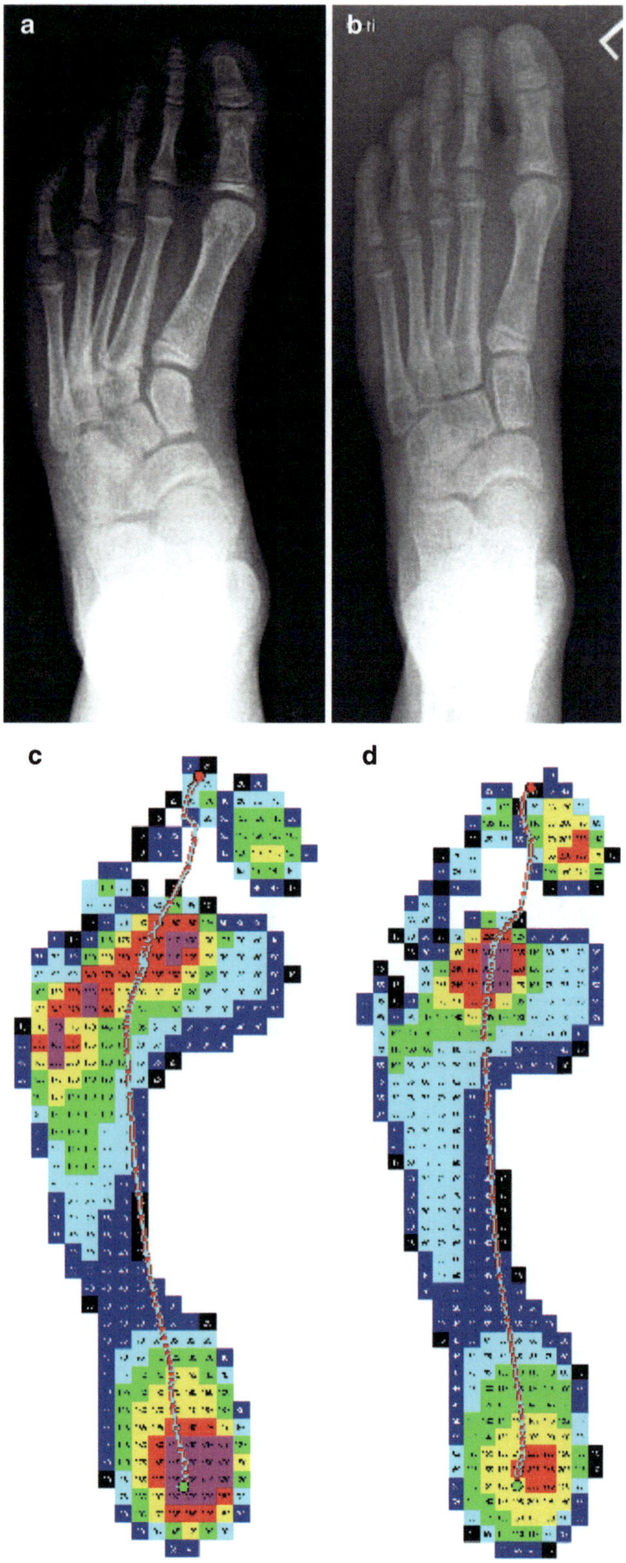

Fig. 2.16 8-Year-old female patient with clinically clear skew foot before (**a**, **c**) and 1 year after (**b**, **d**) surgical correction (metatarsal II–V base osteotomies with epiphysiodesis of an accessory growth plate at metatarsal II, cuboid wedge removal with open-wedge osteotomy of the medial cuneiform, intramuscular lengthening of the M. abductor hallucis). Radiologically, the spontaneous correction of the talonavicular joint is impressively visible (**b**), without the hindfoot eversion having been surgically addressed. Due to the preoperative high load on the lateral midfoot (**c**), the peritalar joint complex was forced into the everted position; this is shown to be normalized postoperatively (**d**)

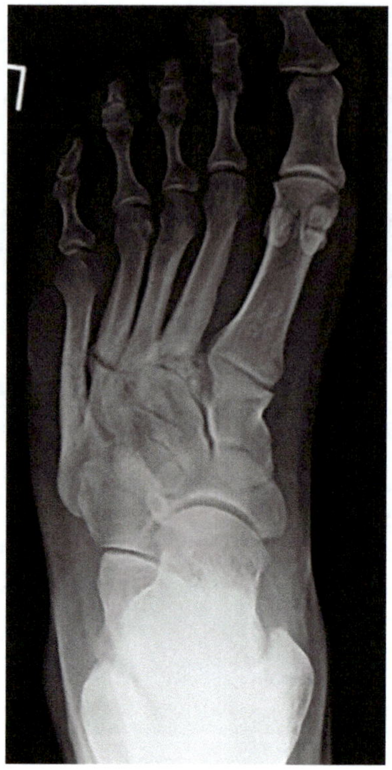

Fig. 2.17 Adult patient with skewfoot, that was treated in the first years of life without sufficient correction. Painful stress fractures were observed at the lateral metatarsals due to chronic overload at this region

osteotomy can be performed as an alternative, taking into account the proximally located growth plate (Fig. 2.15). Napiontek et al. (2003) described a successful osteotomy of the medial cuneiform even in smaller children. The elimination of midfoot adduction may lead to spontaneous improvement of accompanying hindfoot eversion (Fig. 2.16), so that no further surgical intervention might be required in this respect. Similar observations were also described by Feng and Sussmann (2016).

Bony Procedures for Skew/Serpentine Foot

Midfoot adduction
- MT II–V base osteotomy
- Medial cuneiform open-wedge osteotomy (before the fourth year of life alternatively metatarsal-I-osteotomy)
- (Cuboid-closed-wedge osteotomy)

Hindfoot eversion
- Calcaneus lengthening osteotomy
- Calcaneus sliding osteotomy
- Arthroereisis

2.8 Serpentine Foot

In the case of the serpentine foot deformity, in addition to the correction of the adduction as described above, an intervention to reduce the hindfoot eversion should be considered in pronounced cases. Milder hindfoot deformities can correct themselves spontaneously through midfoot osteotomies (Fig. 2.16). For severe hindfoot eversion, a calcaneal lengthening osteotomy (Figs. 2.18 and 2.19), a calcaneal double osteotomy, or tarsal arthroereisis (Fig. 2.20) can be considered (Sect. 4.9). The calcaneus lengthening osteotomy increases the midfoot adduction, which must therefore always be corrected in the same procedure.

However, it must be taken into consideration when deciding on the indication for the surgical procedure: Both malalignment components—midfoot adduction and hindfoot eversion—compensate each other, so that clinically often there is no major obvious deformity. Patients are often completely free of symptoms. A spontaneous correction can be expected at least to a certain extent (Fig. 2.6). The surgical effort is high if both components require correction. Therefore, in less severe cases, it must be carefully considered whether such an intervention is justified or whether a simple medializing calcaneus sliding osteotomy may be sufficient, e.g., if there is a clear valgus deformity of the hindfoot.

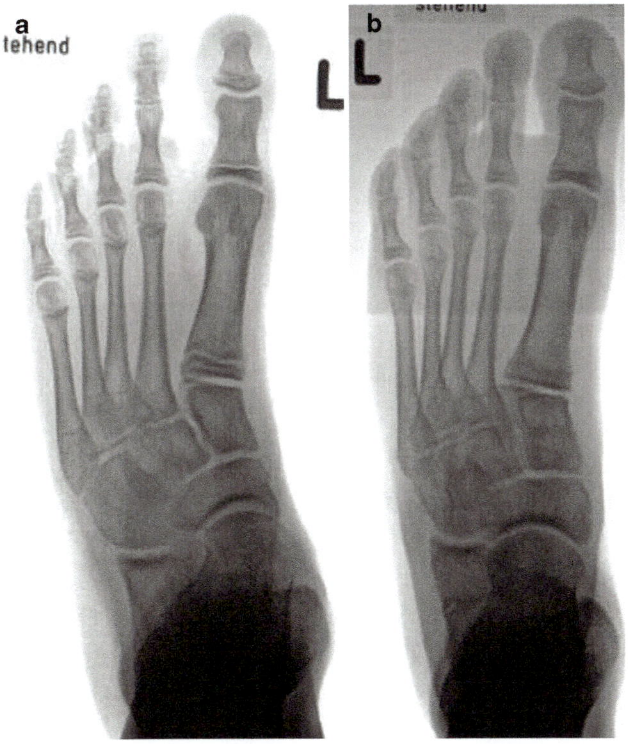

Fig. 2.18 12-Year-old patient with serpentine foot (compensated adductus deformity), mild midfoot adduction with distinct hindfoot valgus (**a**). Lesser tarsus osteotomies with calcaneus lengthening, 2.5 years postoperatively (**b**) good correction result

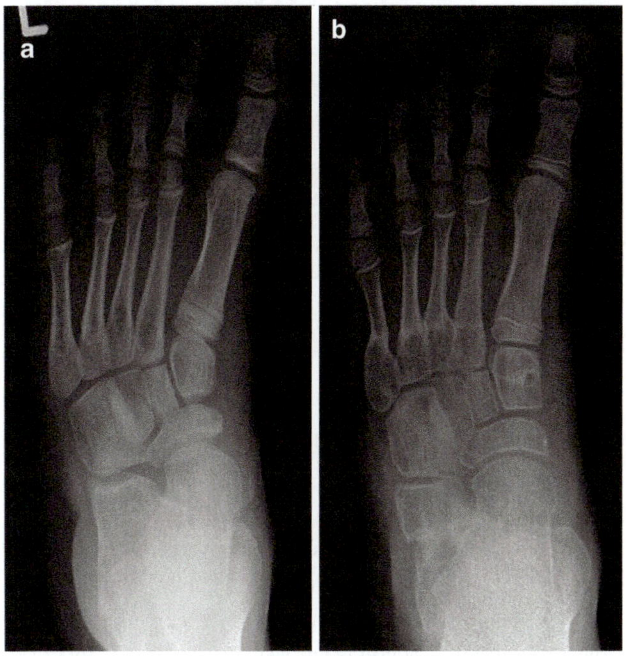

Fig. 2.19 10-Year-old patient with moderate serpentine foot deformity (**a**). After calcaneus lengthening osteotomy, medial cuneiform osteotomy, and metatarsal II–V basal osteotomies, complete repositioning of the talonavicular joint and good overall tarsometatarsal alignment (**b**)

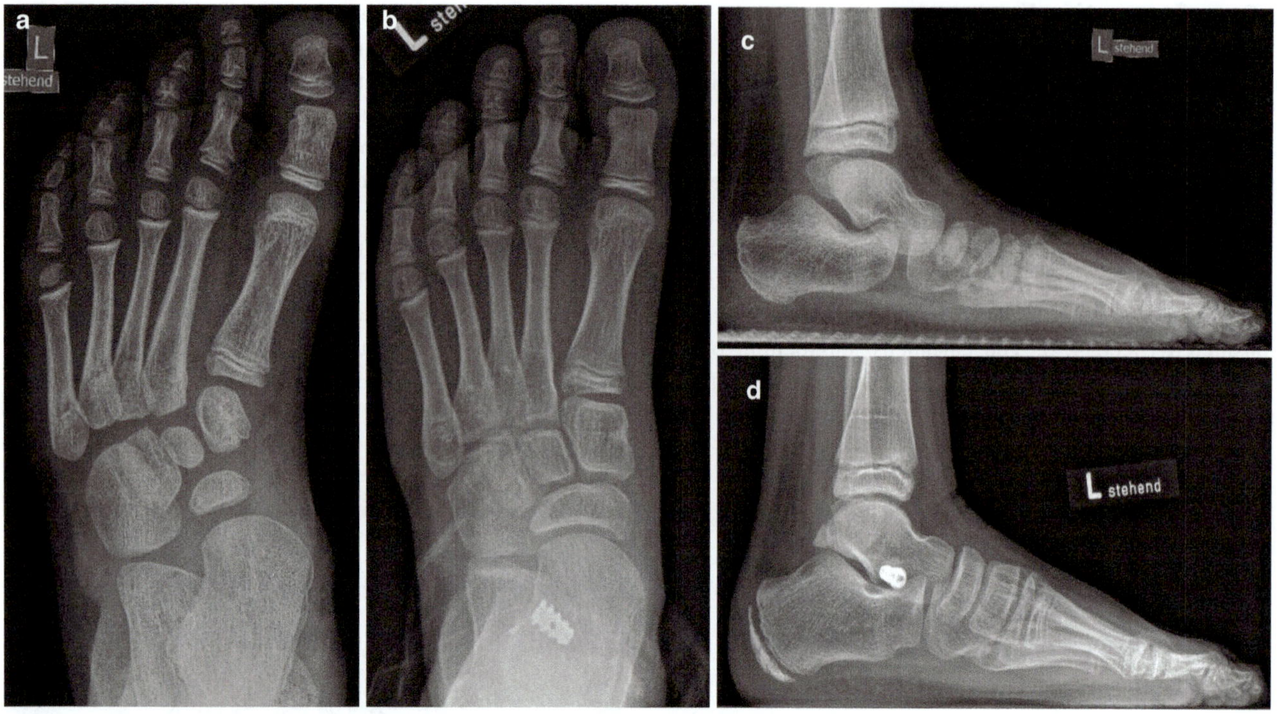

Fig. 2.20 8-Year-old boy with skew foot and hindfoot eversion (**a**, **c**). 2.5 years after metatarsal osteotomies with cuneiforme mediale open-wedge osteotomy and sinus tarsi spacer marked improvement of tarsometatarsal alignment (**b**, **d**)

References

Asirvatham R, Stevens PM (1997) Idiopathic forefoot-adduction deformity: medial capsulotomy and abductor hallucis lengthening for resistant and severe deformities. J Pediatr Orthop 17:496–500

Cahuzac JP, Laville JM, Sales de Gauzy J, Lebarbier P (1993) Surgical correction of metatarsus adductus. J Pediatr Orthop B 2:176–181

Coleman SS (1983) Complex foot deformities in children. Lea & Febiger, Philadelphia

Farsetti P, Weinstein SL, Ponseti IV (1994) The long-term functional and radiographic outcomes of untreated and non-operatively treated metatarsus adductus. J Bone Joint Surg 76-A:257–265

Feng L, Sussmann M (2016) Combined medial cuneiform osteotomy and multiple metatarsal osteotomies for correction of persistent metatarsus adductus in children. J Pediatr Orthop 36:730–735

Ghali NN, Abberton MJ, Silk FF (1984) The management of metatarsus adductus et supinatus. J Bone Joint Surg 66-B:376–380

Knörr J, Soldado F, Pham TT et al (2014) Percutaneous correction of persistent severe metatarsus adductus in children. J Pediatr Orthop 34:447–452

Mosca VS (2014) Principles and management of pediatric foot and ankle deformities and malformations. Wolters Kluwer, Philadelphia

Napiontek M, Kotwicki T, Tomaszewski M (2003) Opening wedge osteotomy of the medial cuneiform before age 4 years in the treatment of forefoot adduction. J Pediatr Orthop 23:65–69

Thompson GH, Abaza H (2010) Metatarsus adductus and metatarsus varus. In: McCarthy JJ, Drennan JC (eds) The child's foot and ankle. Wolters Kluwer, Philadelphia

Talus Verticalis (Vertical Talus)

3

Contents

The congenital rigid flat foot is with an incidence of about 1:10,000 much less frequent than the congenital clubfoot and is often associated with syndromal diseases such as arthrogryposis.

3.1 Therapeutically Relevant Pathomorphology

Pathomorphologically, the vertical talus shows a complete and manually irreducible dislocation of the talonavicular joint (Fig. 3.1). The navicular, which is purely cartilaginous until toddler age, is located dorsolaterally on the neck of the talus, and the talus is in severe plantarflexion in maximum equinus position of the upper ankle joint. The accompanying deformity of the calcaneocuboid joint is somewhat less obvious. Calf muscles, all extensors, and the peroneal muscles are shortened, resulting in a rocker bottom shape of the subtalar footplate. The mid-forefoot complex is in distinct abduction (Drennan 1995).

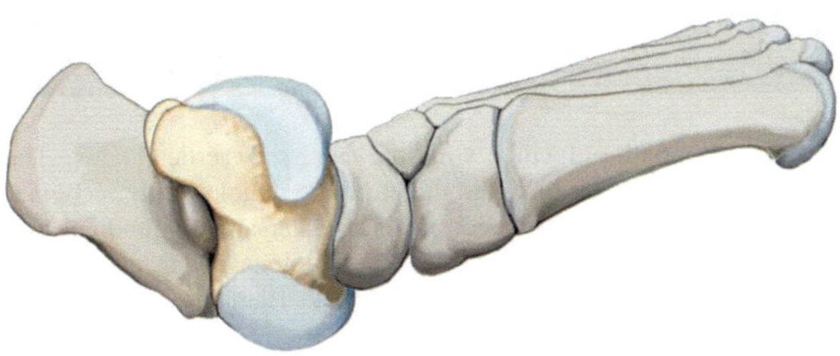

Fig. 3.1 Skeletal pathomorphology of the talus verticalis with rigid, irreducible dislocation of the talonavicular joint. The navicular is located on top of the talar neck, the talus and calcaneus are clearly plantar-flexed, and the calf muscles are always shortened

3.2 Clinical Diagnostics

The extent of muscle-tendon shortening and the degree of remaining flexibility and reducability of the Chopart joints is detected by meticulous manual examination. For this purpose, the grip also used for manual correction is to be applied (Fig. 3.5): By applying pressure from plantar to the medioplantar talar head with the thumb and plantarization and adduction of the mid-forefoot with the other examiner's hand, one gains an impression of the rigidity of the deformity. If the talonavicular joint is almost completely correctable, the deformity is called a talus obliquus (Sect. 4.8). The Achilles tendon (calf musculature) is always significantly shortened in the true vertical talus, an

J. Hamel, *Foot and Ankle Surgery in Children and Adolescents*, https://doi.org/10.1007/978-3-030-58108-4_3

essential distinguishing feature from the infant's flexible planovalgus foot or the harmless but sometimes impressive postural deformity of the newborn child, called talipes calcaneovalgus.

3.3 Imaging

Sonographically a dorsal longitudinal section is used to depict the center of deformity at the talonavicular joint. This is usually possible only after pre-redression. The foot is held in the most corrected position possible as described for the clinical examination (Fig. 3.5). The sonogram shows to what extent a partial reduction of the—not yet ossified—navicular in relation to the talar head is possible, indicating the severity of the deformity (Hamel and Becker 1995) (Fig. 3.2).

Radiological examinations are performed in the lateral and dorsoplantar projection. In the lateral projection, the extension of the metatarsal I axis more or less crosses the talar head in normal feet; however in talus verticalis this line is located dorsally (Fig. 3.3). Informative is an additional lateral functional image taken in the furthest reduced position possible with plantar flexion of the mid-forefoot complex in accordance with the sonographic examination described above. The extent of reducability can be evaluated thereby. In clinically unclear cases, a contracted vertical talus can be confirmed or excluded this way (Fig. 3.4).

Hamanishi (1984) described the TAMBA angle (**t**alar-**a**xis-first-**m**etatarsal-**b**ase **a**ngle) to quantify the malposition on the medial tarsometatarsal ray (normal value close to 0°). It is formed by the longitudinal axis of the talus and a line connecting the anterior talar contour with the metatarsal I base. When comparing the lateral images in spontaneous position and maximum plantar flexion, the difference in the TAMBA angle in both planes gives a measure of the reducability and thus of the severity of the contracture. In pronounced cases, this angle can reach over 120° and is reduced by less than 25° by manual repositioning (Eberhardt et al. 2012). In these cases, according to the experience of these authors, the modern minimally invasive therapeutic approach (Sect. 3.4) is not promising, and repositioning by open surgery is necessary.

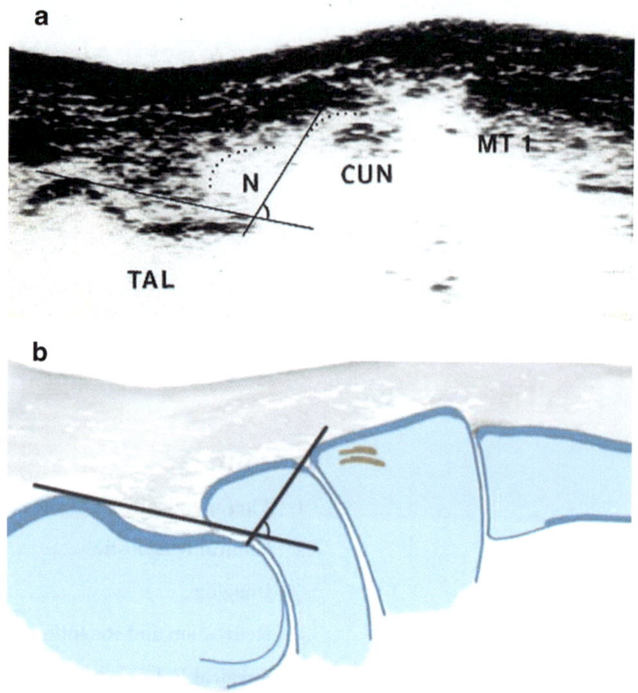

Fig. 3.2 Sonographic dorsal longitudinal section of the medial tarsometatarsal ray in widest possible plantar flexion in talus verticalis in the second year of life after redressing pretreatment (**a**) with explaining drawing (**b**). The marked TnC_P angle (**t**alus-**n**ucleus-**c**uneiforme mediale in **p**lantar flexion) is about 0° at the normal foot (Hamel and Becker 1995). In this case it measures about 70°

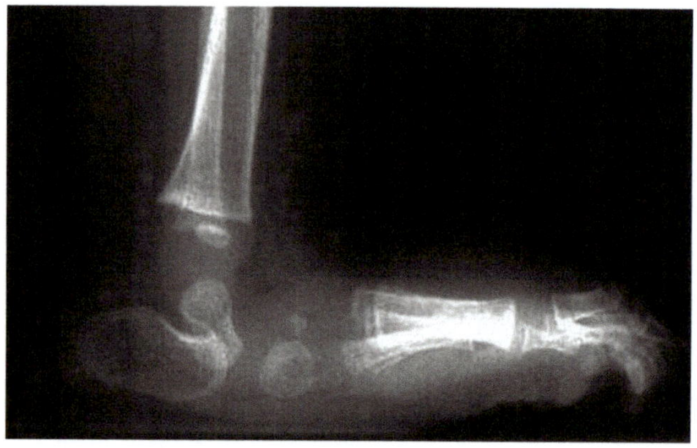

Fig. 3.3 9-month-old child with pre-redressed vertical talus. The navicular is not yet ossified and therefore not radiologically recognizable. The fact that the extension of the metatarsal I longitudinal axis does not hit the talar head proves the severe talonavicular malposition. In this case the TAMBA angle according to Hamanishi (see text) is almost 90°

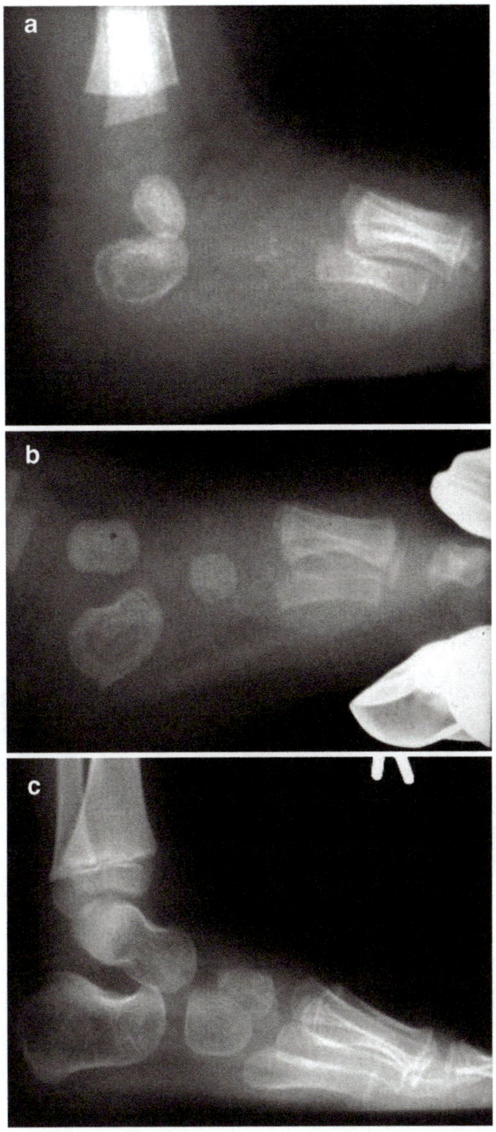

Fig. 3.4 The lateral X-ray of an infant's foot was presented with suspected talus verticalis (**a**). However, the absence of the equinus position of the calcaneus, which is obligatory for the vertical talus, spoke against this diagnosis. An image taken 2 months later in maximum plantar flexion (**b**) confirmed the normal alignment of talus and metatarsal I. The foot developed normally without further treatment until the age of 4 years (**c**)

3.4 Redression and Retention

The primary treatment consists of a manual redression to stretch the contracted soft tissues and to reposition the deformity as much as possible. For this purpose the foot is held in the equinus position. By applying controlled pressure on the medioplantar prominent talar head and manual plantar flexion and adduction of the mid-forefoot complex, the foot is

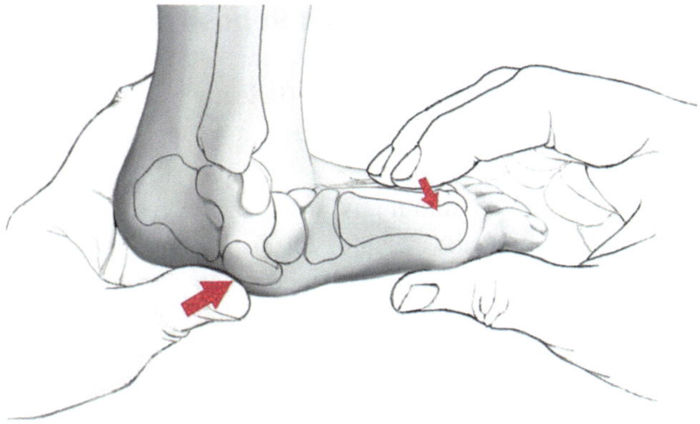

Fig. 3.5 Manual redression of the vertical talus. The midfoot-forefoot complex is mobilized in plantar direction with counter support at the head of the talus from medioplantar. This results in stretching of the shortened soft tissues on the dorsum of the foot

manipulated into the most repositioned status possible in the area of the Chopart line (Fig. 3.5). This is associated with successive stretching of the severely shortened dorsolateral capsular structures and the extensor and peroneal tendons. Long leg redression plasters are applied in the best possible position and changed weekly.

Until recently major surgical release was recommended as the treatment of choice usually around the end of the first year of life and often without any pretreatment. The well-known Cincinnati approach (Krauspe and Raab 2000) or other forms of surgical access (Mosca 2014) were used.

After the Ponseti method for the treatment of idiopathic clubfoot had become generally accepted, Dobbs et al. (2006) described a "reversed Ponseti method" for the early treatment of the vertical talus and further developed the procedure in the following years (Chalayon et al. 2012). Eberhardt et al. (2011) were also able to show that at least the milder cases of vertical talus can in part be repositioned purely conservatively and that temporary K-wire stabilization of the talonavicular joint in a repositioned setting with tenotomy of the Achilles tendon can be sufficient to achieve favorable results (Fig. 3.6). Therefore, a conservative treatment attempt by serial casting today seems justified in any case. Even in cases corrected later by surgery, this manipulative approach serves to pre-stretch the soft tissue and eases the subsequent surgical procedure.

Treatment of the vertical talus is considered extremely difficult, and the results are associated with a high rate of incomplete correction and recurrence. For this reason, once a positional correction has been achieved, it is necessary to secure the results of realignment for the long term with orthoses or complex insole fittings (see Fig. 3.7).

3.5 Surgical Release and Repositioning

If the reduction does not succeed sufficiently by conservative means, different surgical procedures can be applied:

- According to the minimally invasive concept ("reversed Ponseti") by Dobbs et al. (2007), open talonavicular joint reposition via a small medioplantar longitudinal incision and K-wire stabilization as well as relocation of the anterior tibial tendon are often sufficient. The Achilles tendon is tenotomized percutaneously. If necessary, further muscle-tendon units must be lengthened intramuscularly.
- Traditionally, peritalar release via a semicircular Cincinnati incision was recommended (Krauspe and Raab 2000) and is still appropriate in severe cases. The release includes the posterior soft tissue structures (Achilles tendon, upper ankle joint capsule), the peroneal tendons, as well as the extensor tendons. Talonavicular, calcaneocuboid, and subtalar joints are repositioned under direct view and stabilized by capsuloplasty and temporary Kirschner wire fixation. The tendon of the anterior tibial muscle is repositioned on the medioplantar capsule of the talonavicular region.
- Mosca (2014) and previously Coleman (1983) describe an equally extensive soft tissue release via a transverse incision on the dorsum of the foot, through which the contracted extensor tendons and also the talonavicular joint can be easily accessed. In addition, a percutaneous tenotomy of the Achilles tendon is performed. Ramanoudjame et al. (2014) also address more the talonavicular and calcaneocuboid region than the subtalar joint without peritalar release and partly without Achilles tendon lengthening.

The first two forms of access offer advantages in capsuloplasty of the talonavicular joint, while the dorsal access allows a more direct approach to the contracted soft tissue structures. An essential component of surgical treatment is the soft tissue stabilization of the talonavicular joint after its reduction. This involves capsuloplastic surgery with reinforcement of the severely overstretched medioplantar capsular structures using non-resorbable sutures combined with a (partial) rerouting of the anterior tibial tendon attachment to the capsular structures of the medioplantar talonavicular joint. Frequently, a tightening or distalization of the posterior tibial tendon attachment is also advisable. This corresponds approximately to the soft tissue surgery historically described by Schede (1929). The rerouting of the anterior tibial tendon attachment eliminates its deformity-promoting effect on the talonavicular joint and acts as a suspension for the talar head. The associated slight weakening of the dorsal extension power is often advantageous.

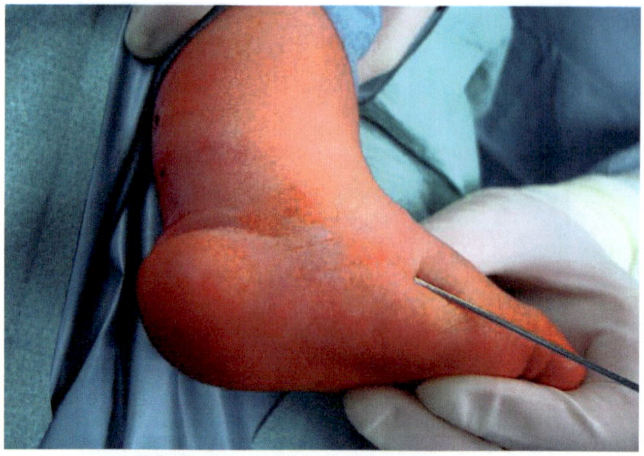

Fig. 3.6 After conservative redressive pretreatment of a moderately severe vertical talus, the talonavicular joint is temporarily stabilized in the reduced position with a percutaneously inserted Kirschner wire and the Achilles tendon is tenotomized percutaneously

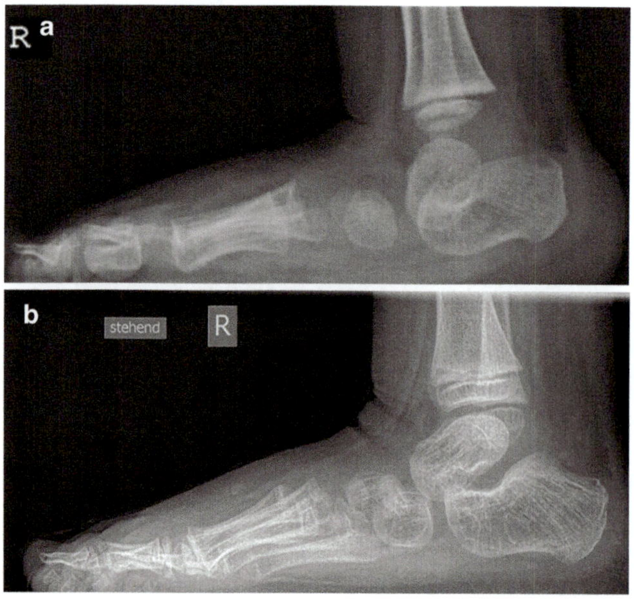

Fig. 3.7 Moderate talus verticalis deformity at the age of 3 years (**a**). 26 months after open Achilles tendon lengthening with capsuloplasty of the talonavicular joint and temporary K-wire stabilization, a largely but not completely corrected position of the medial tarsometatarsal ray (**b**) is observed. Postoperatively, after 3 months of plaster immobilization, the patient was treated in an ankle foot orthosis for 6 months, followed by prescription of a molded insole with sufficient support for the longitudinal arch

Today, in contrast to the earlier practice (Drennan 1995), it seems to make sense in general, as in the case of idiopathic clubfoot in infancy, to first follow the concept of reversed Ponseti concept, including a closed or open talonavicular joint reduction with percutaneous Achilles tendon lengthening before walking age. Particularly the arthrogrypotic and syndromal forms of the vertical talus, however, require extensive surgical repositioning either subsequently or primarily in larger numbers. This raises the question of the optimal time for surgery, which must also be considered in the context of the overall disability and the necessary follow-up treatment.

3.6 Treatment Results and Case Studies

Long-term treatment results after early primary correction of the vertical talus are hardly found in the literature. Predominantly satisfactory short- to medium-term results are reported in about 80% of cases (Ricco et al. 2014), but with sometimes significant residual deformities. Of particular importance is the question of the optimal time of surgery for the primary intervention. Corrections are often performed at the age of 6–18 months or after the onset of walking ability (see Figs. 3.8 and 3.9), in order to positively influence the further development of the bone and joint structures. Napiontek (1995) described medium- to long-term results in 32 cases of treatment of partly older children with 53% good and very good results. Eberhardt et al. (2012) found complete primary correction in 70% of the 20 children treated with the reversed Ponseti concept, while in Chalayon et al. (2012) this was observed in all 15 treated cases of syndromal vertical talus. Yang and Dobbs (2015) demonstrated the superiority of the minimally invasive approach over the more extensive release procedures.

Undesirable results are often incomplete corrections or loss of correction in the area of the talonavicular joint. In addition to renewed soft tissue corrections, depending on the individual findings and age of the patient, extra-articular talocalcaneal arthrodesis according to Grice (1952) (Fig. 3.10) or resection of the entire navicular and later also fusion procedures in the Chopart line region (Fig. 3.12) may be considered.

Figures 3.7, 3.8, 3.9, 3.10, 3.11, and 3.12 show examples of surgically treated talus verticalis cases, which reveal some of the typical sequelae and accompanying problems in the therapy of this clinical entity: the often incomplete correction in the further course of the disease, the necessity of intensive orthotic aftercare (see Fig. 3.7), and the frequently required renewed surgical correction (see Fig. 3.10).

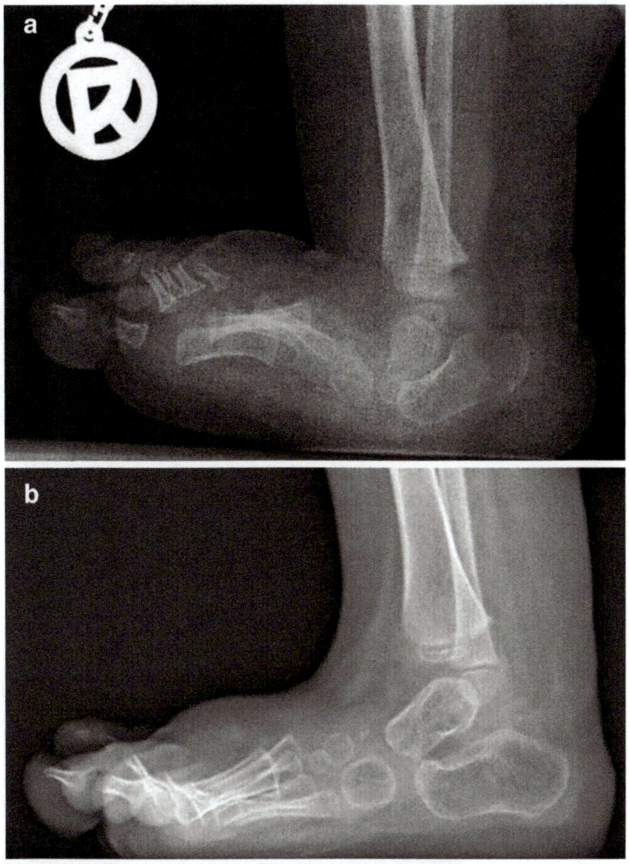

Fig. 3.8 Severe vertical talus (**a**), surgical correction at 15 months in the form of a peritalar release: lengthening of the Achilles tendon and peroneus brevis tendon, rerouting of the anterior tibial tendon and capsuloplasty of the talonavicular joint. 7 months postoperatively (**b**) significant but not complete reduction

Often the question arises beyond infancy as to whether remaining talonavicular malalignment should be tolerated or again be treated surgically. In these cases, the situation at the upper ankle joint in particular must be taken into account: If the dorsal extension of the ankle is clearly limited (lateral X-ray in maximum dorsal extension) and sagittal mobility is more likely to occur in the talonavicular joint, a further correction with soft tissue stabilization of the talonavicular joint, anterior tibial tendon rerouting, and lengthening of the Achilles tendon should be considered in younger age groups in order to optimize the further development of the ankle (Fig. 3.11). Later, the given range of motion of the upper ankle joint must be respected (Fig. 3.12).

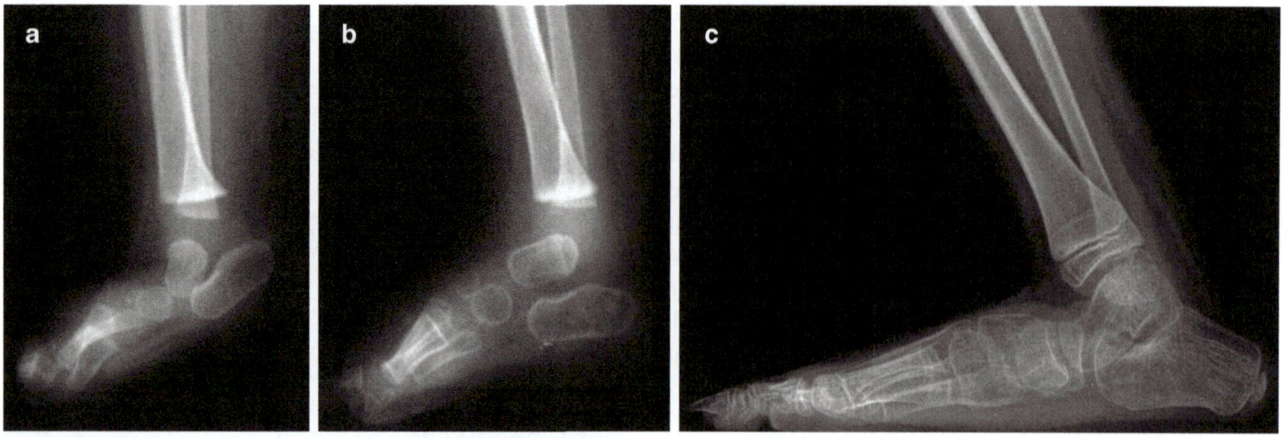

Fig. 3.9 Talus verticalis in syndromal underlying disease (**a**). Surgical peritalar release at 9 months (lengthening of Achilles tendon, peroneal tendons, and toe extensor tendons as well as rerouting of the anterior tibial tendon). 5 months postoperatively complete, even slightly excessive correction (**b**). 7 years postoperatively loss of correction, but clinically still sufficiently stable conditions at the medial foot ray in an image in maximum dorsal extension of the upper ankle joint (**c**)

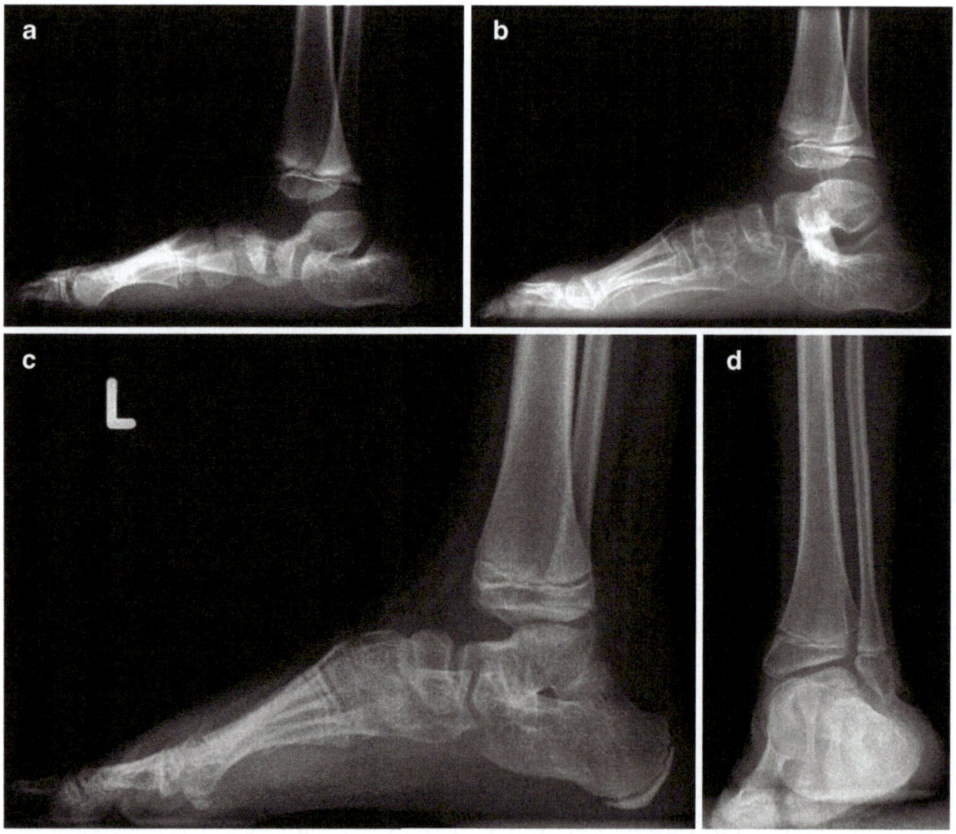

Fig. 3.10 Recurrence of a non-syndromal talus verticalis at the age of 6 years after surgery (**a**). Hindfoot correction and stabilization of the talocalcaneal joint with extra-articular Grice arthrodesis (Fig. 6.13) and anterior tibial tendon rerouting, 2 years postoperatively good talonavicular alignment (**b**). In the further course of time, a distinct supramalleolar valgus deformity developed (see Chap. 8) with largely stable conditions of the hindfoot and slight cavus deformity 6 years postoperatively (**c, d**)

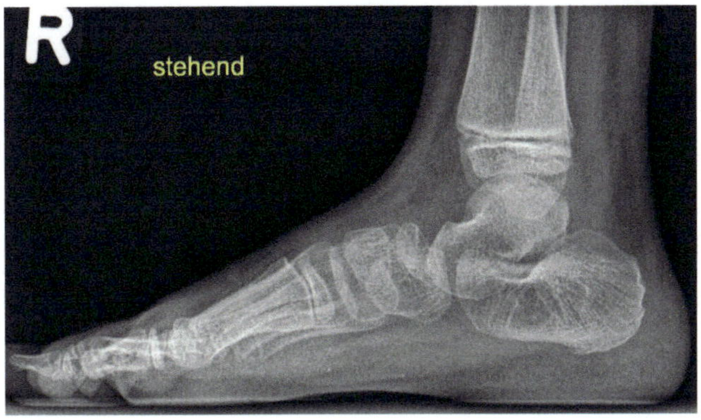

Fig. 3.11 Talus verticalis in a 7-year-old patient, treated as an infant with redression and medial soft tissue release, no Achilles tendon lengthening, clinically acceptable position. The shape of the talonavicular joint indicates pathological mobility in the sagittal plane. If the trochlea tali is properly formed, a soft tissue correction with rerouting of the anterior tibial tendon, possibly in combination with a Grice arthrodesis, could be considered at this age

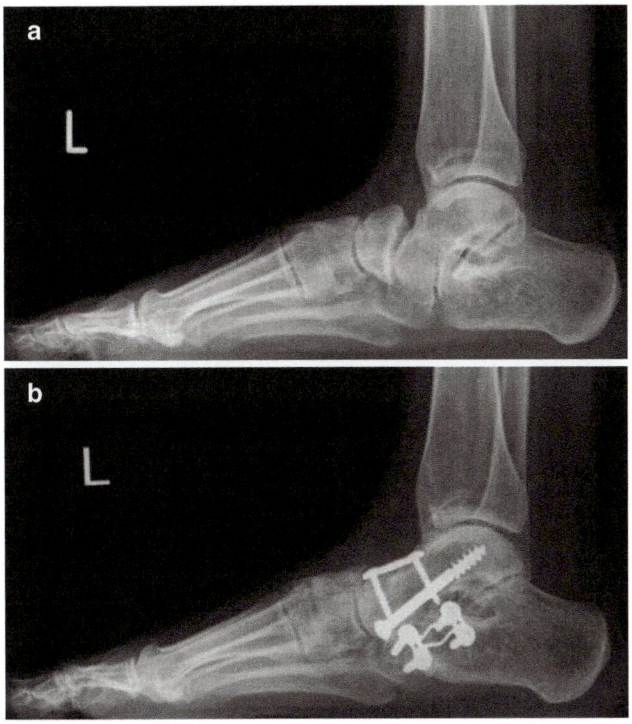

Fig. 3.12 Adult female patient with increasing talonavicular complaints (**a**). The formation of the trochlea tali should be considered in conjunction with Chopart arthrodesis. Due to incomplete repositioning of the talonavicular joint and Notchplasty at the talus, a sufficient dorsal extension of the upper ankle joint could be obtained (**b**)

References

Chalayon O, Adams A, Dobbs MB (2012) Minimally invasive approach for the treatment of non-isolated congenital vertical talus. J Bone Joint Surg 94-A:e73

Coleman SS (1983) Complex foot deformities in children. Lea & Febiger, Philadelphia

Dobbs MB, Purcell DB, Nunley R, Morcuende JA (2006) Early results of a new method of treatment for idiopathic congenital vertical talus. J Bone Joint Surg 88A:1192–1200

Dobbs MB, Purcell DB, Nunley R, Morcuende JA (2007) Early results of a new method of treatment for idiopathic congenital vertical talus. Surgical technique. J Bone Joint Surg 89-A:111–121

Drennan JC (1995) Congenital vertical talus. J Bone Joint Surg 77-A:1916–1923

Eberhardt O, Fernandez FF, Wirth T (2011) Die Behandlung des Talus verticalis mit der Methode nach Dobbs. Z Orthop Unfall 149:219–224

Eberhardt O, Fernandez FF, Wirth T (2012) The talar axis-first metatarsal base angle in CVT treatment: a comparison of idiopathic and non-idiopathic cases treated with the Dobbs method. J Child Orthop 6:491–496

Grice DS (1952) An extra-articular arthrodesis of the subastragalar joint for correction of paralytic flat feet in children. J Bone Joint Surg 34-A:927–940

Hamanishi C (1984) Congenital vertical talus: classification with 69 cases and new measurement system. J Pediatr Orthop 4:318–326

Hamel J, Becker W (1995) Sonographische Diagnostik bei Talus verticalis im Säuglings- und Kleinkindesalter. Ultraschall Klein Prax 9:185–189

Krauspe R, Raab P (2000) Die Operation des Talus verticalis congenitus. Oper Orthop Traumatol 12:154–170

Mosca VS (2014) Principles and management of pediatric foot and ankle deformities and malformations. Wolters Kluwer, Philadelphia

Napiontek M (1995) Congenital vertical talus: a retrospective and critical review of 32 feet operated on by peritalar reduction. J Pediatr Orthop B 4:179–187

Ramanoudjame M, Loriaut P, Seringe R, Glorion C, Wicart P (2014) The surgical treatment of children with congenital convex foot (vertical talus). Bone Joint J 96:837–844

Ricco AI, Richards BS, Herring JA (2014) Chapter 23: Disorders of the foot. In: Tachdjian's pediatric orthopaedics. Elsevier Saunders, Philadelphia

Schede F (1929) Die Operation des Plattfußes. Z Orthop Chir 50:528–538

Yang JS, Dobbs MB (2015) Treatment of congenital vertical talus: comparison of minimally invasive and extensive soft-tissue release procedures at minimum five-year follow-up. J Bone Joint Surg 97-A:1354–1365

The Flexible Planovalgus Foot

4

Contents

Flexible planovalgus deformity is the most common condition in pediatric foot and ankle clinic. Many questions related to this problem such as the range of the normal, expected further development, long-time prognosis, and necessity of treatment will arise in the discussion with the parents. Therefore, some propaedeutical remarks are necessary for further understanding. Obviously, circumstances related to our modern lifestyle, such as increasing physical inactivity and excess weight in childhood and adolescence are in favor of persisting planovalgus deformity. Those youngsters with active and sportive lifestyle will be found less frequently in a flatfoot clinic. However, cause and effect of this observation remain unclear.

J. Hamel, *Foot and Ankle Surgery in Children and Adolescents*, https://doi.org/10.1007/978-3-030-58108-4_4

Recommended Overview Literature on the Flexible Planovalgus Foot in Growth Age

- Döderlein L et al. (2002) Der Knickplattfuß – Extensive lexical work, child and adult age group (in German).
- Mosca VS (2010a) Flexible flatfoot and skewfoot. In: The child's foot and ankle
- Mosca VS (2010b) Flexible flatfoot in children and adolescents—Perspective of American pediatric orthopedics
- Mahan KT, Flanigan KP (2013) Flexible valgus deformity. In: Mc Glamry's comprehensive textbook of foot and ankle surgery—Aspects of American Podiatry

4.1 Stages of Development: Natural Course

The human foot undergoes certain developmental stages until complete maturity at the end of growth. In order to differentiate pathologic conditions from physiologic variants of the age-related norm, it is important to regard these developmental aspects. Children at the beginning of walking age and toddlers normally exhibit the morphologic characteristics of planovalgus feet with valgus heel and absence of a medial arch. During early childhood up to the age of 8–10 years, the foot shape changes spontaneously to a more or less straight or slightly valgus heel position and the development of a medial arch (Fig. 4.1). This process decelerates after the age of 8–10, so that spontaneous correction to any greater extent cannot be expected later on. Spontaneous correction is based mainly on the following morphologic features.

Developmental Factors of Spontaneous Correction of the Planovalgus Foot in Infants

- Reduction of plantar fat pad still present in newborn age and around the beginning of walking age at the medial plantar region.
- Reduction of supramalleolar valgus alignment of early childhood.
- Reduction of hypermobility due to ligamentous laxity and flexibility of the cartilaginous structures of the tarsal skeleton.
- Increasing muscular power of the long and short muscles acting on the foot and ankle.
- Presumably skeletal shaping processes in the tarsometatarsal region (e.g., at the calcaneus) play an additional role, which so far have not been examined in more detail.

Due to these maturation processes after verticalization, and as an effect of weight-bearing, surgical interventions in flexible flatfoot before the age of about 8 years are indicated only in rare, exceptional cases.

Prognostically Unfavorable Factors for Spontaneous Correction

- Shortened gastrocnemius muscle
- Painful os tibiale externum
- Marked genu valgum deformity
- Generalized joint hypermobility
- High body mass index

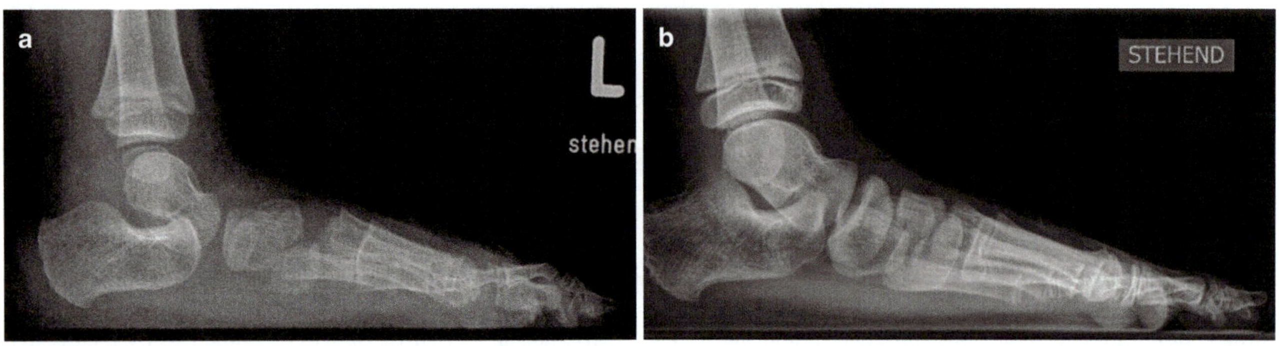

Fig. 4.1 3.5-Year-old patient with infantile planovalgus deformity (**a**) and natural course up to the age of 9.5 years (**b**). Here, a certain spontaneous correction—as can be seen, for example, at the talar inclination angle and at the talus-metatarsal-I angle—was observed without treatment. However, this correction remained incomplete

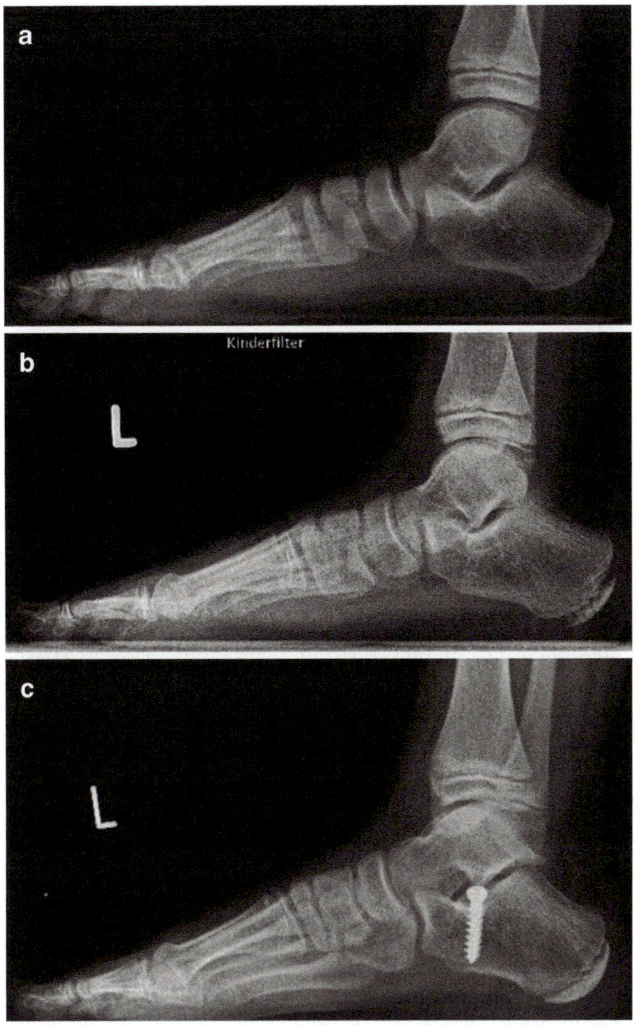

Fig. 4.2 In this boy, no spontaneous positional correction was observed between the age of 7 (**a**) and 10 years (**b**). After arthroereisis at the age of 10 years, significant improvement of tarsometatarsal alignment at the age of 12 years (**c**)

It is not completely clear at which exact age or developmental status further spontaneous correction to any additional significant extent is unlikely. The age of 8–10 is supposed to be the relevant age limit. Park et al. (2013) determined an average spontaneous correction rate of the talometatarsal I angle in the lateral projection by 0.7° per year until the end of growth in a comprehensive study of flat-footed children. Reduction in the TMT-I angle in ap projection were 6.3° in the 5-year period between 3 and 8 years of age and only 1.8° between 10 and 15 years of age. Choi et al. (2020) found about 4°–5° improvement of TMT-I angle in the lateral projection between 10 years of age and maturity with and without treatment with insoles. Own observations of the author in children with radiologic follow-up, who later were treated surgically, showed no significant progress of spontaneous correction in most cases beyond the age of 8–10 (Figs. 4.2 and 4.3). On the other hand, further deterioration could be observed in several cases.

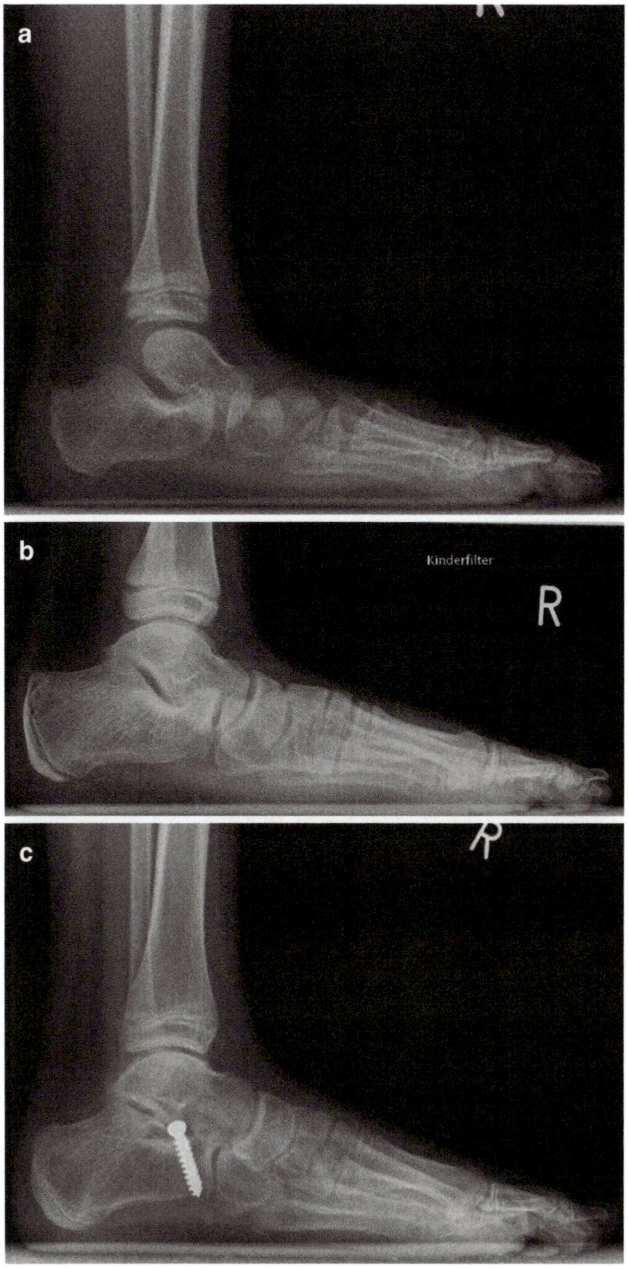

Fig. 4.3 This boy only showed a small extent of spontaneous straightening between the age of 6 years (**a**) and 12 years (**b**). 3 years after calcaneostop arthroereisis, significant positional correction (**c**)

4.2 Long-Term Prognosis

Whether or not planovalgus deformity of childhood will necessarily cause symptoms later on in life is not completely predictable. There is no scientific evidence that static pain will occur frequently in this patient group after adolescent age. However, our own experience shows—in agreement with Hansen (2010), who has also worked on children's and adults' feet for decades—that it is not uncommon for patients with severe planovalgus deformities to be presented for surgical correction as young adults or in later life (Fig. 4.4). Also, the

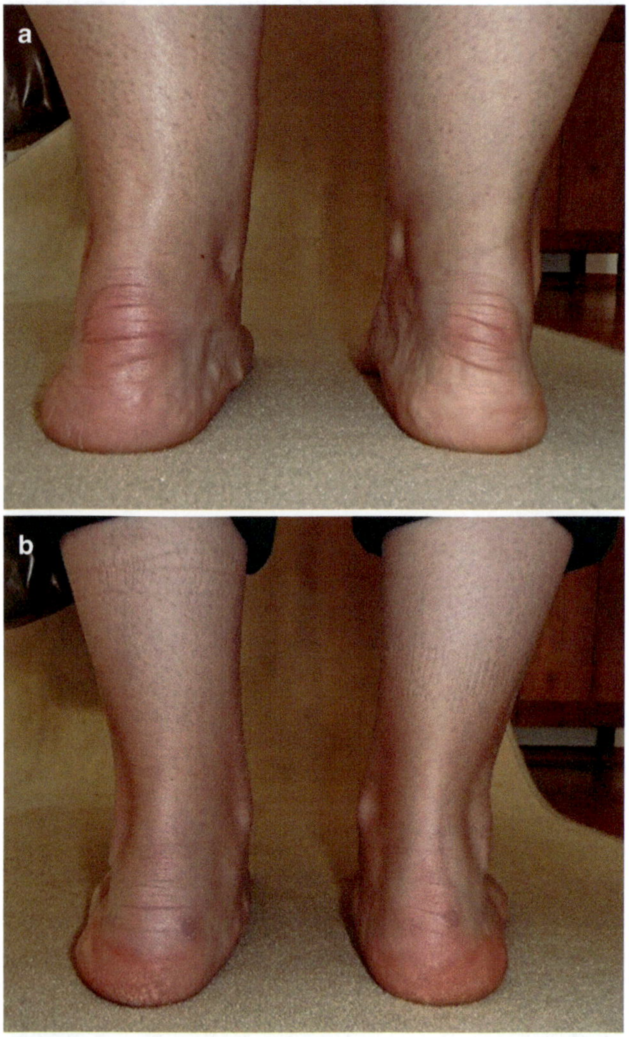

Fig. 4.4 Mother (a) and daughter (b) at the age of 56 and 18 years, respectively, both presenting with chronic strain complaints on the left side in clinically significant hindfoot valgus deformity

connection between planovalgus deformity persisting from childhood and the occurrence of soft tissue degeneration at the medial tarsal region, known as adult acquired flatfoot deformity (AAFD) of older patients with degeneration of capsular tissue around the talonavicular joint and rupture of posterior tibial tendon, remains unclear. However, the degenerated soft tissue structures nowadays are looked at more as "victims" rather than as "committers" of the progressive deformity. Therefore, the assumption seems justified that at least a loose connection does exist between severe planovalgus deformity in childhood and later problems caused by this static insufficiency.

4.3 Surgically Relevant Pathomorphology of the Planovalgus Deformity

Clinically, the planovalgus deformity represents a three-dimensional deformity observed in a weight-bearing position, consisting of a hindfoot valgus component, mid-forefoot abduction, and flattening of the medial longitudinal arch.

The flexible planovalgus deformity can be pathomorphologically understood as a combination of an excessive eversion of the talocalcaneal-navicular joint complex and a destabilization of the medial foot ray under load. Both phenomena are mutually dependent and cannot occur in isolation from each other. These two "regions of interest" are also the targets of therapeutic approaches for stabilization. Gait analysis has shown significant functional abnormalities in children with a flexible planovalgus condition (Hösl et al. 2014).

In many cases of pronounced planovalgus deformities, there is an isolated gastrocnemius shortening. It remains unclear whether this is the cause or consequence of the planovalgus malalignment. It is not uncommon to find a painful os tibiale externum associated with the planovalgus deformity (Fig. 4.18), which is in a sense the juvenile form of posterior tibial tendon dysfunction. The tendon itself is not altered in childhood and adolescence. Surgical removal of the os tibiale externum with refixation of the tendon is indicated in case of therapy-resistant complaints (Mosca 2014).

4.3.1 Excessive Hindfoot Eversion

In the case of excessive eversion of the hindfoot complex, the osteoligamental chain of calcaneus, cuboid, and navicular takes up a position under load in relation to the talus, which can be described as abduction (transverse plane), valgus deformity (frontal plane), and extension (sagittal plane) (Fig. 4.5b) (Inman 1976). In the view from the weight-bearing foot (closed kinetic chain), the position of the talus shows an inward rotation and plantar flexion versus the fixed calcaneus. This positional relationship can be observed most pronounced at the talonavicular joint, which has the greatest range of motion of the tarsal joints.

The motion axis of the subtalar joint complex runs from lateral-plantar to medial-dorsal through the center of the talocalcaneal joint (Fig. 4.6). It is important to note that the course of this joint axis can vary greatly from person to person, especially in the sagittal plane (Isman and Inman 1968): If the course of the joint axis is flat, the deformity in the frontal plane (hindfoot valgus) with a pronounced flattening of the medial longitudinal arch and hindfoot valgus deformity is more impressive; if the joint axis is steeper, the deformity in the transverse plane (mid-forefoot abduction) with a less pronounced flattening of the longitudinal arch is dominant. This condition is referred to as "planar dominance" (Mahan 1992) and explains the quite different clinical manifestations of planovalgus deformity, where in some cases the mid-forefoot abduction is more dominant, in others the hindfoot valgus deformity. The variations in planar dominance are also the reason why only radiological imaging in two planes is suitable for meaningful evaluation of the extent of the deformity (Sect. 4.5). This phenomenon of planar dominance is also expressed in the

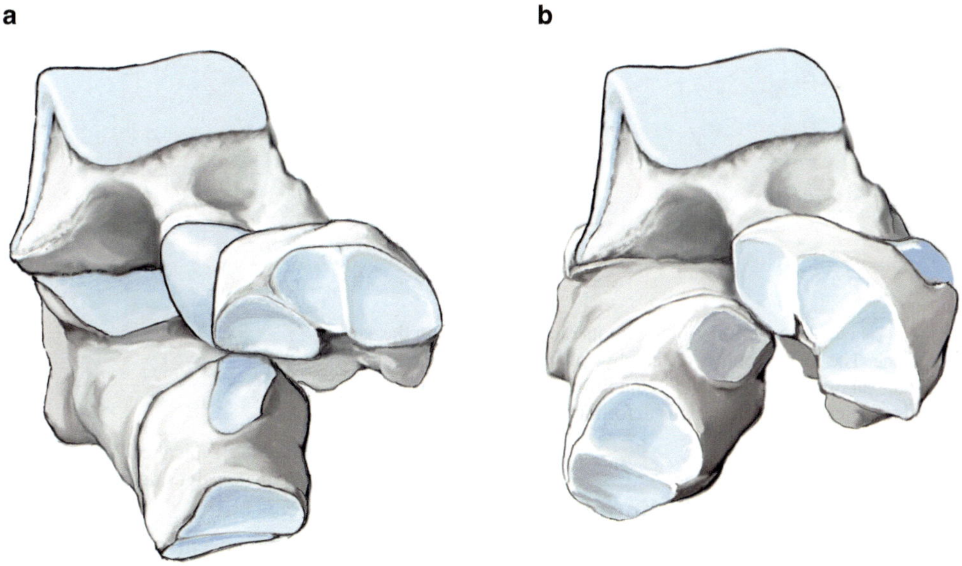

Fig. 4.5 The hindfoot complex in inverted (**a**) and everted (**b**) position (see text). The functional unit of the osteoligamental chain consisting of calcaneus, cuboid, and navicular bone generally executes a movement in relation to the talus in the depicted sense. Thereby, in the inverted position, a stable locking of the hindfoot complex occurs; in everted position, the joint axes of the talonavicular and calcaneocuboid joint assume a more parallel position to each other. This puts the system in a mobile state

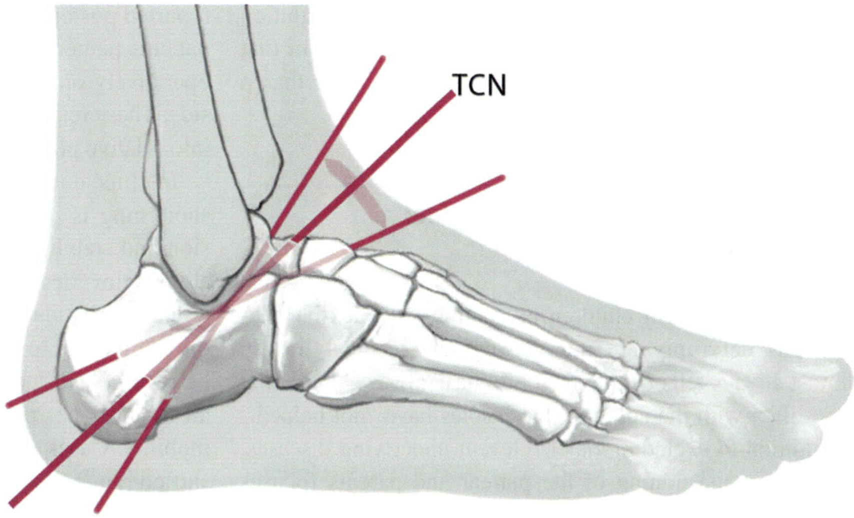

Fig. 4.6 Individually differing joint-axis course of the talocalcaneal-navicular complex (TCN) in the sagittal plane

radiological analysis by Bourdet et al. (2013), who distinguish the "subtalar pes planus type" from the "midtarsal pes planus type."

Pathological changes in the area of the posterior tibial tendon or the medially stabilizing soft tissues as in the adult planovalgus deformity are not present in children and adolescents, apart from a certain laxity of the spring ligament and the medial talonavicular capsule. However, a painful os tibiale externum is often seen in conjunction with a planovalgus deformity and can be considered an infantile form of posterior tibial dysfunction. The active stabilizer of the hindfoot complex is the posterior tibial muscle, whose—e.g., traumatic—loss of function in childhood leads to a severe planovalgus deformity.

4.3.2 Destabilization of the Medial Ray

The second pathomorphologically significant phenomenon, the destabilization of the medial column—which is relatively stable in the normal foot (Roling et al. 2002)—affects the talonavicular and especially the naviculo-cuneiform joint line ("naviculo-cuneiform sag") in childhood and adolescence to varying degrees, less so the tarsometatarsal joints. Figure 4.7 shows the movement behavior of the cylindrically shaped naviculo-cuneiform joint, which tends towards hypermobility in planovalgus deformity (Hamel 2016) with excessive mobility in the sagittal plane. The most important active stabilizer of the medial column is the long peroneal muscle with its powerful plantar-flexing effect on the medial foot ray.

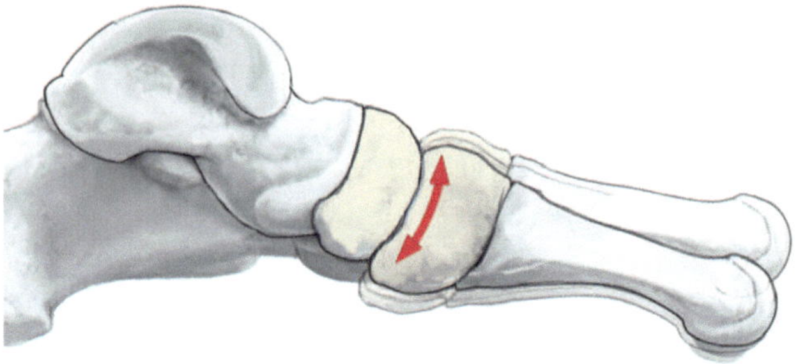

Fig. 4.7 Naviculo-cuneiform joint with its range of motion in the sagittal plane. The main mobility of the physiologically stable medial tarsometatarsal ray is in the naviculo-cuneiform joint line and can reach a considerable extent in planovalgus deformity

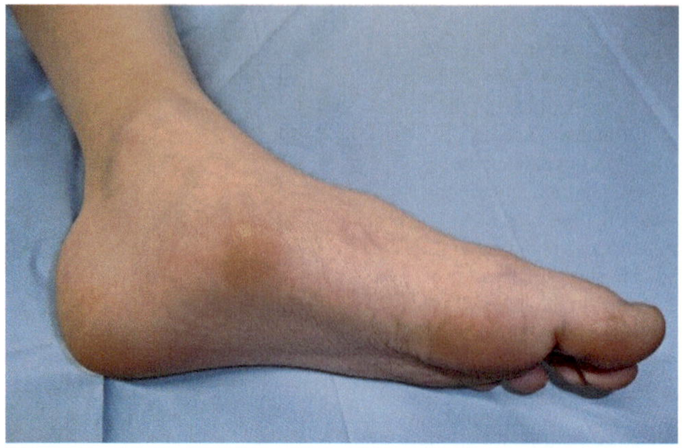

Fig. 4.8 Typical callosity above the talonavicular region in hypermobile planovalgus deformity

4.3.3 The Isolated Hindfoot Valgus Deformity

Isolated valgus deformities of the hindfoot are a special case, in which the clinical and radiological signs of excessive eversion and destabilization of the medial column are at least significantly less impressive, but a pronounced—isolated—valgus component of the hindfoot exists. The recognition of such a constellation is therapeutically important in that a motion-limiting arthroereisis is less indicated here than a corrective osteotomy of the calcaneus (Sect. 4.11.1).

4.4 Medical History and Clinical Examination

When the parents of children presenting with flexible planovalgus deformity are interviewed, the medical history almost always tells us that the child has "always" had a flat foot, often with the addition that insoles have "not helped." In addition to excluding other relevant underlying diseases, the further questioning of the patient and parents focuses on performance. Here, very specific questions have to be asked about longer walking distances, standing for long periods, "foot fatigue," and early fatigue in general. Often, the patients concerned are children who are less keen to move and hardly active in sports, although it is sometimes difficult to distinguish between cause and effect.

Pain actively expressed by the child is rather rare and then usually diffuse in the region of the longitudinal arch. Other causes of pain, such as a symptomatic os tibiale externum or a coalition, should be excluded by palpation, pain localization, or motion testing and may require other surgical measures. According to Mosca (2010a) painfulness and calf muscle shortening are closely related. In pronounced cases, pressure points with increased callus formation in the area of the medial longitudinal arch are observed, often reinforced by supporting insoles (Fig. 4.8).

A retrospective survey after arthroereisis of the patients and their parents in our own medical inventory showed that only in 35% of the cases "considerable complaints" had been present preoperatively, i.e., from the point of view of the parents or the patient, the extent of the deformity was more important. A reduction in performance capacity was also less frequently mentioned preoperatively, but in 62% of cases, a significant increase in performance capacity was reported postoperatively. Frequently, the juvenile-adolescent patients perceive the increase in performance capacity postoperatively only in comparison with the untreated opposite side. These results place the significance of preoperative data into relative perspective.

In clinical examination, the assessment of gastrocnemius shortening is particularly important. With full knee extension and stabilization of the hindfoot complex in neutral or slightly inverted position, a dorsal extension of the foot of at least 10° should be possible. When testing for flexibility of the hindfoot to exclude a coalition, a limitation can easily be overlooked due to hypermobility of adjacent joints. Not all infantile pes planovalgus deformities show tarsal hypermobility. Cases are also observed which show a normal but shifted range of motion towards the direction of eversion.

The straightening (shifting into varus position) of the heel when actively moving into forefoot stance and the formation of a longitudinal arch during passive dorsal extension of the big toe when standing are more indicative of the flexibility of the hindfoot than of the severity of the planovalgus deformity. Even in severe infantile planovalgus deformity, an active varization of the hindfoot is usually preserved.

4.5 X-Ray Diagnostics

As with other orthopedic relevant malpositions of the locomotor system, standardized X-ray diagnostics under relaxed loading of the foot in a bilateral stance and thus with the elimination of muscular forces is the appropriate method to quantify the deformity of the osteoligamentary system "foot" in severe cases. The importance of full weight-bearing for the positional relationships shown should be emphasized (Fig. 4.9). X-ray diagnostics always comprises

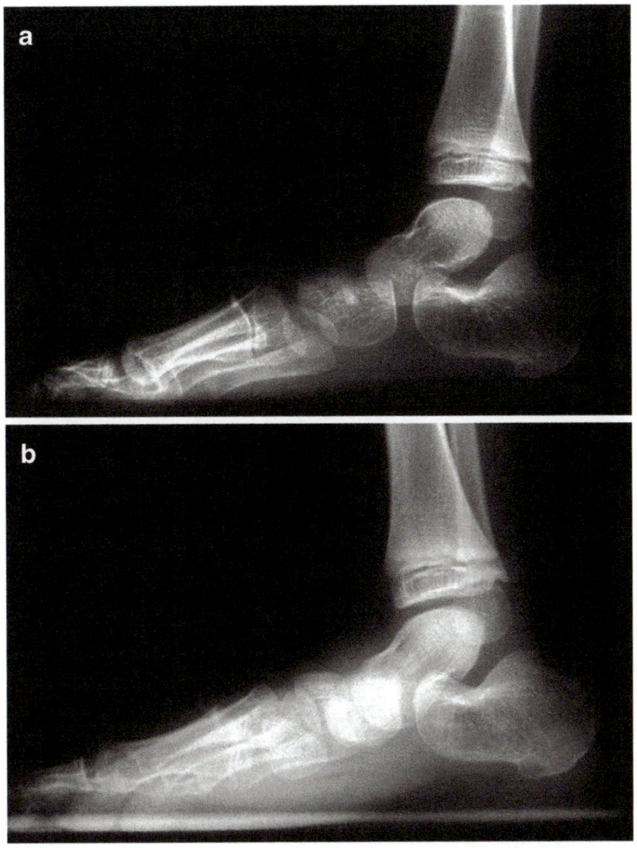

Fig. 4.9 Lateral X-ray image in a "weight-bearing position" in a 7-year-old boy. Both images were taken on the same day. In the first one (**a**), the child obviously only partially loaded carefully, whereas in the repetition (**b**) full loading in the bilateral position was observed. The different projected talar positions in particular are clearly visible

a lateral image and a dorsoplantar image with the tube tilted by approx. 20°. At least if a supramalleolar valgus component is suspected (see Chap. 8), an ankle ap image has to be added. In the literature there are numerous suggestions for quantification of radiological imaging of the infantile foot and planovalgus deformity. Some important studies should be mentioned in their essential statements:

- Vanderwilde et al. (1988) and Davids et al. (2005) recorded normal ranges for individual X-ray angles. A considerable change depending on age and a particularly large spreading range in infancy was found.
- The talocalcaneal angles in both projection planes show broad variations and seem to be of minor practicability in comparison to talometatarsal angles. The addition of both talocalcaneal angles (TC index), e.g., can discriminate much better between clubfeet and normal feet (Beatson and Pearson 1966) than the single values do.
- The TMT-I angle in the lateral projection ("TMT-I angle lat.") proved to be a well-defined parameter with a rather smaller range of variation for many authors. The same is true for the Costa-Bartani angle (Vontey 1978).
- Several authors have made suggestions for the recording of the talonavicular positional relationship in the ap X-ray image ("hyperpronation" according to Gould (1983), "talar head uncovering" according to Alman et al. (1993), "talonavicular angle" according to Giannestras (1976)).

In the following, the author's approach will be presented, which partly takes up the abovementioned results from the literature: Because of the three-dimensionality and "planar dominance" (Sect. 4.3.1), at least two planes of projection are always required for quantitative assessment and—as in clubfoot (Beatson and Pearson 1966)—no single angle measure is suitable for reliably defining the severity of the malposition. The tarsometatarsal index (TMT index) according to Hamel and Kinast (2006) has proven in practice to be an easily determined measure for quantifying planovalgus deformity. It is formed from the sum of the known TMT-1 angle in the lateral projection ("TMT-I angle lat.") and the "TMT-I base angle" in the dorsoplantar image with vertical alignment of the central beam to the mid-forefoot (Fig. 4.10). This biplanar angle index thus includes both the excessive eversion of the talocalcaneal-navicular complex and the destabilization of the medial column as pathomorphological factors of planovalgus deformity (Sect. 4.3). However, validation of this index for different age groups is still pending. For the TMT-1 angle lat. in the lateral projection, Davids et al. (2005) give normal values of –13° (s = 7.5°) for 10-year-old children. The TMT-I base angle in the transversal plane was preferred to the talus-metatarsal-I angle in the dorsoplantar image (see Fig. 1.18) which is more common in the literature, to form the TMT index. The reason is because it cannot be influenced by an additional adduction (serpentine foot or severe hallux valgus) or abduction in the Lisfranc line that may exist in addition to the hindfoot eversion.

Recently an S2 Guideline for pediatric flatfoot, published by a group of German experts (Hell et al. 2018), recommended nine angles for the quantification of planovalgus deformity. In a statistical analysis of the author's group (Hamel et al. 2020), severe planovalgus feet of children and adolescents from age 10–14 were compared to age-matched normal feet, and a statistical analysis of these nine parameters was undertaken. The parameter that discriminated best between the two groups was the TMT index (Hamel and Kinast 2006), which takes into account both projections.

Additionally, the following radiological parameters are important in the assessment of planovalgus deformity:

- The flattening of the calcaneal pitch angle shows a certain correlation with the shortening of the calf muscles (Fig. 4.20).

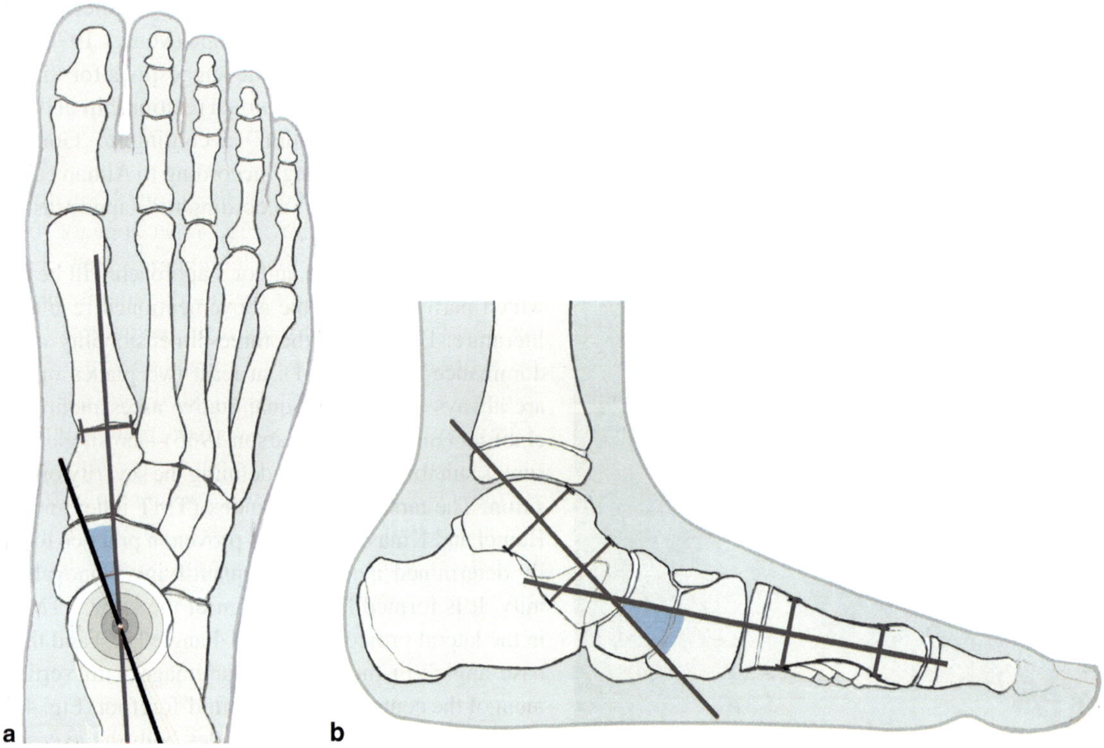

Fig. 4.10 The TMT index according to Hamel and Kinast (2006), which has been proven to be reliable for the quantification of planovalgus deformity, as the sum of the TMT-I base angle (**a**) and the TMT-I lat. angle (**b**). The TMT-I base angle is formed by the longitudinal axis of the talus, which is oriented parallel to the medial contour of the talus and a second line connecting the geometric center of the talar head with the center of the first tarsometatarsal joint

- The increased talus inclination angle is an important measure of the excessive eversion of the talocalcaneal-navicular complex and at the same time of the equinus adjustment of the ankle joint.
- The MASA angle ("medial arch sag angle") between the proximal joint surface of the navicular and metatarsal I in the lateral image (see Figs. 4.27b and 4.49a, b), according to Aiyer et al. (2016), records the conditions at the naviculo-cuneiform joint but is only meaningful for assessing stability if the medial ray is loaded. Therefore, it does not significantly exceed the indication of the talometatarsal I angle in the lateral projection.
- The height of the medial longitudinal arch can be estimated on the basis of the distance of the os naviculare to the loading surface. Since it is a measure of length, this parameter is size-dependent.

Radiological Parameters for the Quantification of Planovalgus Deformity in School Children
(specified "normal ranges" according to own experience)

TMT index (according to Hamel and Kinast)	Normally about −10 to −30°
– TMT-I angle (lat.)	Normally −10° to −20°
– TMT-I-base angle (ap)	Normally about −10°
Calcaneal pitch angle	Normally 10–20°
Talar inclination angle	Normally up to about 30°
MASA angle ("medial arch sag angle")	Normally near 0°
Height of the longitudinal arching at the navicular	(Size dependent)

4.6 Pedography

Static measures of flexible flatfoot by radiography should be supplemented by assessment of foot function (Böhm et al. 2019). Pedography (cf. Sect. 1.4.3) can be used to impressively document severe planovalgus conditions—even during the course of the disease by repeated examination (Fig. 4.11). Overloading of the medial tarsometatarsal ray, lack of indentation of the loaded sole surface, and increased (compensatory) use of the toes in the late stance phase are some of the typical characteristics of flexible planovalgus deformity. The pre- and post-operative course provides information about the achieved functional improvement (e.g., Figs. 4.19, 4.30, 4.34, 4.45, and 4.46). For the indication to perform a surgical correction however, pedography has not proven very successful, especially in borderline cases, as the recorded load phases can often differ considerably from each other depending on the—spontaneously changing—use of the stabilizing muscles, e.g., the long toe flexors and the long peroneal muscle.

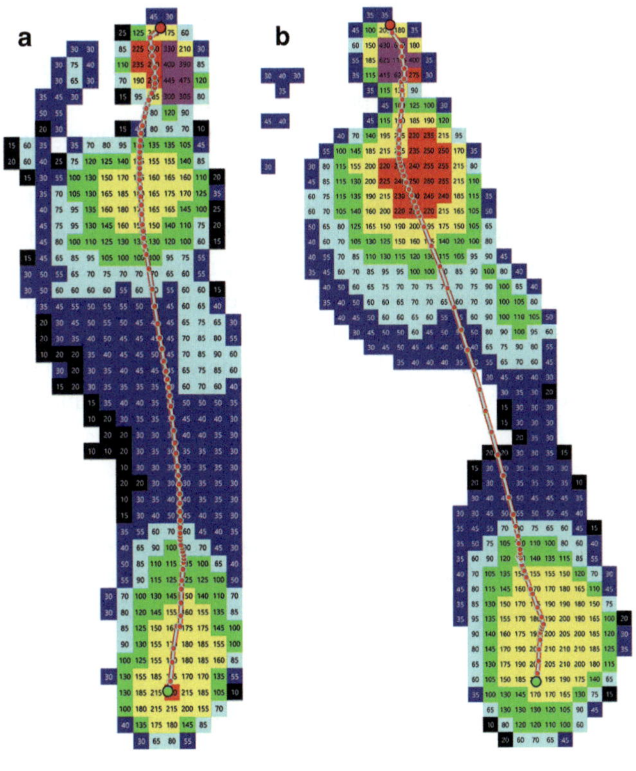

Fig. 4.11 Pedographic follow-up of an untreated patient with a pronounced planovalgus deformity at the age of 11 (**a**) and 15 years (**b**). The distinct functional deterioration is clearly visible, especially in comparison to the surgically treated opposite side (Fig. 4.19)

Pedographic Characteristics of Planovalgus Deformity

- Missing medial indentation in the footprint
- Shifting of the metatarsal pressure and force distribution towards medial
- Reduced maximum force of the forefoot
- Compensatory increased use of the toe imprint
- Missing medial-convex curvature of the gait line after initial contact

4.7 Indication for Surgical Treatment

The recommendations of the literature and corresponding guidelines for the surgical treatment of pes planovalgus in childhood and adolescence have changed considerably in the past decades: In the middle of the twentieth century, soft tissue interventions were predominant (Niederecker 1959), and, for instance, Imhäuser warned strongly against bony interventions. This had an effect right up to the German 2001 AWMF guidelines, in which the now widely used bony correction procedures did not yet play any role at all. Due to mass screenings of young adults, which did not show any performance limitations of patients with planovalgus feet on one side, and due to poor late results on patients corrected by tarsal partial arthrodeses (Ricco et al. 2014) on the other side, surgical treatment in pediatric orthopedics was generally discredited. In contrast, Mosca (1995) propagated the calcaneus lengthening osteotomy for particularly pronounced and symptomatic cases, Wagner (1986) the calcaneus sliding osteotomy in Germany. Furthermore, the American podiatrists and later de Pellegrin (2007) developed various arthroereisis techniques, some of which were very generously indicated. A recently published S2 guideline propagates arthroereisis and osteotomies in severe cases (Hell et al. 2018). In the following, an attempt will be made to redefine the indication limits.

After verticalization of the child, the flexible planovalgus foot position without contracture of the tarsal joints should initially only be observed and only in particularly severe cases supported with orthotics, possibly from the age of about 3–4 years. A supramalleolar valgus component still present at this age, the general ligament laxity of this stage of life, age-related low strength of the stabilizing musculature, and a pronounced fat pad in the area of the longitudinal arch often result in impressive deformities in the standing position at the beginning of walking (see Sect. 4.1). In principle, all these phenomena have a tendency to spontaneous correction. For this reason, the soft tissue interventions that were often recommended in the past (e.g., Schede (1929), Niederecker (1959)) are now almost obsolete at this age group.

There are—rarely—cases of talus obliquus that need to be treated differently (Sect. 4.8). Pathomorphologically, they assume an intermediate position between the flexible planovalgus deformity and the vertical talus (Chap. 3): shortening of the calf muscles, incomplete repositionability of the talonavicular joint, thus a minor form of slight contracture.

Surgical growth-modifying measures (arthroereises) are usually considered, if sufficient straightening has not taken place by about the age of 9–11 years. There is still insufficient knowledge about the extent to which further spontaneous correction phenomena can be expected after the age of 10 years. However, these are of minor degree (Park et al. 2013; Choi et al. 2020), and the question arises in each individual case as to whether the last years of foot development should be used for guided growth in order to improve foot statics and further maturation—also of the ankle joint—with a limited surgical intervention. If there is not enough time left until the end of growth (of the foot) to achieve sufficient effect through guided growth, bony corrections are generally considered. The indications for both procedures differ significantly in that the arthroereises are age-related and minimally invasive procedures, while the osteotomy procedures are not tied to a specific age group and are more complex in surgical terms. Recently, a tendency could be observed to combine both procedures in order to extend the traditional age limits of arthroereisis into adolescent age (Sect. 4.11.3).

The discussion on the benefits of surgical planovalgus corrections in the growth age is characterized by very different points of view, the extreme positions of which will be briefly outlined here.

Position 1

As a matter of principle, surgery is only performed in the case of "complaints" or contractures (although the gastrocnemius shortening, which is almost always encountered, is evaluated differently), since there is not enough evidence that the affected children and adolescents will later develop secondary damage and pain (e.g., in the sense of posterior tibial tendon dysfunction). Experts such as Vince Mosca, for example, generally continue to reject arthroereises, especially if there are no symptoms (Mosca 2010a).

Position 2

It is worthwhile to treat even minor malpositions—or even only at the request of the parents (the parents are usually satisfied with the results of the arthroereisis)—as otherwise one has to assume later complaints. In the discussion about the case of the adult planovalgus deformity (AAFD), it has been increasingly emphasized in recent years that the insufficiency of the talonavicular capsular structures and the posterior tibial tendon is more the result than the cause of this widespread clinical entity. This would attribute more significance to the remaining abnormal statics during growth than previously assumed.

The author takes a middle position between the two statements presented here and takes a more differentiated view of the indication, which will be explained in more detail: **anamnesis, extent of deformity, and clinical aspects** should be considered in combination in the decision for surgery (Fig. 4.12). The possible complications should also be addressed in the clarification process (Sects. 4.10.2.3 and 4.10.3.3). It has proved to be useful to clarify when informing patients and parents that surgery is not "necessary" as such. Instead, the question should be asked when deciding on the indication, which treatment is likely to produce the best prognostic result.

The indication for surgical stabilization of the growing foot is based on the extent of the malposition in combination with clinical findings such as gastrocnemius shortening, callus formation, and shoe wear. A shortening of the gastrocnemius and a pronounced tarsal hypermobility rather suggest a stabilizing (and thus motion-limiting) intervention. Anamnestic expressed complaints and limitations in performance (de Pellegrin et al. 2014), which can often only be assessed more precisely in retrospect, are important additional parameters.

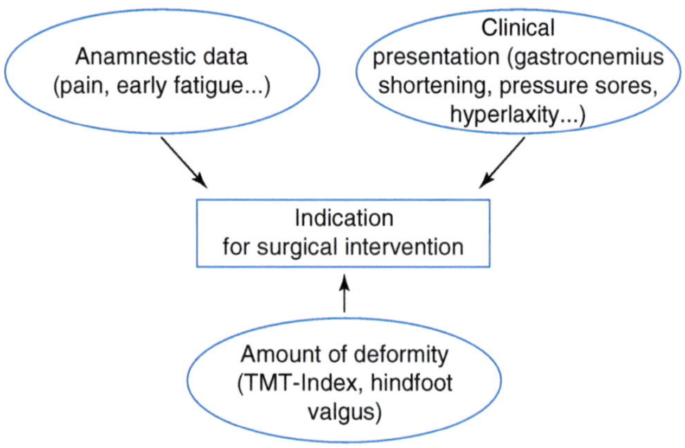

Fig. 4.12 Decision criteria for surgical intervention in pediatric flexible planovalgus deformity

The extent of the deformity is determined radiologically (TMT index) as in all other areas of orthopedics and the extent of the hindfoot valgus component by clinical evaluation. If there is a high degree of deformity, treatment may be carried out even in the absence of “complaints”; if the degree of deformity is lower, treatment is carried out only if the anamnestic clinical parameters (see above) suggest this. De Pellegrin et al. (2014) report in only 16% of the children treated with an arthroereisis of preoperatively expressed performance limitations (“fatigue”), and only in 11% of them pain was a problem. This means that it was mainly the extent of the malposition that was decisive for the indication. Our own retrospective survey also showed that the performance limitations were often less clearly stated preoperatively and are only named retrospectively (Sect. 4.10.2.2).

The conservative physiotherapeutic and orthopedic treatment methods offered are not the subject of this book. With regard to passive or active correction by means of supporting or sensorimotor insoles, there is still no proof of effectiveness despite decades of use. Recently Choi et al. (2020) observed nearly the same limited radiological improvement in flatfoot patients from 10 to 11 year of age until the end of growth with and without supporting insoles. From a physiotherapeutic point of view, spiral dynamics could probably offer the best approach, provided that the corresponding strengthening exercises with activation of the posterior tibial muscle and the long peroneal muscle, the most important active stabilizers of the foot, are performed to a sufficient degree. Due to the lack of personal experience, we refer to the special literature.

4.8 Soft Tissue Correction in Infancy

Older textbooks contain various suggestions for soft tissue correction procedures with capsuloplasty and tendon transfers in the area of the insertions of the tibial musculature (see Schede (1929), Niederecker (1959)). These procedures—carried out as an isolated intervention—are today regarded as largely obsolete apart from the resection of the painful os tibiale externum, as they were associated with frequent recurrences, but also secondary problems. Arthroereisis techniques performed at a somewhat later age appear clearly superior. Rare exceptions for purely soft tissue early corrections already in infancy and early school age are limited to:

- Talus obliquus (extreme and mostly partial slightly contracted inclined position of the talus, abortive cases of the vertical talus (Chap. 3) without extensive contracture of the talonavicular joint)
- Planovalgus deformities with particularly pronounced calf muscle shortening (Fig. 4.13)

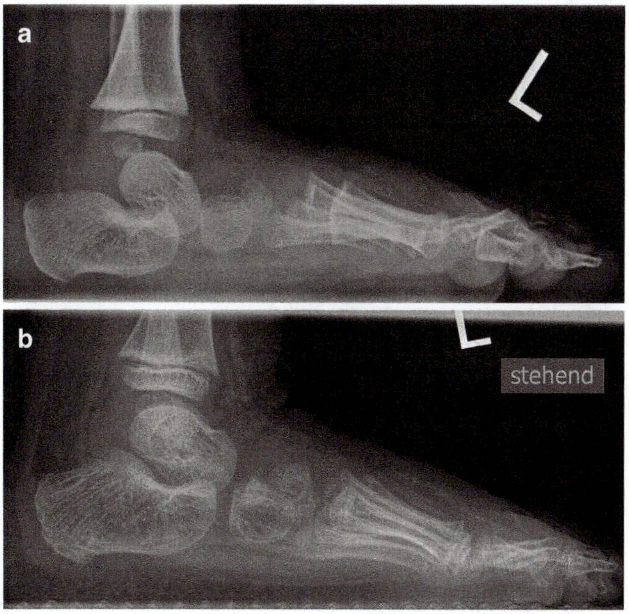

Fig. 4.13 3-Year-old child with significant calf muscle shortening (**a**). Assuming that the calf muscle shortening negatively affects spontaneous straightening of the foot, an open Achilles tendon lengthening was combined with capsuloplastic surgery of the talonavicular joint and temporary K-wire stabilization. 26 months postoperatively significantly improved hindfoot position (**b**)

Technique

A longitudinal incision medially at the talonavicular region exposes the tendon insertions of the anterior and posterior tibial muscles and the overstretched talonavicular capsule. The posterior tibial tendon is severed in a Z-shape and, after slightly shortening both tendon halves, is sutured in a stable manner with shortening. Alternatively, a distalization of the posterior tibial attachment to the medial cuneiform bone (“advancement”) has been described. From the talonavicular capsule, either an oval section is resected and stably sutured or the capsule is sutured in an overlapping fashion after incision, resulting in the repositioning of the talonavicular joint. Temporary stabilization can be achieved with a talonavicular-transfixing K-wire. In addition, the distal half of the split anterior tibial tendon can be relocated proximally to the talonavicular capsule and the posterior tibial tendon insertion. This corresponds approximately to the soft tissue intervention historically described by Schede in 1929 (Hamel et al. 1994) (Fig. 4.14).

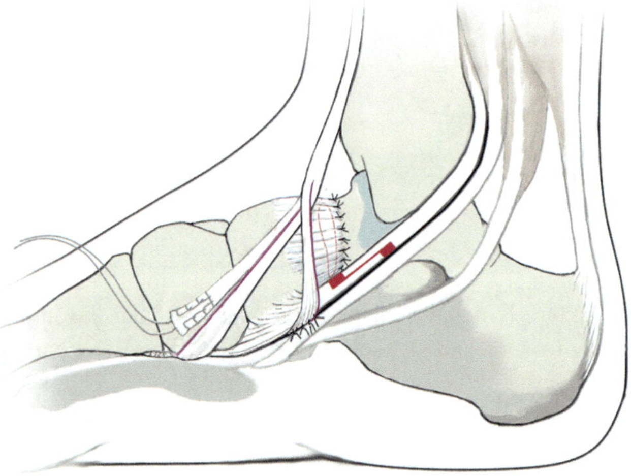

Fig. 4.14 The purely soft tissue stabilization of the planovalgus deformity includes a capsule retightening of the talonavicular joint capsule, a shortening of the posterior tibial tendon and a relocation of the distal half of the split anterior tibial tendon attachment to the medioplantar navicular pole

2014; Coleman 1983), has not proven to be effective. If a painful os tibiale externum exists in connection with or possibly also as a contributory cause of a planovalgus deformity, a resection and posterior tibial reinsertion at the medioplantar navicular pole should be performed as part of the surgical correction of the planovalgus deformity.

Soft tissue corrections can also be considered, such as the relocation of the anterior tibial tendon insertion and the distalization of the posterior tibial tendon insertion ("advancement"), but always only as an addition to the stabilization of the hindfoot (see Hamel et al. 1994). The argument repeatedly derived from the work of Basmajian and Stecko (1963), that muscular forces have no influence on the integrity of the foot architecture, is only valid in a standing position without regarding dynamic effects. For example, the rerouting of the anterior tibial tendon insertion has its biomechanical justification, among other aspects, in the fact that the impact of the antagonistic M. peroneus longus, which stabilizes the medial column, is increased. This effect contributes to its higher efficiency due to the hindfoot straightening.

4.9 Principles of Stabilization in School Children's Age

Surgical correction of juvenile planovalgus deformities can basically be carried out at the hindfoot complex and/or the medial tarsometatarsal ray, depending on the pathomorphology (Sect. 4.3). In most cases, a bony intervention at the hindfoot in the form of an arthroereisis, osteotomy, or arthrodesis should be considered first. However, the situation at the medial tarsal ray must always be taken into consideration: In younger children, a certain spontaneous stabilization potential under the dynamic influence of the peroneus-longus effect can be assumed during further development, for example, after an arthroereisis. In later childhood and adolescence, an additional stabilizing measure by osteotomy or arthrodesis in the area of the naviculo-cuneiform joint should always be considered. From the experience with the adult foot, it can be concluded that successful stabilization of the medial ray has an independent, straightening effect on the hindfoot (Benthien et al. 2007). Thus, it can be concluded that the stabilization of the talocalcaneal-navicular complex and the medial column can be regarded as complementary, mutually supportive measures. In contrast, stabilization exclusively via the medial ray, as described in the form of a naviculo-cuneiform arthrodesis in childhood (Ricco et al.

4.10 Guided Growth Through Arthroereisis

Arthroereises are motion-limiting interventions to reduce the excessive eversion of the talocalcaneal-navicular complex. They are intended to bring about stabilization by growth modification, a stabilization that remains permanent even after removal of the implants after growth has been completed. Arthroereisis procedures are minimally invasive procedures that allow immediate loading of the foot and therefore do not lead to long-term postoperative impairment of the child. As a rule, a remaining growth period of approx. 2–3 years is required as a prerequisite for performing an arthroereisis. However, favorable results are also observed in later procedures, and, in combination with other procedures, arthroereises are now successfully used even after growth has been completed. Two competing techniques are common in childhood and will be described in more detail. Presumably, the mode of action of arthroereisis contains both a purely mechanical component and sensomotoric effects. A high concentration of sensory organs in the area of the sinus tarsi with proprioceptive-active receptors has been proven (Rein et al. 2013). Under the influence of the arthroereisis, the development of subtalar joint surfaces and soft tissue stabilizers is modified, so that after removal of the implant, no recurrence can be observed.

Arthroereises have no direct effect on the destabilization of the medial ray besides their hindfoot-stabilizing effect. It is assumed that in further development, the stabilizing effect of the long peroneal muscle in particular will be sufficient to bring about adequate stability here as well (cf., e.g., pedographic course in Fig. 4.19). In cases where a plantarizing measure is added on the medial ray, the advantage of immediate full weight-bearing is lost.

4.10.1 Indication Criteria for Arthroereisis

A TMT index of about −35° has proven to be a practical threshold value for the indication for an arthroereisis. The criterion for shortening of the gastrocnemius part of the calf muscles is a passive dorsal extension of less than 10° with the knee joint extended. Complaints are indicated—if present—diffusely in the area of the longitudinal foot arch (a painful os tibiale externum should be excluded here) or also in the medial knee joint area. This must be actively inquired about. It is not uncommon for pediatric patients after successful correction, to report that they previously had diffuse stress pain, which they did not consciously register. Parents often notice an increase in performance, for example, when walking for long distances or report that their child has become "more active" after surgery.

If a TMT index is clearly below −35° after careful X-ray diagnostics, the indication for an arthroereisis does not seem to apply. However, if a pronounced hindfoot valgus component is clinically observed, a calcaneus sliding osteotomy should be considered as an alternative.

In the presence of a coalition (rigid planovalgus deformity), an arthroereisis is indicated at best after resection of the bony bridge (see Fig. 5.32). If the coalition is overlooked or if it only becomes apparent later after the arthroereisis, the desired correction effect and pain relief will not be achieved (Fig. 4.29).

Arthroereisis can be performed at the age of 7–8 years in case of special indications; however, as a rule, one will rather wait because of the spontaneous correction potential in this age group (de Pellegrin et al. 2014). The ideal age for girls is about 10–11 years and for boys about 10.5–12 years, depending on their "biological age" (ossification status, height, menarche, secondary sexual characteristics, etc.). The upper age limit is controversial; positive results have also been reported in significantly older patients (pers. communication Dr. G. Mindler, Wien-Speising), especially in syndromal clinical entities with delayed development and delayed skeletal age (de Pellegrin et al. 2014).

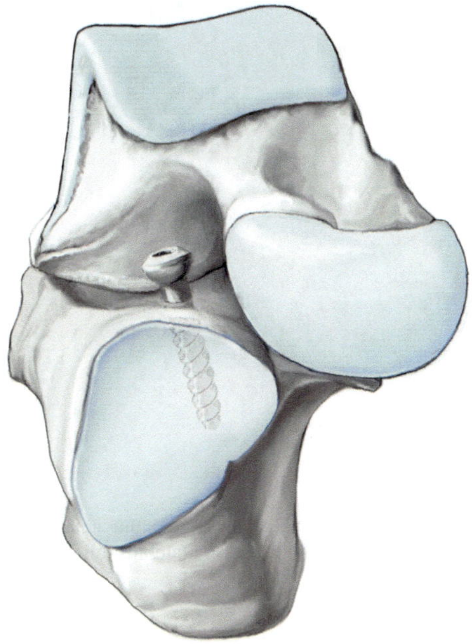

Fig. 4.15 Position of the calcaneostop screw with impingement of the screw head at the processus lateralis tali. The effect can be dosed by turning the screw back and forth

4.10.2 Calcaneostop Arthroereisis

The calcaneostop arthroereisis was introduced in Central Europe, following earlier precursors, in particular by De Pellegrin (2007). A 6.0–7.0 mm screw is placed in the anterior calcaneal section in such a way that its screw head provides a stop for the lateral processus tali, thereby mechanically limiting the eversion (Fig. 4.15). In addition, proprioceptively mediated effects appear to be effective. A high density of sensory receptors in the area of the sinus tarsi has been proven (Rein et al. 2013). In the Anglo-American region, this form of arthroereisis seems to be hardly known.

4.10.2.1 Surgical Procedure

Among the users of this procedure, there are three main differences in the approach: unilateral or bilateral surgery, with or without calf muscle lengthening, and with or without temporary immobilization in hard casts. The author—like de Pellegrin et al. (2014)—usually performs the procedure unilaterally but in most cases combines it with an intramuscular gastrocnemius lengthening (Sect. 6.3.1) and immobilizes for 4 weeks in a hard cast of the lower leg with primary full weight-bearing. The effect of the hindfoot straightening is usually visible immediately after cast removal (Fig. 4.17).

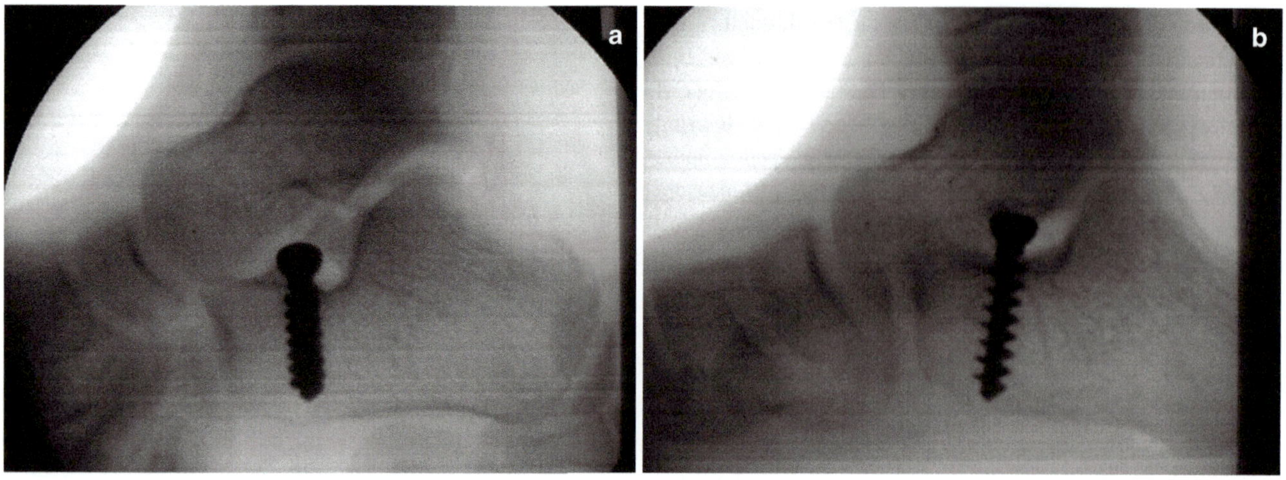

Fig. 4.16 Intraoperative image converter documentation in inversion (**a**) and eversion (**b**) of the talocalcaneal-navicular complex with impingement of the screw head on the processus lateralis tali in everted position (**b**)

Technique

An incision of 1.5 cm length is made above the sinus tarsi along the skin lines. To protect the branches of the sural nerve, the subcutaneous soft tissue is incised parallel to their presumed course and the wound is spread until the cranial surface of the calcaneus is palpated with the elevatorium. A K-wire is inserted at the lowest point of the cranial indentation of the calcaneus or slightly distally at maximum inversion of the hindfoot, slightly oblique from dorsal-cranial to anterior-plantar, and its position is checked in the image intensifier. The K-Wire lies tight against the anterior edge of the fibula. Alternatively, the access can be widened slightly so that a 2.0 mm K-Wire can be drilled in and also be removed under visual control. A thinner K-Wire, which is bent over at the end, is inserted into the prepared canal, and thus the effect of the planned screw position can be checked. When the bent K-Wire gets in contact with the processus lateralis tali as desired in everted hindfoot position, a 3.2 mm drill bit is used, and a 25–30 mm long, 6.5 mm fully threaded cancellous screw is inserted (Fig. 4.15). Injury to the skin, which is penetrated very tangentially, should be avoided by slightly widening the incision and protecting the tissue. Alternatively a cannulated screw can be used and should be inserted after radiologic control of the K-wire-position. The effect of the eversion inhibition can be dosed by turning the screw back and forth. A "stop" should be noticeable in a very slight eversion, near the neutral position. The impingement phenomenon can be tested in the image intensifier by inversion and eversion (Fig. 4.16). The screw must not be inserted too far lateral, as otherwise there is no contact of the screw head with the lateral process (see Fig. 4.24). In principle, a primary full load is possible. Since in many cases an additional intramuscular gastrocnemius lengthening is performed (see Sect. 6.3.1), the application of a hard lower leg cast is therefore necessary anyway. In the author's experience, it is also advisable even without this procedure for practical reasons in childhood (school attendance, rapid remobilization, protection against occasional injuries).

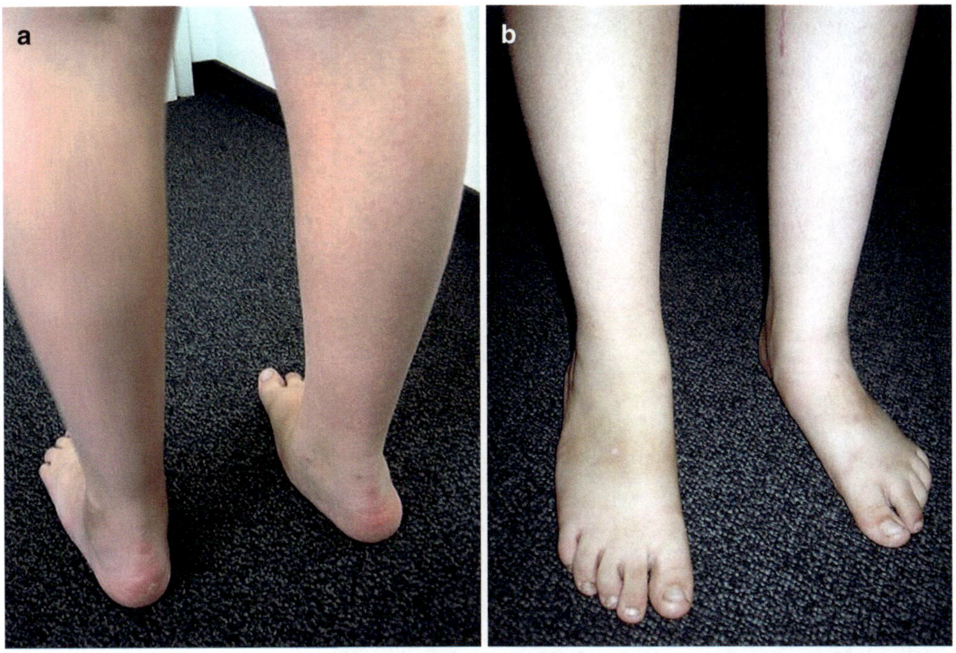

Fig. 4.17 10-Year-old female patient, 4 weeks after calcaneostop arthroereisis with gastrocnemius lengthening on the left side (**a**), a complete clinical correction can be seen compared to the opposite side (**b**), which was less affected preoperatively

4.10.2.2 Results and Treatment Examples

De Pellegrin et al. (2014) have the most experience with the calcaneostop procedure. Based on earlier communications from other authors, de Pellegrin has been propagating this approach since the 1990s and can be regarded as an inaugurator of the method. He reports 93.7% good results 3 months after the procedure in a large number of otherwise healthy children but also in patients with syndromal diseases. The angles in the lateral projection measured by de Pellegrin et al. (2014) improved in the short-term course by 17° (Costa-Bartani angle), 18° (talar inclination angle), and 3° (calcaneal pitch angle) and were thus in the respective normal range postoperatively. A subgroup of these patients showed even more pronounced angle corrections 2.9 years after screw removal. Unfortunately, a second X-ray projection plane was not considered, so that the achieved alignment correction can only be assessed to a limited extent (see Sect. 4.5). Abbara-Czardybon et al. (2014) found an average correction of the TMT index according to Hamel and Kinast (2006) of 19.3° in 68 cases and clinically predominantly favorable results; Arbab et al. (2017) found an average correction of 15.2° after 30.6 months of observation in the partially identical patient population (73 cases).

Since 2004, the author has applied the procedure in over 200 cases, most of which have also shown good and very good results. A retrospective survey (not published) of 37 patients on average 26 months after the procedure showed that about 35% of the patients had preoperative stress-related complaints in the stricter sense. An increase in the activity level after surgery was reported in 62% of the cases by the parents. Slight or occasional pain during sports activities was reported postoperatively in 27% of cases and seemed to depend on the amount of correction achieved (Fig. 4.22). 86.5% of the patients were "very satisfied" and 13.5% "satisfied," and no patient was dissatisfied.

The radiologically assessed TMT index (Hamel and Kinast 2006) showed an alignment improvement of 22.8° (from –42.3° to –19.5°) in a group of 26 consecutive patients, which was slightly less than the correction of 29.8° achieved with the calcaneus lengthening during the same period (Hamel 2010a). Especially in the transverse plane, the correction effect of the calcaneus lengthening with an average of 13.8° was higher than that of the arthroereisis with 8.7° on average.

Six representative examples of treatment will be presented: Figs. 4.18 and 4.19 show two typical cases with good alignment, recognizable especially by the postoperative talar inclination in the lateral projection. In Fig. 4.19, the plane of the subtalar joint is also significantly more horizontal postoperatively than before surgery, which is likely to be associated with a reduced thrust of the talus towards medioplantar. The pedographic course shows a near normalization of the forces involved in the stance phase of gait with an increase in the maximum force in the forefoot area. The case in Fig. 4.20 is characterized by a particularly pronounced shortening of the calf muscle, which preoperatively hardly allowed heel loading (Fig. 4.20c) and required Achilles tendon lengthening. Even very severe deformities can be successfully corrected by arthroereisis, as the examples in Figs. 4.21, 4.22, and 4.23 show, the latter in a patient with trisomy. Postoperative pain at the screw site seems to be more likely in severe deformities (Fig. 4.22).

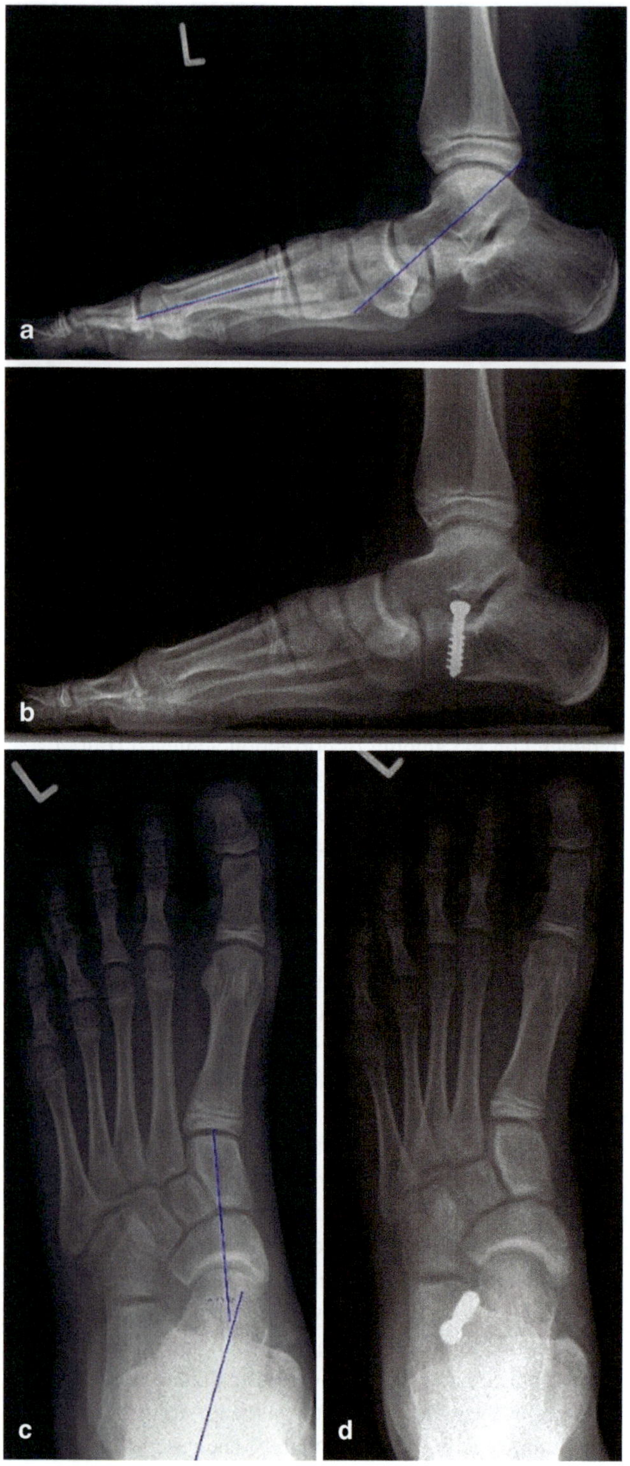

Fig. 4.18 9-Year-old girl with planovalgus deformity and asymptomatic os tibiale externum before (**a**, **c**) and 5 months after calcaneostop arthroereisis with gastrocnemius lengthening (**b**, **d**). The complete correction in both planes is clearly visible. The TMT index could be improved from about −45° to about −18°

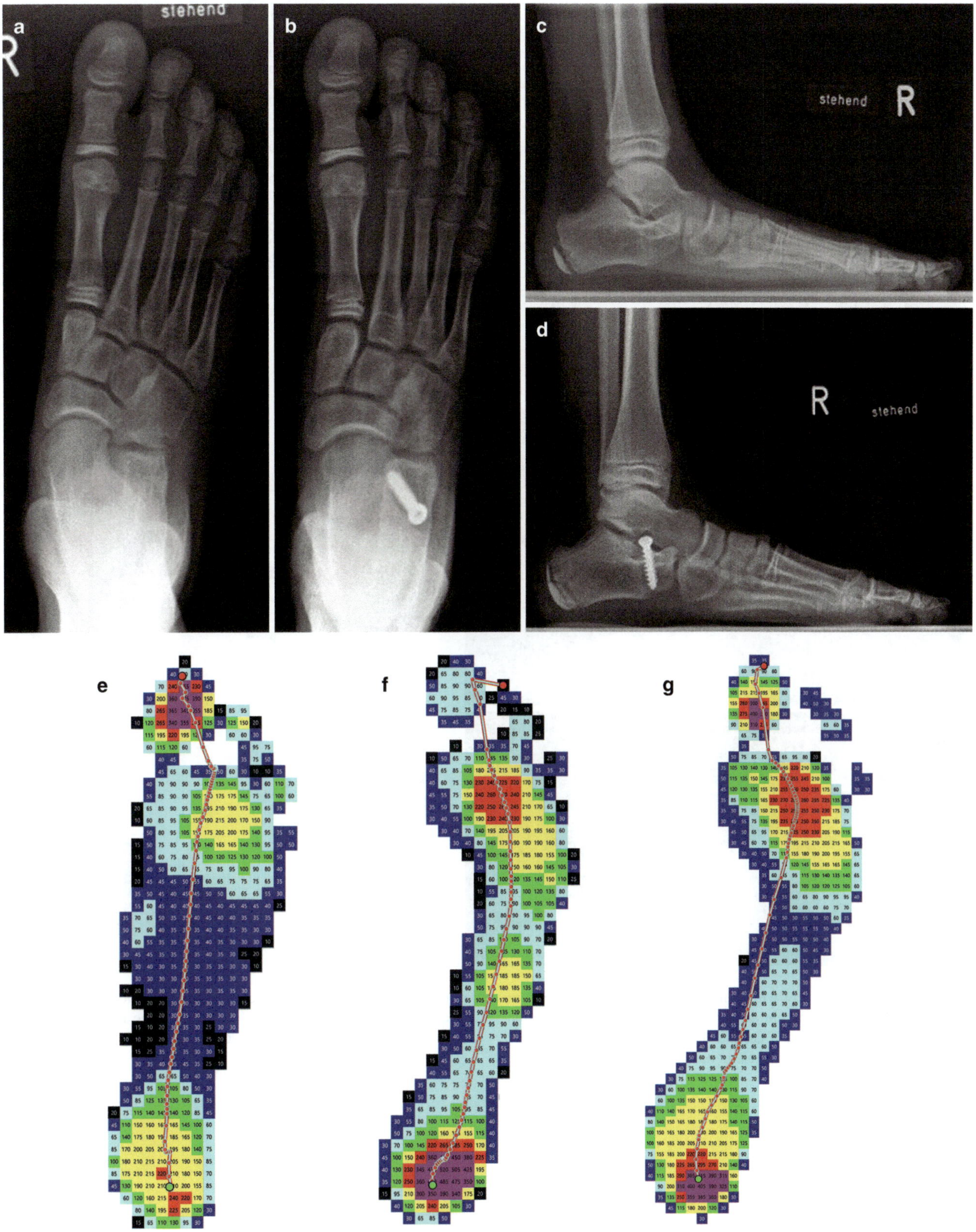

Fig. 4.19 12-Year-old male patient before (**a**, **c**, **e**), 18 months (**f**) and 4 years after calcaneostop arthroereisis with gastrocnemius lengthening (**b**, **d**, **g**). The articular surface of the subtalar joint, which appears inclined in the lateral preoperative image (**c**), is much more horizontally oriented postoperatively (**d**). The pedographic course shows 1.5 years postoperatively (**f**) still an increased load on the lateral metatarsus of the foot compared to preoperatively (**e**), which recedes over 4 years postoperatively (**g**). The body weight-related maximum force in the forefoot area increases significantly postoperatively after 1.5 (**i**) and 4 (**j**) years compared to the preoperative situation (**h**) with a significant reduction in the preceding compensatory increased use of toes before surgery. Figure 4.11 shows the pedographic development of the non-treated left opposite side in the same course over 4 years with clear functional deterioration

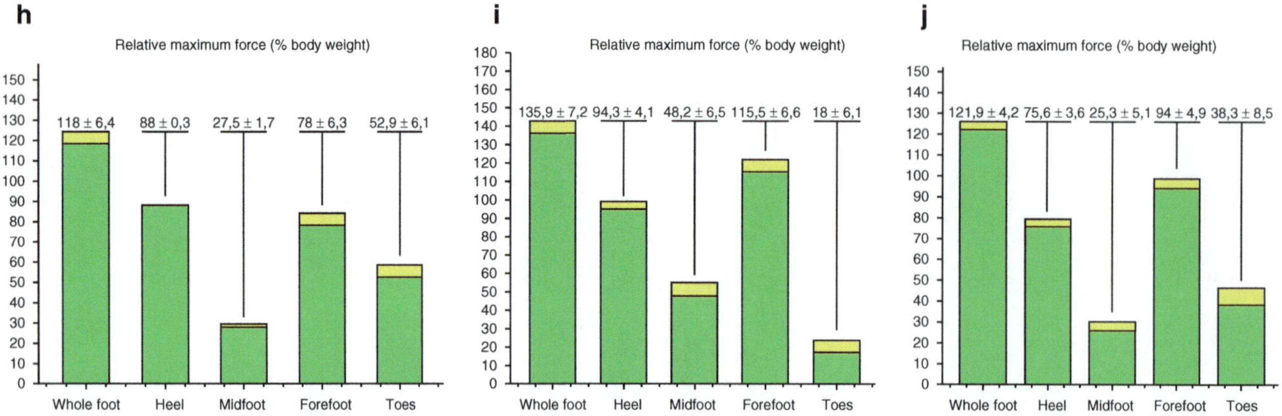

Fig. 4.19 (continued)

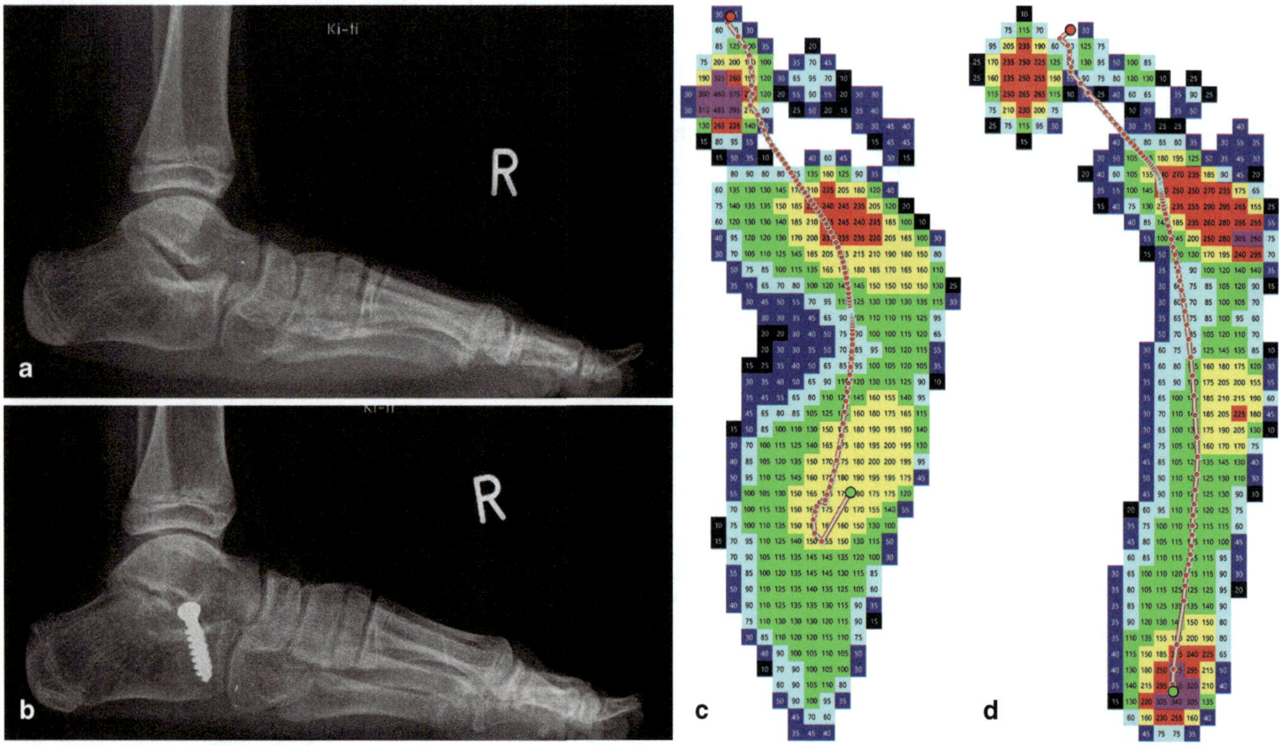

Fig. 4.20 11-Year-old boy with Chiari malformation and preoperatively (**a**, **c**) particularly severe calf muscle shortening, also recognizable by the slightly negative calcaneal pitch angle. 7 months after calcaneostop arthroereisis with gastrocnemius recession and additional dosed Z-shaped Achilles tendon lengthening (**b**, **d**), loading of the heel is recognizable. The postoperative elevation of the medial ray is still clearly visible radiologically and pedographically

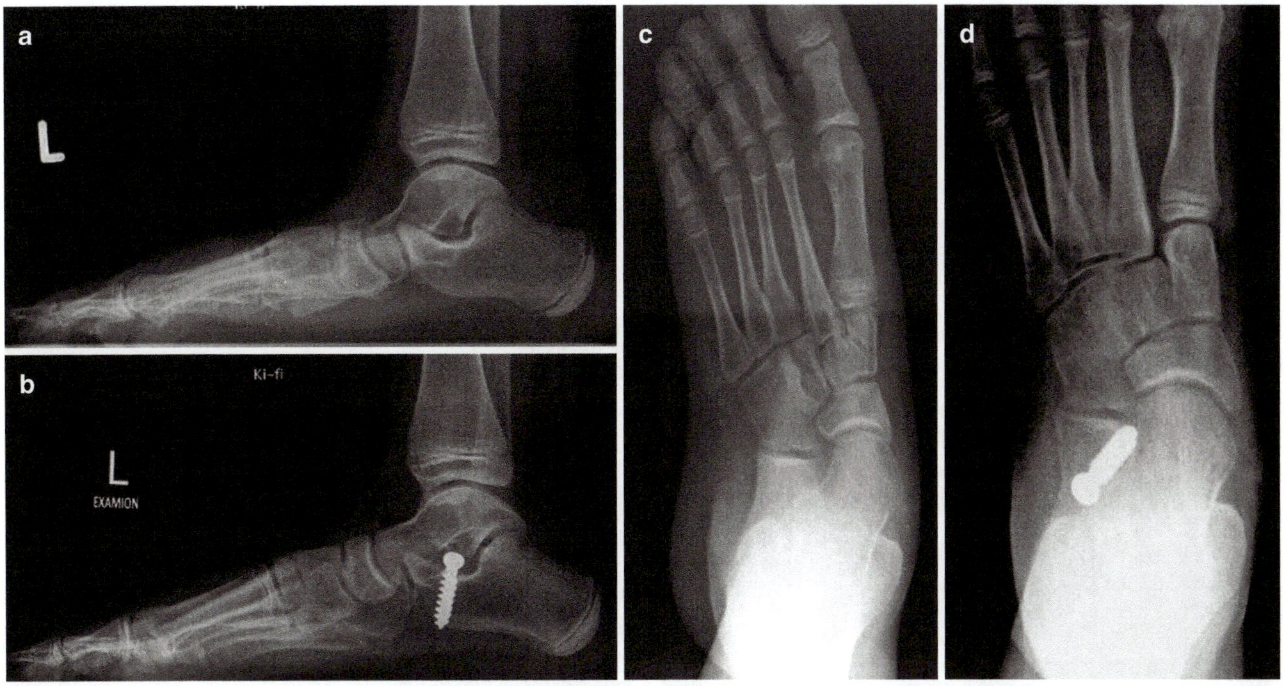

Fig. 4.21 Particularly severe hypermobile planovalgus deformity in an 11-year-old boy pre- (**a**, **c**) and postoperatively (**b**, **d**). The realignment of the talus is clearly visible, the TMT index was reduced from –60° to –28°

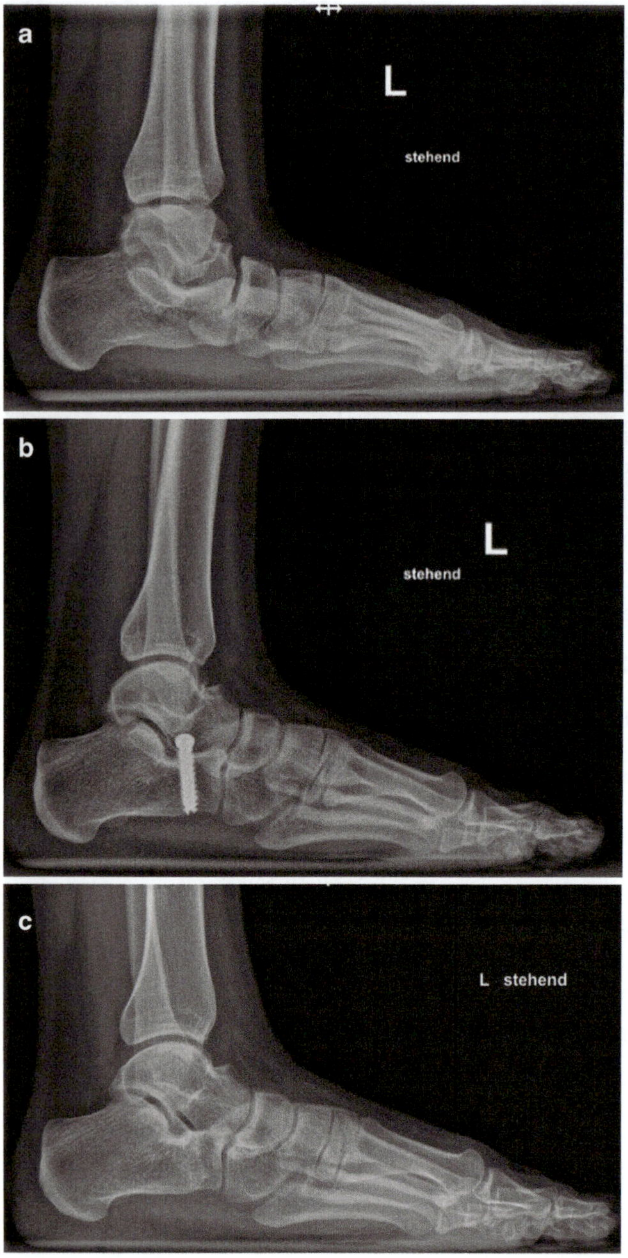

Fig. 4.22 12-Year-old girl with particularly pronounced inclination of the talus preoperatively (**a**), postoperatively complete correction (**b**), however the patient had several months of pain until the screw was well tolerated. The peritalar complex remained stable after removal of the screw (**c**)

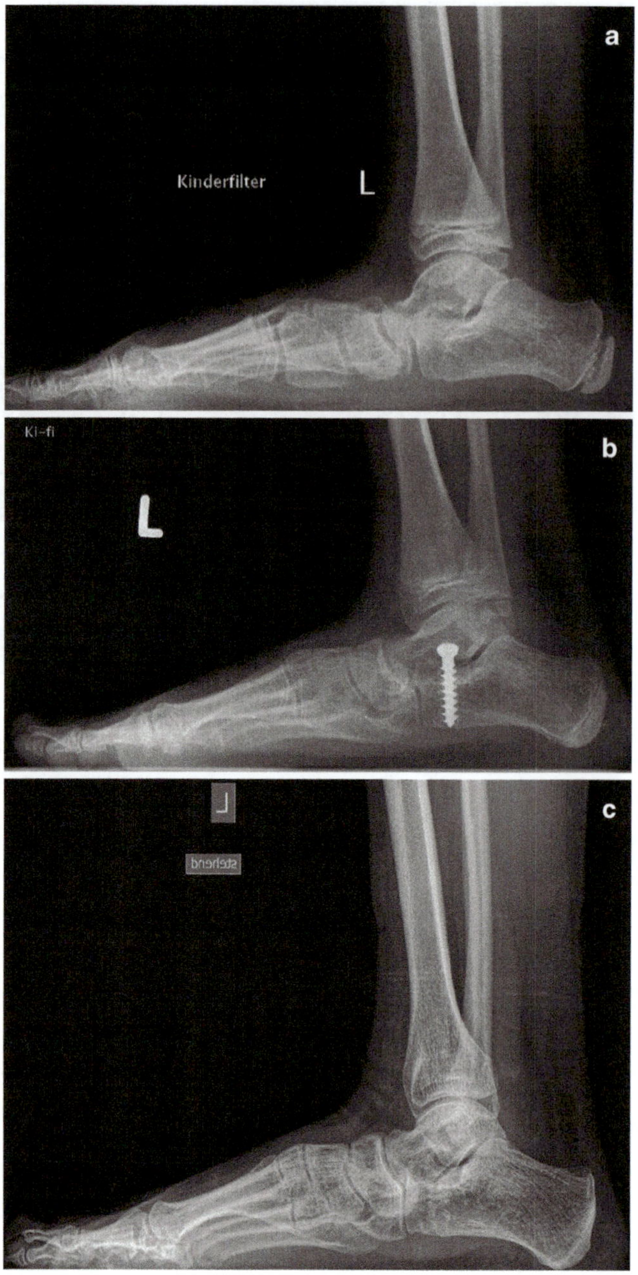

Fig. 4.23 12-Year-old boy with trisomy 21 and extreme planovalgus deformity (b). Significant positional improvement 9 months after calcaneostop arthroereisis (**b**) and 5 years postoperatively after screw removal (**c**)

4.10.2.3 Errors, Problems, and Complications

The calcaneostop arthroereisis is a minimally invasive procedure that does not irreversibly damage any joint structures. However, it is not completely free of complications, which must be pointed out especially in borderline indications. In the literature, hardly any undesirable results are reported in detail. De Pellegrin et al. (2014) give a complication rate of 6.3% in the short-term course. Hamel (2010b) described in a first communication good positional corrections with, however, a larger proportion of at least temporary undesirable phenomena. In the majority of these patients, the problems were of a temporary surgery or correspond to the learning curve of the author with this procedure. In the following, some examples of undesirable outcomes will be presented, some of which are due to incorrect performance.

Problems and Complications of the Calcaneostop Arthroereisis

- Incorrect positioning of the screw
- Painful impingement
- Peroneal spasm
- Undercorrection
- Coalition, which was diagnosed later

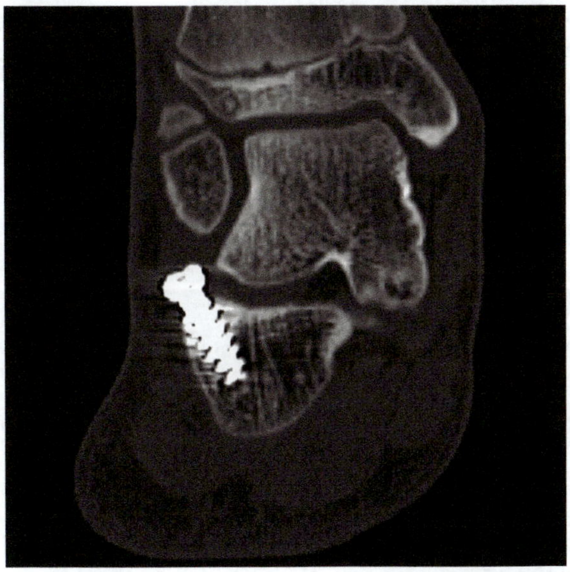

Fig. 4.24 Externally performed mispositioned calcaneostop screw without any effect on the processus lateralis tali (CT frontal section)

As this is a method with at least predominantly mechanical effect, the positioning of the screw is of considerable importance for the result. The principle of the procedure is that the screw head comes in contact with the processus lateralis tali at a certain level of eversion and prevents further eversion. Therefore, the position of the screw (see Figs. 4.24 and 4.57) and also the insertion depth are important. If the eversion is too severely limited by excessive protrusion of the screw (overcorrection, "impingement"), pain and very persistent peroneal spasm may occur (Figs. 4.25 and 4.26), which in some cases can be corrected by local corticoid application; if it is screwed in too deeply, the effect of the hindfoot realignment will be too small ("undercorrection"). However, practical experience shows that even a suboptimal screw position can be compatible with a favorable result. Further information on screw positioning can be found at Hamel (2010b).

However, uncertainties remain in the assessment of unfavorable results. For example, it is not clear why the desired correction did not occur in the cases shown in Figs. 4.27 and 4.28 due to the screw positioning. Turning back the screw to increase the effect could possibly be considered in the cases mentioned. Possibly the age, the conditions at the naviculo-cuneiform line, and the fact that the destabilization of the medial column is generally not treated in the hindfoot arthroereisis play a role. A combination of the arthroereisis with a stabilization of the medial ray (cuneiform-medial osteotomy or naviculo-cuneiform arthrodesis) in the case of a clearly pathological MASA angle would probably have led to a better correction (see Sect. 4.11.3). A practical solution may be to change the procedure to a spacer arthroereisis (Fig. 4.28).

If an arthroereisis is carried out by mistake in the presence of a rigid planovalgus deformity with an undetectable or unrecognized coalition, a favorable result cannot be expected (Fig. 4.29). On the other hand, in suitable cases the arthroereisis can be used in combination with a coalition resection (Chap. 5).

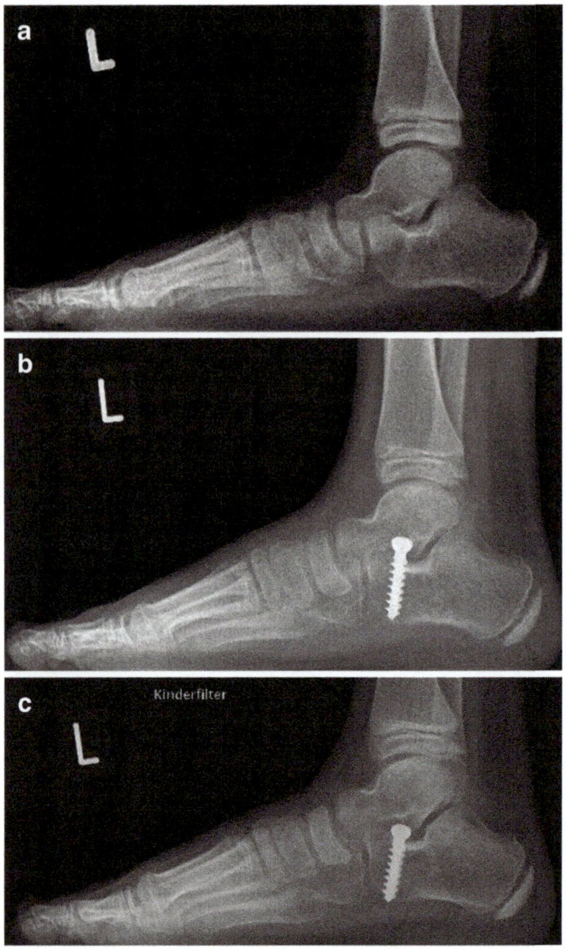

Fig. 4.25 10-Year-old boy with planovalgus deformity (**a**). After arthroereisis and gastrocnemius lengthening, there was a considerable correction (**b**), but with significant pain at the screw. After driving the screw deeper into the calcaneus 4 months postoperatively, good functional result with complete correction (**c**)

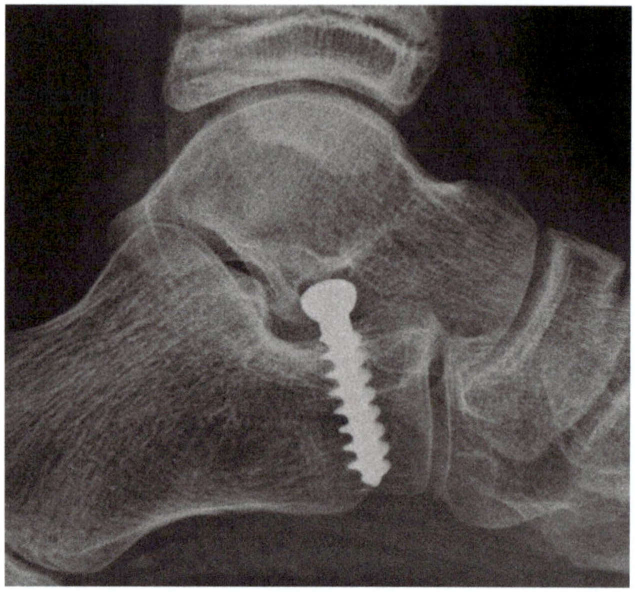

Fig. 4.26 Significant screw impingement with pain and prolonged peroneal spasm. A bony arrosion developed at the processus lateralis. The case presented in Fig. 5.32 shows, that bony arrosion is not always connected with pain

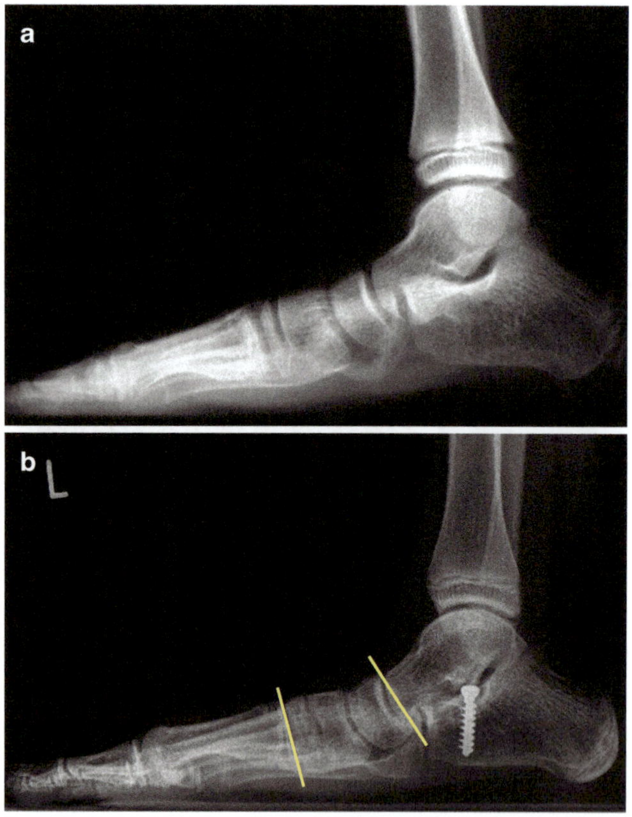

Fig. 4.27 9-Year-old boy before (**a**) and after calcaneostop arthroereisis with gastrocnemius lengthening (**b**). A clear correction did not occur. A relatively distinct naviculo-cuneiform instability is conspicuous, recognizable by the MASA angle ("medial arch sag angle" according to Aiyer et al. 2016) of about 17°

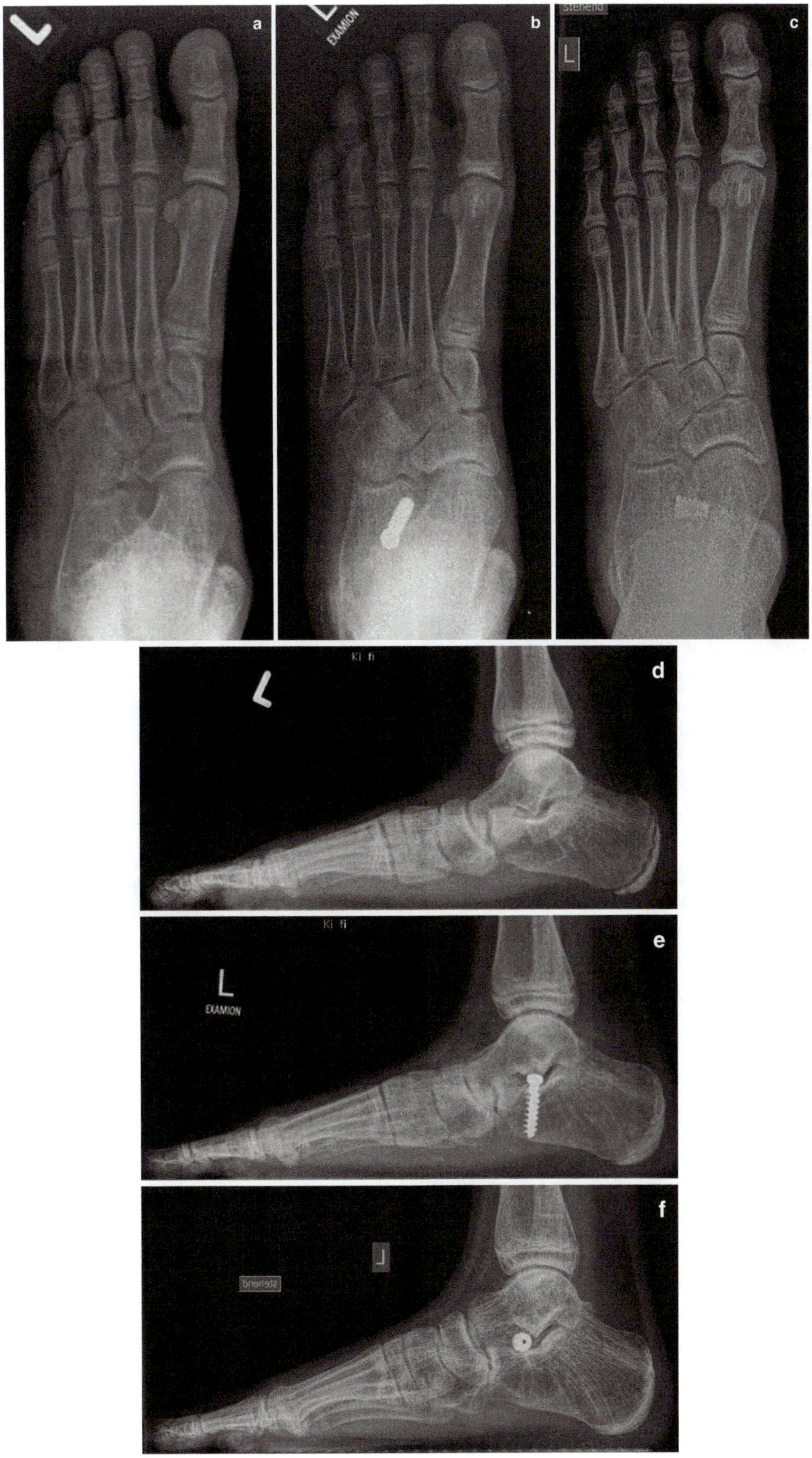

Fig. 4.28 12-Year-old boy with distinct planovalgus deformity (**a**, **d**). After calcaneostop arthroereisis with gastrocnemius lengthening, the desired correction did not occur, although the screw head clearly hits the processus lateralis tali (**b**, **e**). 9 months postoperatively, the screw was removed, and a spacer arthroereisis was performed with good correction after 15 months (**c**, **f**)

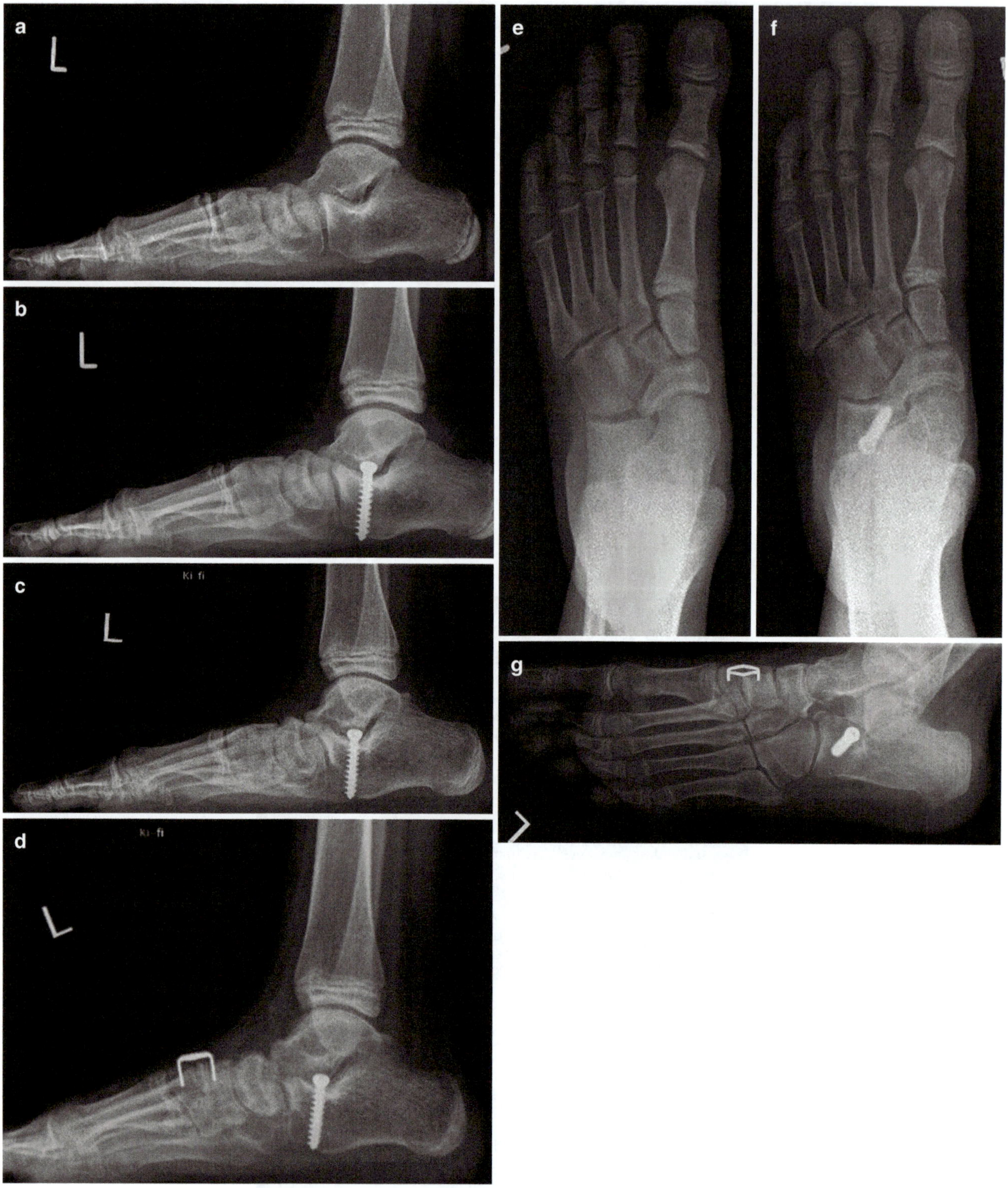

Fig. 4.29 Arthroereisis in an 11-year-old boy with planovalgus deformity (**a**, **e**) without significant correction (**b**, **c**, and **f**). Only at the age of 15 years a calcaneonavicular coalition became obvious as the cause of the lacking correction (**c**, **f**). After resection of the coalition (**g**) with lengthening of the peroneus brevis tendon and a plantarizing cuneiform medial and intermedial osteotomy (**d**), a sufficient correction of the position is evident. The arthroereisis screw was left in place

4.10.3 Sinus Tarsi Spacer

Sinus-tarsi spacers were already used in the 1970s (Smith and Millar 1983; Green and Williams 2013). By spreading the sinus tarsi, which collapsed completely in the planovalgus deformity, by means of a conical-shaped threaded spacer, the talocalcaneal joint is repositioned. Spacers with different designs are offered by the industry (Needleman 2005). In Anglo-American literature, this form of arthroereisis has been used by representatives of podiatry for a long time but continues to be largely rejected by pediatric orthopedists due to the lack of long-term results and the rather favorable spontaneous course of the pediatric planovalgus deformity (e.g., Ricco et al. 2014).

4.10.3.1 Surgical Procedure

Technique

A guide wire is inserted into the sinus tarsi via a 1.5–2 cm long skin incision above the sinus tarsi, so that it can be palpated in the medial tarsal region and later removed here after a counter-incision. The slightly oblique course of the sinus tarsi from lateral-anterior to medial-posterior must be taken into account. Using the guide wire, the sinus tarsi is spread with trial specimens until the desired correction and stabilization of the previously hypermobile talocalcaneal joint are achieved. This must be checked in the image intensifier in both planes. The determined implant size is now inserted. In the dorsoplantar X-ray projection, the spacer should end laterally exactly with the contour of the talar neck (Figs. 4.30 and 4.50). According to Vulcano et al. (2016) it should be placed about 4 mm further medially. The guide wire is pulled out medially. Postoperatively, immobilization in the hard cast of the lower leg can be maintained for about 2–6 weeks under full load to avoid early dislocation. However, this is not considered necessary by other surgeons.

4.10.3.2 Results and Treatment Examples

A good overview of the pediatric orthopedic literature on the—predominantly positive—published results with sinus tarsi implants in children is given by Needleman (2005) and Metcalfe et al. (2011). Gutierrez and Lara (2005) report good clinical and radiological results. However, leading pediatric orthopedic foot specialists continue to reject the procedure and question the indication (Mosca 2010b; Ricco et al. 2014). In contrast, the podiatric literature on the subject is immense (e.g., Tompkins et al. 1993). Here, the spacer arthroereisis is commonly used. In the German-speaking countries, retrospective studies have been published on smaller case numbers, which also describe predominantly good results (Schröder et al. 2006; Kuhn et al. 2010; Arnold and Weber 2010). Recently Indino et al. (2020) described statistically significant improvement of all measured radiologic parameters in 112 consecutively treated moderate pediatric planovalgus deformities. The author's initial experiences are also positive, and in particular the application in combination with other procedures seems to represent a promising enrichment of the therapeutic spectrum (Sect. 4.11.3, e.g., Figs. 4.54 and 4.55).

Usually, the spacer arthroereisis leads to an immediate correction of the position without a significant loss of mobility of the talocalcaneal joint (see Figs. 4.28, 4.30, and 4.31). In the author's experience, a spacer arthroereisis can be particularly successful if no relevant elevation of the medial ray persists postoperatively. This is ensured by the high flexibility of the child's foot and the expected adaptation and strengthening of the long peroneal muscle. If, on the other hand, the mid-forefoot supination persists, there is a torque towards valgus on the hindfoot complex in the late stance phase with the risk of pain in the sinus tarsi area or spacer dislocation.

4.10.3.3 Errors, Problems, and Complications

When using an image intensifier, the procedure is technically simple. Difficulties may be caused by the choice of implant size; over- and undercorrections are possible. As with the—often only additive and temporary—use of sinus tarsi spacers in adults, a considerable proportion of patients experience symptoms. A dislocation of the spacer is quite often observed (Fig. 4.32). The shape of the selected implant obviously plays a role here. On the other hand, cases of dislocation have also been observed in which the desired alignment correction was nevertheless achieved. A critical aspect is the use of sinus tarsi spacers in clubfoot overcorrection (Fig. 4.33).

4.10.4 Summarized Assessment of the *Arthroereisis* Procedures

According to the current state of knowledge and the author's experience, the arthroereisis procedures are effective interventions for growth control with a minimally invasive character, which can be recommended if the indication is suitable. However, neither of these procedures is completely free from complications, which should limit their use to pronounced planovalgus deformities.

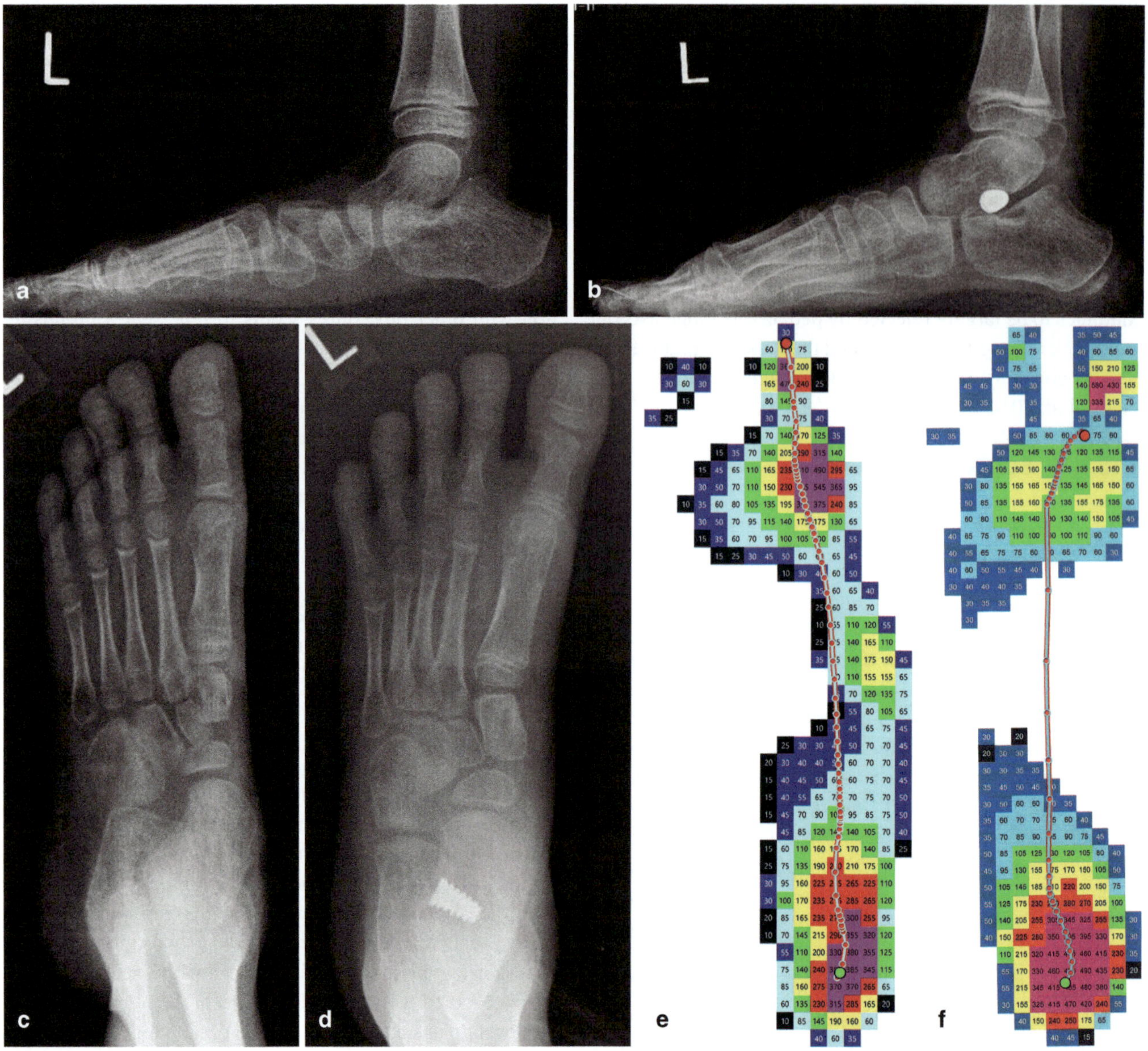

Fig. 4.30 8.5-Year-old patient with very pronounced planovalgus deformity (**a**, **c**), recognizable especially by the preoperative pedogram (**e**). Postoperatively (**b**, **d**) complete correction. The preoperatively strongly planar flexed talus (**a**) appears clearly repositioned postoperatively, recognizable by the corrected TMT-lat angle. In the ap projection (**d**), the spacer exactly matches the lateral contour of the talar neck (**d**). 20 months postoperatively (**f**) the pressure distribution has largely normalized

As in adult foot surgery, spacer arthroereises are increasingly used in combination with other procedures today (Sect. 4.11.3). For example, the additional stabilization of the medial foot ray is often considered (Fig. 4.29). In the future, combined procedures, in which the arthroereisis is only one component of the overall intervention, will probably be increasingly used in children's feet (Fig. 4.53). A combination with calcaneus sliding osteotomy is also possible for the correction of the hindfoot (Figs. 4.54 and 4.55).

Which form of arthroereisis is preferable does not seem to be decided yet on the basis of the available literature. The calcaneostop method offers the advantage that the soft tissue structures of the sinus tarsi (interosseous ligaments, proprioceptive receptors) are not affected. It is not known, whether this can lead to long-term disadvantages when using spacers. The author up to now recommends the removal of arthroereisis implants after the end of growth, whereas others do so only in case of localized pain at the implant.

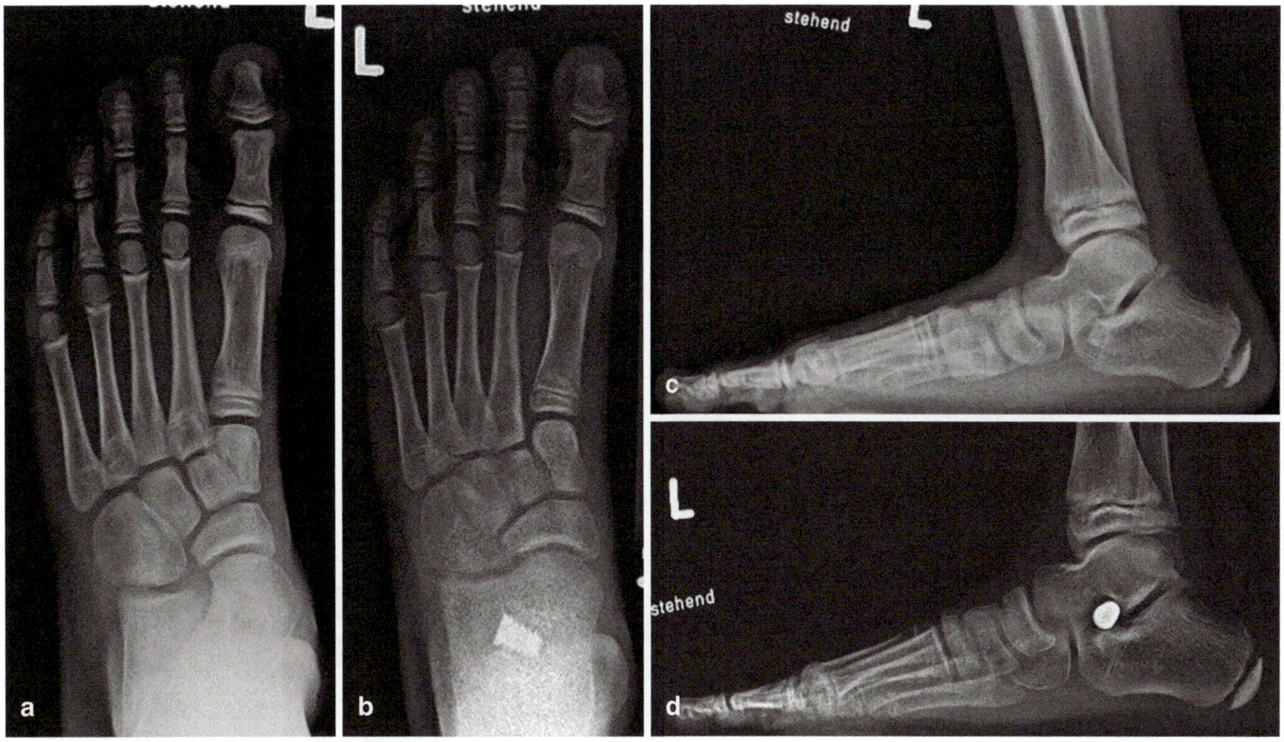

Fig. 4.31 11-Year-old patient before (**a**, **c**) and after spacer arthroereisis (**b**, **d**) without gastrocnemius lengthening with good correction effect

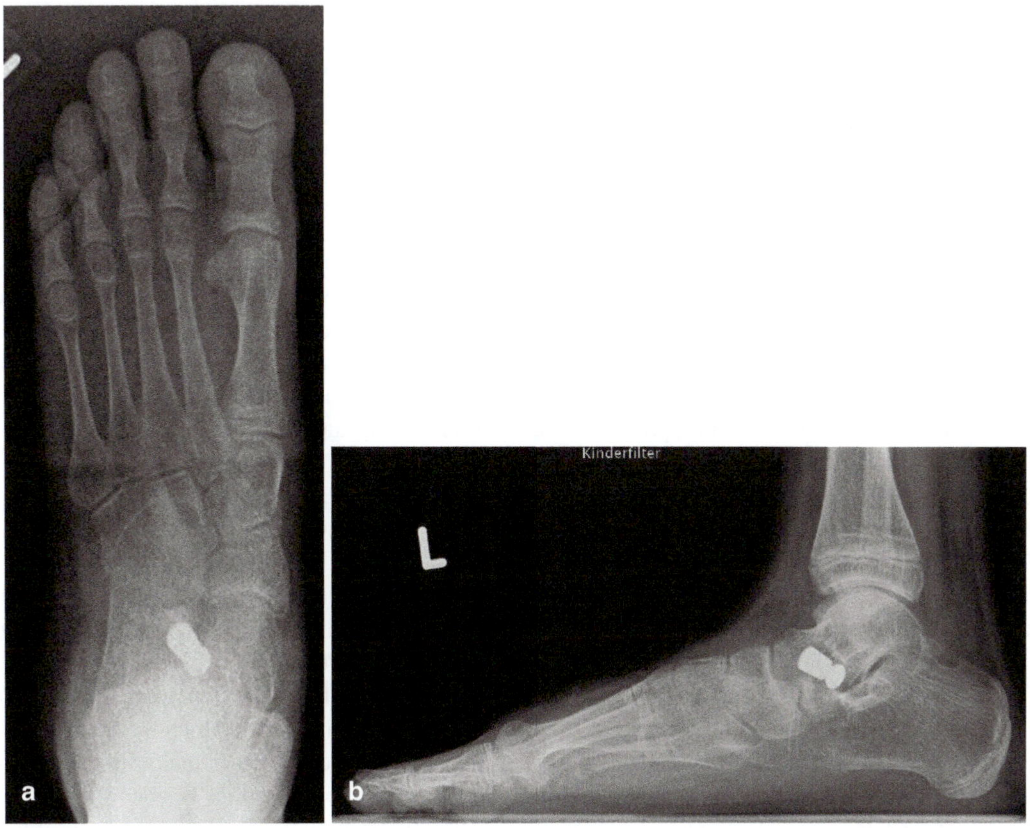

Fig. 4.32 In the case of an externally implanted sinus tarsi spacer, there was a clear postoperative dislocation of the spacer, that is located outside the sinus tarsi (**a**, **b**)

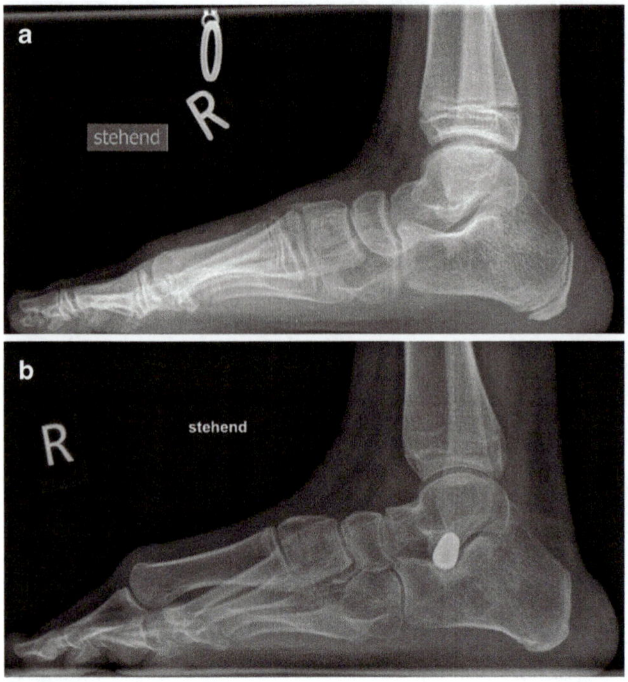

Fig. 4.33 An 11-year-old girl with clubfoot overcorrection (**a**) received a sinus tarsi spacer implanted externally. The patient had persistent pain at the implant and developed a clear dorsal-bunion deformity within 2.5 years (**b**), possibly due to overactivity of the anterior tibial muscle to avoid pain

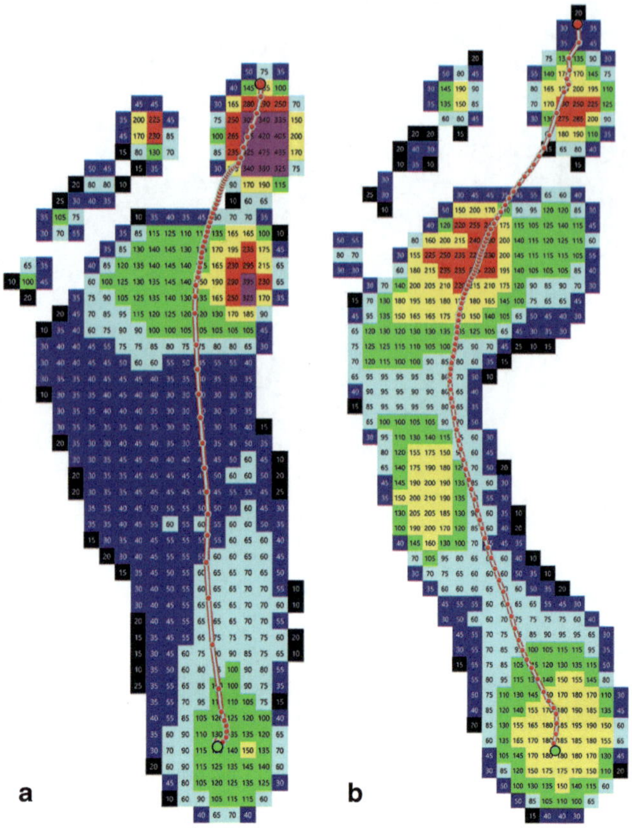

Fig. 4.34 Pre- (**a**) and 22 month postoperative pedography (maximum pressure image) (**b**) after calcaneus sliding osteotomy with gastrocnemius lengthening in a 12-year-old boy. In the quantitative analysis of the pedography, it is particularly noticeable that the maximum force is only reached postoperatively in the late stance phase (**b**), an expression of the good stabilization of the foot under the influence of the effect of the posterior tibial muscle

4.11 Corrective Osteotomies and Combined Procedures in Older Children and Adolescents

The indication for corrective osteotomies—some of which are much more complex—is determined in a similar way as described above for arthroereisis (see Sect. 4.7). Osteotomies are considered if there is not enough time left until full maturation to expect sufficient stabilization by an arthroereisis as a single procedure. In addition, experience in our own clinical practice has shown that the average correction potential of a calcaneus lengthening osteotomy exceeds that of arthroereisis, although this can vary considerably in individual cases (Hamel 2010a). The improvement of the calcaneal pitch angle was also more clearly evident in calcaneal lengthening compared to arthroereisis (see Fig. 4.47). Therefore, osteotomies seem to have an advantage in the case of particularly pronounced malalignment. It should also be remembered that arthroereisis—usually performed in isolation—basically only affect the hindfoot, while osteotomies can also be used to stabilize the medial ray (which in most cases is indicated).

In principle, corrective osteotomies can also be performed at a later age, beyond adolescence. Arguments in favor of an early intervention at the end of the growth period are the better healing tendency and adaptability of the young foot to the postoperatively altered condition. Two procedures have proven to be successful, which are described below, the calcaneus sliding osteotomy and the tarsal triple osteotomy. An isolated calcaneal lengthening osteotomy has not been performed by the author for many years.

4.11.1 Calcaneus Sliding Osteotomy

The isolated calcaneus sliding osteotomy (Wagner 1986) is a very proven and effective procedure for correction of the hindfoot in the frontal plane without negative effects on midfoot and forefoot supination. It is therefore particularly indicated in cases in which the hindfoot valgus clearly predominates over the other malposition components (Sect. 4.3.3). An additional effect besides the positive influence on the hindfoot statics is the increase in efficiency of the posterior tibial muscle. As shown in Fig. 4.34, a significant normalization of the load distribution can occur from a functional point of view. The procedure is increasingly being performed using minimally invasive techniques.

Technique

A 3–4 cm long oblique skin incision exposes the lateral corpus-tuber junction of the calcaneus subperiostally. The incision is clearly dorsal-plantar of the N. suralis, and this nerve should remain in the soft tissue layer during the procedure without exposure. The incision is made directly down to the corticalis without a layered preparation. The periosteum is mobilized anterior-cranially without weakening the attachment of the fibulocalcaneal ligament, and the bone is circumvented subperiostally on both sides with Hohmann hooks. Using the oscillating saw (especially cranial and caudal, close to the Hohmann hooks), various chisels and again the saw, the calcaneus is completely severed. The technique of working alternately with the oscillating saw and chisel described below makes it possible to protect the soft tissues and avoids severe overheating of the bone due to the saw action. The tuber fragment is then moved medial until the hindfoot valgus component is fully corrected (Fig. 4.40). The osteosynthesis in the child is carried out with two percutaneously placed Kirschner wires, which are left in place for about 4 weeks.

Technical Procedure for Calcaneus Sliding Osteotomy (Principle)

- Oscillating saw up to the opposite corticalis (cooling with irrigation!)
- Chisel for slight expansion of the still incomplete osteotomy
- Osteotomy of the opposite corticalis with the saw (very carefully)
- Distraction of the osteotomy by rotating the inserted chisel
- Inserting the osteotomy spreader with the chisel in a transverse position
- Widening of the osteotomy (loosening of the periosteal structures medially)
- Correction and fixation

4.11.2 Tarsal Triple Osteotomy (TTO)

The calcaneal lengthening osteotomy according to Evans (1975) with complete severance of the calcaneus between the middle and anterior joint facet, which has been particularly well established by Mosca (1995) since the 1990s, is an effective correction procedure for planovalgus deformity in later childhood and adolescence. Oh et al. (2011) combined it routinely with a medializing calcaneal osteotomy. Hintermann (2015) places the osteotomy further posterior between the posterior and middle joint facet as an incomplete open-wedge osteotomy (Fig. 4.35). The direction of the latter osteotomy is located slightly from anterolateral to posterior medial. The calcaneal lengthening particularly corrects midfoot-forefoot abduction in the transverse plane but also has a corrective effect on the hindfoot valgus. It is not clear in which way the mid-forefoot supination is influenced. Overall, the calcaneus lengthening osteotomy can be considered a form of arthroereisis in that it limits the extent of movement of the peritalar complex in the direction of eversion. Based on experience with planovalgus corrections in childhood and adulthood, pedographic observations and the reception of more recent literature, especially from the group around Deland (e.g., Oh et al. 2013), the author has developed the tarsal triple osteotomy (TTO) (Fig. 4.36) (Hamel and Nell 2016; Hamel et al. 2014), which has successively replaced the isolated calcaneal lengthening osteotomy in his own practice since 2008. The main considerations in this regard are explained in the following.

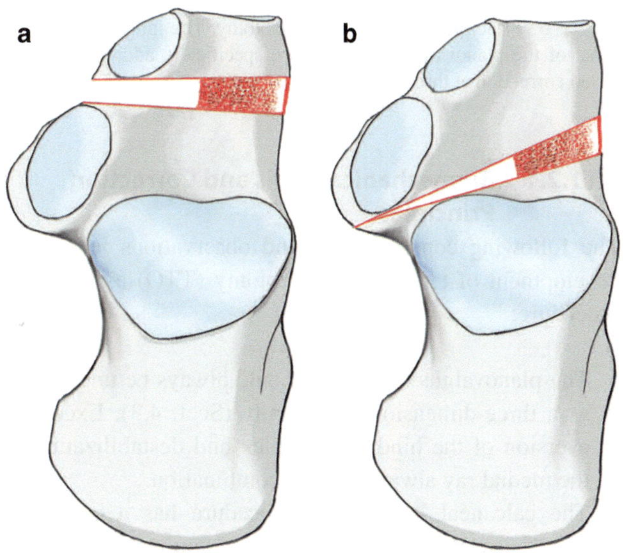

Fig. 4.35 Forms of calcaneal lengthening: Evans osteotomy with complete severing of the calcaneus (**a**) and Hintermann osteotomy as open-wedge osteotomy further posterior (**b**)

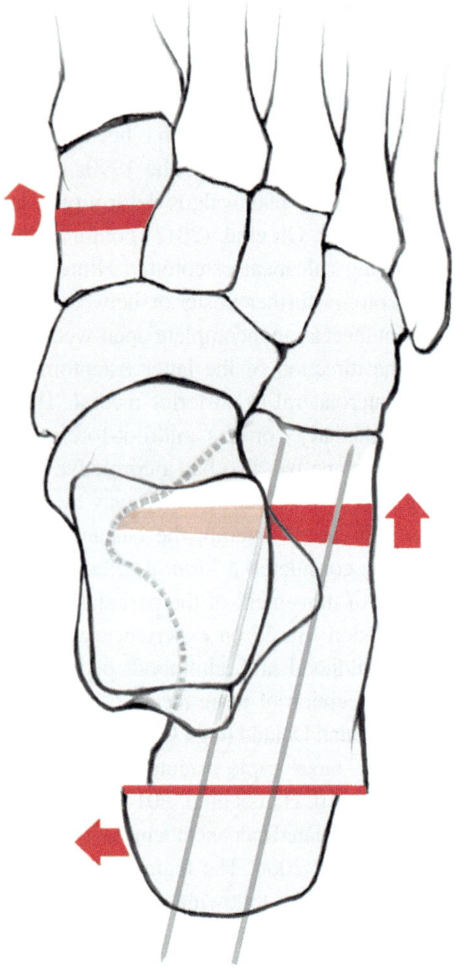

Fig. 4.36 Principle of tarsal triple osteotomy. The individual components of the planovalgus deformity are specifically addressed by the dosed correction at three localizations

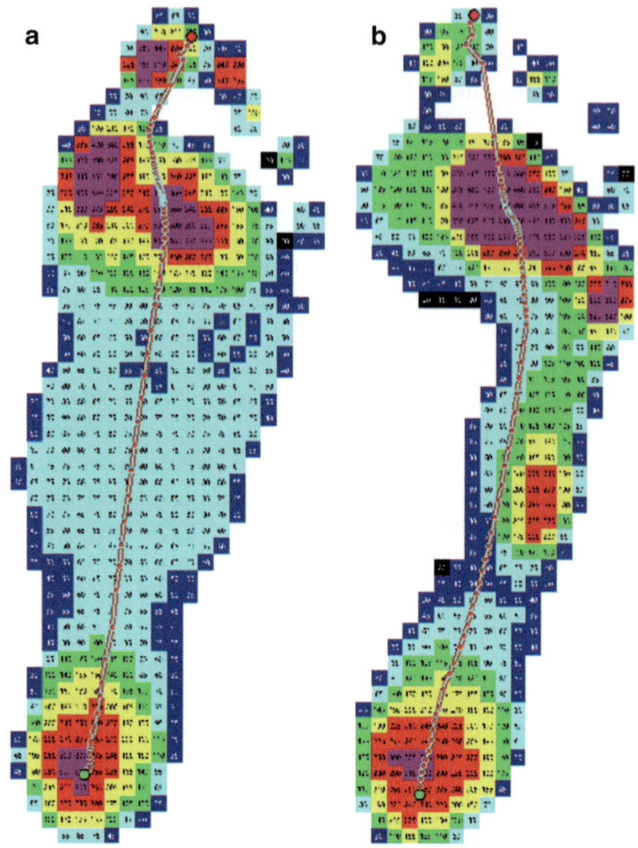

Fig. 4.37 Before (**a**) and after (**b**) correction of a severe planovalgus deformity in adolescence. After isolated calcaneal lengthening, the lateral foot rim was overloaded, causing extensive reduction of pressure at the metatarsal I

4.11.2.1 Biomechanical Basis and Correction Principles

The following considerations and observations led to the development of tarsal triple osteotomy (TTO) as a routine procedure:

- The planovalgus deformity should always be understood as a three-dimensional deformity (Sect. 4.3). Excessive eversion of the hindfoot complex and destabilization of the medial ray always exist in combination.
- The calcaneal lengthening procedure has a corrective effect also of the hindfoot valgus component. However, this effect is limited, so that excessive lengthening would be necessary to correct the hindfoot valgus component sufficiently.
- Lengthening to a greater extent may result in a pronounced reduction in subtalar mobility and also in the risk of bothersome and persisting overloading of the lateral foot rim (Figs. 4.37 and 4.38) (Davitt et al. 2001) and excessive pressure at the calcaneocuboid joint (Xia et al. 2013). All these effects are dose-related.
- In particular with pronounced calcaneal lengthening, subluxation of the calcaneocuboid joint often occurs (Moraleda et al. 2012), which clinical significance is not fully clarified.
- The influence of calcaneus lengthening on midfoot supination is controversial. According to the author's observation, this component is usually not sufficiently corrected. Therefore, an additional plantarization at the medial ray is usually necessary (Fig. 4.41).

The following consequences were derived from these findings:

- The calcaneal lengthening is required as a component of the TTO because of its correction potential in the transverse plane but can be dosed much lower than usually required for isolated applications with a base length of the inserted graft of up to 15 mm (Döderlein et al 1998). In not too severe cases, it can therefore be designed in the sense of an open-wedge osteotomy as suggested by Hintermann (2015).

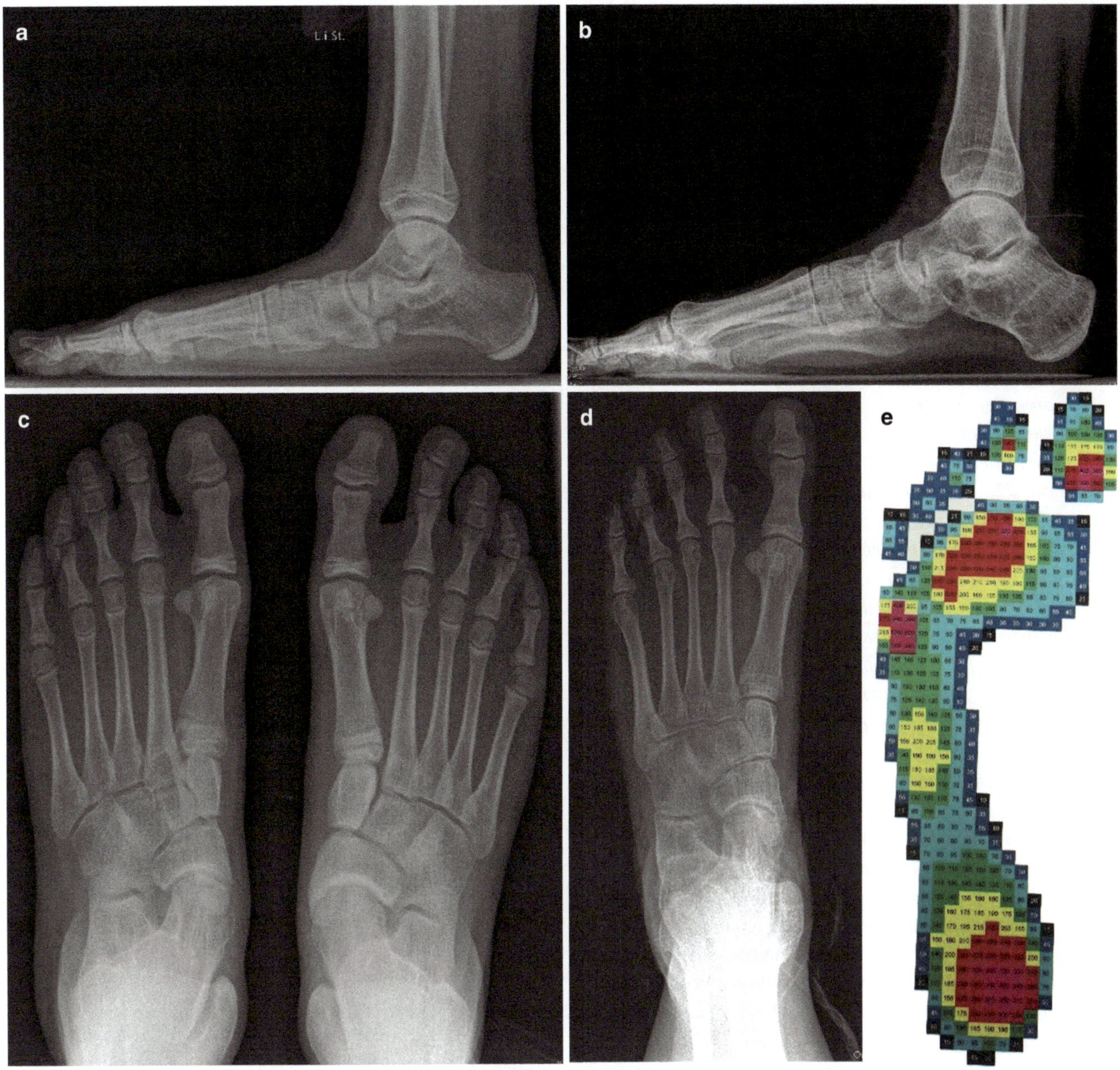

Fig. 4.38 11-Year-old girl with very pronounced planovalgus deformity accentuated on the left side (**a**, **c**). 3 years after double calcaneal osteotomy with lengthening of 10 mm, good hindfoot correction (**b**, **d**). However, pedographic analysis shows a significant overloading of the lateral foot rim with extensive reduced pressure at the medial ray (**e**). This also persisted in the following years. In this case, a more moderate calcaneal lengthening and the addition of a plantarizing measure to the medial ray would have been more beneficial

- As a rule, a calcaneus sliding osteotomy has to be added in order to completely correct the biomechanically important hindfoot valgus component in the frontal plane.
- Since hindfoot eversion is inevitably associated with an elevation of the medial ray in the sagittal plane, a plantarizing measure should always be included. In hypermobile cases, an open-wedge osteotomy of the medial cuneiform seems to be useful because of its stabilizing effect on the naviculo-cuneiform joint line (Cotton 1936; Hirose and Johnson 2004); in non-hypermobile conditions (e.g., rigid planovalgus deformity in case of coalition), a closed-wedge osteotomy is preferable (Rathjen and Mubarak 1998; Mosca 2014), which additionally slightly shortens the (overlong) medial ray of the foot.

Apparently similar experiences led to the development of the "Triple C" procedure (Rathjen and Mubarak 1998), in which, however, an open wedge osteotomy of the cuboid is carried out instead of the calcaneal lengthening. This also lengthens the lateral foot rim but does not reduce the eversion and thus cannot achieve stabilization of the talocalcaneal navicular complex. Moraleda et al. (2012) found in a radiological analysis that—as expected—the talonavicular alignment is corrected by this method significantly less than with a calcaneal lengthening.

4.11.2.2 Surgical Technique

In the following, the technique of the TTO via three separate incisions is presented as it was described in 2016 (Hamel 2016). The calcaneal lengthening can—in very pronounced cases—be carried out in the Mosca technique (Mosca 1995), otherwise rather in the Hintermann version (Hintermann 2015) (Fig. 4.35b). The calcaneus sliding osteotomy can generally also be performed minimally invasively as an alternative. On the medial ray, a closed-wedge osteotomy is preferable for rigid feet, an open-wedge osteotomy (Cotton) for hypermobile feet.

Technique

The procedure is carried out in a supine position with the ipsilateral buttocks raised and pelvic support on the opposite side. A tourniquet is applied, and the ipsilateral anterior iliac crest is prepared. The surgery begins with a gastrocnemius lengthening (see Sect. 6.3.1), which usually shows sufficient effect. Otherwise, a percutaneous Achilles tendon lengthening can be added at the end. The first skin incision follows the split lines of the skin diagonally above the anterior calcaneal region (Fig. 4.39a). In the plantar aspect of the approach, the sural nerve is to be exposed in a short section and protected in its further course; in the dorsal aspect of the approach, attention must be paid to the dorsal sural branch and the branches of the superficial peroneal nerve. The origin of the M. extensor digitorum brevis is partially detached in an L shape directly above the peroneus brevis tendon (Figs. 4.39a and 4.42a), and the calcaneus is circumvented subperiostally about 6 mm distal to the posterior facet of the subtalar joint and thus about 15–20 mm proximal to the calcaneocuboid joint, for the Evans variant with complete severance a little further distal. On both sides of the planned osteotomy, two strong K-Wires are placed to anchor a bone distractor. The distractor (e.g., Hintermann distractor) with 1.6 mm K-wires is placed in such a way that it later allows the planned osteotomy to be spread open; however, it is removed again for the osteotomy itself. The osteotomy is first performed with the oscillating saw, then with the chisel. Depending on whether in very pronounced cases a complete osteotomy or—as a rule—only an open-wedge osteotomy is planned, the calcaneus is also carefully severed on the medial side or left intact. The Hintermann-osteotomy runs from anterolateral to posteromedial (Fig. 4.35b). The distractor is now used to spread the calcaneus so that an opening with a width of 5 to a maximum of 8 mm is created on the lateral side (Fig. 4.39b). In dorsoplantar projection control, the talonavicular joint should not be overcorrected in the transverse plane but rather still show a slight abduction in passive eversion. An appropriately large tricortical iliac crest graft mounted with a K-wire like a shashlik is inserted (Fig. 4.39b) and fixed from the distal side with a 1.6 mm K-wire (Fig. 4.40a). Transfixation of the calcaneocuboid joint does not appear necessary if the calcaneus is only slightly lengthened.

Via a separate incision (Figs. 4.40a and 4.42b), a calcaneus sliding osteotomy (see Sect. 4.11.1) is then performed. The extent of the shift is selected so that the hindfoot valgus component appears completely corrected. The already inserted K-wire is advanced further, so that it exits the skin at the heel and is supplemented by a parallel placed second K-wire to prevent malrotation (Fig. 4.40b).

After the double osteotomy of the calcaneus, the relationship between the hindfoot and the forefoot is carefully inspected. As a rule, a mid-forefoot supination in need of correction with elevation of the medial foot ray can be recognized. If in doubt, the plantarizing osteotomy should rather be performed. A 4–5 cm long longitudinal incision is made above the medial cuneiform on the dorsum of the foot, protecting the skin nerve branches and the tendon of the extensor hallucis longus muscle. Now two 1.6 mm K-wires are inserted vertically proximal and distal into the medial cuneiform. Using an image intensifier control in the dorsoplantar projection, the position of the planned osteotomy between the two K-wires is precisely checked. This osteotomy is in many cases extended laterally into the intermediate cuneiform bone. However, it is essential to protect the second tarsometatarsal joint. The osteotomy is now spread with the osteotomy distractor, which is attached to the two positioned K-wires (Figs. 4.41 and 4.42c). A second graft taken from the iliac crest with a base width of about 4–6 mm is fitted into the osteotomy. Scott et al. (2016) determined 1.9° angular correction per millimeter of base width of the inserted graft in a cadaver study. The extent of the plantarization of the medial ray can be dosed by driving in the wedge-shaped graft more or less deeply. An osteosynthesis is not necessary here. Alternatively, the Cotton osteotomy can be fixed with a dorsomedially positioned small bar plate after spreading (Fig. 4.53) in conjunction with cancellous bone grafting from the lateral bony projection on the calcaneal main fragment after the calcaneus sliding osteotomy. Especially if the anterior iliac crest does not have to be exposed anyway for calcaneal lengthening, which is replaced by a sinus tarsi spacer (Sect. 4.11.3), this avoids harvesting bone from the iliac crest.

In individual cases it is possible to refrain from cuneiform osteotomy after close clinical evaluation. Alternatively to the Cotton osteotomy, the plantarization of the medial ray at the level of the cuneiformia can be performed as a closed-wedge osteotomy (Fig. 4.43). In principle, the closed wedge variant is the obvious choice for planovalgus deformity in that it slightly shortens the extra-long medial column. This procedure is therefore

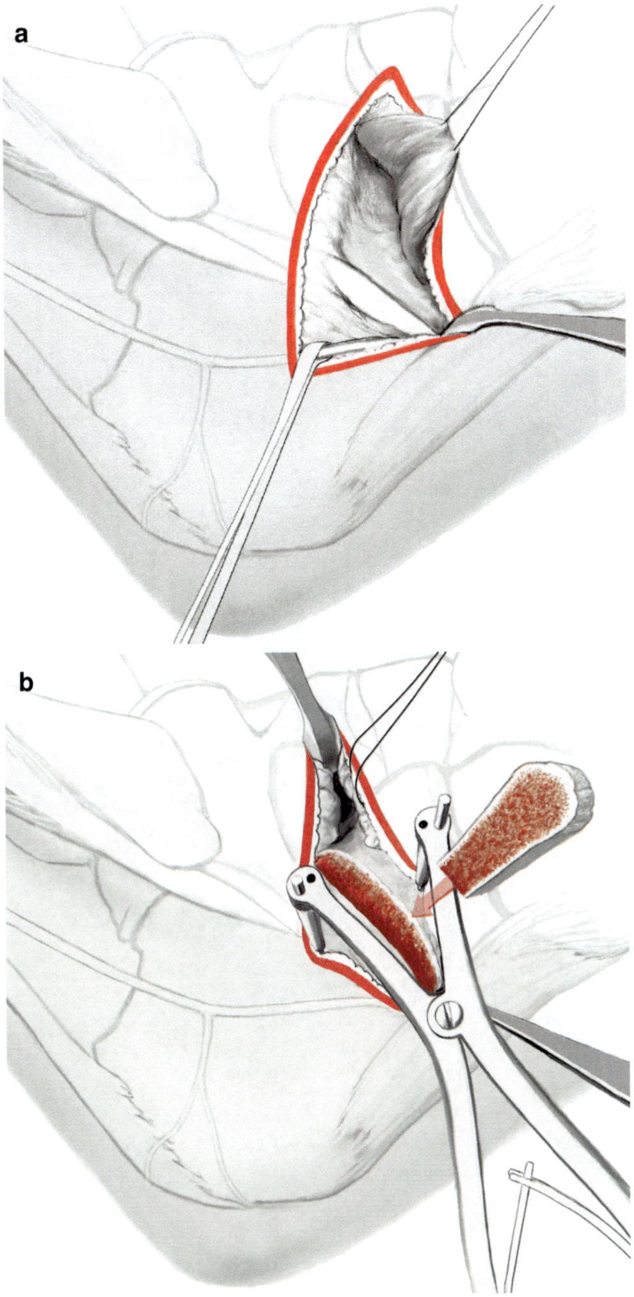

Fig. 4.39 Calcaneal lengthening osteotomy via a lateral oblique skin incision with L-shaped detachment of the extensor-digitorum-brevis origin (**a**) and insertion of a tricortical graft after osteotomy of the calcaneus (**b**)

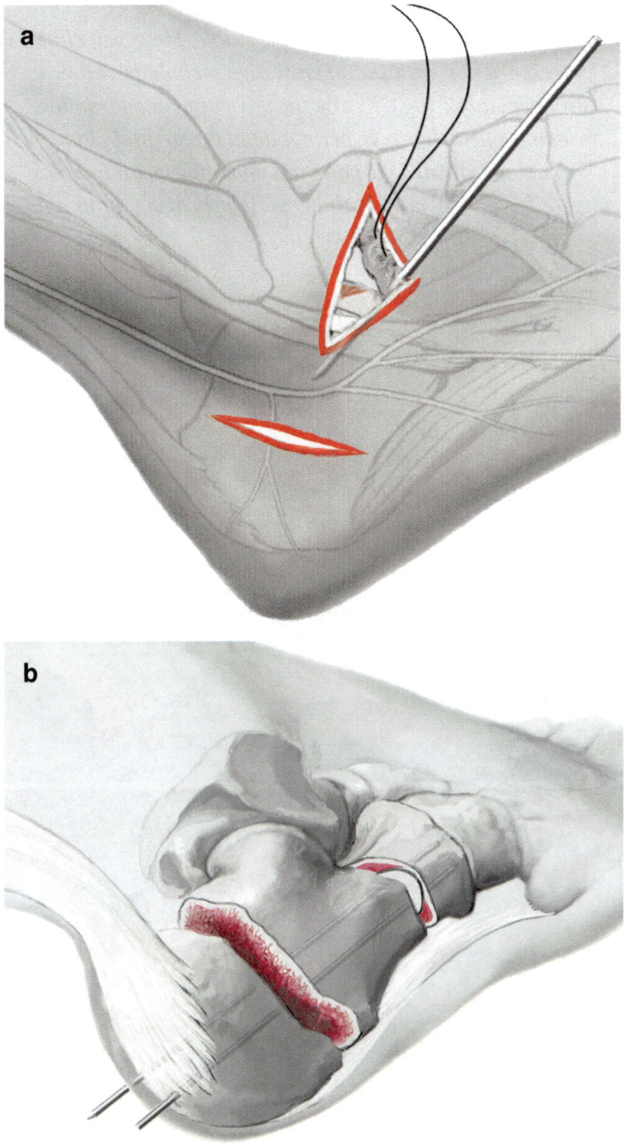

Fig. 4.40 The dosed calcaneal lengthening is supplemented by a calcaneus sliding osteotomy through a separate incision (**a**) and fixed with two Kirschner wires (**b**)

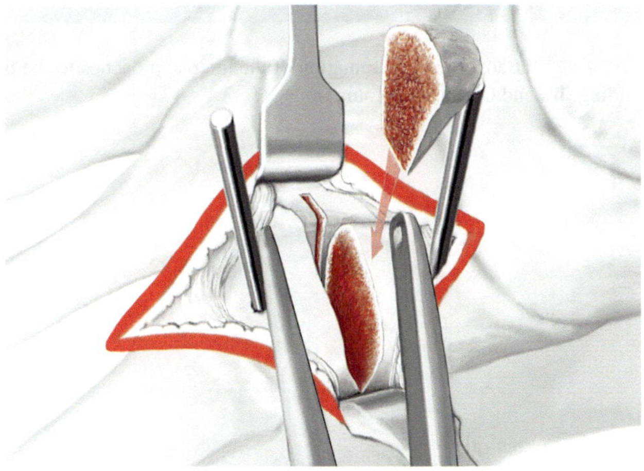

Fig. 4.41 Open-wedge osteotomy of the medial cuneiform from the extensor side with osteotomy of the intermediate cuneiform

preferable when the medial ray is stable. However, clinical experience with the open-wedge technique shows a stronger stabilizing effect on the naviculo-cuneiform line, which is often clearly hypermobile in the sagittal plane.

Postoperatively, the patient is immobilized for 6 weeks in a lower leg cast without weight-bearing until the Kirschner wires are removed from the heel. Afterwards, successive loading in the lower leg walker is possible until full loading is achieved about 10 weeks postoperatively. For about 6–8 weeks, a slightly heel-encompassing insole with support of the longitudinal arch should be worn after initiation of full weight-bearing.

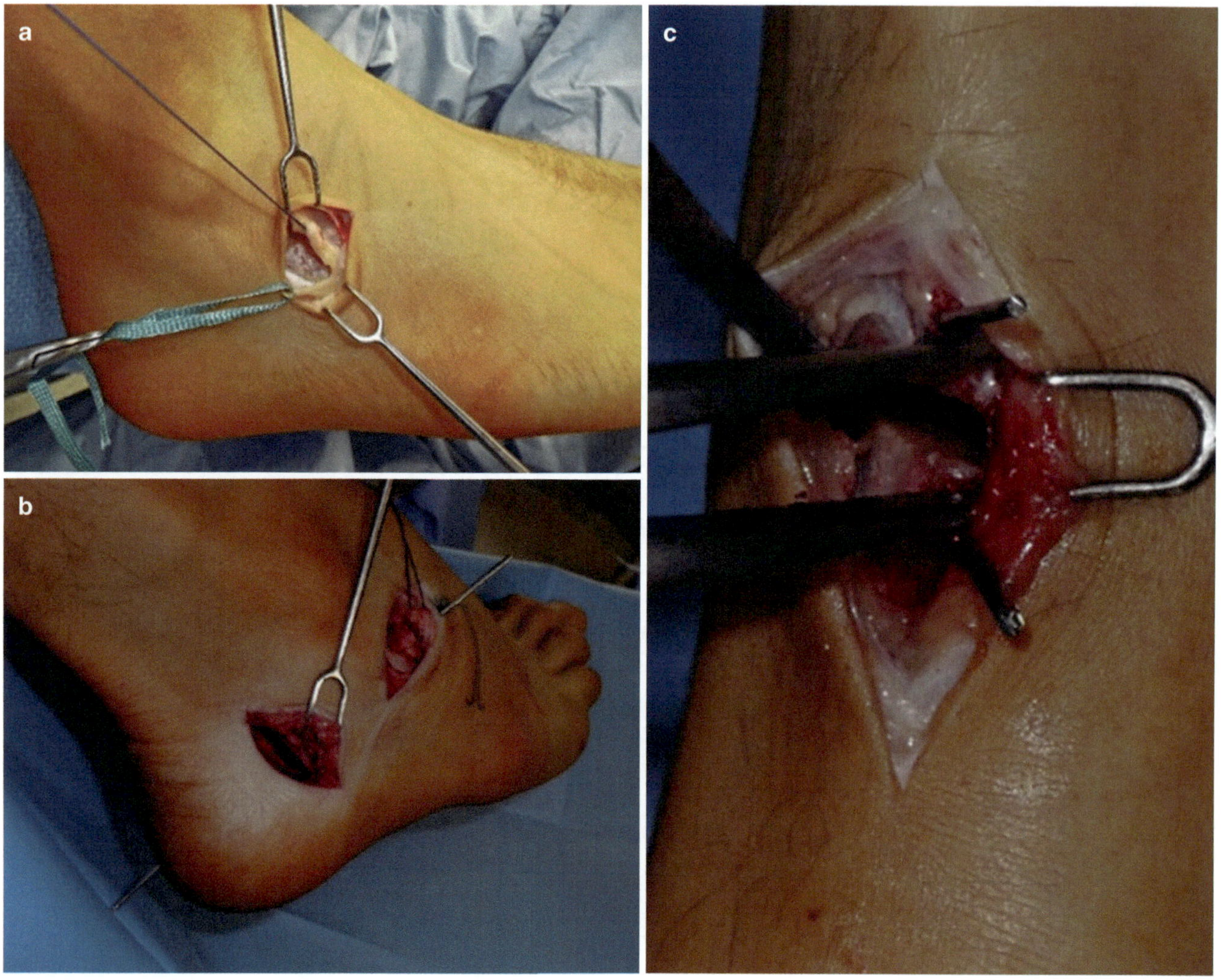

Fig. 4.42 Intraoperative presentation of the three approaches to the three osteotomy localizations of TTO, calcaneal lengthening (**a**), calcaneus sliding (**b**), and Cotton osteotomy (**c**)

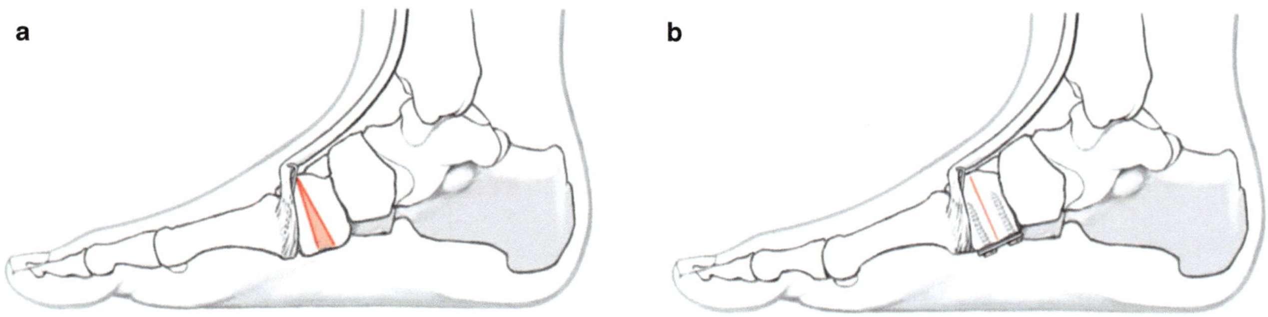

Fig. 4.43 Closed-wedge osteotomy of the medial cuneiform bone (**a**) with plantar plate fixation (**b**)

4.11.2.3 Results and Treatment Examples

The clinical results after TTO are usually very satisfactory. Often a slight pes planus component persists with good correction in the frontal and transverse planes. Compared to the isolated calcaneus lengthening performed frequently by the author before 2008, the pressure distribution in the midfoot area is more harmonious, as shown by quantitative pedographic analyses (Fig. 4.44). The significant increase in the force transmitted to the ground via the forefoot in the late stance phase (Fig. 4.47) appears remarkable, despite the gastrocnemius lengthening performed simultaneously. The values for the relative maximum force and the relative force-time integral in the area of the forefoot are approaching the normal values determined for adults (Fig. 4.44). In particular, the lateral midfoot area, which is largely relieved in a severe pes planovalgus, is again included in the load transfer during the late stance phase after TTO (Hamel et al. 2014). Two examples of maximum pressure images demonstrate how the dynamic footprint normalizes after TTO without excessive lateral overload (Figs. 4.45 and 4.46).

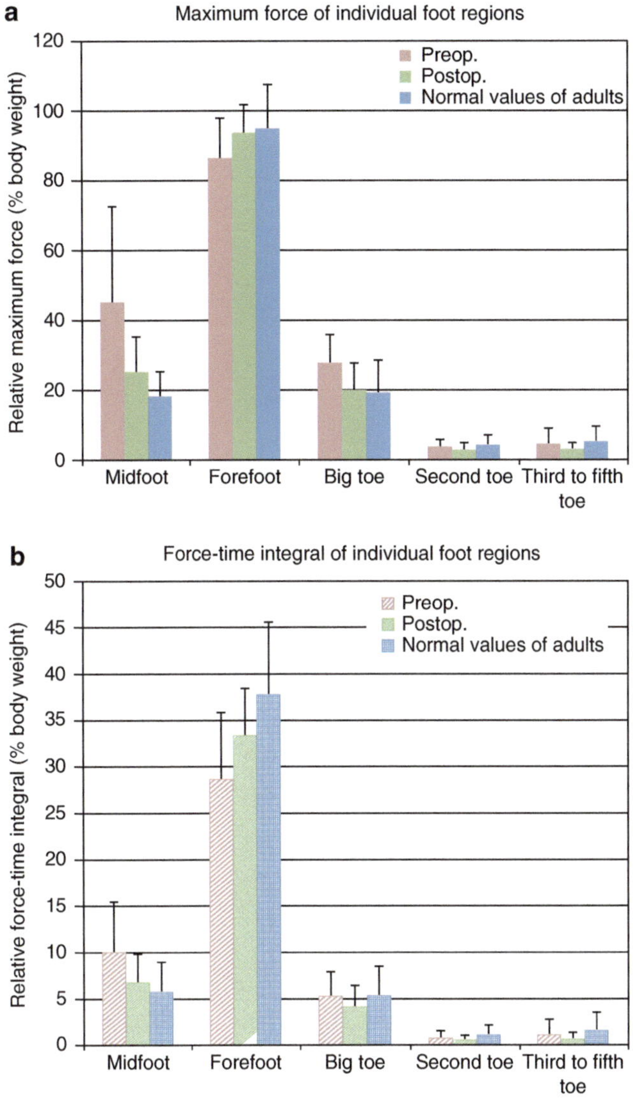

Fig. 4.44 The values of the relative maximum force (**a**) and the force-time integral (**b**) of the individual foot regions in ten cases of adolescent patients before (red bars) and after (green bars) tarsal triple osteotomy postoperatively approach the normal values determined in adults (blue bars) (from Hamel et al. 2014)

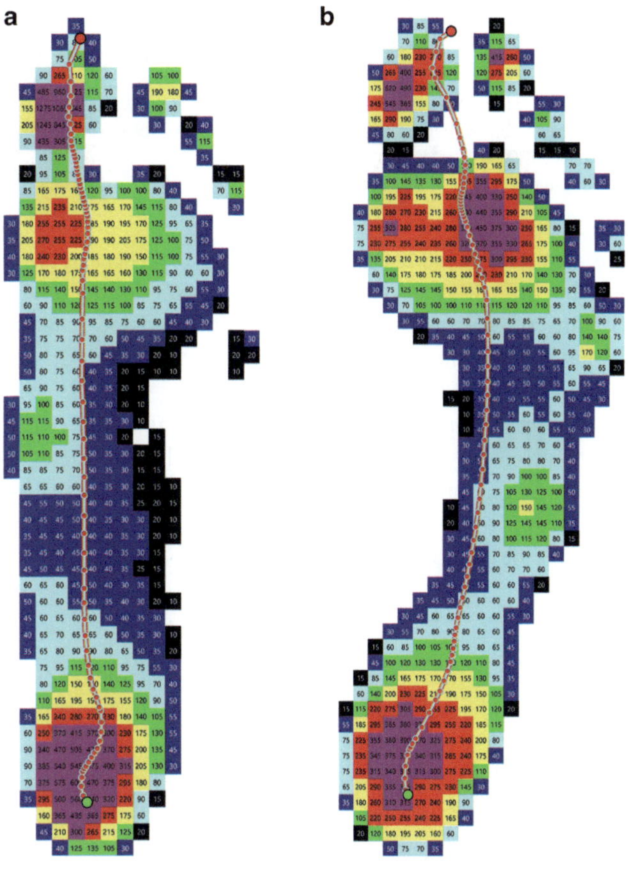

Fig. 4.45 Pre- (**a**) and 22 months postoperative (**b**) pedography in a 14-year-old patient before and after TTO with only slight overload at the lateral midfoot

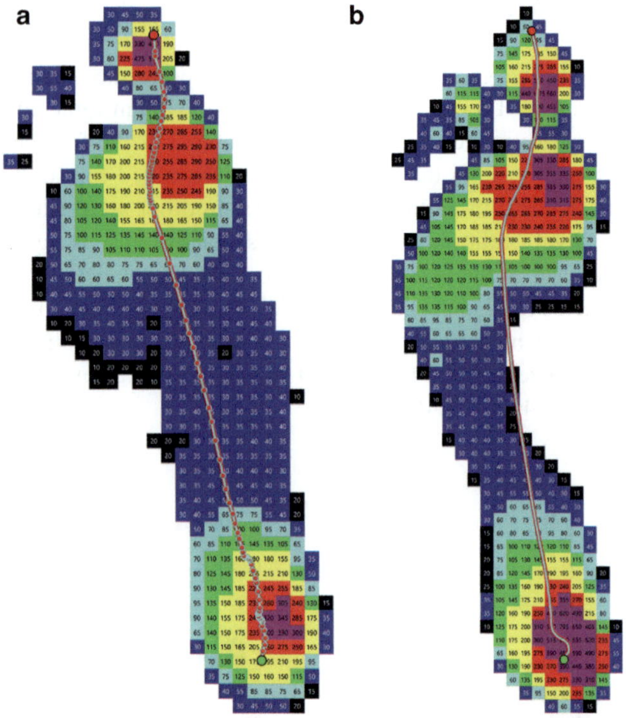

Fig. 4.46 Pre- (**a**) and 26 months postoperative (**b**) pedography in a 13-year-old patient before and after TTO

Radiologically, a correction of the TMT index from an average of −47.7° to −23.7° was demonstrated in a group of ten treatment cases (Hamel et al. 2014). The average correction of the TMT-I angle lat. was 12.8°, that of the TMT-I base angle 11.2°. The calcaneal pitch angle increased on average by 4.9°. A later evaluation of 19 treatment cases of adolescent patients showed a correction of the MASA angle as a measure of stabilization of the naviculo-cuneiform region in the sagittal plane of 9.4° on average. Three treatment examples before and after TTO demonstrate the extensive deformity correction, especially at the talonavicular joint (Figs. 4.47, 4.48, and 4.49). Good clinical results after multiple tarsal osteotomies in a comparable patient population but with a significantly lower initial deformity are found in the literature in Oh et al. (2011).

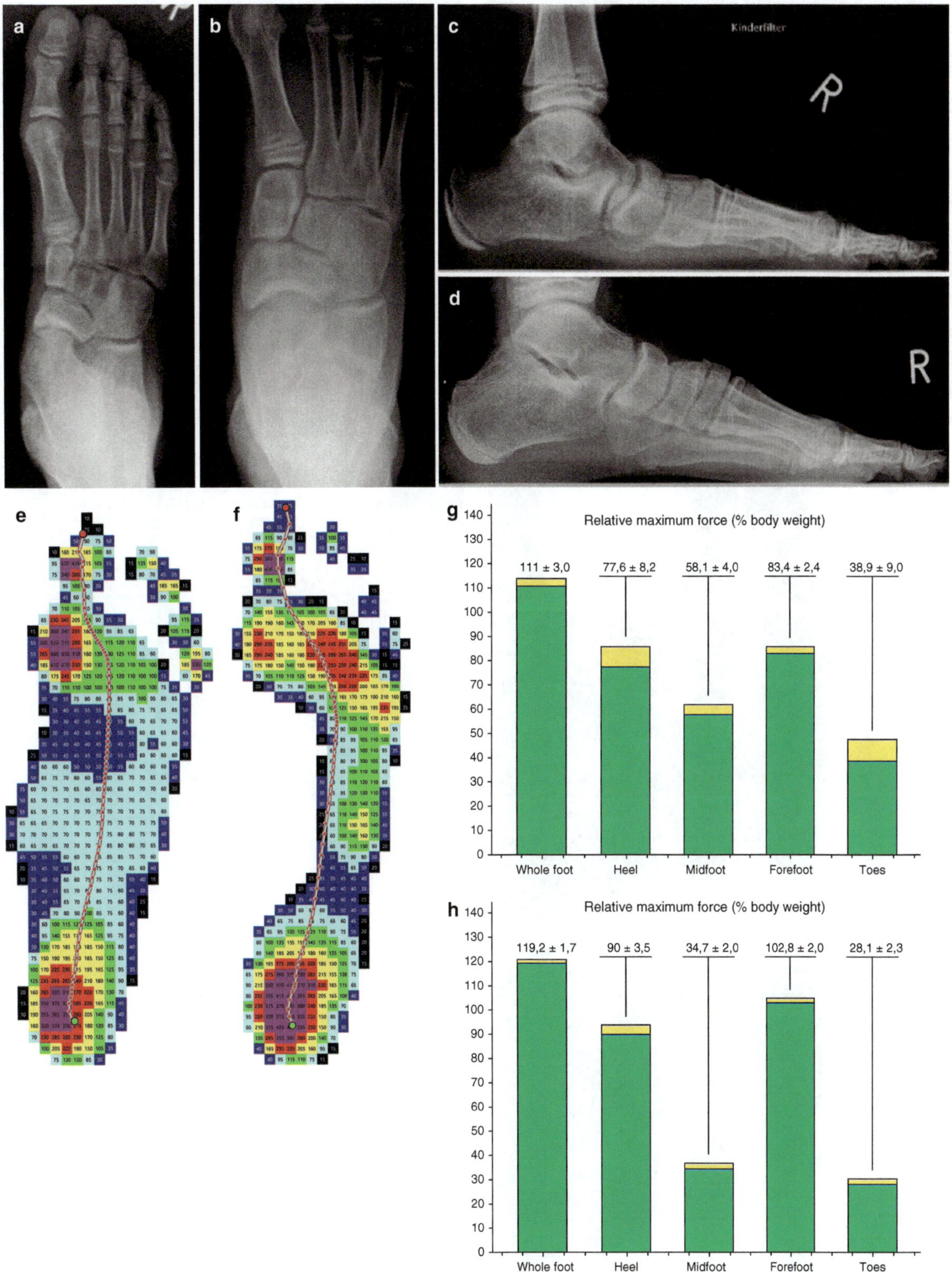

Fig. 4.47 A 13-year-old boy before (**a**, **c**, **e**) and 20 months after TTO (**b**, **d**, **f**) with severe planovalgus deformity. Radiologically complete correction with TMT index of –23° versus –58° preoperative. Pedographically postoperative (**f**) largely normalized pressure distribution with harmonious loading of medial and lateral midfoot. The analysis of the forces shows postoperatively (**h**) a clear increase in force of the forefoot in the late stance phase with reduced force application of the toes compared to preoperatively (**g**). ("Midfoot" refers to the anatomical region of the lesser tarsus, not the metatarsal head region)

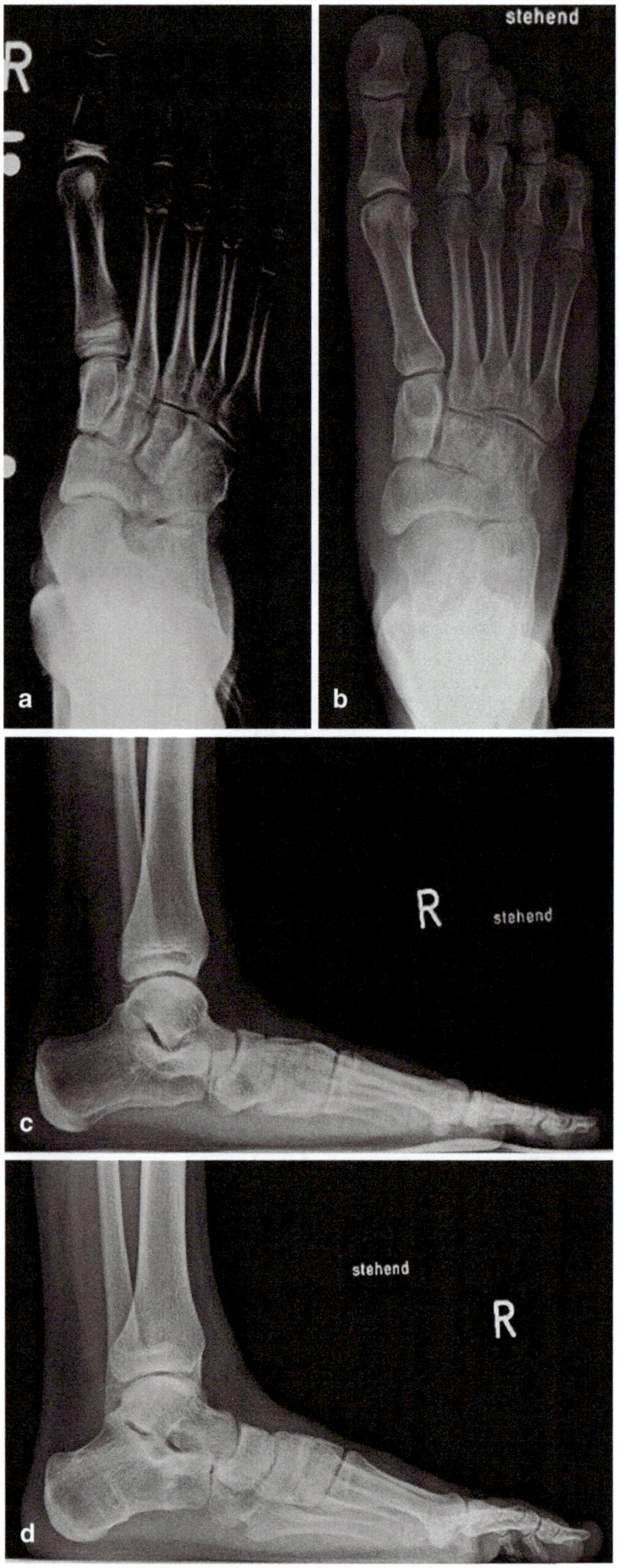

Fig. 4.48 13-Year-old boy before (**a**, **c**) and after (**b**, **d**) TTO with gastrocnemius lengthening

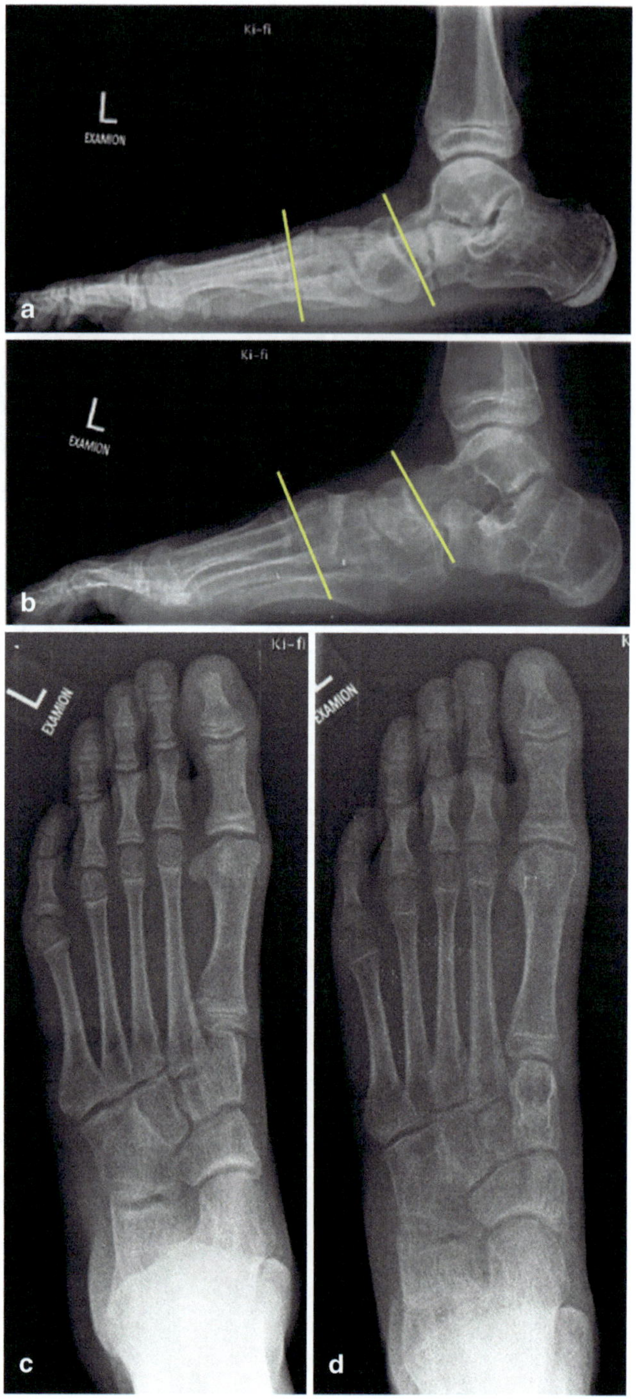

Fig. 4.49 13-Year-old boy before (**a**, **c**) and after (**b**, **d**) TTO with gastrocnemius lengthening. The MASA angle (proximal articular surfaces of the navicular and metatarsal I base) has been significantly corrected by the Cotton osteotomy (from about 15° to about 5°), the naviculo-cuneiform joint is in maximum dorsal extension in the pre- (**a**) and post-operative lateral projection (**b**)

4.11.2.4 Undesirable Results and Limits of TTO

In individual cases, the dosed calcaneal lengthening in the course of a TTO can also lead to an overload of the lateral foot rim in the metatarsal V region and the metatarsal V head itself. In adolescent patients, this often adjusts itself in the further course of the procedure. Otherwise, a re-osteotomy of the calcaneal neck can raise the distal fragment slightly and rotate it in the frontal plane around the center of the talar head as a pivotal point with a (limited) pronating effect on the mid-forefoot.

Individual cases of undercorrection with TTO have been observed by the author (Fig. 4.50). This is probably a question of the dosage of the individual correction components. In extremely hypermobile cases, a purely joint-preserving procedure is not sufficient, as an example from the initial period of the learning curve shows (Fig. 4.51). Here, partial arthrodesis should have been used (Sect. 4.12).

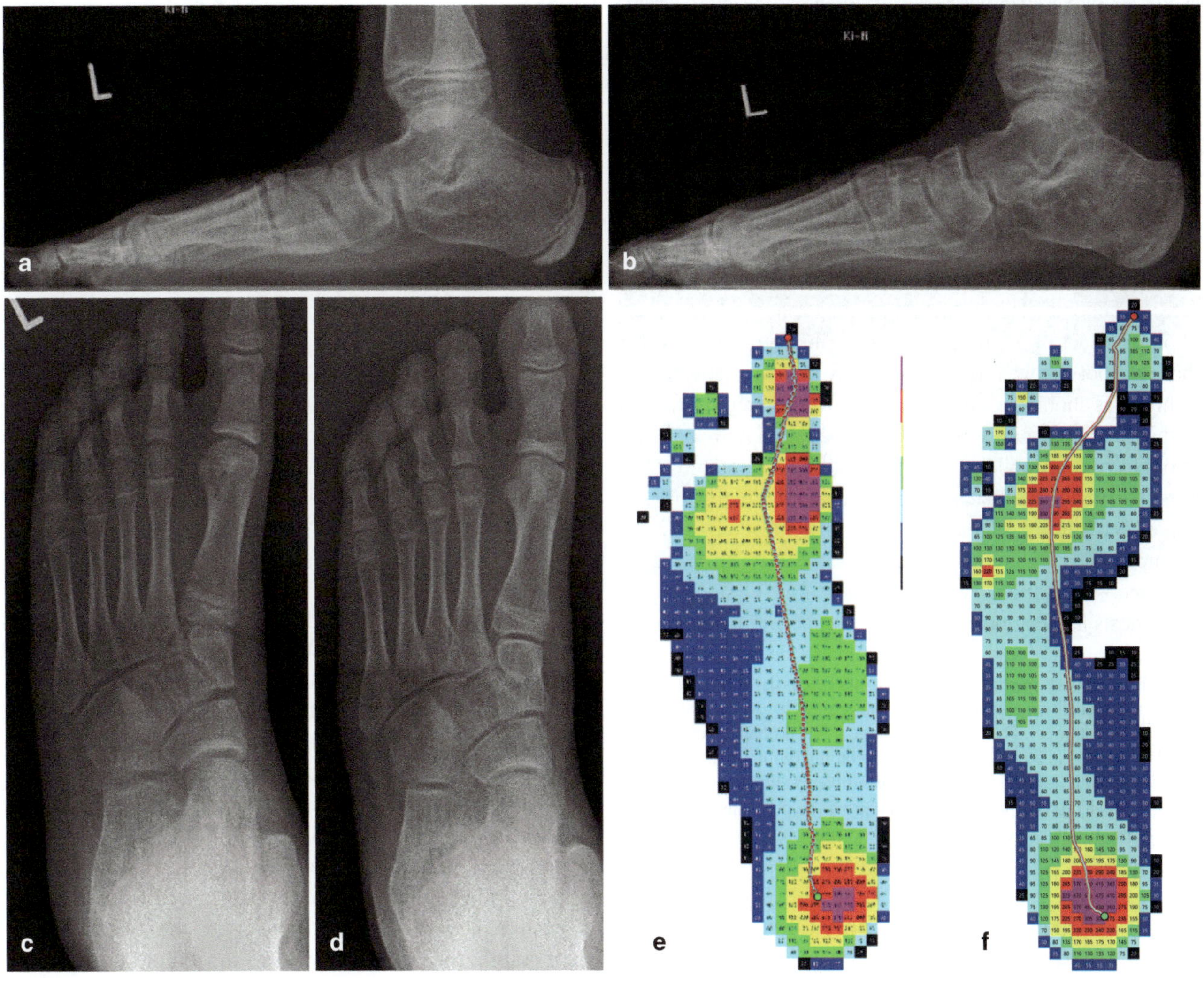

Fig. 4.50 13-Year-old boy with distinct planovalgus deformity before (**a**, **c**, **e**) and after TTO with gastrocnemius lengthening (**b**, **d**, **f**). A calcaneal lengthening of 7 mm, a shift of 11 mm, and a cuneiform medial correction of 5 mm were performed. Especially the postoperative pedogram (**f**) shows an incomplete correction

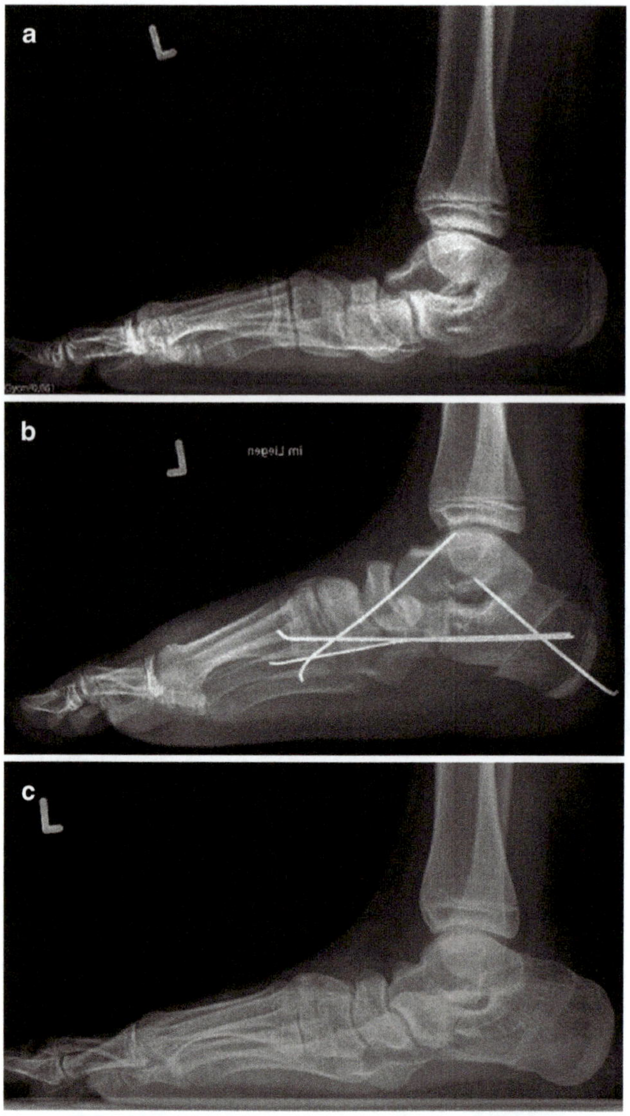

Fig. 4.51 12-Year-old boy with extreme planovalgus deformity and calcaneonavicular coalition before (a), immediately after (b), and two years after surgical correction (c). The resection of the coalition probably increased the tarsal instability, so that the tarsal triple osteotomy (with Z-shaped lengthening of the Achilles tendon and the peroneus brevis tendon and a capsuloplasty at the talonavicular joint) could not provide a permanent correction. In this case, fusion surgery in the naviculo-cuneiform area and of the talocalcaneal joint would have been appropriate

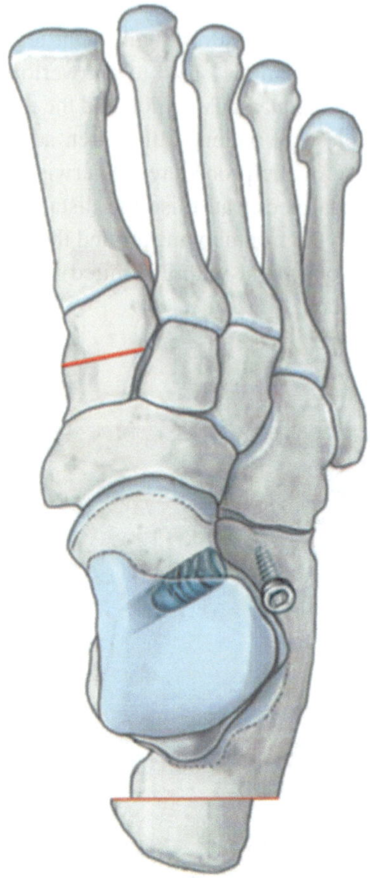

Fig. 4.52 Both forms of arthroereisis (sinus tarsi spacer or calcaneostop arthroereisis) can alternatively be combined with calcaneal sliding osteotomy and cuneiform mediale osteotomy

4.11.3 Arthroereisis-Osteotomy Combination (AOC)

Different combinations of arthroereisis with tarsal osteotomies can be considered depending on the initial findings and age (Fig. 4.52). If there is some growth reserve, a calcaneostop arthroereisis can be combined, for example, with a plantarizing osteotomy on the medial ray (Fig. 4.53). After completion of growth, the calcaneal lengthening osteotomy of the TTO can be replaced by a spacer arthroereisis (Fig. 4.54). Even in severe deformities, the spacer can replace calcaneal lengthening procedure in order to correct mid-forefoot abduction in the transversal plane (Fig. 4.55). The author has had good experiences with this procedure, denoted as "AOC", in cases which already seemed too old or too pronounced for an isolated arthroereisis. The three components unfold their stabilizing effect in the three dimensions of the space to varying degrees and thus act in a complementary way to each other. The forces acting on the spacer or the arthroereisis screw seem to be reduced, so that the danger of pain or dislocation can be minimized.

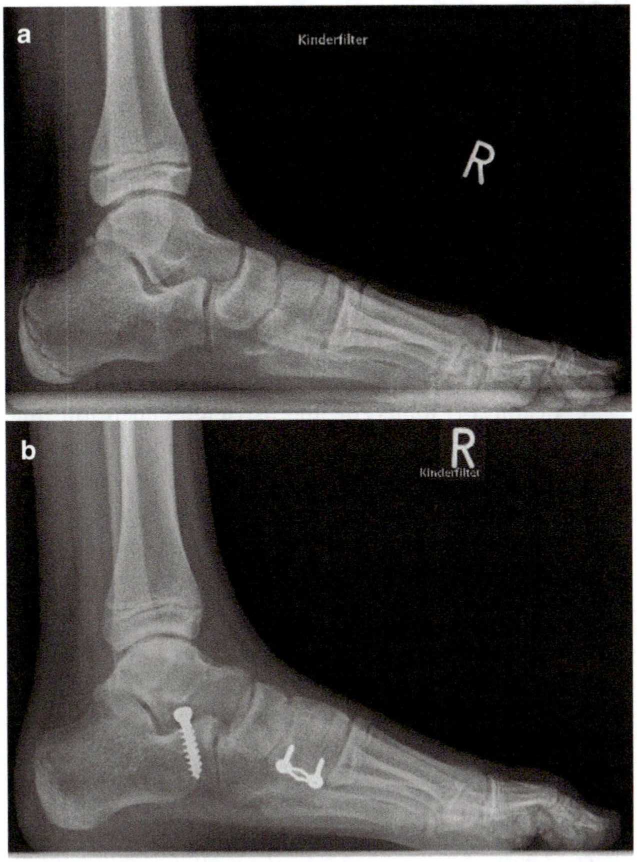

Fig. 4.53 12-Year-old boy before (**a**) and after calcaneostop arthroereisis with calf muscle lengthening and plantarizing medial cuneiform osteotomy (**b**)

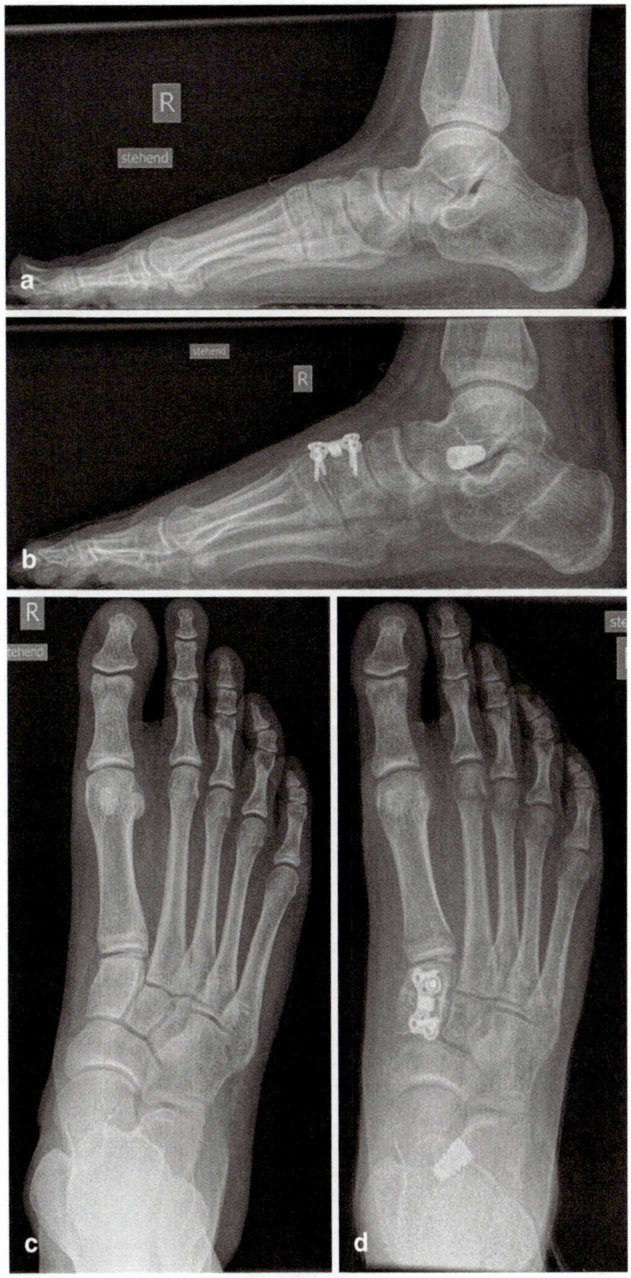

Fig. 4.54 14-Year-old female patient with static complaints with distinct planovalgus deformity before (**a**, **c**) and after (**b**, **d**) tarsal osteotomies (calcaneus sliding and Cotton osteotomy) in connection with a spacer arthroereisis

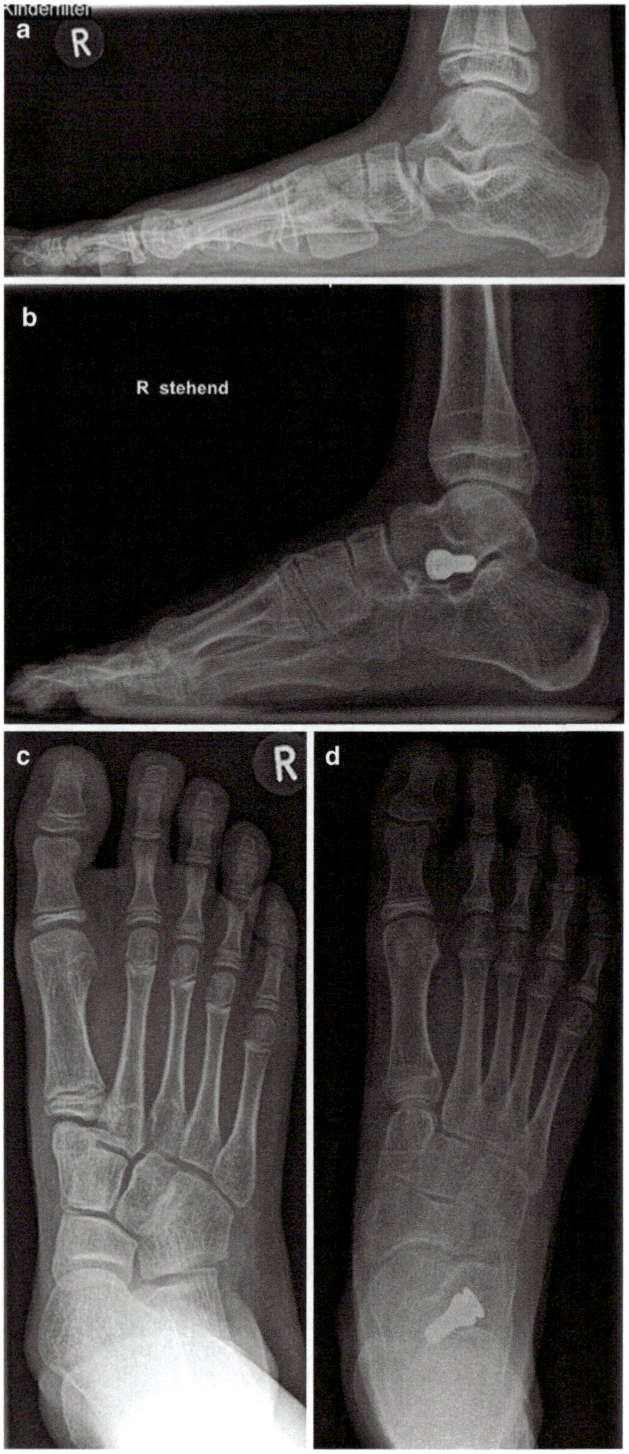

Fig. 4.55 12-Year-old boy with severe flexible planovalgus deformity before (**a**, **c**) and two years after AOC (**b**, **d**) including calcaneal sliding osteotomy and closed-wedge osteotomy at the medial cuneiform bone

4.12 Tarsal Corrective Fusions

In the case of higher degrees of instability in schoolchildren, a (partial) fusion should also be considered. The positive stabilizing effect usually clearly outweighs the resulting loss of function. However, the "hierarchy" of the hindfoot joints (Sect. 6.2.2) must always be taken into account, especially the high functional importance of the talonavicular joint. Isolated fusions of the naviculo-cuneiform joint line, talocalcaneal fusion, or fusion with inclusion of the Chopart joint are possible solutions. This will be demonstrated using different treatment examples.

A fusion of joints of the naviculo-cuneiform line (Fig. 4.56), which at the normal foot has only slight mobility in the sagittal plane but may be severely hypermobile in planovalgus deformity, does not cause a significant loss of function. However, exact alignment of the hindfoot-forefoot relationship is essential here for optimal load distribution at the midfoot. Figures 4.57, 4.58, and 4.59 show further examples.

Technique

From a medial incision the naviculo-cuneiform joint line is opened and distracted with a bone distractor with careful protection of the anterior tibial tendon. The cartilage is removed from the medial and intermediate chamber, and the subchondral bone is prepared by multiple drilling. The mounted bone distractor can be used with rotational movements to achieve the optimal alignment in a plantarized position, which is held by K-wires. For osteosynthetic stabilization three compression screws are placed under control with the image intensifier (Figs. 4.56).

Pronounced tarsal hypermobility can also be stabilized in growth age by talocalcaneal arthrodesis, e.g., in the extra-articular technique according to Grice (1952) (Figs. 4.60 and 4.63) or Denneyson and Fulford (1976), to such an extent that a useful partial mobility is maintained in the functionally important Chopart line (Fig. 6.15). Overcorrection must be avoided, and a plantarizing measure on the medial ray is usually necessary to eliminate the thus unmasked midfoot and forefoot supination.

Extreme deformities such as those shown in Figs. 4.51 and 4.61a, c should be stabilized from the age of about 10–12 years by tarsal arthrodeses involving the talonavicular joint (Fig. 4.61b, d; 4.62b); otherwise, a definitive deformity correction cannot be expected. In such cases, the functional improvements are impressive, as can be seen from the increase in strength of the calf muscles and thus the forefoot load.

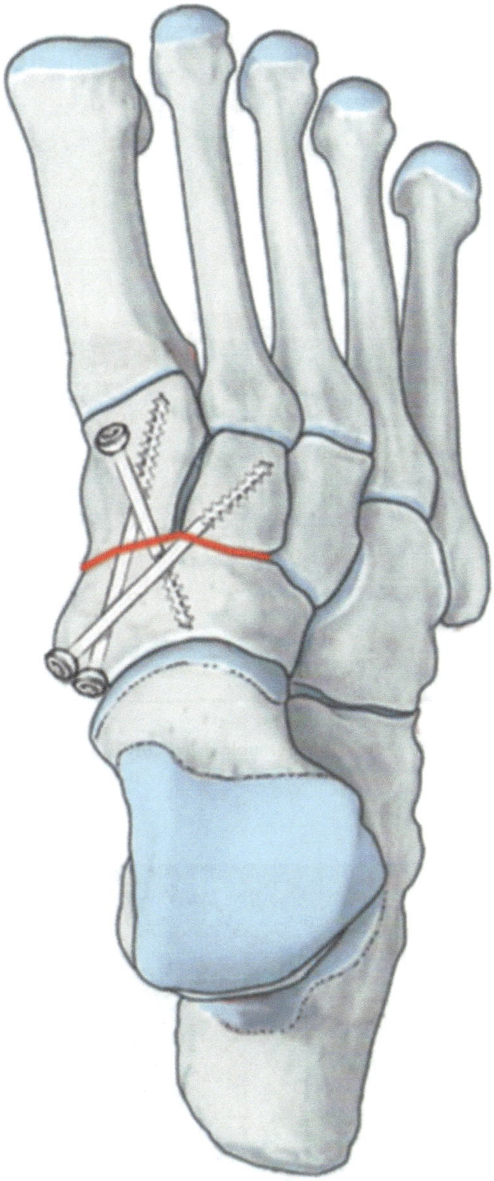

Fig. 4.56 Fusion of the medial and intermediate chamber of the naviculo-cuneiform joint line. For osteosynthetic stabilization three compression screws are used. Two of these screws are inserted at the medial navicular pole. The screw crossing the medial naviculo-cuneiform joint is placed plantar

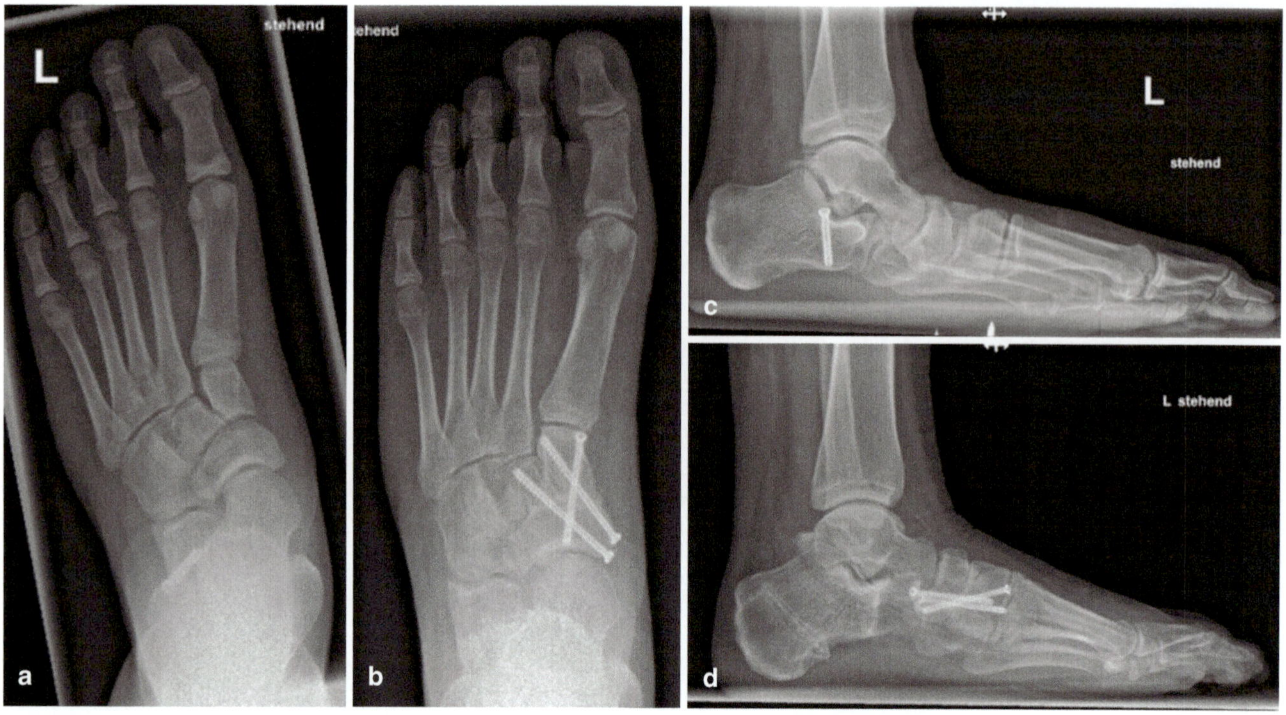

Fig. 4.57 15-Year-old patient with insufficient arthroereisis performed in another hospital earlier (**a**, **c**). Double osteotomy of the calcaneus was combined with naviculo-cuneiform fusion (**b**, **d**)

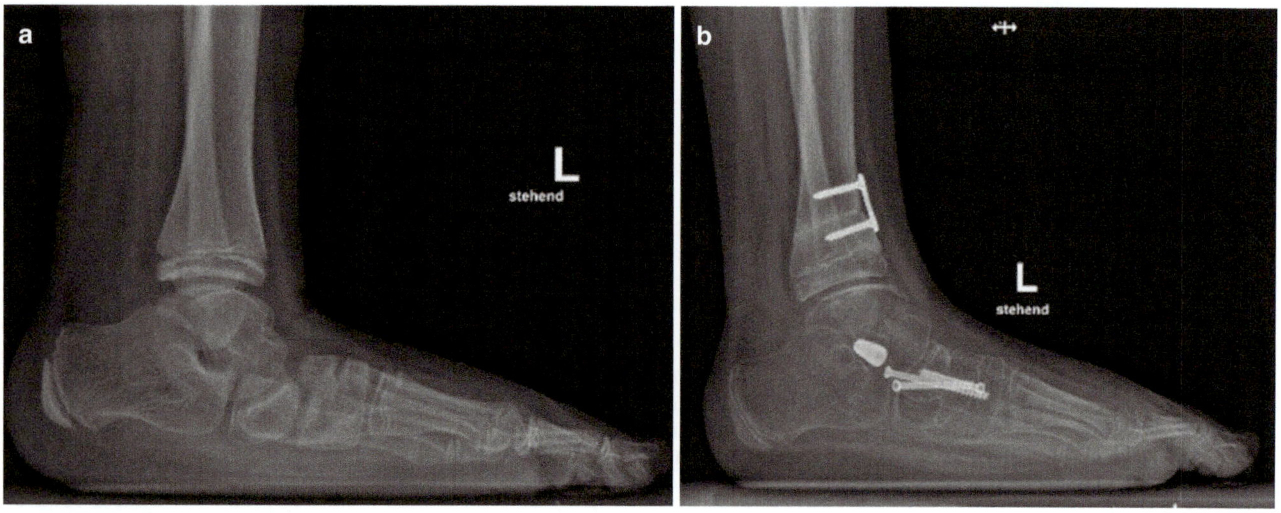

Fig. 4.58 15-Year-old boy with extreme deformity at the naviculo-cuneiform joint line (**a**). The medial tarsometatarsal ray was corrected and stabilized with naviculo-cuneiform fusion (**b**). A supramalleolar extension osteotomy was added in order not to overstrain the compensation capacity of the tibiotalar joint

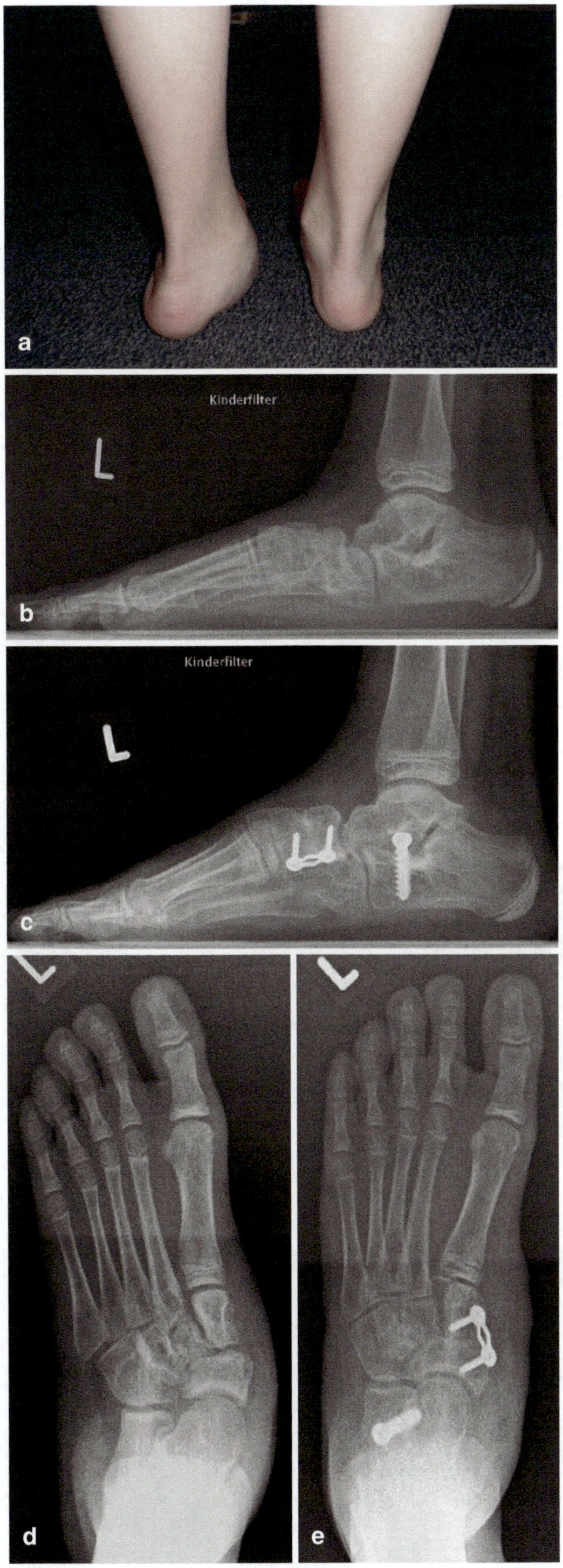

Fig. 4.59 10-Year-old girl with unilateral severe planovalgus deformity in neurofibromatosis. The extreme deformity on the left side (**a**, **b**, **d**) was optically enhanced by a plexiform neurofibroma in the medial tarsal region. The hindfoot could be stabilized by a calcaneostop arthroereisis, the naviculo-cuneiform line was corrected three-dimensionally by arthrodesis (**c**, **e**)

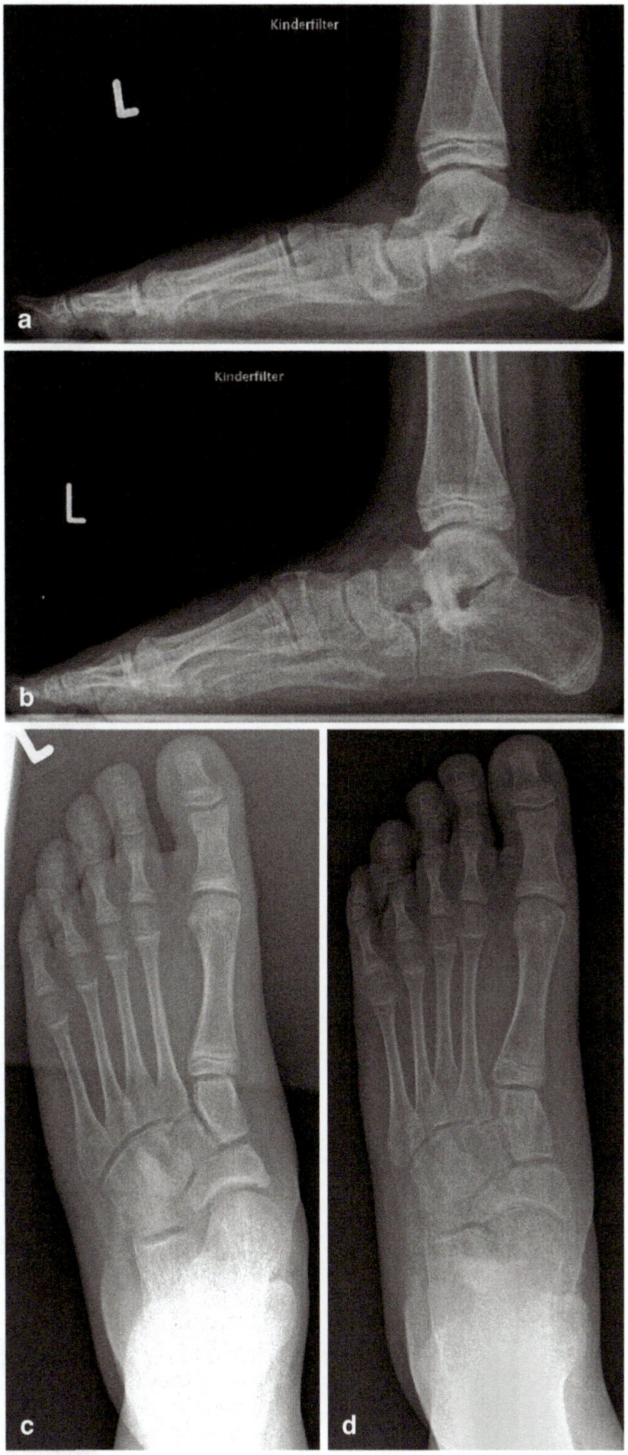

Fig. 4.60 11-Year-old boy with extreme tarsal hypermobility and pronounced plantar flexion of the talus (**a**, **c**). Here, stabilization was achieved with an extra-articular arthrodesis according to Grice, and the midfoot-forefoot supination was additionally corrected by plantarizing medial cuneiform osteotomy. An open Achilles tendon lengthening was performed (**b**, **d**)

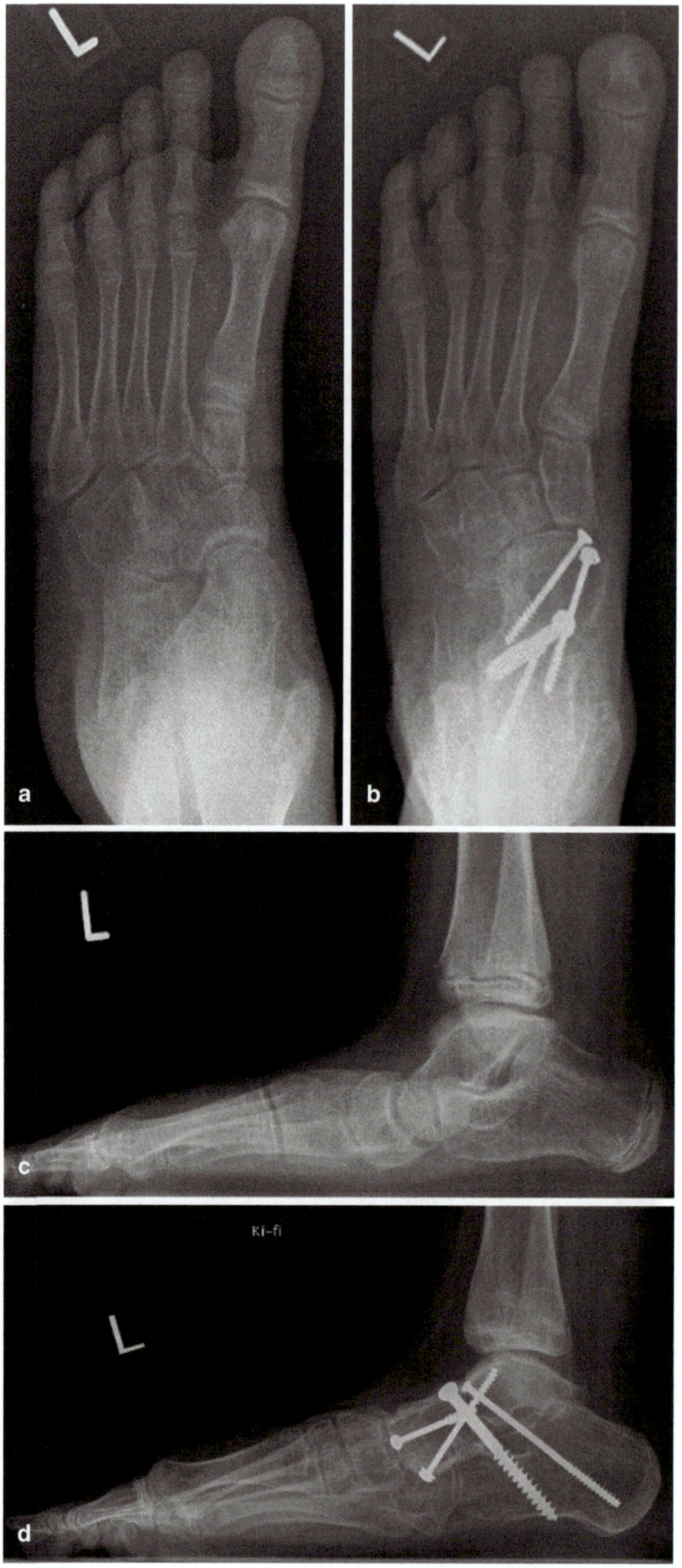

Fig. 4.61 11-Year-old boy, underlying syndromal disease with severe hypermobile planovalgus deformity (**a** and **c**). In this case only talonavicular and talocalcaneal arthrodesis seemed suitable to stabilize the severe deformity permanently (**b** and **d**). Additionally, osteotomies were performed in the lesser tarsal region to correct the mid-forefoot adduction component. The slight incongruity of the ankle joint after distinct talar correction in the sagittal plane is visible (**d**). The persistent elevation of the medial ray could have been corrected by a medial cuneiform osteotomy

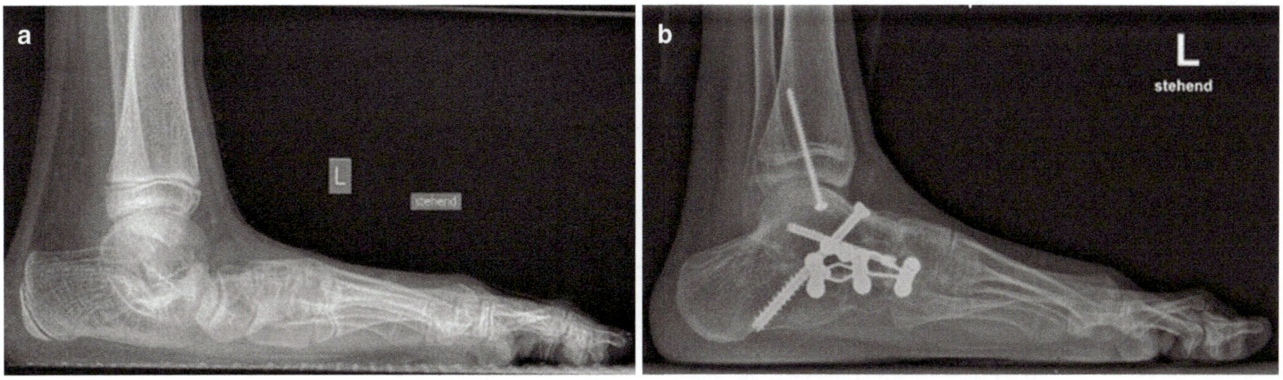

Fig. 4.62 14-Year-old male patient with Marfan syndrome and extreme tarsal instability (**a**). Triple fusion with additional stabilization of naviculo-cuneiform joint line was necessary to achieve permanent realignment (**b**). Hemiepiphysiodesis at the distal tibia was added to correct supramalleolar valgus deformity

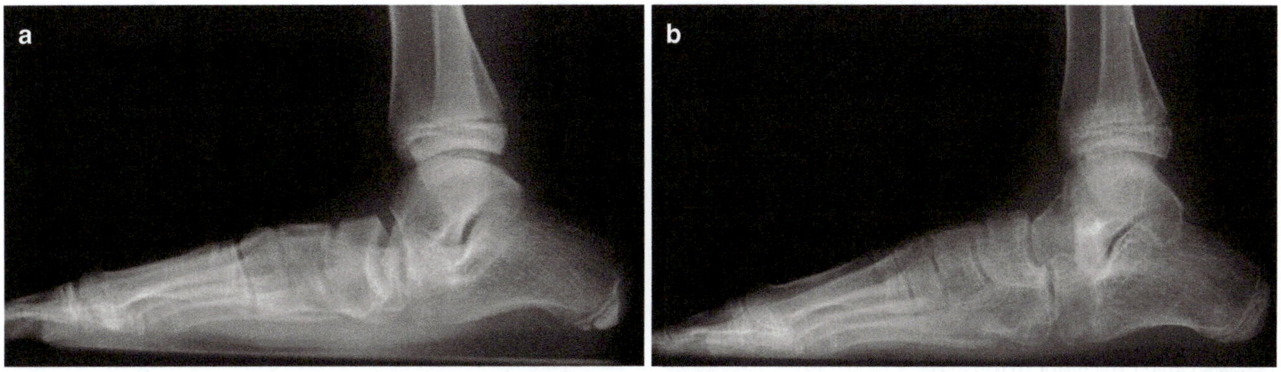

Fig. 4.63 In this case of an already 12-year-old female patient, a partial tarsal correction with an extremely plantar-flexed talus (**a**) was carried out by Grice arthrodesis, deliberately leaving a moderate plantar flexion of the talus (**b**) in order not to overtax the compensatory capacity of the ankle joint.

In cases with severe plantarflexion of the talus, the compensatory capacity of the ankle joint must always be considered (Figs. 4.58 and 4.61). Partial tarsal correction may be preferable in order to avoid incongruity and early degenerative changes in the anterior ankle joint (Fig. 4.63, see Fig. 6.14).

4.13 Differential Indication

Figure 4.64 shows a rough algorithm for the surgical treatment of severe pes planovalgus in schoolchildren and adolescents. The planning of borderline indications and combined interventions requires special consideration. The dosage and fine adjustment of individual measures has received little attention in the literature to date. Due to the different tarsal-mechanical conditions (planar dominance), a very individual approach is often necessary. Bourdet et al. (2013) favor arthroereisis for the "subtalar" planovalgus type and calcaneal lengthening for the "midtarsal planovalgus type." A further refinement of the therapeutic algorithm can be expected in the future. In particular, it seems possible to replace the calcaneal lengthening with a temporarily inserted sinus tarsi spacer in the context of tarsal corrective osteotomies in cases where the mid-forefoot abduction is not too pronounced, thus dispensing with the bone harvesting on the iliac crest.

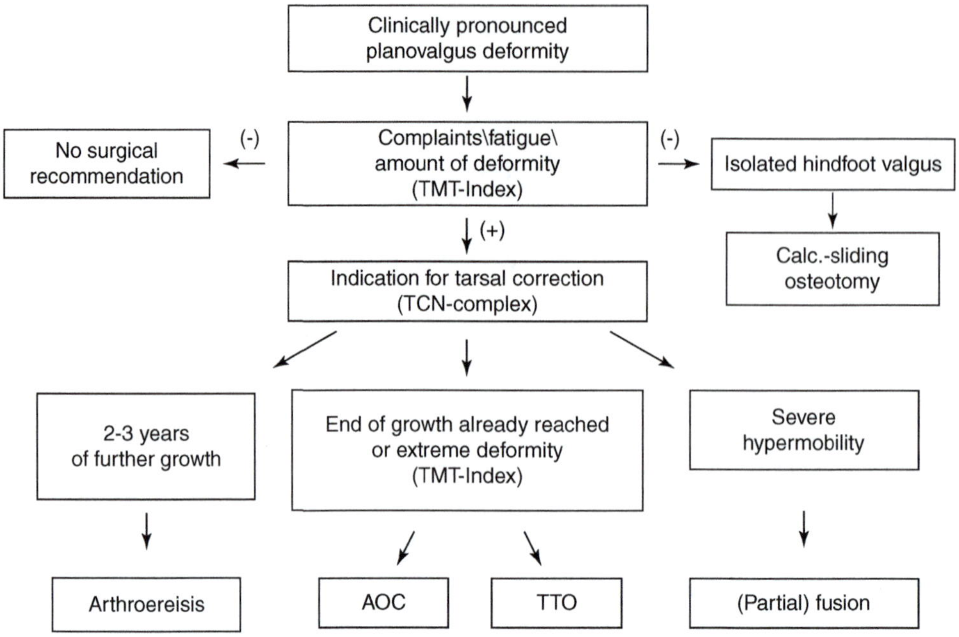

Fig. 4.64 Algorithm of surgical stabilization in flexible pes planovalgus in later age of schoolchildren and adolescents (*TCN complex* talocalcaneonavicular complex, *AOC* arthroereisis-osteotomy combination, *TTO* tarsal triple osteotomy)

References

Abbara-Czardybon M, Frank D, Arbab D (2014) Die Talus-Stopp-Schraubenarthrorise beim flexiblen kindlichen Pes planovalgus. Oper Orthop Traumatol 26:625–631

Aiyer A, Dall GF, Shub J, Myerson MS (2016) Radiographic correction following reconstruction of adult acquired flat foot deformity using the Cotton medial cuneiform osteotomy. Foot Ankle Int 37:508–513

Alman BA, Craig CL, Zimbler S (1993) Subtalar arthrodesis for stabilization of valgus hindfoot in patients with cerebral palsy. J Pediatr Orthop 13:634–641

Arbab D, Frank D, Bouillon B, Lüring C, Wingenfeld C, Abbara-Czardybon M (2017) Die subtalare Schraubenarthrorise zur Behandlung des symptomatischen, flexiblen Pes planovalgsu—Ergebnisse und eine aktuelle Literaturübersicht. Z Orthop Unfall 156:93–99

Arnold H, Weber J (2010) Die subtalare Arthrorise mittels Endorthese zur Behandlung des "idiopathischen" kindlichen Pes planovalgus—Indikation und Ergebnisse. FussSprungg 8:253–258

Basmajian JV, Stecko G (1963) The role of muscles in arch support of the foot. J Bone Joint Surg 45-A:1184–1190

Beatson TR, Pearson JR (1966) A method of assessing correction of clubfoot. J Bone Joint Surg 48-B:40–50

Benthien RA, Parks BG, Guyton GP, Schon LC (2007) Lateral column calcaneal lengthening, flexor digitorum longus transfer and opening wedge medial cuneiform osteotomy for flexible flatfoot: a biomechanical study. Foot Ankle Int 28:70–77

Böhm H, Döderlein L, Fujak A, Dussa CU (2019) Is there a correlation between static radiographs and dynamic foot function in pediatric foot deformities? Foot Ankle Surg. https://doi.org/10.1016/j.fas.2019.10.006

Bourdet C, Seringe R, Adamsbaum C, Glorion C, Wicart P (2013) Flatfoot in children and adolescents. Analysis of imaging findings and therapeutic implications. Orthop Traumatol 99:80–87

Choi JY, Lee DJ, Kim SJ, Suh JS (2020) Does the long-term use of medial arch support insole induce the radiographic structural changes for pediatric flat foot? A prospective comparative study. Foot Ankle Surg 26(4):449–456. https://doi.org/10.1016/j.fas.2019.05.017

Coleman SS (1983) Complex foot deformities in children. Lea & Febiger, Philadelphia

Cotton FJ (1936) Foot statics and surgery. N Engl J Med 214:353–362

Davids JR, Gibson W, Pugh LI (2005) Quantitative segmental analysis of weight-bearing radiographs of the foot and ankle for children—normal alignment. J Pediatr Orthop 25:769–776

Davitt JS, Williams BAM, Armstrong PF (2001) Plantar pressure and radiographic changes after distal calcaneal lengthening in children and adolescents. JPO 21:70–75

Denneyson WG, Fulford GE (1976) Subtalar arthrodesis by cancellous grafts and metallic internal fixation. J Bone Joit Surg 58-B:507–510

Döderlein L, Wenz W, Mau H, Axt M (1998) Die Behandlung des Knick-Plattfußes mit der Kalkaneusverlängerungsosteotomie. Oper Orthop Traumatol 10:219–231

Döderlein L, Wenz W, Schneider U (2002) Der Knickplattfuß. Springer Verlag, Berlin, Heidelberg, New York

Evans D (1975) Calcaneo-valgus deformity. J Bone Joint Surg 57-B:270–278

Giannestras NJ (1976) Foot disorders, Second edition. Lea & Febiger, Philadelphia

Gould N (1983) Evaluation of hyperpronation and pes planus in adults. Clin Orthop 181:37–45

Green DR, Williams ML (2013) Arthroereisis. In: Southerland JT et al (eds) Mc Glamry's Comprehensive textbook of foot and ankle surgery. Wolters Kluwer Lippincott Williams & Wilkins, Philadelphia

Grice DS (1952) An extra-articular arthrodesis of the subastragalar joint for correction of paralytic flat feet in children. J Bone Joint Surg 34-A:927–940

Gutierrez PR, Lara MH (2005) Giannini prosthesis for flatfoot. Foot Ankle Int 26:918–926

Hamel J (2010a) Radiologisch-dokumentierte Korrektureffekte beim kindlichen Pes planovalgus mit der Calcaneostop-Arthrorise und der Calcaneus-Verlängerungsosteotomie. FussSprungg 8:42–46

Hamel J (2010b) Die Calcaneostop-Arthrorise—eine retrospective klinische Studie mit Komplikations-Analyse. FussSprungg 8:35–41

Hamel J (2016) Planovalguskorrektur durch tarsale Triple-Osteotomie (TTO). In: Hamel J, Zwipp H (eds) Sprunggelenk und Rückfuß. Springer-Verlag, Berlin, Heidelberg
Hamel J, Hörterer H, Harrasser N (2020) Der Talometatarsalindex ("TMT-Index"), Orthopäde. https://doi.org/10.1007/s00132-020-03954-0.
Hamel J, Kinast C (2006) Der TMT-Index zur radiologischen Quantifizierung von Planovalgus-Deformitäten. FussSprungg 4:221–226
Hamel J, Nell M (2016) Instabilität und Deformität in der Naviculo-Cuneiforme-Gelenklinie—fußchirurgische Bedeutung und eigene Beobachtungen bei Planovalgus-Korrekturen. FussSprungg 14:195–203
Hamel J, Kissling C, Heimkes B, Stotz S (1994) A combined bony and soft-tissue tarsal stabilization procedure (Grice-Schede) for hind-foot valgus in children with cerebral palsy. Arch Orthop Trauma Surg 113:237–243
Hamel J, Nell M, Kalpen A (2014) Das Konzept der Tarsalen Triple-Osteotomie (TTO) zur 3-D-Korrektur schwerer Pes planovalgus-Deformitäten—erste radiologisch-pedographische Ergebnisse im Adoleszentenalter. FussSprungg 12:160–169
Hansen ST (2010) Adult consequences of pediatric foot disorders. In: McCarthy JJ, Drennan JC (eds) Drennan's the child's foot and ankle, second edition. Lippincott, Philadelphia, pp 526–530
Hell A, Döderlein L, Eberhardt O et al (2018) S2-Guideline: pediatric flat foot. Z Orthop Unfall 156:306–315
Hintermann B (2015) Laterale Verlängerungsosteotomie des Kalkaneus. Oper Orthop Traumatol 27:298–307
Hirose CB, Johnson JE (2004) Plantarflexion opening wedge medial cuneiforme osteotomy for correction of fixed forefoot varus associated with flatfoot deformity. Foot Ankle Int 25:568–574
Hösl M, Böhm H, Multerer C, Döderlein L (2014) Does excessive flatfoot deformity affect function? A comparison between symptomatic and asymptomatic flatfeet using the Oxford Foot Model. Gait Posture 29(1):23–28
Indino C, Villafane JH, D'Ambrosi R et al (2020) Effectiveness of subtalar arthroereisis with endorthesis for pediatric flexible flat foot: a retrospective cross-sectional study with final follow up at skeletal maturity. Foot Ankle Surg 26:98–104
Inman VT (1976) The joints of the ankle. Williams & Wilkins, Baltimore
Isman RE, Inman VT (1968) Antropometric studies of the human foot and ankle. Biomechanics Laboratory, University of California, San Francisco and Berkeley. Technical Report 58. The Laboratory, San Francisco
Kuhn H, Zuther W, Heine A, Küster HH (2010) Die subtalare Arthrorise mittels Kalix-Implantat beim flexiblen Knick-Senkfuß. FussSprungg 8:48–54
Mahan KT (1992) Pes planovalgus deformity. In: Mc Glamry ED, Banks AS, Downey MS (eds) Comprehensive textbook of foot surgery, second edition, vol 1. Williams & Wilkins, Baltimore
Mahan KT, Flanigan KP (2013) Flexible valgus deformity. In: Southerland JT et al (eds) Mc Glamry's Comprehensive textbook of foot and ankle surgery. Wolters Kluwer/Lippincott Williams & Wilkins, Philadelphia
Metcalfe SA, Bowling FL, Reeves ND (2011) Subtalar joint arthroereisis in the management of pediatric flexible flatfoot: a critical review of the literature. Foot Ankle Int 32:1127–1139
Moraleda L, Salcedo M, Bastrom TP, Wenger DR, Albinana J, Mubarak SJ (2012) Comparison of the calcaneo-cuboid-cuneiform ostotomies and the calcaneal lengthening osteotomy in the surgical treatment of symptomatic flexible flatfoot. J Pediatr Orthop 32:821–829
Mosca VS (1995) Calcaneal lengthening for valgus deformity of the hindfoot. Results in children who had severe, symptomatic flatfoot and skewfoot. J Bone Joint Surg 77-A:500–512
Mosca VS (2010a) Flexible flatfoot and skewfoot. In: McCarthy JJ, Drennan JC (eds) The child's foot and ankle. Wolters Kluwer/Lippincott Williams & Wilkins, Philadelphia
Mosca VS (2010b) Flexible flatfoot in children and adolescents. J Child Orthop 4:107–121
Mosca VS (2014) Principles and management of pediatric foot and ankle deformities and malformations. Wolters Kluwer, Philadelphia
Needleman RL (2005) Current topic review: Subtalar arthroereisis for the correction of flexible flatfoot. Foot Ankle Int 26:336–346
Niederecker K (1959) Der Plattfuß. Ferdinand Enke Verlag, Stuttgart
Oh I, Williams BR, Ellis SJ, Kwon DJ, Deland JT (2011) Reconstruction of the symptomatic idiopathic flatfoot in adolescents and young adults. Foot Ankle Int 32:225–232
Oh I, Imhauser C, Choi D, Williams B, Ellis S, Deland J (2013) Sensivity of plantar pressure and talonavicular alignment to lateral column lengthening in flatfoot reconstruction. J Bone Joint Surg 95-A:1094–1100
Park MS, Kwon SS, Lee SY, Lee KM, Kim TG, Chung CY (2013) Spontaneous improvement of radiographic indices for idiopathic planovalgus with age. J Bone Joint Surg 95-A:e193; (1–8)
De Pellegrin M (2007) 15-jährige Erfahrung mit der subtalaren Schrauben-Arthrorise beim kindlichen Plattfuß. FussSprungg 5:12–20
De Pellegrin M, Morahamzadeh D, Strobl WM, Biedermann R, Tschauner C, Wirth T (2014) Subtalar extra-articular screw arthroereisis (SESA) for the treatment of flexible flatfoot in children. J Child Orthop 8:479–487
Rathjen KE, Mubarak SJ (1998) Calcaneal-cuboid-cuneiform osteotomy for the correction of valgus foot deformities in children. J Pediatr Orthop 18:775–782
Rein S, Hanisch U, Zwipp H et al (2013) Comparative analysis of inter- and intraligamentous distribution of sensory nerve endings in ankle ligaments: a cadaver study. Foot Ankle Int 34:1017–1024
Ricco AI, Richards BS, Herring JA (2014) Chapter 23: Disorders of the foot. In: Tachdjian's pediatric orthopaedics. Elsevier Saunders, Philadelphia
Roling BA, Christensen JC, Johnson CH (2002) Biomechanics of the first ray. Part IV: The effect of selected medial column arthrodesis. A three-dimensional kinematic analysis in a cadaver mode. J Foot Ankle Surg 41:278–284
Schede F (1929) Die Operation des Plattfußes. Z Orthop Chir 50:528–538
Schröder S, Ihme N, Kochs A, Niedhart C (2006) Subtalare Arthrorise mittels Kalix-Schraube beim Knick-Senkfuß. FussSprungg 4:214–220
Scott RT, Bussewitz BW, Hyer CF, Berlet GC, Philbin TM (2016) The corrective power of the Cotton osteotomy. FussSprungg 14:9–13
Smith SD, Millar EA (1983) Arthrorisis by means of a subtalar polyethylene peg implant for correction of hindfoot pronation in children. Clin Orthop Relat Res 181:15–23
Tompkins MH, Nigro JS, Mendicino S (1993) The Smith STA-peg: a 7-year retrospective study. J Foot Ankle Surg 32:27–32
Vanderwilde R, Staheli LT, Chew DE, Malagon V (1988) Measurements on radiographs of the foot in normal infants and children. J Bone Joint Surg 70-A:407–415
Vontey H (1978) Manuel de chirurgie orthopedique et de reeducation du pied. France Publisher, Paris, Masson
Vulcano E, Maccario C, Myerson MS (2016) How to approach pediatric flatfoot. Word J Orthop 7:1–7
Wagner H (1986) Calcaneus displacement osteotomy in pediatric flatfoot. Orthopade 15:233–241
Xia J, Zhang P, Yang YF, Zhou JA, Li QM, Yu GR (2013) Biomechanical analysis of the calcaneocuboid joint pressure after sequential lengthening of the lateral column. Foot Ankle Int 34:261–266

Tarsal Coalitions and Rigid Planovalgus Deformity

5

Contents

Recommended Literature

- Downey MS, DeWaters AM (2013) Tarsal coalition. In: Mc Glamry's comprehensive textbook of foot surgery, 4. Ed., Vol. 1 (Hrsg.: Southerland JT et al) Wolters Kluwer, Lippincott, Williams & Wilkins, Philadelphia
- Cass AD, Camasta CA (2010) A review of tarsal coalition and pes planovalgus: clinical examination, diagnostic imaging and surgical planning. J Foot Ankle Surg 49: 274–293

Coalitions are fairly often observed segmentation disorders of single joint connections in the tarsal region. Very early, during the delimitation of the later skeletal elements, approximately in the 8th to 9th week of embryonic development, the incomplete separation of the pre-stages of two later tarsal bones occurs (Kawashima and Uhthoff 1990). The total frequency is stated very divergent in the literature but is presumably at least 1–2%, whereby both feet are affected in about half of the cases. Mosca (2015) even indicates a frequency of 2–13%. In addition to two more or less equally frequent forms, which together account for at least 95% of all cases, a wide variety of sometimes very rare forms have been described (atypical coalitions, Sect. 5.3). The talocalcaneal form of coalescence concerns a real joint with cartilaginous joint surfaces, whereas in the calcaneonavicular form, the bone bridge partly exists in the area of a physiologically localized ligament connection (ligamentum bifurcatum). Both more frequent forms are associated with a deformity in some cases, mostly in the planovalgus sense Hamel (2013). If tarsal skeletal elements are completely fused without

J. Hamel, *Foot and Ankle Surgery in Children and Adolescents*, https://doi.org/10.1007/978-3-030-58108-4_5

a residual joint area, this is referred to as synostoses and should be dealt with separately.

5.1 Talocalcaneal Coalition

The talocalcaneal coalition accounts for about 45% of all cases in the author's surgically treated patients' base. It is manifested in a variety of forms and raises numerous diagnostic and differential therapeutic questions. Also, the results of surgical treatment are by no means always favorable, so that a particularly careful consideration of the procedure in the individual case seems necessary.

5.1.1 Therapeutically Relevant Pathomorphology and Pathophysiology

The anatomical localization and pathomorphology of the talocalcaneal coalitions will be presented according to the principle of "regions of interest." The coalescences are always located in the medial area of the talocalcaneal joint (Fig. 5.1). The medial facet region of the joint (Fig. 5.2) is most frequently affected by the segmentation disorder ("medial facet coalition"), but mostly in addition also further posterior located parts of the talocalcaneal joint in the area of the sustentaculum tali and the posterior facet of the joint are affected. Hamel (2008) described after earlier sporadic reports in the literature a dorsomedial form of the talocalcaneal coalition in which the medial facet and the sustentacular region are completely normally developed (Fig. 5.3), corresponding to type V of Rozansky et al. (2010). Also, purely posterior localizations were observed especially in younger children (Fig. 5.4), and sometimes, there seems to be an overlap or a combination with the os trigonum syndrome (Hamel 2008). A distinction is made between completely ossified coalitions (Fig. 5.2) and incomplete forms with a fibrous gap (Fig. 5.13). The shape of the coalition itself can differ greatly. In addition to a horizontal course of the gap formation, overlapping forms are also observed (Sect 5.1.3). Abortive forms are described as well (El Rassi et al. 2005).

Lateral talocalcaneal coalitions have not yet been described. However, the typical, apparently secondary, often pain-inducing phenomenon of the "anterolateral subtalar impingement" occurs in this area: The reduced mobility of the talocalcaneal joint due to the medial coalition leads to a disturbed joint mechanism with reduction of the sliding motion of the lateral processus tali on the inclined joint surface of the posterior subtalar facet. The center of rotation of the subtalar joint in coalition patients is no longer located centrally in the region of the interosseous ligament connections but in the coalition itself. This causes characteristic adaptic anatomical changes in the anterolateral area of the joint during growth. The processus lateralis tali acts as if "buried" in the cranial saddle-shaped indentation of the calcaneus (Fig. 5.5), which shows

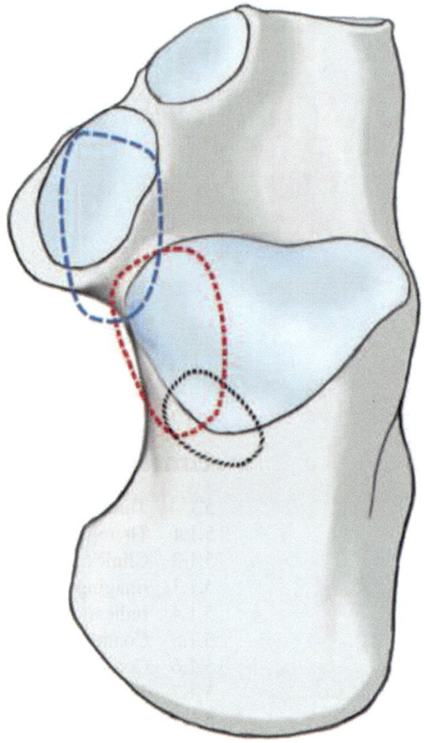

Fig. 5.1 Localization of the talocalcaneal coalitions in relation to the three joint facets: medial (blue), dorsomedial (red), and posterior (black)

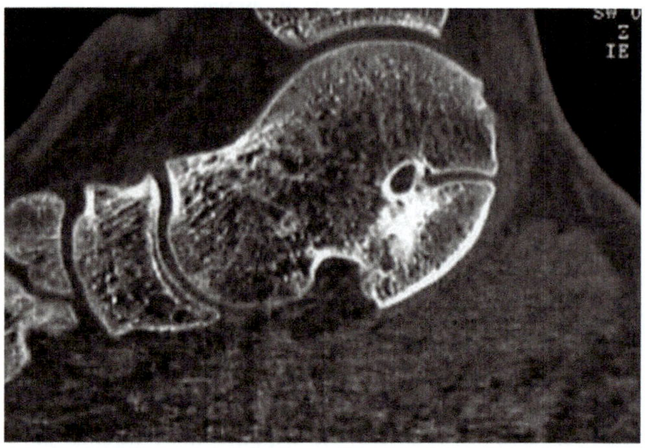

Fig. 5.2 CT of a complete medial facet coalition in a 17-year-old patient

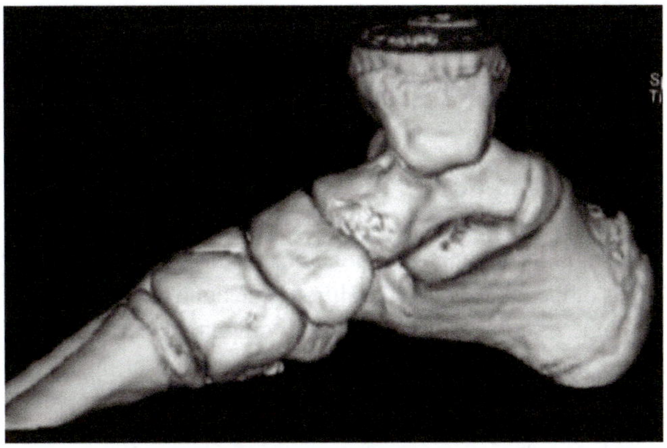

Fig. 5.3 Three-dimensional reconstruction of a dorsomedially located, incomplete talocalcaneal coalition in an 11-year-old female patient

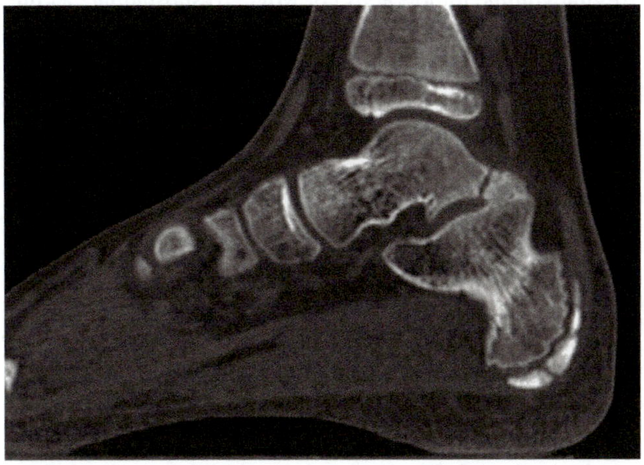

Fig. 5.4 Localized posterior talocalcaneal coalition in a patient at the age of 7 years (CT)

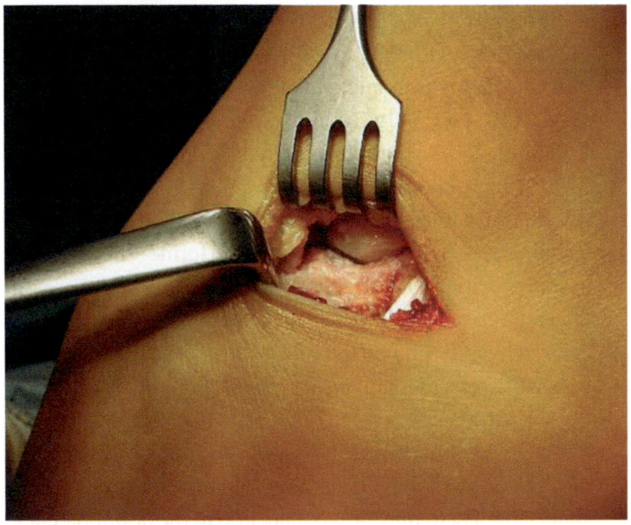

Fig. 5.5 Intraoperative image of anterolateral subtalar dysmorphy in a patient with talocalcaneal coalition. The processus lateralis tali appears as if "buried" in the cranial surface of the calcaneus. The minimal residual mobility of the talocalcaneal joint that is still preserved despite the coalition causes painful anterolateral subtalar impingement

a strong cortical hypertrophy (Figs. 5.10, 5.11, and 5.12). This is most obvious in cases where planovalgus deformity is additionally present and the talocalcaneal-navicular complex is contracted in everted position and is referred to here as "anterolateral subtalar dysmorphy" (see Sect. 5.1.3).

In up to 50% of cases, a rigid planovalgus deformity develops in patients with talocalcaneal coalition. This is apparently caused on the basis of, or in connection with, a more or less strongly developed peroneal spasm. It is not clear why this phenomenon occurs in some cases, while other patients with talocalcaneal coalition do not develop planovalgus deformity.

5.1.2 Clinic

Typical is the occurrence of a rather diffuse pain in the area of the hind foot at the age of 10–13 years, especially during or after exercise, in temporal connection with increasing ossification. Often a trauma is the (presumed or actual) initial reason for the onset of the symptoms. Pressure pain can often be triggered above the medially situated coalition but often also or exclusively in the sinus tarsi area, corresponding to the anterolateral subtalar impingement (see Sect. 5.1.1).

The increasing stiffening of the talocalcaneal joint is usually not noticed by the patient or the parents. Due to the formation of an excessive mobility in the Chopart joint line, it can easily be overlooked if not examined thoroughly. A strong hypermobility and the appearance of enhanced joint opening of the calcaneocuboid joint visible from outside should raise the diagnostic suspicion of restricted motion of the talocalcaneal joint. Inversion of the peritalar complex appears markedly limited (Fig. 5.6). When looking at the patient from behind, it is noticeable that there is no physiological varus inclination of the hindfoot when lifting the heel to stand on tiptoes, as in the case in patients with mobile tarsus.

In the case of passive inversion, the examiner notices a clear counter-tension of the peroneal muscles in some of the cases. In extreme cases, the inversion is also completely blocked in the area of the Chopart joint line by the strongly tensed peroneal tendons (Fig. 5.7), and the attempt to passively overcome this tension is clearly unpleasant and painful for the patient. An active tensioning of the tibialis posterior muscle, the antagonist of the peroneal muscles, is not possible for the affected patients. This "peroneal spasm" is characteristically completely eliminated immediately after the anesthesia is administered, indicating that it is not a structural muscle-tendon shortening but rather a reflex-like event. A pronounced peroneal spasm blocks the entire talocalcaneal-navicular complex in a functionally unfavorable everted position and is therefore significantly more impairing than the articular rigidity of the talocalcaneal joint caused by the coalition itself. However, a peroneal spasm is not pathognomonic for tarsal coalitions and is also observed

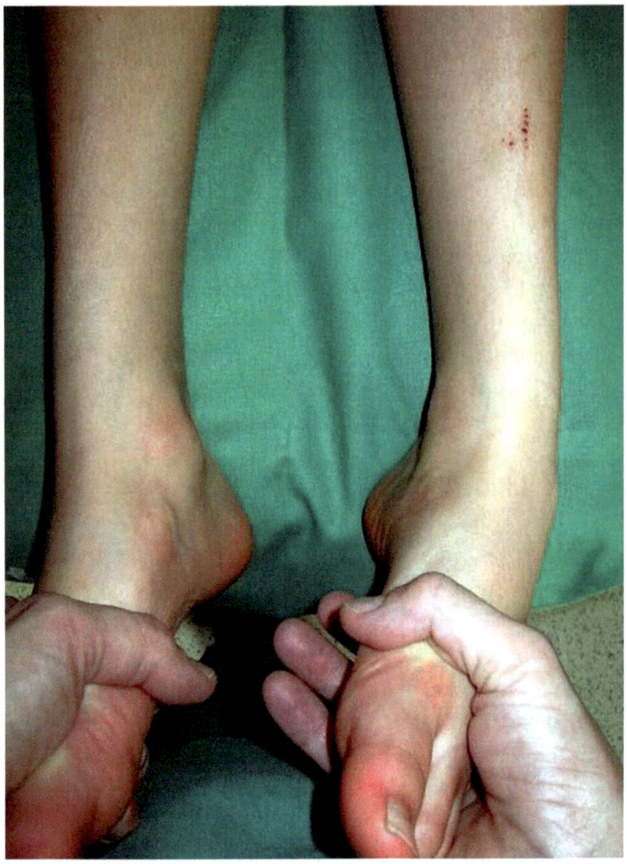

Fig. 5.6 11-Year-old female patient with dorsomedial talocalcaneal coalition on the right and the resulting significant limitation of inversion during passive motion testing (same patient as in Fig. 5.3)

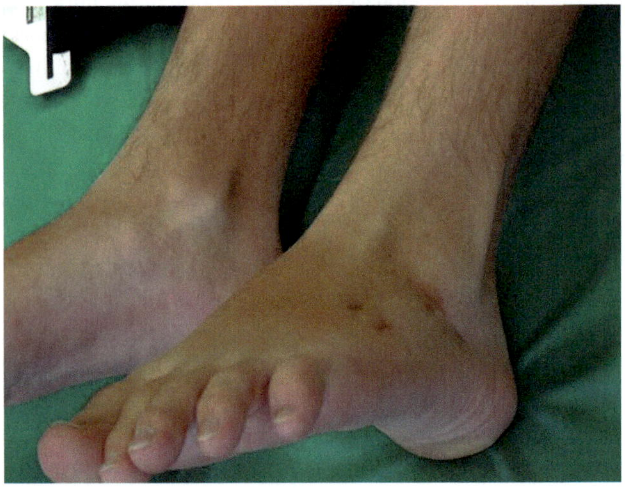

Fig. 5.7 12-Year-old patient with severe peroneal spasm after coalition resection and calcaneal lengthening osteotomy. The severely tensed peroneal tendons are clearly visible. After induction of general anesthesia, completely free motion was immediately apparent, an indication that it is not an anatomical shortening of the peroneal muscle-tendon units but a pain-induced muscle spasm

in other entities (Cass and Camasta 2010; Mosier and Asher 1984). The calf muscles, especially the M. gastrocnemius, are generally shortened in rigid pes planovalgus.

5.1.3 Imaging

In imaging, a distinction is made between *direct* and *indirect* signs of the talocalcaneal coalition. The bone bridge itself can in some cases be recognized radiographically in the lateral projection, e.g., by the missing representation of the medial facet or in the ankle ap projection or the posteroplantar oblique image ("Harris view")—which is no longer used frequently and more or less replaced by three-dimensional imaging modalities. However, the more precise assessment is carried out in case of suspicion by (weight-bearing) CT, DVT (digital volume tomography) or MRI. To substantiate a clinical suspicion, three indirect X-ray signs are of importance:

Indirect Radiological Signs of Talocalcaneal Coalition

- C-sign
- "Talar beak"
- Anterolateral subtalar dysmorphy

- The C-sign (Lateur et al. 1994) is a continuous contour line of the trochlea tali and the sustentaculum tali ossis calcanei, which is characteristic for extensive talocalcaneal coalitions (Fig. 5.8), but is also observed in severe planovalgus deformities.
- "Talar beaking" represents a traction osteophyte located dorsolaterally at the head of the talus, which should not be confused with a sign of degenerative arthritis but rather corresponds to a capsular reaction on compensatory pathological motion behavior of the talonavicular joint and is almost pathognomonic for the talocalcaneal coalition (Fig. 5.9) and only rarely observed in CN-coalition. Luhmann and Schoenecker (1998) found talar beaking in 52% of their talocalcaneal cases.
- The anterolateral subtalar dysmorphy—which is observed in a similar way in the calcaneonavicular form—shows a close spatial proximity of a widened and rounded lateral processus tali and the calcaneal neck in the lateral projection, a distinct cortical hypertrophy on the calcaneal side, as well as a radial trabecular orientation of the calcaneal spongious bone below the hypertrophic area (Fig. 5.10). This apparently is due to an impingement phenomenon as a result of the disturbed joint mechanics and a possible source of pain in the area of the sinus tarsi. There may be a connection to the development of peroneal spasm (Fig. 5.11). However, similar anterolateral

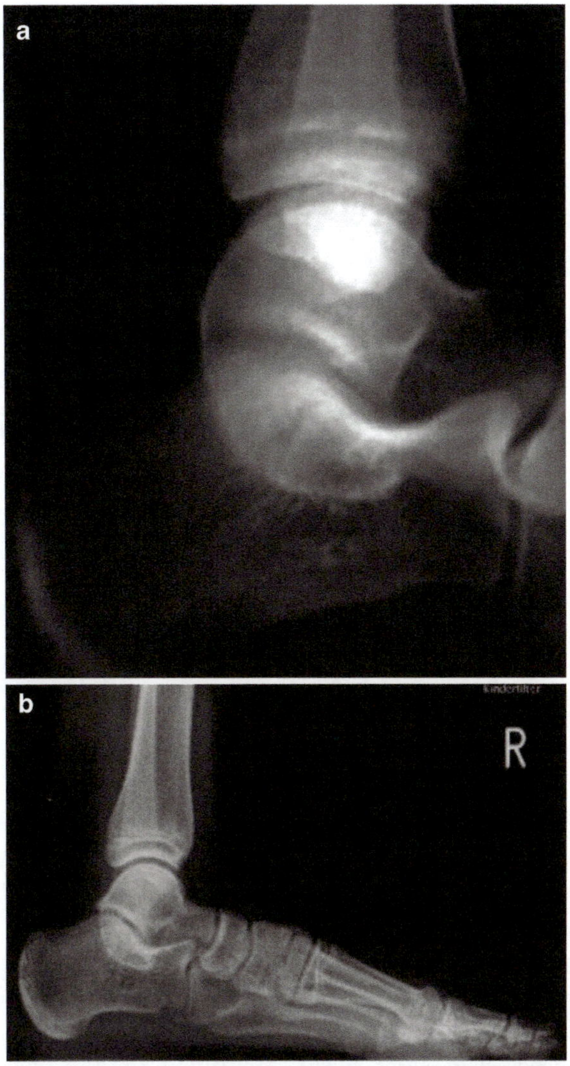

Fig. 5.8 C-sign in 13- (**a**) and 14-year old patients (**b**) as an indirect X-ray sign of a talocalcaneal coalition confirmed by CT and intraoperatively

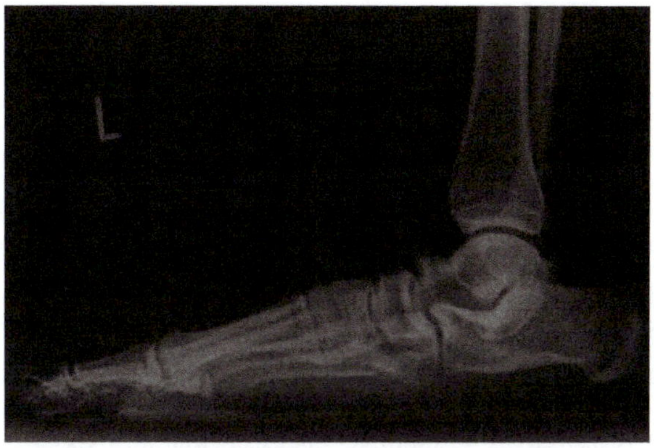

Fig. 5.9 "Talar beaking" in a 16-year-old female patient with talocalcaneal coalition, confirmed by CT. This "traction osteophyte" dorsally at the head of the talus corresponds to a bony reaction at the capsule attachment and should be distinguished from a degenerative osteophyte in osteoarthritis

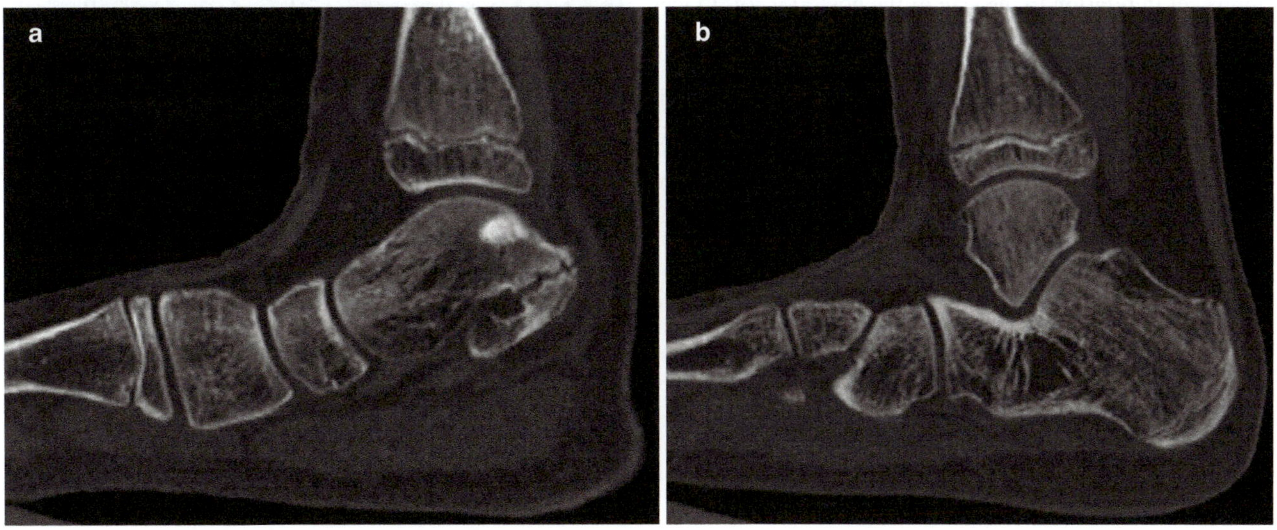

Fig. 5.10 10-Year-old patient with dorsomedial talocalcaneal coalition (**a**) and marked hypertrophy of the cranial calcaneal corticalis due to anterolateral subtalar impingement (**b**). This "anterolateral subtalar dysmorphy" is often already visible in a conventional X-ray projection

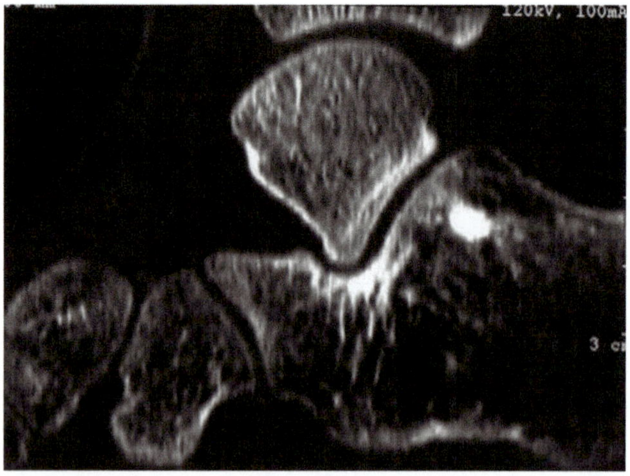

Fig. 5.11 13-Year-old patient with talocalcaneal coalition and clinically marked peroneal spasm due to anterolateral subtalar impingement

subtalar dysmorphy is occasionally observed without coalition (Fig. 5.12) and may be associated with the formation of an additional joint facet (Martus et al. 2008; Niki et al. 2015; Vossen et al. 2020) (Fig. 5.12).

In three-dimensional diagnostics, the MRI is suitable for imaging not only the coalition itself but also the cartilage conditions of the non-affected remaining joint and intraosseous changes (e.g., bone marrow edema in the calcaneus, corresponding to the anterolateral subtalar impingement), as well as accompanying pathologies; however, the CT is clearly superior for assessing the size, expansion, position, and course of the gap of the coalition itself (Fig. 5.13). The longitudinal and transverse expansion is determined in the CT sagittal and frontal sections. In most cases, values of approx. 15–25 mm are found for the longitudinal expansion and 10–20 mm for the transverse expansion. In the literature, the coalition cross-section is set in relation to the size of the posterior joint facet (Wilde et al. 1994). The frontal sections are placed vertically on the plane of the sole of the foot in order to avoid misleading imaging section phenomena and should reach far to the posterior side in order not to overlook isolated localized forms here.

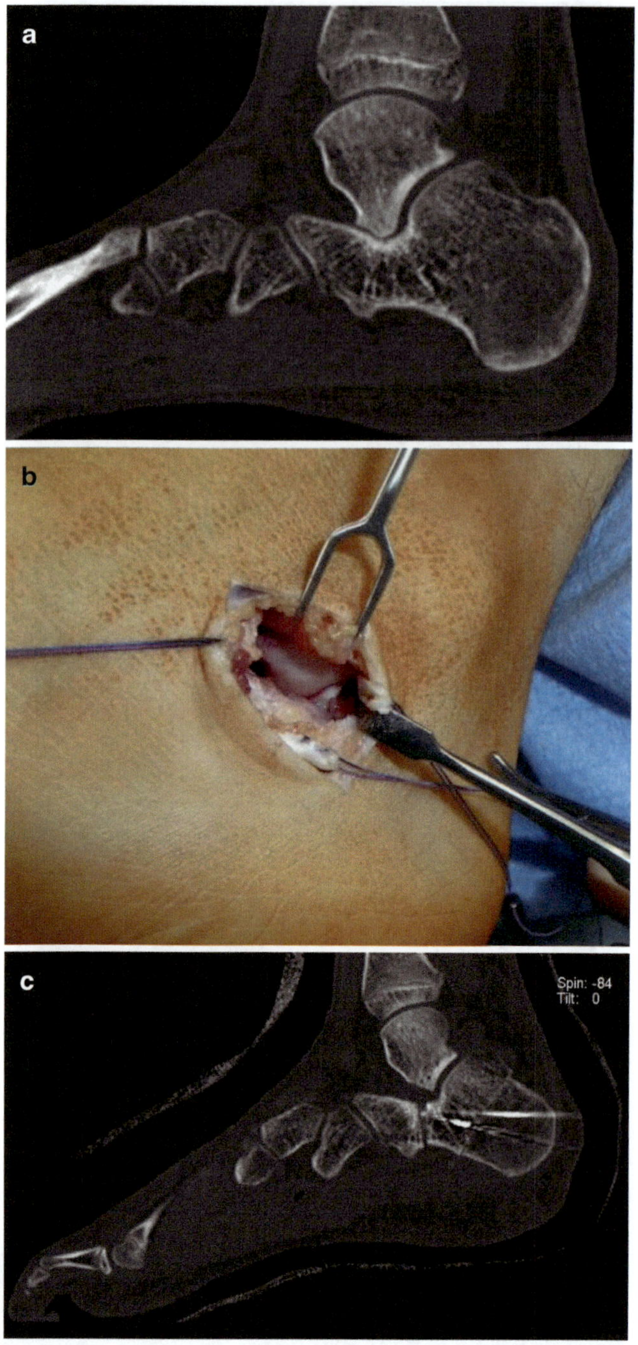

Fig. 5.12 13-Year-old patient with pronounced pain in the area of the sinus tarsi. The CT showed signs of anterolateral impingement with the formation of an accessory articular surface (**a**), confirmed intraoperatively (**b**). No talocalcaneal coalition was found medially during the intraoperative inspection. The accessory articular surface was carefully resected and a calcaneal lengthening osteotomy was additionally performed due to planovalgus deformity, which at the same time prevents the continuation of bony impingement (**c**)

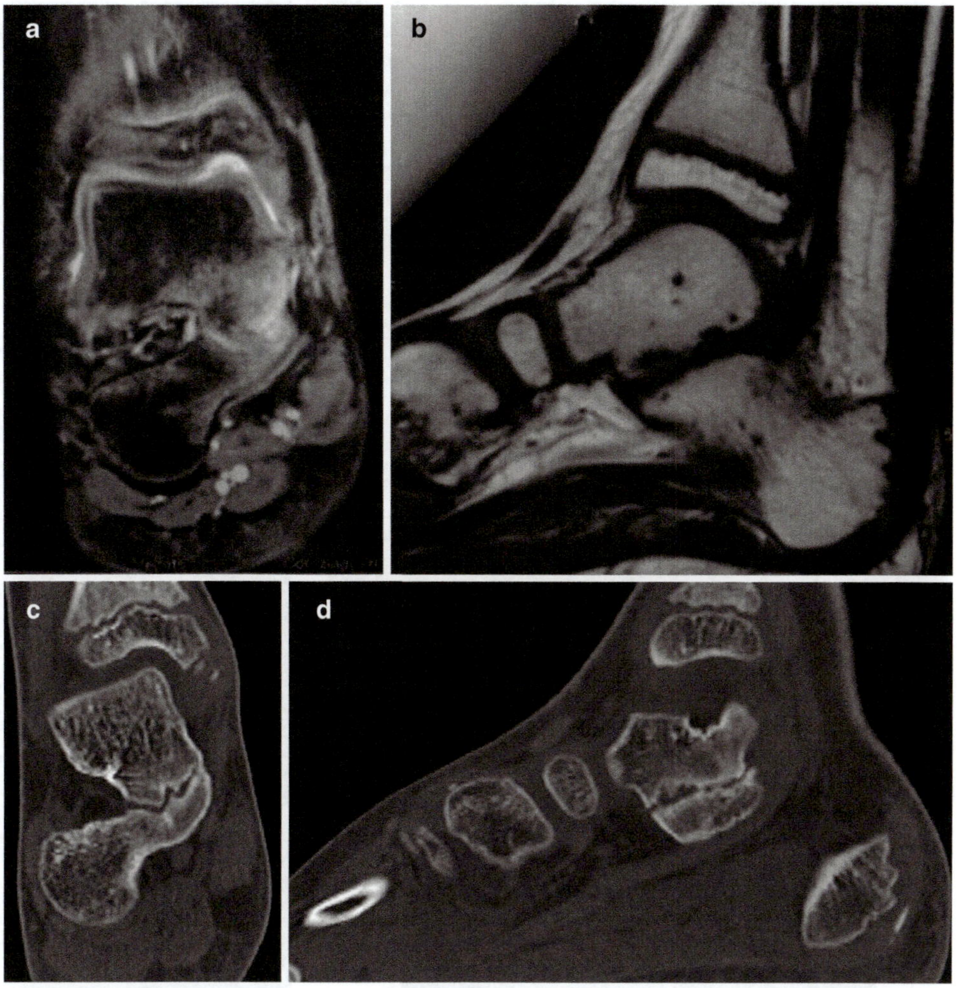

Fig. 5.13 8-Year-old patient with large, incomplete talocalcaneal coalition. The comparison of MRI (**a**, **b**) and CT (**c**, **d**) shows that, e.g., the cartilaginous parts of the skeletal elements and also certain intraosseous changes (bone marrow edema) can be visualized in the MRI, whereas the bony microstructure and, e.g., the extent and course of the coalition gap can be assessed much more conclusively in the CT

Rozansky et al. (2010) distinguish five forms based on 3-D CT investigations. In addition to the horizontally configured forms (Fig. 5.13), strongly medioplantar "shingled" oblique forms of the medial facet coalition are observed (Fig. 5.20). This may be important intraoperatively for the desired preservation of the sustentaculum tali. Kernbach and Blitz (2010) derive the extent of the degenerative changes in the area of the subtalar joint from the CT frontal section.

An important parameter for treatment planning is the joint space width of the posterior facet of the subtalar joint in the (weight-bearing) CT. A comparison with the joint space width of the upper ankle joint allows conclusions concerning the condition of the joint cartilage in that part of the subtalar joint, that is not affected by the bony bridge formation of the coalition (Figs. 5.14 and 5.15) and thus about the chances of success of a joint-preserving surgical procedure. Degenerative changes, such as subchondral sclerosis and cyst formation represent relevant parameters already in adolescents (Blitz 2010).

When assessing planovalgus deformities in connection with coalitions (rigid planovalgus deformities), standard X-ray diagnostic is used in two planes under weight-bearing conditions (see Sect. 4.5). Quantification is possible with the TMT index according to Hamel and Kinast (2006). The CT frontal plane section perpendicular to the sole of the foot can show the extent of the indicatively important hindfoot valgus deformity (Fig. 5.16b) and in pronounced cases indicates a fibulocalcaneal impingement as well (Blitz 2010). The CT also permits the creation of a three-dimensional reconstruction, which clearly shows the location and expansion of the coalition (Figs. 5.3 and 5.16c) for preoperative planning. The DVT (digital volume tomogram) can further be used to quantitatively assess the deformity under load by means of corresponding angle measurements (Fig. 5.17). DVT has gained more and more importance in pre- and postoperative coalition imaging especially in younger patients because of less radiation exposure compared to CT. It has proven to be especially helpful in case of persisting pain after coalition resection.

Diagnostics may reveal to be challenging in cases, which clinically raise the suspicion of a coalition, but cannot be confirmed clearly by means of imaging modalities. Such abortive forms are also described in the literature (El Rassi et al. 2005). They pose considerable problems for indication and can sometimes only be clarified by surgical inspection. Cass and Camasta (2010) speak of a "gray zone" in the patient

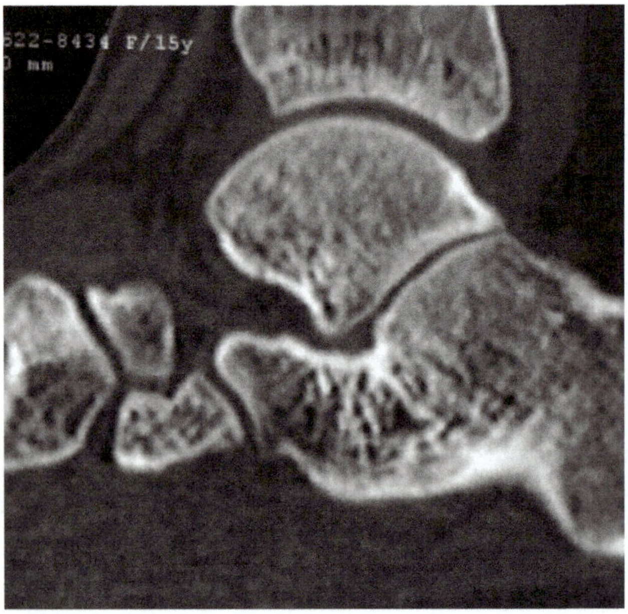

Fig. 5.14 15-Year-old female patient with talocalcaneal coalition. The joint space of the posterior chamber of the subtalar joint is clearly narrowed compared to the tibiotalar joint, which indicates a deficient cartilage coverage

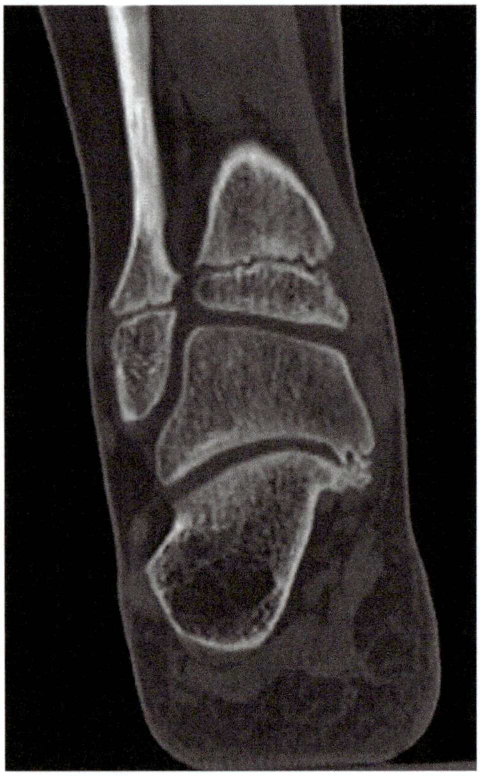

Fig. 5.15 10-Year-old female patient with small medial talocalcaneal coalition and wide joint space of the non-affected part of the subtalar joint, also compared to the upper ankle joint

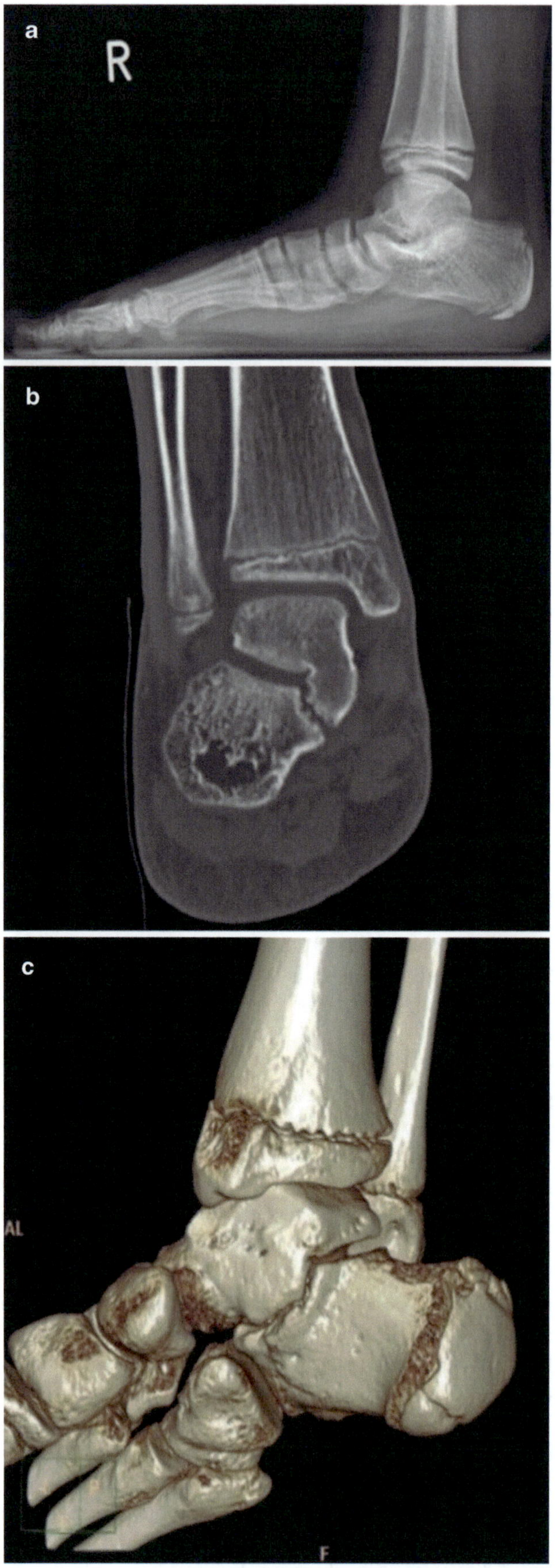

Fig. 5.16 14-Year-old patient with rigid planovalgus deformity (**a**). The extent of the valgus component in the frontal plane can be estimated on the basis of the CT (**b**); the morphology of the coalition can be well evaluated in the 3-D reconstruction (**c**)

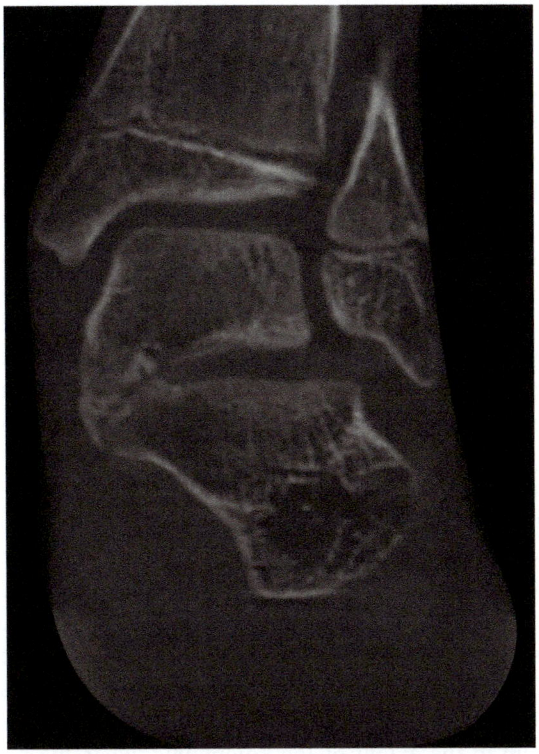

Fig. 5.17 12-Year-old patient with talocalcaneal coalition. The digital volume tomogram (DVT) allows the combination of coalition imaging and evaluation of hindfoot alignment under weight-bearing conditions

spectrum, i.e., cases that are clinically appearing as coalition syndromes but lack the evidence of a coalition. It is not uncommon for these patients to be obese adolescents who have previously exhibited a flexible pes planovalgus (Cass and Camasta 2010) and develop a secondary peroneal spasm.

5.1.4 Indication for Surgical Treatment

The indication criteria for the surgical treatment of a talocalcaneal coalition are the patient's level of distress and the prognosis to be expected after surgical treatment. The degree of suffering is often difficult to assess and the anamnesis for patients in childhood age includes the information provided by the parents. In the case of a talocalcaneal coalition, until recently, the somewhat simplistic rule propagated in the literature applies, apart from few exceptions, that no surgical intervention should be performed without distress, i.e., in the case of accidental findings. However, this might not to be maintained any longer, if the prognosis of surgery is especially favorable in small coalitions of young children. The following factors must be considered when assessing the prognosis after resection of the coalition:

Factors of Prognostic Relevance for the Indication for Resection

- Age of the patient
- Extension of the coalition
- Morphological factors (fibrous, cartilaginous, bony, complete, incomplete)
- Peroneal spasm
- Deformity (hindfoot valgus, planovalgus)
- Condition of the not involved part of the subtalar joint
- Intraoperatively observed mobility of the subtalar joint after resection
- Previous surgery

There is no single criterion that can be used solely to estimate the prospects of success after resection. The following prognostic relevant factors are partly documented in the literature, partly based on the author's experience:

- The younger the patient is at the time of the resection and the longer the period of the remaining joint development, the more adjustment processes, and thus a favorable result can be expected.
- The size expansion (cross section) of the coalition is certainly of prognostic importance. In the literature, the threshold value for a still resectable coalition is given as 50% of the size of the posterior facet (Wilde et al. 1994). In individual cases however, a resection can also be successful with more expansive coalitions (Luhmann and Schoenecker 1998).
- The lesser the coalition shows a complete bony bridging, the more favorable the prognosis can be, particularly favorable are purely fibrous coalitions.
- Unfavorable prognostic factors are the presence of a longstanding peroneal spasm, which can often persist postoperatively, and the presence of a planovalgus deformity.
- Of particular prognostic importance are the condition of the remaining joint not affected by the coalition (Mosca and Bevan 2012; Kernbach and Blitz 2010), the mobility achieved intraoperatively, and the motion behavior after resection, as it can be observed intraoperatively.
- According to the author's experience, secondary resections are often unsuccessful, and an arthrodesis is usually preferable.

Little is known about the *spontaneous course* and effectiveness of conservative treatment measures, and also the author can contribute little experience on this. In the literature, a conservative treatment attempt for chronic complaints

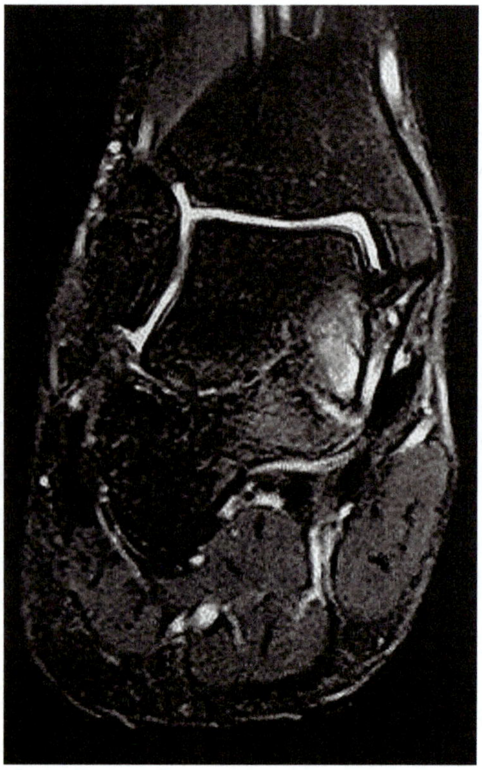

Fig. 5.18 14-Year-old female patient with condition after severe distortion trauma with local pain persisting for months. A previously undiagnosed large talocalcaneal coalition was obviously disrupted. The symptoms subsided after prolonged immobilization

is sometimes recommended (e.g., Luhmann and Schoenecker 1998; Mosca 2014), but is not considered promising by other authors (e.g., Gantsoudes et al. 2012). In the case of acute symptoms arising for the first time due to trauma however, an attempt of immobilization for a limited period of several weeks may be promising (Fig. 5.18).

The literature on the prognosis after *coalition resection* is hardly surveyable, and it is up to the therapist to weigh the abovementioned indication criteria in the individual case and thus compare the patient's level of suffering with the expected result, when considering the indication for resection. In an ideal case, resection can achieve the usable and pain-free partial mobility of the subtalar joint in the long term (Fig. 5.33). However, there are sobering findings in gait analysis, that regained subtalar mobility is hardly ever used functionally (Hetsroni et al. 2008).

In the author's experience, the prognosis after isolated *talocalcaneal arthrodesis* is generally favorable at least in the medium term, so that in the case of a non-resectable coalition, it is exclusively a question of the current level of suffering, whether the advice for fusion should be given. As a rule, the symptomatic patient in nearly all cases is satisfied with the result after arthrodesis.

In the literature, resection of the coalition with the option of secondary arthrodesis in case of persistent complaints is generally recommended as a primary treatment for young patients (e.g., Luhmann and Schoenecker 1998). According to the author's experience however, it should be assessed carefully before the primary intervention, whether a resection is really promising, in order to avoid prolonged periods of persisting pain until a definitive surgical solution is considered. The following practical strategy for therapy planning has proved to be successful (Fig. 5.19): In the case of confirmed symptomatic talocalcaneal coalition, an initial assessment is made on the basis of the abovementioned indication criteria as to whether a resection is generally an option or whether primary arthrodesis is more likely. If the constellation is favorable, early resection is recommended, even if the current complaints are rather moderate. If only an arthrodesis is to be considered, it is up to the extent of the complaints, when the patient decides to undergo surgery. In case of doubt, a decision can be made even intraoperatively, observing the achieved mobility and the condition of the remaining subtalar joint after coalition resection.

5.1.5 Coalition Resection

When planning a coalition resection, the location and shape of the coalition is assessed from the CT or DVT. The localization (medial, dorsomedial, posterior) is relevant for the chosen approach. The—possibly very different—course of the coalition gap in the CT frontal section (Fig. 5.20) provides information on how to proceed with the sustentaculum tali, which should be protected as much as possible as an important fulcrum for the flexor hallucis longus tendon. A fracture of the sustentaculum can be observed as a complication, for example, when the subtalar joint is forcefully distracted by a laminar spreader. In larger, far dorsally located coalitions, the glide channel and the glide path of the FHL tendon can be altered by resection in such a way, that a relative excess length of the tendon and a weakness of the active plantar flexion of the big toe can occur at least temporarily.

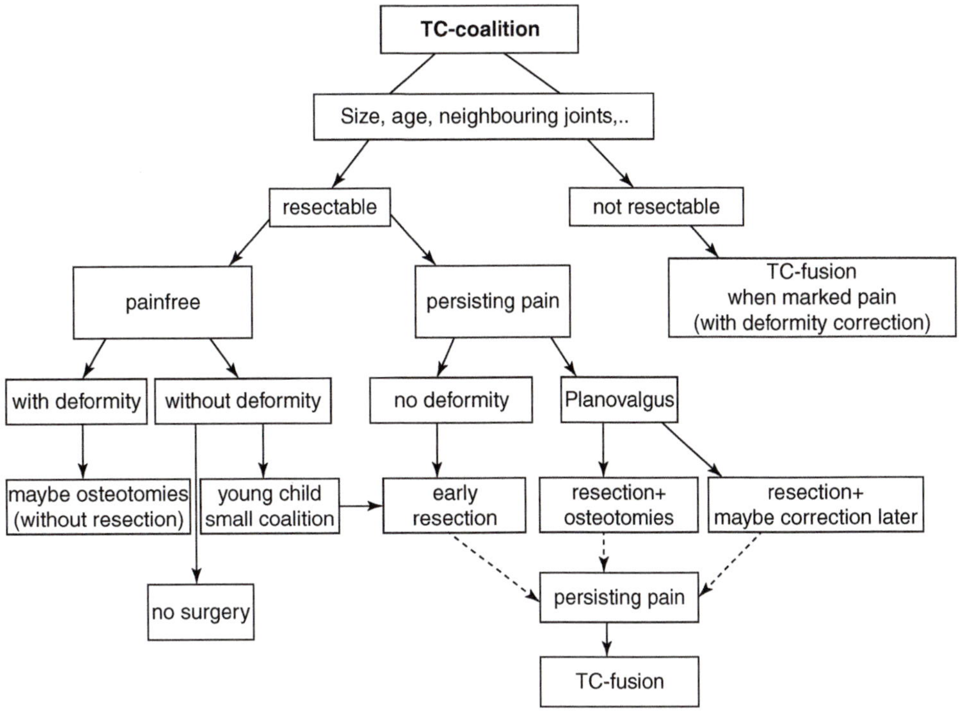

Fig. 5.19 Flow chart of the therapeutic procedure for talocalcaneal coalition. In symptomatic cases, a distinction is made between resectable and non-resectable coalition (see text)

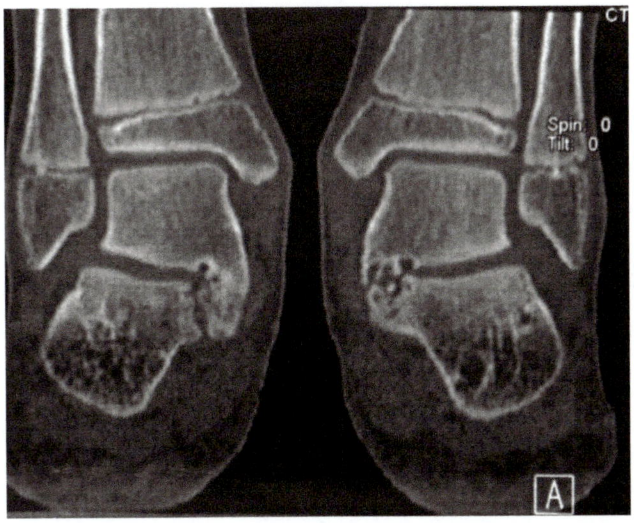

Fig. 5.20 DVT of a 10-year-old patient with bilateral talocalcaneal coalition. Notice the very different course of the coalition gap, on the left side shown overhanging, on the right horizontal

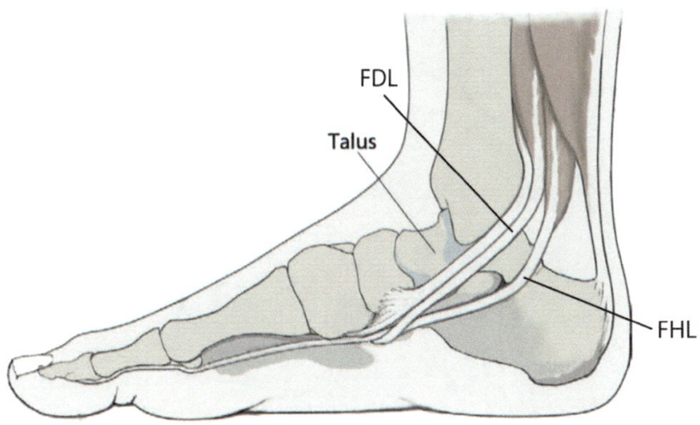

Fig. 5.21 Course of the flexor tendons in the medial tarsal region. Depending on the location of the coalition, the tendon of the flexor digitorum longus muscle is held away either caudally or cranially

5.1.5.1 Technique

A longitudinal incision is made in the medial tarsal area between the tendons of the posterior tibial muscle and the flexor hallucis longus muscle (Fig. 5.21) above or below the flexor digitorum longus tendon, and the coalition is exposed with Kirschner wires for soft tissue retraction (Fig. 5.22). Resection is performed with the oscillating saw, various chisels, and the power-burr, if necessary after marking with an image intensifier. As soon as joint cartilage tissue of the posterior facet of the subtalar joint becomes visible, this can serve as orientation for further resection, which should be continued in the total expansion of the coalition up to a resection width of at least 8–10 mm (Fig. 5.23).

Finally, the subtalar joint can be carefully distracted with the laminar spreader or a Kirschner wire-anchored spreader for some millimeters (Fig. 5.24) so that all parts of the posterior subtalar facet which are not affected by the coalition can be inspected and—after removal of the spreader—the degree and way of motion can be assessed, be it physiological gliding or unphysiological pure angulating. Extreme spreading should be avoided in order not to overstretch the tibial nerve or its branches.

If the coalition resection is left as it is, the cancellous resection surfaces are covered with bone wax, a fat tissue

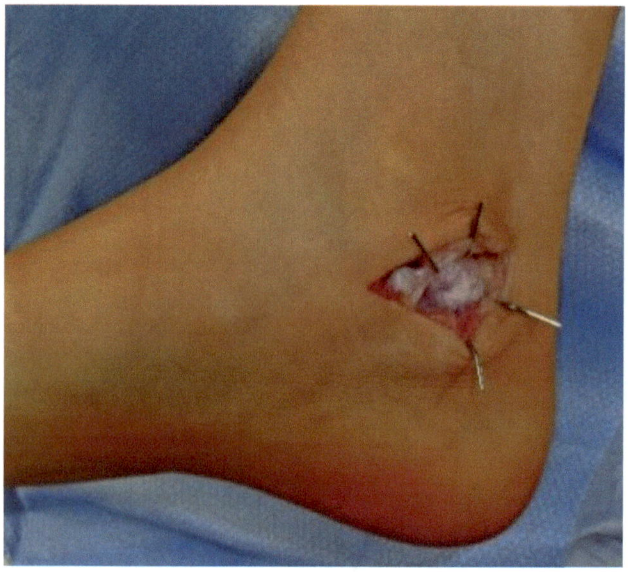

Fig. 5.22 Intraoperative situs of a talocalcaneal coalition resection using Kirschner wires for soft tissue retraction

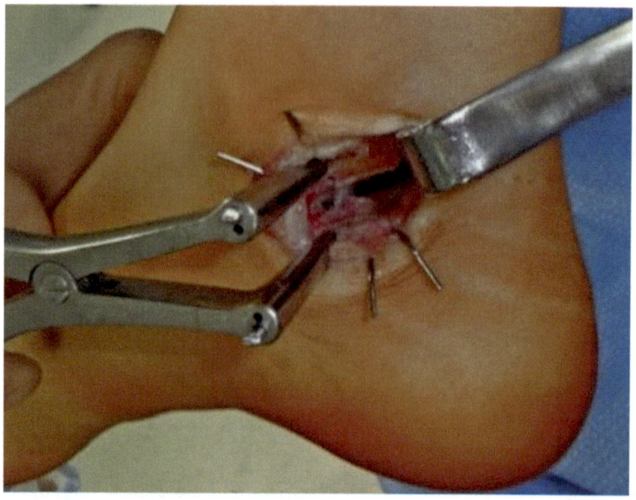

Fig. 5.24 Careful distraction of the subtalar joint after complete resection of the coalition using a K-wire fixed spreader

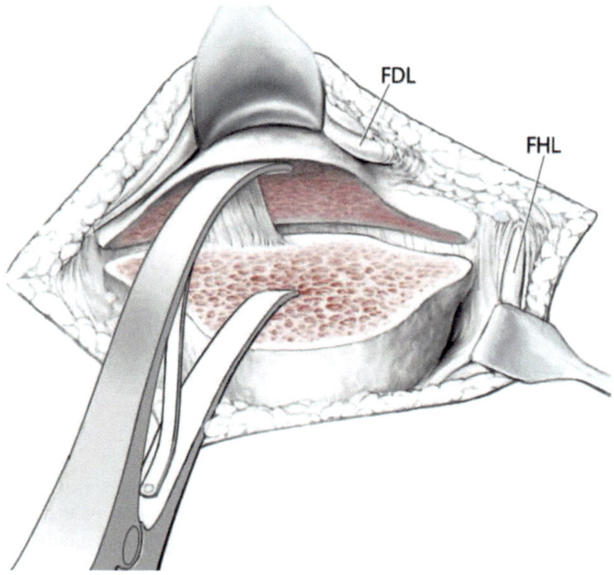

Fig. 5.23 Condition after resection of the coalition up to a distance of 8–10 mm between the resection surfaces. With an osteotomy spreader the mobility and thus the completeness of the resection can be checked. A fracture of the sustentaculum tali (bottom of the picture) must be carefully avoided. In this case the tendon of the flexor digitorum longus muscle (FDL) was mobilized cranially. The tendon of the flexor hallucis longus muscle (FHL) should be carefully protected in the dorsal aspect of the resection area

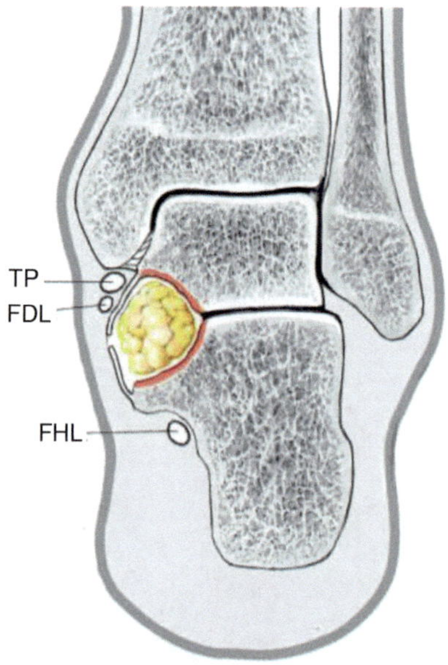

Fig. 5.25 After resection of the coalition, the cancellous resection surfaces are covered with bone wax (red) and a free fat tissue graft is inserted (yellow). The anatomical relationship of the resection area to the flexor tendons (tendons of the posterior tibial muscle (TP), flexor digitorum longus (FDL), and flexor hallucis longus (FHL)) is indicated.

graft (popliteal region, groin, buttocks) is inserted (Fig. 5.25), and the wound is closed in layers with readaptation of severed parts of the periosteum and ligamentum deltoideum. If in borderline cases of the indication the impression is acquired, that the quality of the residual joint and its motion behavior after mobilization do not give rise to the expectation of painless function, the surgeon can proceed with isolated talocalcaneal arthrodesis performed from the same access (see Sect. 5.1.7).

Figure 5.26 shows intraoperative images of resection and fat interposition in dorsomedial talocalcaneal coalition. In cases with a pronounced anterolateral subtalar dysmorphy (see Sect. 5.1.1), arthroplastic resection and, if necessary, a molding of the calcaneal neck to eliminate the impingement are generally considered after resection of the medial coalition in order to further improve the mobility of the joint; however, experience has only been gained in individual cases (Fig. 5.27). In the case of a very pronounced "talar beak," the removal of this traction osteophyte located dorsolaterally at the head of the talus should be considered, as it can irritate the soft tissues.

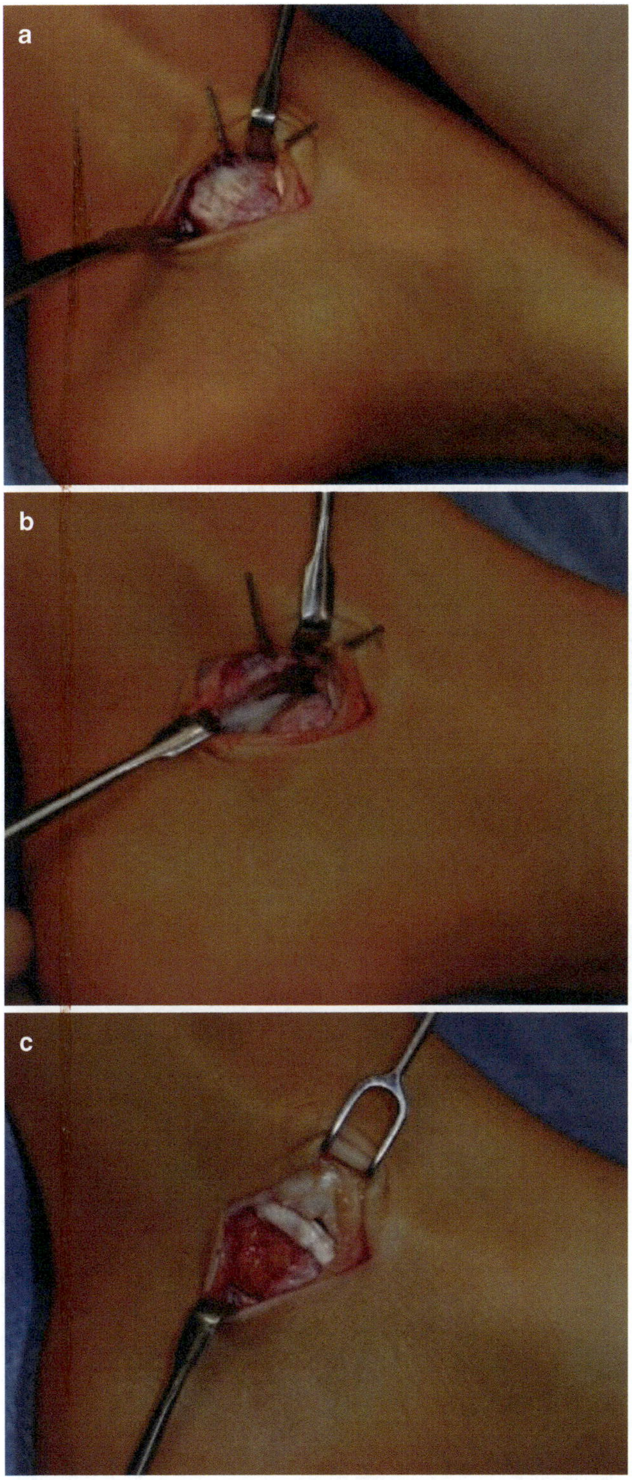

Fig. 5.26 Exposition (**a**), post-resection status (**b**), and fat interposition (**c**) in dorsomedial talocalcaneal coalition of an 11-year-old patient

In the follow-up treatment after coalition resection, an early mobilization of the subtalar joint with intensive physiotherapeutic treatment should always be strived for. However, practical experience has shown that this is often only pos-

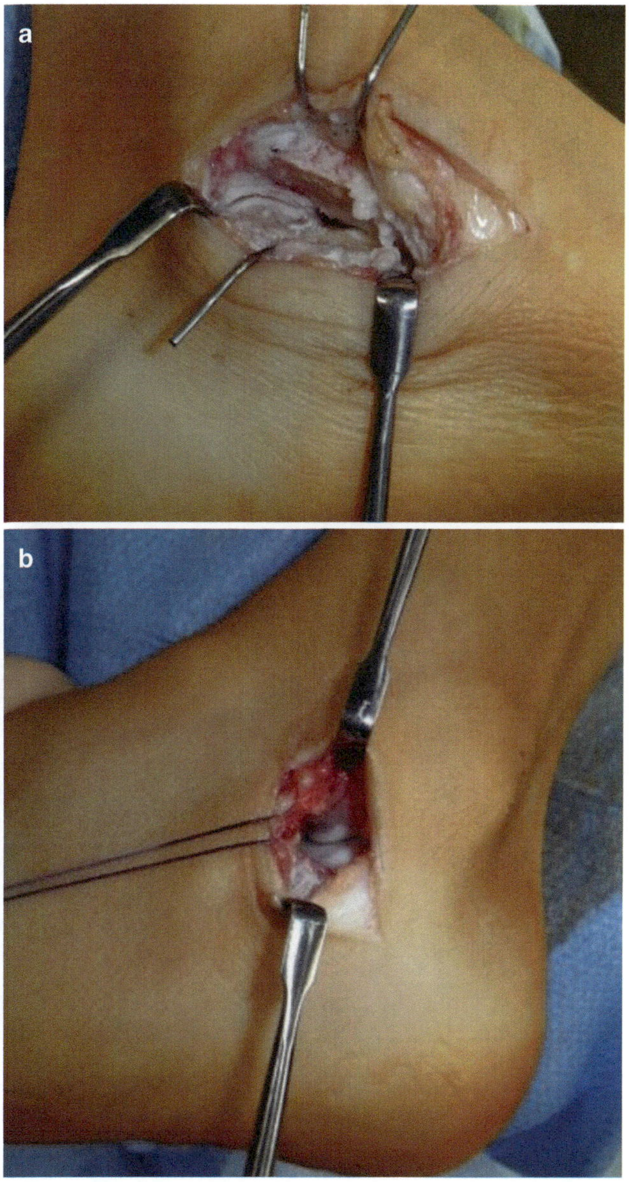

Fig. 5.27 12-Year-old patient, intraoperative situs after resection of the talocalcaneal coalition (**a**) and before calcaneal lengthening with significant anterolateral impingement (**b**). Same patient as in Fig. 5.17

sible after approx. 3–4 weeks due to the postoperative pain and swelling symptoms, and immobilization until then does bring advantages. Good results of subtalar mobility were also observed by the author despite several weeks of postoperative immobilization and subsequent initiation of passive and active range of motion exercises by physiotherapists and parents with emphasis on mobilization toward inversion.

5.1.5.2 Results

The results after isolated resection of a talocalcaneal coalition in childhood and adolescence show a wide range in the literature of between 50% and up to 100% favorable courses (according to Luhmann and Schoenecker 1998). In the largest retrospective study in recent years of 49 treatment cases from the study group of Mubarak and coworkers, 85% good and very good results were reported after an average observation period of 42.6 months (Gantsoudes et al. 2012), although with 37% re-interventions (mostly secondary deformity correction). Luhmann and Schoenecker (1998) report 76% favorable results in 25 treatment cases.

In the own patient population, the medium-term results were predominantly favorable in younger patients. In a retrospective evaluation based on the medical records, in 31 cases of isolated coalition resection, four cases (13%) showed an undesirable result, including one with the necessity of secondary talocalcaneal arthrodesis (Fig. 5.42) (Hamel et al. 2016). These favorable results compared to the literature can be explained, among other factors, by the fact that, from the age of about 13 years, primary fusion was indicated in cases with unfavorable prognostic factors.

Almost all reported results refer to medium-term observation periods. There are hardly any meaningful long-term studies available; McCormack et al. (1997) found no significant clinical deterioration by degenerative changes in the 10-year course. Khoshbin et al. (2013) also describe good long-term functional results. In the evaluation of results, distinctions must be made regarding cases with persistent complaints that can be explained by incomplete resection (Figs. 5.28 and 5.29). Since DVT is available and in regular use in the postoperative period instead of X-ray, an increasing number of incomplete resection of coalitions can be observed in those patients with incomplete pain relief.

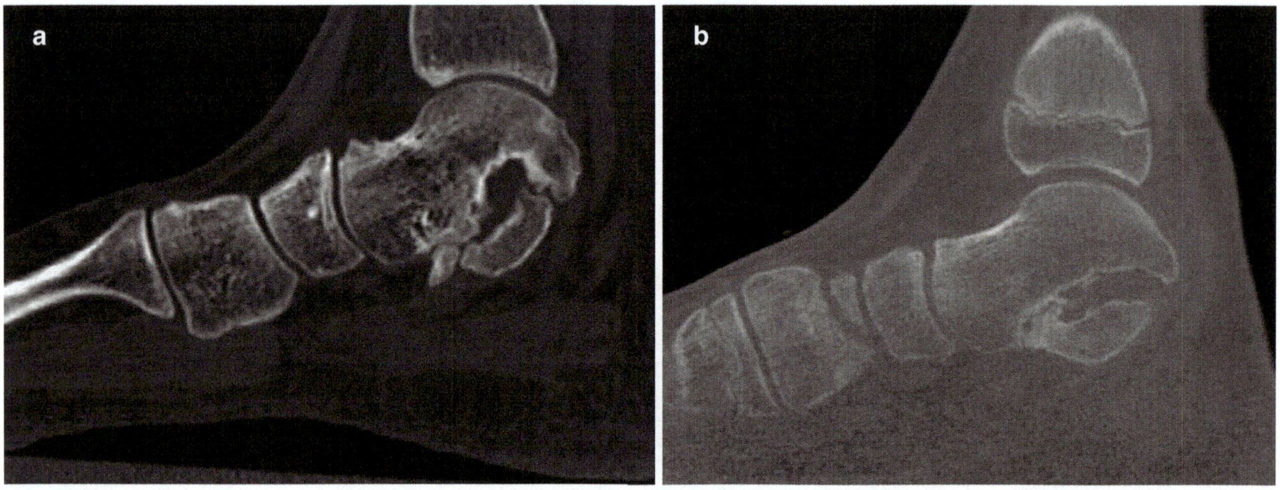

Fig. 5.28 Two different cases of incomplete coalition resection especially in the anterior part of the coalition in externally pre-operated adolescent patients with persistent complaints. Diagnosis was made by CT (**a**) or DVT (**b**)

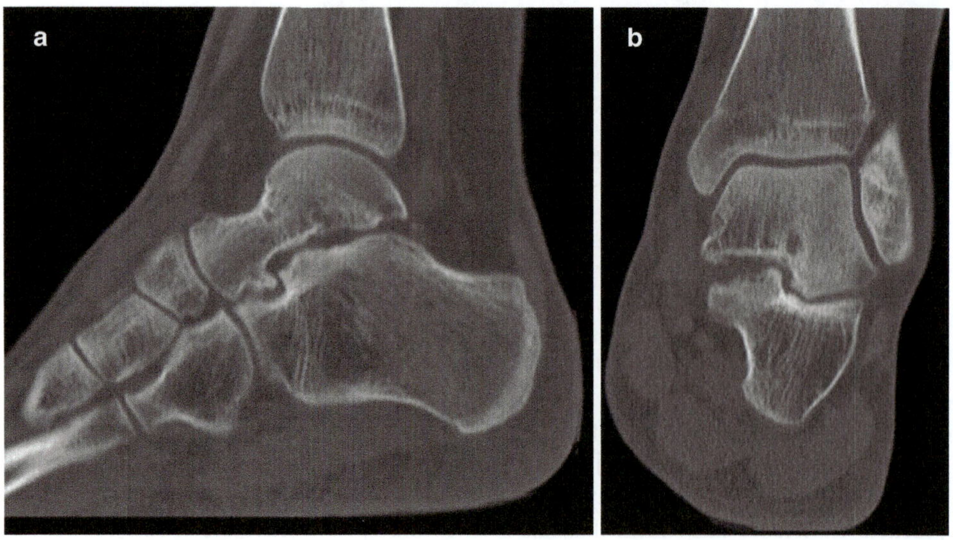

Fig. 5.29 Weight-bearing DVT of a 13-year-old female patient with status after externally performed resection of a large talocalcaneal coalition and persisting symptoms (**a**, **b**). The resection has obviously not been performed sufficiently rigorously on the calcaneal side

5.1.6 Coalition Resection and/or Deformity Correction in Rigid Planovalgus Deformity

In about 50% of all cases, the talocalcaneal coalition is combined with a planovalgus deformity (rigid planovalgus deformity). In this constellation, an isolated resection of the coalition often does not lead to a sufficient improvement of the deformity. In recent years, different therapeutic concepts have been propagated for these patients:

Therapeutic Options for Rigid Planovalgus Deformity

- Resection of the coalition, deformity correction later if necessary
- Deformity correction without resection of the coalition
- Simultaneous coalition resection with deformity correction

For example, the group of Mubarak and coworkers primarily recommends an isolated resection of the coalition without correction of the malposition and, if necessary, plans a secondary intervention to correct the deformity (Gantsoudes et al. 2012). This was necessary in their patient population in as many as 34% of the cases without specifying the exact indication. In individual cases, the deformity may even be exacerbated by resection of the coalition (Fig. 5.30). The shear forces associated with the malposition are likely to have a negative effect on the prognosis of the subtalar joint.

Mosca and Bevan (2012) point out that the complaints in rigid planovalgus deformity may be caused more by the deformity than by the coalition itself. They report favorable results in nine cases in which a calcaneal lengthening osteotomy was performed in conjunction with soft tissue interventions, leaving the coalition unaffected and thus accepting the restricted subtalar motion to persist.

At about the same time, the study group around Blitz (Kernbach et al. 2008; Blitz 2010), Lisella et al. (2011), and Hamel (2009 and 2012) published first experiences with simultaneous resection of the talocalcaneal coalition and deformity correction by tarsal osteotomies. Here, the disadvantage of delayed mobilization of the subtalar joint is accepted. This concept will be explained in more detail below. Alternatively, deformity correction in younger children can also be achieved using arthroereisis techniques in selected cases.

5.1.6.1 Technique and Indication

After resection of the coalition as described in Sect. 5.1.5.1, all components of the planovalgus deformity (see Chap. 4) are corrected by osteotomies (for surgical technique of tarsal triple osteotomy, see Sect. 4.11.2). The (moderate) calcaneal lengthening osteotomy addresses in particular the middle forefoot abduction. At the same time, it can effectively eliminate the anterolateral subtalar impingement (Fig. 5.31) if it is applied directly anterior to the joint surface boundary of the posterior facet. Excessive lengthening should be avoided, as with the flexible planovalgus foot, also because this would further reduce subtalar mobility. In individual cases, the coalition material, resected in one block, can also be used as a bone graft for the lengthening. The remaining hindfoot valgus component is corrected by a calcaneal sliding osteotomy. In the case of a relevant elevation of the medial ray, a closed-wedge osteotomy of the medial cuneiform is recom-

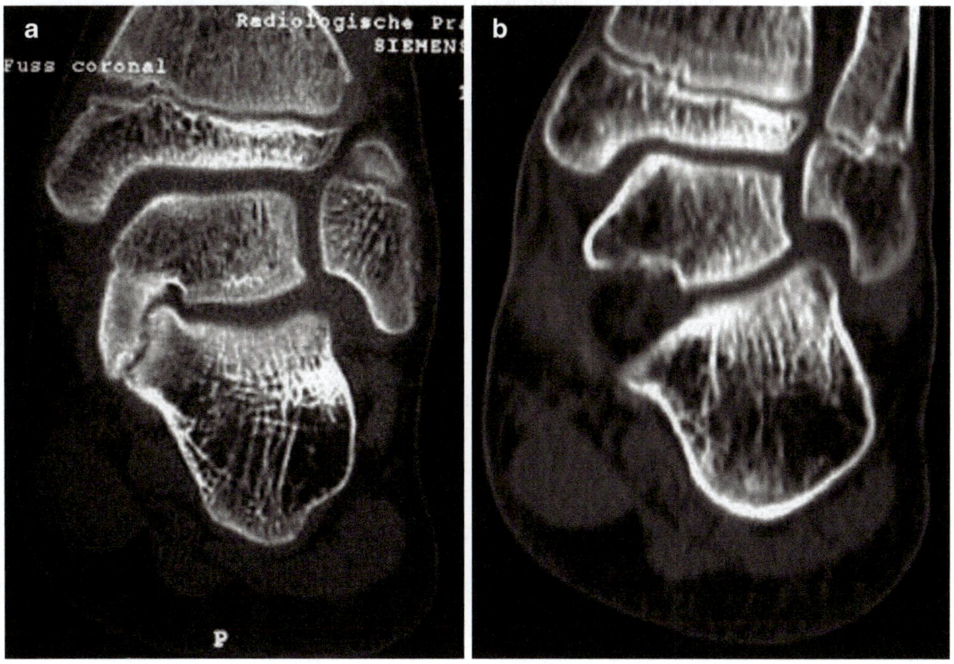

Fig. 5.30 CT frontal section before (**a**) and after (**b**) resection of a talocalcaneal coalition in a 12-year-old patient. The resection seems to have led to destabilization with valgus decompensation

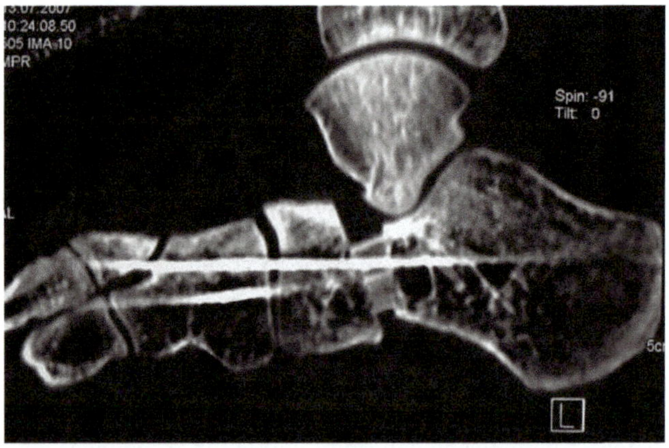

Fig. 5.31 Condition after calcaneal lengthening in the context of a correction of a rigid pes planovalgus in a 14-year-old patient. The anterolateral subtalar impingement indicated by the marked hypertrophy of the calcaneal corticalis could be addressed additionally by the lengthening procedure

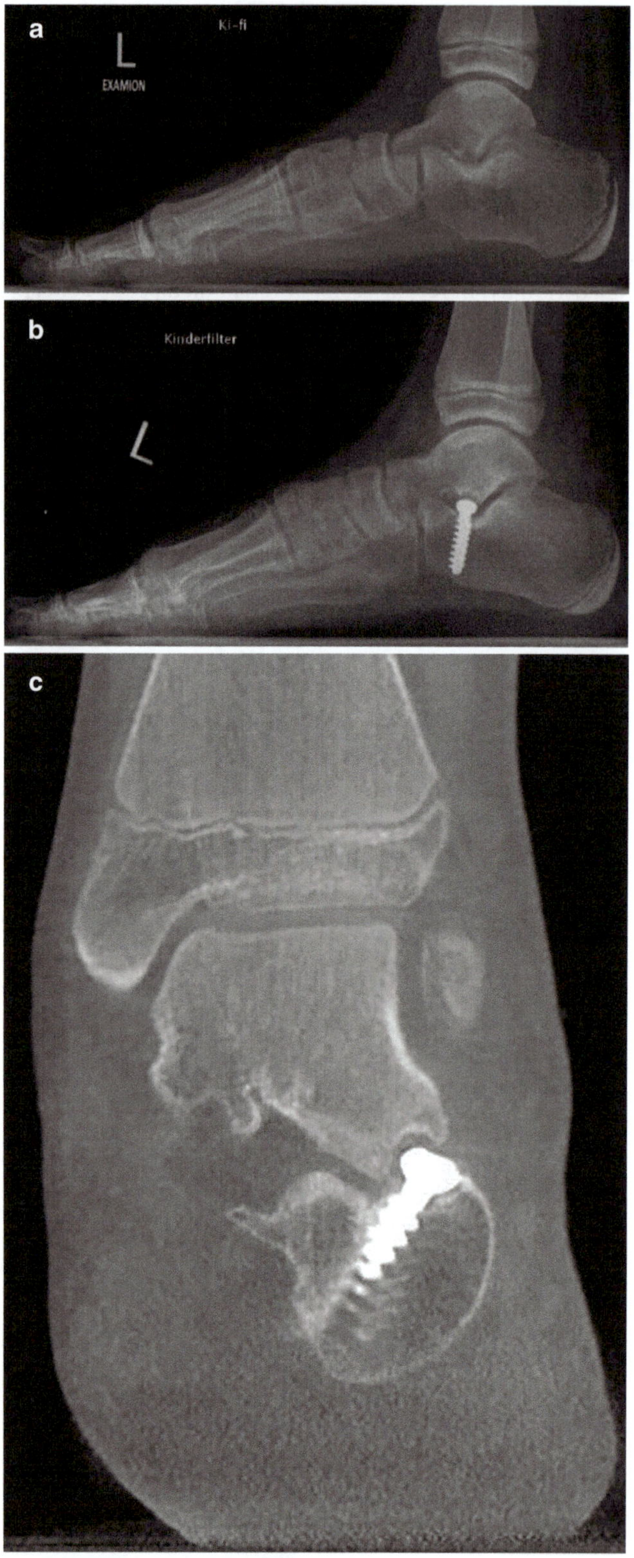

Fig. 5.32 10-Year-old patient with talocalcaneal coalition and moderate planovalgus deformity (same patient as in Fig. 5.20) before (**a**) and after (**b**) resection of the talocalcaneal coalition and calcaneostop arthroereisis with marked improvement of hindfoot alignment. 3 years after surgery, the foot was mobile and pain-free; however, an asymptomatic bony arrosion is visible in the DVT (**c**)

mended, since these are more likely contracted feet without pronounced hypermobility (Fig. 5.34). A calf muscle or gastrocnemius lengthening is often required, as in the case of a flexible pes planovalgus (Sect. 6.2.1). The simultaneous performance of osteotomies does not permit early mobilization, as recommended in the literature after coalition resection. According to the author's experience, this does not represent a significant disadvantage with regard to subsequent mobility.

At the age of 9–12 years, deformity correction by arthroereisis (guided growth) after resection of the coalition may be considered as an alternative procedure to corrective osteotomies. Giannini et al. (2003) recommend the implantation of a sinus tarsi spacer for deformity correction in conjunction with coalition resection up to the age of 14 years. Figure 5.32 shows an example with calcaneostop arthroereisis.

5.1.6.2 Results and Treatment Examples

Kernbach et al. (2008) and Lisella et al. (2011) report of good results in six or eight cases of simultaneous coalition resection and tarsal osteotomies. Hamel et al. (2016) achieved currently in the short to medium term 77% favorable results in 26 cases of simultaneous resection of a talocalcaneal coalition and corrective osteotomies. In four cases distinct complaints persisted; in two others a secondary arthrodesis was performed. In one patient treated bilaterally by Mosca and Bevan (2012), stress pain on both sides remained. Masquijo et al. (2017) report on eight cases with different tarsal osteotomies (including cases with tarsal triple osteotomy) and good results.

The four cases presented in Figs. 5.33, 5.34, 5.35, and 5.36 show exemplary treatment courses. In a patient

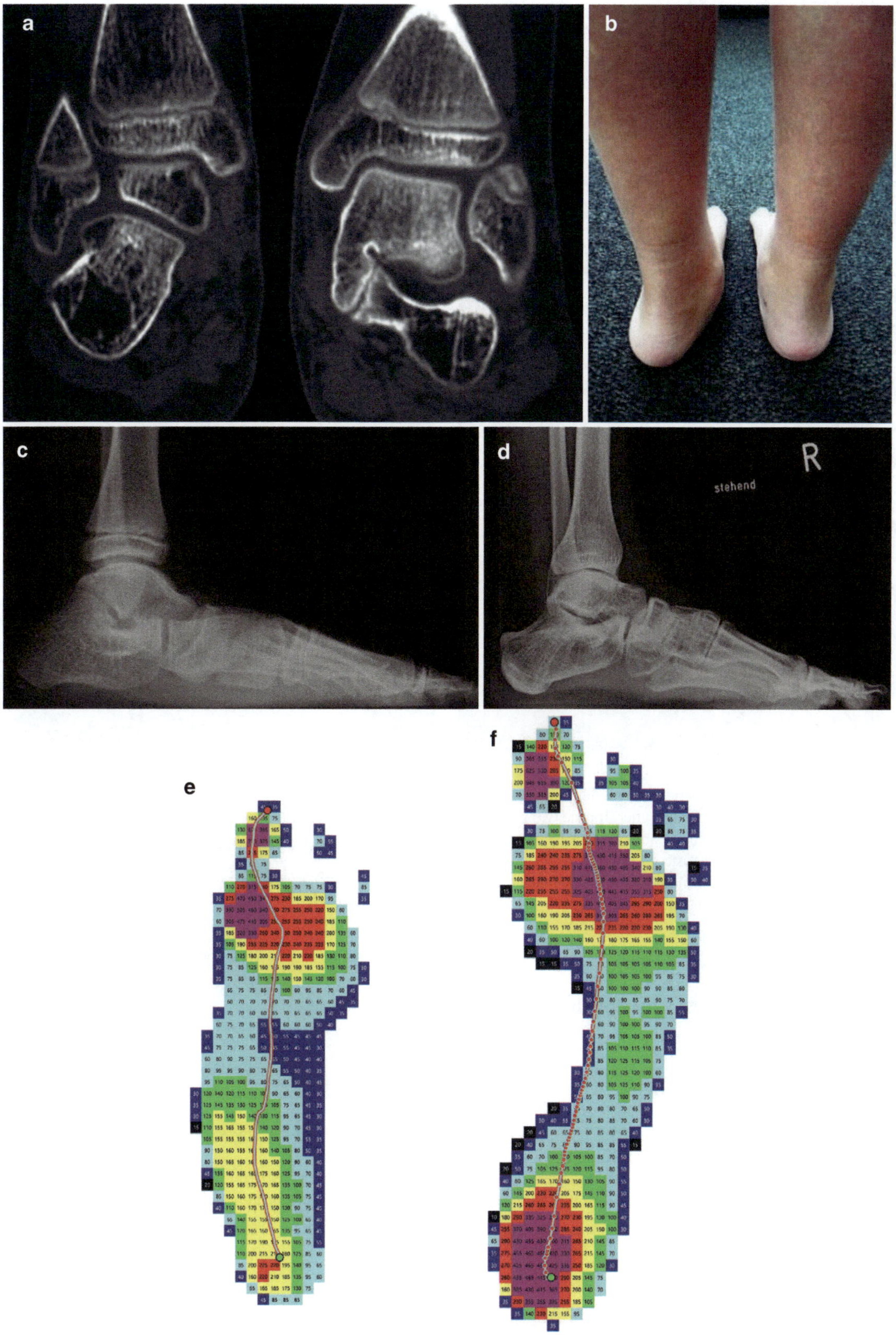

Fig. 5.33 9-Year-old patient with bilateral rigid planovalgus deformity. Talocalcaneal coalition was detected on both sides (**a**, the coalition is shown only on the right side of this CT scan). Initially, surgery was performed on the right side with clinically good hindfoot correction (**b**). The preoperative deformity (**c**) could be completely corrected by calcaneal lengthening osteotomy with gastrocnemius lengthening and the tarsal skeleton developed favorably, as the image 9 years postoperatively shows (**d**). The pedography shows a clear functional improvement postoperatively (**f**) compared to preoperatively (**e**) with physiological pressure distribution and normalized gait line. The medial-convex course of the gait line after initial heel contact indicates good shock absorption of the clinically flexible hindfoot complex

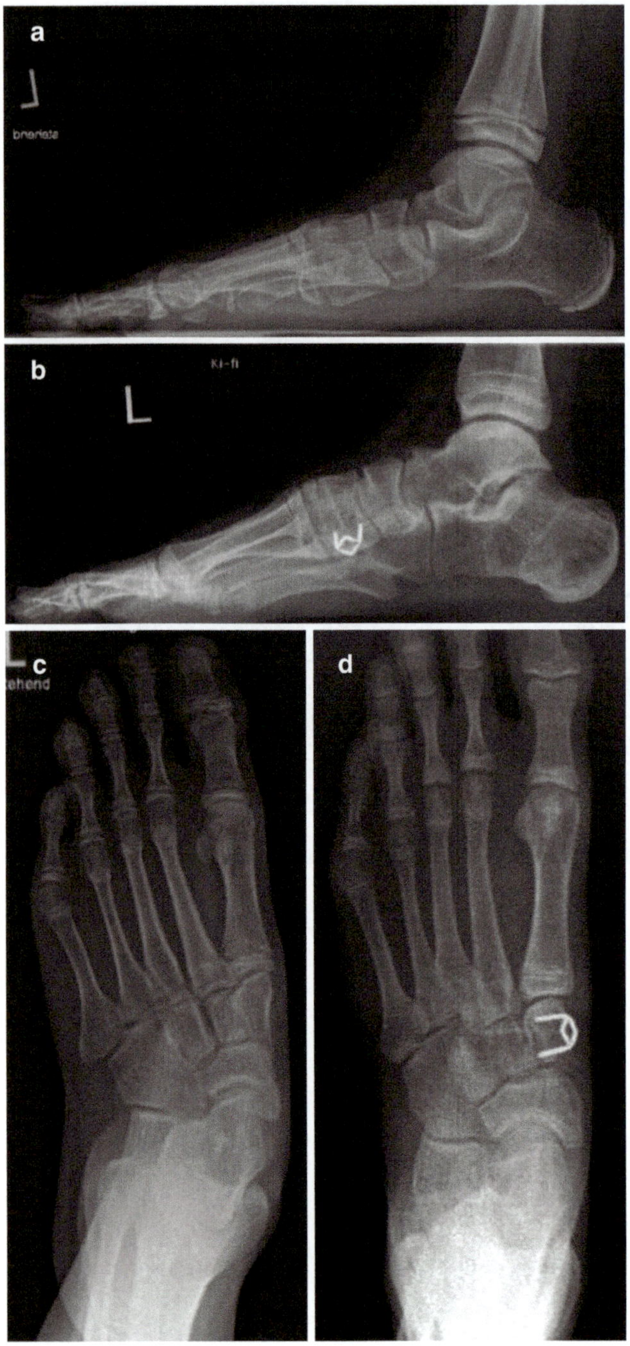

Fig. 5.34 Pre- (**a**, **c**) and postoperative images (**b**, **d**) of a 15-year-old patient with rigid planovalgus deformity. The resection was combined with a tarsal triple osteotomy (see Sect. 4.11.2) and gastrocnemius lengthening. The medial cuneiform was osteotomized using the closed-wedge technique

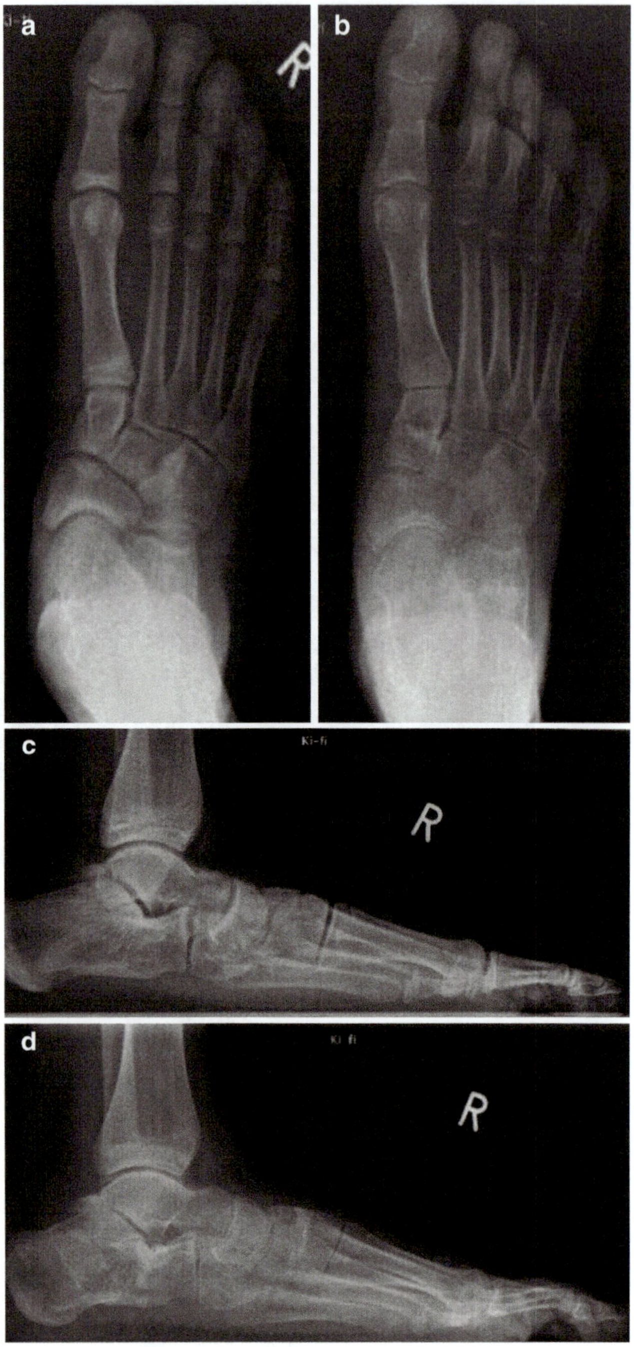

Fig. 5.35 15-Year-old boy with dorsomedial coalition and rigid planovalgus deformity (**a**, **c**). After resection of the coalition, a tarsal triple osteotomy with gastrocnemius lengthening was performed in the same procedure. 6 months postoperatively (**b**, **d**), residual mobility and good alignment correction, but the subtalar joint space appears significantly narrowed

who underwent surgery at a very young age, a combined coalition resection and calcaneal lengthening achieved an optimal, also long-term, result (Fig. 5.33). Two adolescent patients only to be assessed in the short term, with resection and tarsal triple osteotomy (cf. Sect. 4.11.2), showed a complete deformity correction (Fig. 5.34 and 5.35). If this primarily joint-preserving procedure does not eliminate the complaints, a talocalcaneal in situ fusion provides a good option as a salvage procedure (Fig. 5.36).

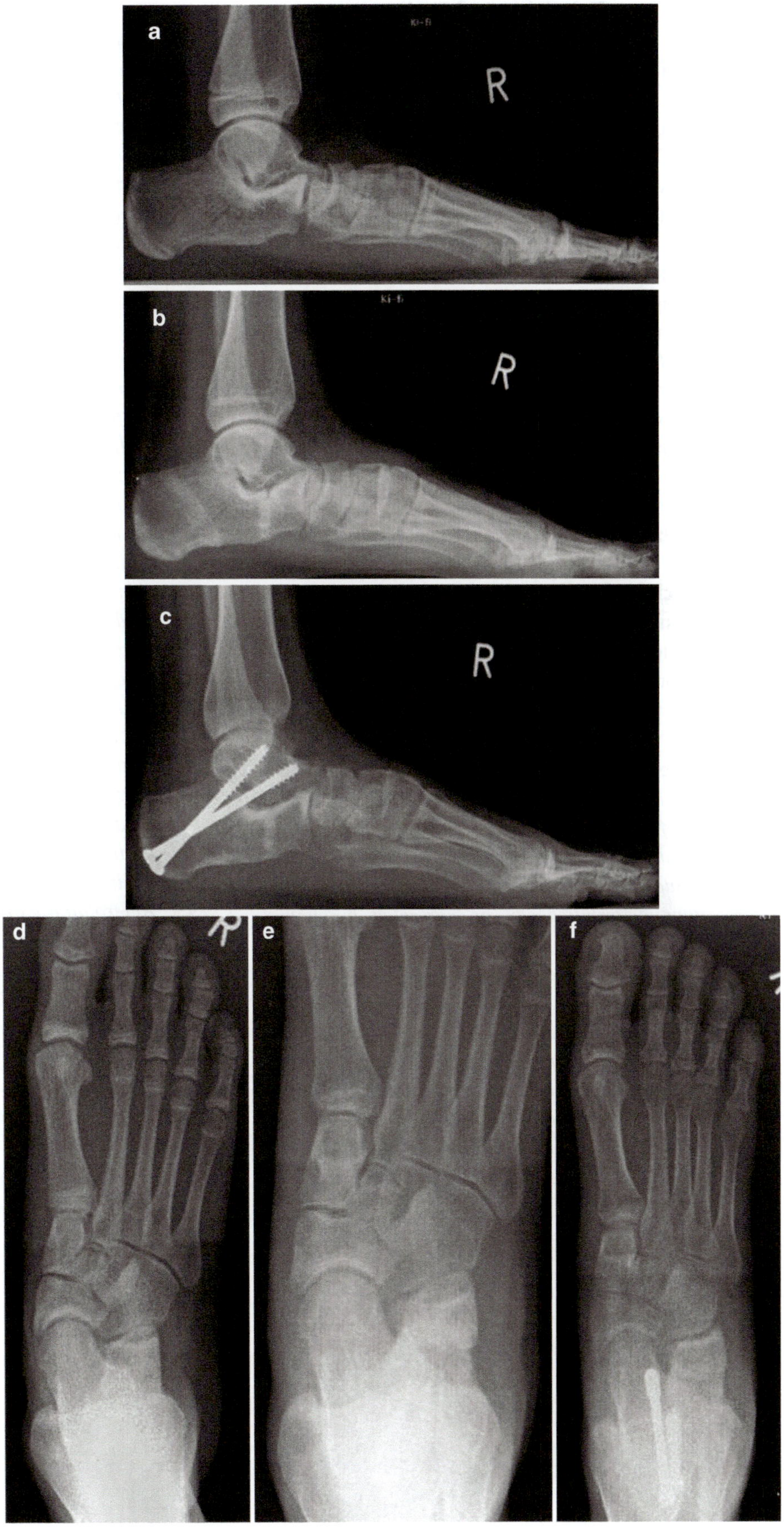

Fig. 5.36 16-Year-old patient with talocalcaneal coalition (**a**, **d**). After resection of the coalition and tarsal triple osteotomy (**b**, **e**), subtalar complaints persisted with incomplete alignment correction, so that a subtalar fusion was performed 1 year later (**c**, **f**)

5.1.7 Primary Talocalcaneal Fusion

In the literature, triple arthrodesis is usually indicated as a therapy for a non-resectable coalition (e.g., Downey and DeWaters 2013), especially in cases of rigid planovalgus deformity (Cowell and Elener 1983). The author, however, has never seen an indication for the regular inclusion of the Chopart joint line into the fusion area in adolescent age. In the more recent literature, a primary (talocalcaneal) arthrodesis in childhood and adolescence is rarely discussed due to the expected long-term degenerative changes in the neighboring joints and is regarded more or less as a possibility of salvage only in case of persistent complaints after coalition resection. In the author's experience, however, there are also prognostically unfavorable cases at a younger age (Fig. 5.37), for which a primary talocalcaneal fusion appears to be advantageous and prolonged periods of pain with multiple interventions can thereby be avoided. A balanced discussion can be found in Blitz (2010) and Cass and Camasta (2010).

5.1.7.1 Technique

If the assessment of the indication criteria shows that a primary talocalcaneal arthrodesis is preferable to resection, it can be performed in different ways

Technique

1. *The medial approach (Fig. 5.38) with prior resection of the coalition is the most common access. This allows bony material from the coalition to be obtained for a spongious bone graft; mild hindfoot valgus deformities can be corrected by medial resection of the joint surfaces. The medial approach is particularly advantageous for cases that have an unclear indication preoperatively, since a decision can be made intraoperatively between resection of the coalition and primary fusion. After spreading with the K-wire-anchored distractor, cartilage is removed as much as possible with curettes and raspatories. To prepare the arthrodesis surfaces, power-burrs are helpful, which are controlled by a guiding sleeve. If the calcaneal growth plate is closed, the osteosynthesis can be stabilized with two strong cannulated compression screws; the lateral screw is placed in the corpus tali, the medial screw in the corpus-neck junction. In younger children, Kirschner wires are used. The superficial parts of the delta ligament are slightly weakened by the access and should be sutured carefully. Relevant instabilities were never observed.*
2. *The posterior approach is chosen for dorsomedial or posterior localized forms of coalition (Fig. 5.39). The coalition is then osteotomized from the posterior side. The main advantage lies in the possibility of using a posteriorly inserted wedge-shaped bone graft to additionally shift the talus into a more inclined position and thereby treat an existing or threatening anterior upper ankle joint impingement, or at least not further worsen it. The disadvantage is the required prone position for any additional procedures that may be necessary. The skin incision is made directly lateral to the Achilles tendon, and the sural nerve is carefully protected. Through the Kager fat triangle, the joint capsule is reached, which is opened after identification of the subtalar joint and the FHL tendon. The K-wires for the distractor are placed under image intensifier control and the joint is spread open. After osteotomy of the coalition, the cartilage of the posterior joint facet is removed, and a wedge-shaped tricortical bone graft is molded precisely and inserted for interpositional fusion.*
3. *Anterolateral arthrodesis usually requires a graft and can be performed in the form of an extra-articular Grice procedure (Fig. 6.15) with a corticospongious tibia or fibula graft (Fig. 5.42), but also after cartilage removal from the posterior joint facet of the subtalar joint, osteotomy of the medial coalition, and interposition of a corticospongious iliac crest graft. Also, a cartilage removal with cancellous bone grafting is possible while leaving the coalition and without osteosynthesis, if no deformity correction is necessary (Cass and Camasta* 2010*).*

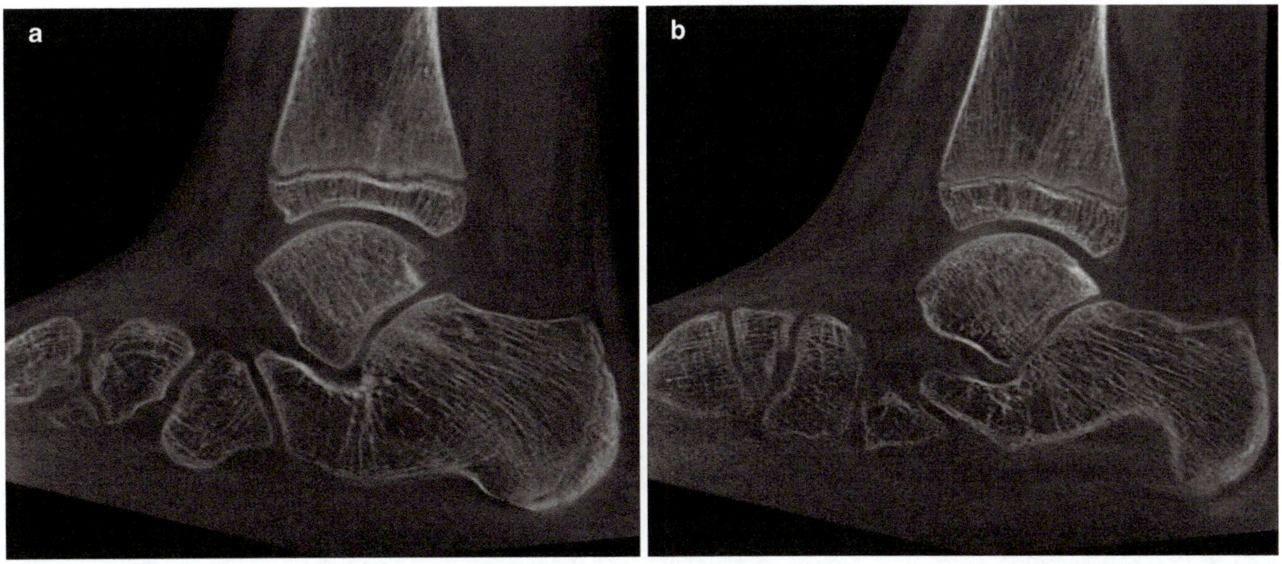

Fig. 5.37 DVT of a 13-year-old male patient with bilateral rigid planovalgus deformity. Whereas on the right side (**a**) resection of the coalition with tarsal osteotomies was indicated and the subtalar joint was preserved, on the left side (**b**) primary fusion seemed appropriate because of severe joint space narrowing.

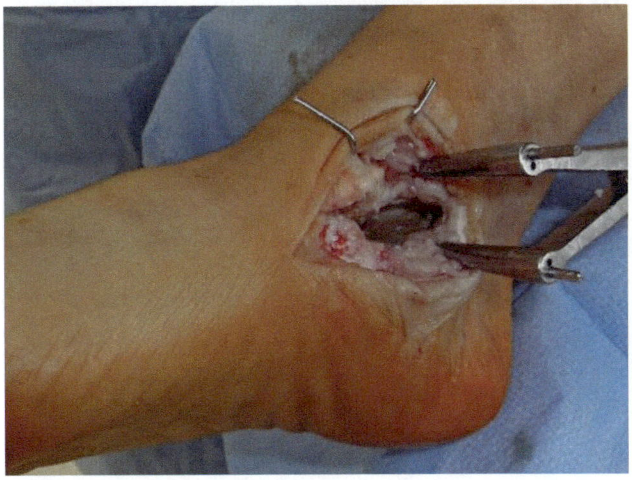

Fig. 5.38 Access to perform talocalcaneal arthrodesis after coalition resection from a medial approach

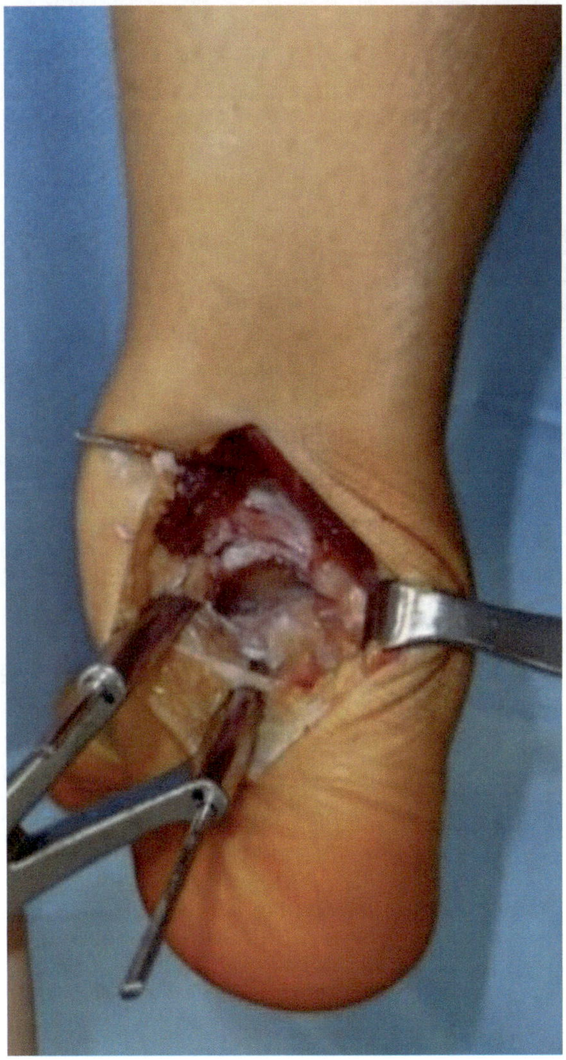

Fig. 5.39 Dorsal access for performing an (interposition) arthrodesis in talocalcaneal coalition

5.1.7.2 Results and Treatment Examples

Data on the performance and results of talocalcaneal arthrodesis in coalition patients are almost non-existent in the more recent literature. The author has primarily performed fusion in 26 cases in patients under 18 years of age (Hamel et al. 2016). Cases of pseudarthrosis were not observed; however, a routine CT examination was not performed. In three cases, additional osteotomies were performed to correct the position. In three cases, there were still moderate complaints, partly in connection with massive overweight. As a general rule, the patients were very satisfied at least in the medium term and did not register any significant loss of mobility, since the coalition already had resulted in a significant reduction of the range of motion preoperatively. In cases of preoperative peroneal spasm, this improved in some cases only in the course of several months. Two typical cases with additional correcting tarsal osteotomies are presented in Figs. 5.40 and 5.41.

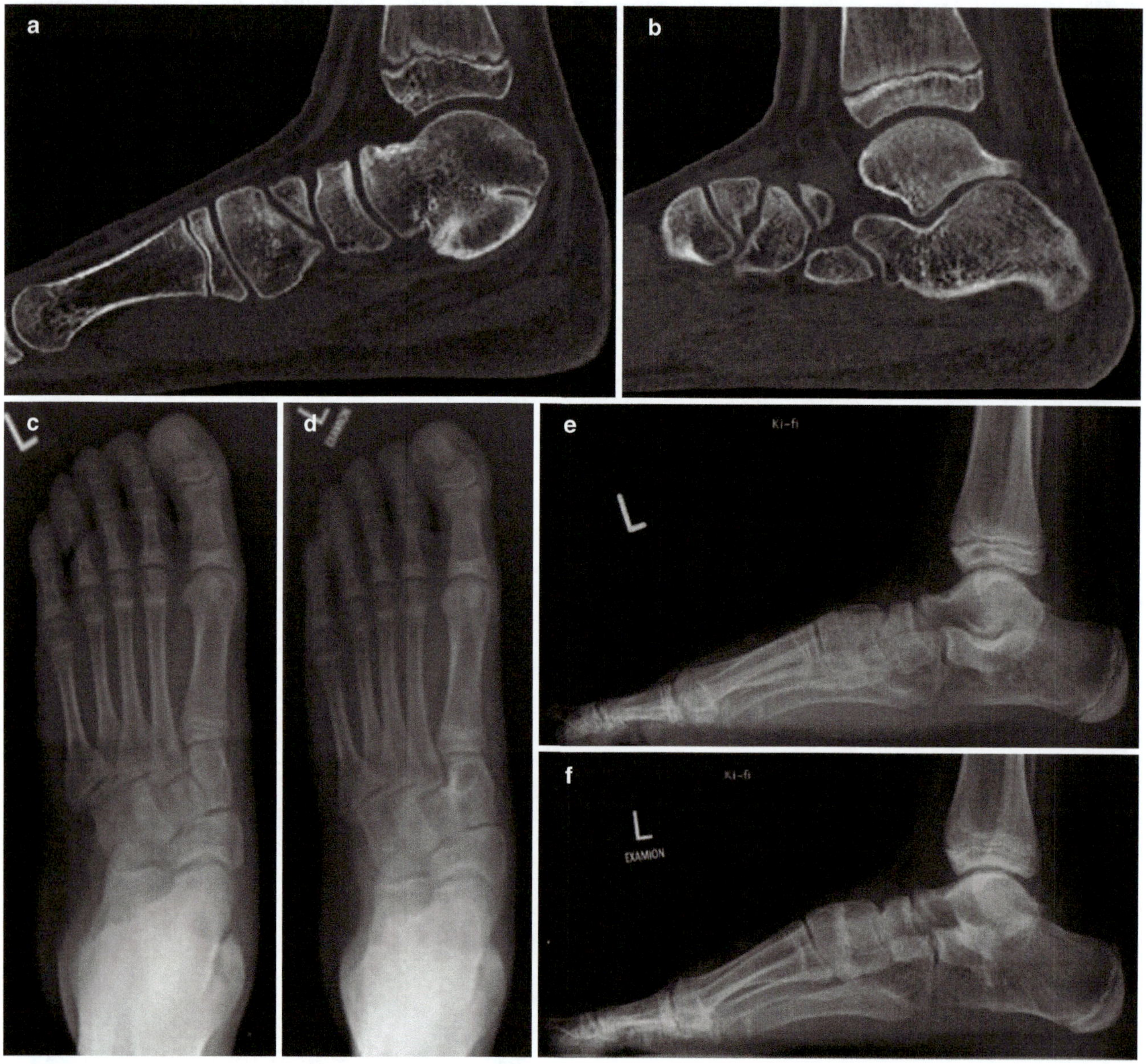

Fig. 5.40 13-Year-old patient with large, complete talocalcaneal coalition (**a**) and partially distinct subtalar joint space narrowing (**b**). Clinically and radiologically moderate planovalgus deformity (**c**, **e**) and distinct peroneal spasm. Intraoperatively, only minimal talocalcaneal residual mobility in the sense of an angular tilting movement was observed after resection of the coalition. It was therefore decided to perform a primary talocalcaneal arthrodesis. Malalignment components were additionally corrected by slight calcaneal lengthening and cuneiform osteotomy, supplemented by a gastrocnemius lengthening, 9 months postoperatively good alignment correction (**d**, **f**)

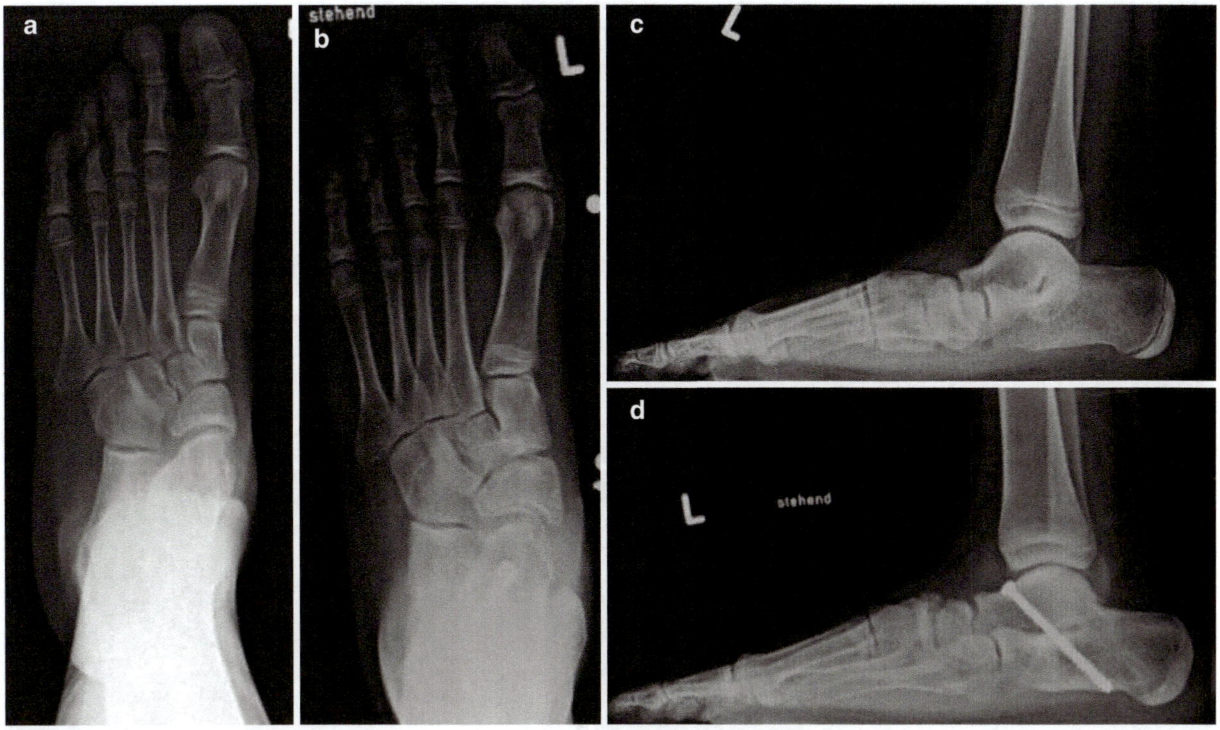

Fig. 5.41 13-Year-old patient with severe planovalgus deformity (**a, c**) and large talocalcaneal coalition. A corrective talocalcaneal arthrodesis was combined with further osteotomies (calcaneal lengthening and cuneiform osteotomy) and a lengthening of the gastrocnemius and peroneus brevis tendon and resulted in a good postoperative realignment (**b, d**)

5.1.8 Secondary Interventions After Coalition Resection

After a talocalcaneal coalition resection, symptoms can persist for months before a definitive result may be assumed. It must be taken into account that, apart from the coalition itself, these are not normally developed subtalar joints, instead joint surface configuration and capsule-ligament apparatus could not develop normally with the existing movement limitation by the coalition. Permanently remaining complaints can have different causes.

Possible Causes for Persisting Pain After Coalition Resection

- Incomplete resection (Figs. 5.28, 5.29, and 5.43)
- Reossification at the former coalition site
- Persisting deformity
- Anterolateral subtalar impingement
- Additional coalition left untreated
- Degenerative changes at the subtalar joint (exaggerated indication, Fig. 5.42)

Some experiences with patients, who are not complaint-free after coalition resection, are: complete freedom from pain should always be rated higher than mobility (cf. Fig. 5.42). Functionally very unfavorable is a persistent peroneal spasm that locks the entire talocalcaneal-navicular complex in an unfavorable everted position. Nevertheless, the aversion to a secondary fusion is often high on the patient's (and parent's) side, even with a functionally severe impairment, and requires longer clarification talks. As a rule, a surgical revision, e.g., with repeated resection, does not appear promising, except in the case of clearly incomplete previous surgery, and a fusion should preferably be considered. Two examples of secondary arthrodesis are presented in Figs. 5.42 and 5.43.

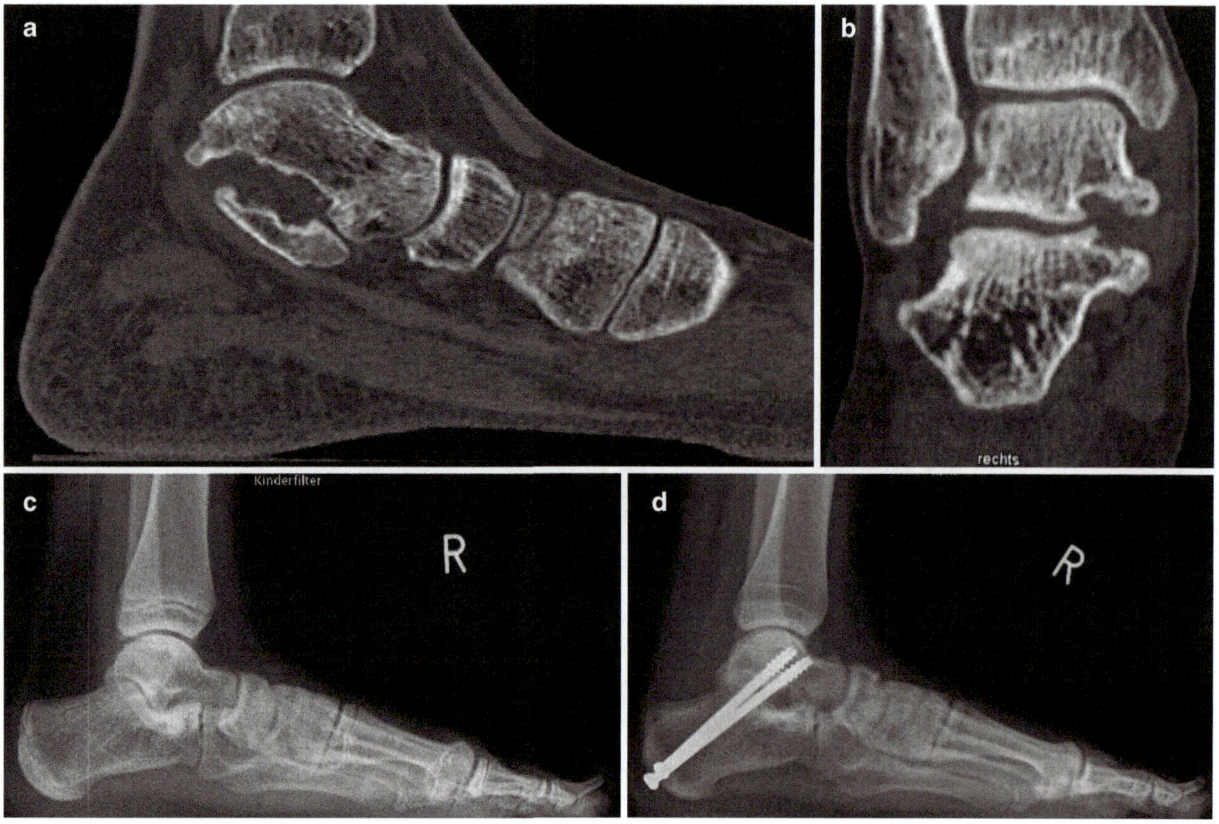

Fig. 5.42 In a 12-year-old female patient, a medium-sized talocalcaneal coalition was completely resected (**a**, **b**), and a good clinical mobility of the subtalar joint could be achieved. Nevertheless, considerable complaints persisted, so that 2.5 years postoperatively, a secondary talocalcaneal fusion was performed (**d**). Retrospectively, a clear narrowing of the subtalar joint space is noticeable in the preoperative X-ray (**c**), possibly as an indication of already extensive damage to the residual joint not affected by the coalition

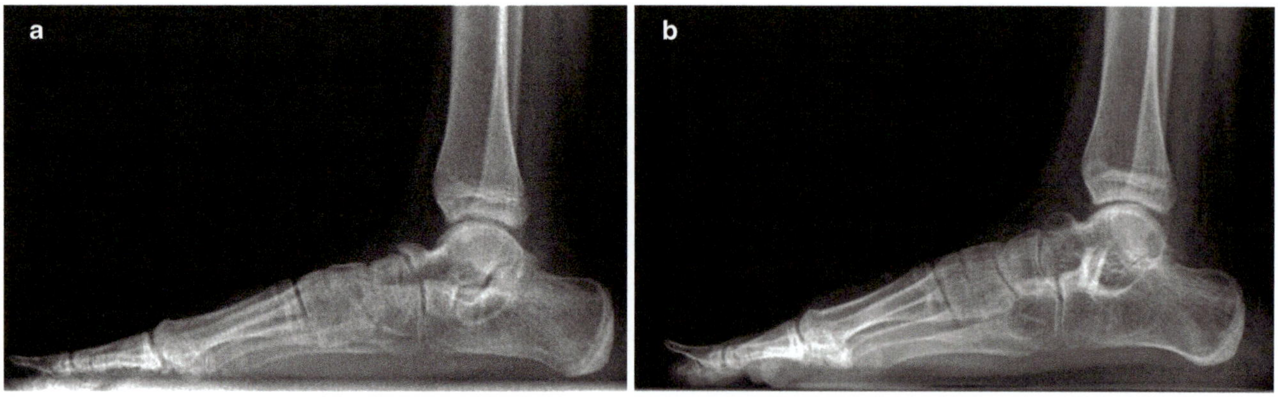

Fig. 5.43 Externally preoperated female patient with incomplete resection and persistent, quite severe complaints. At the age of 12 years (**a**), a Grice arthrodesis was performed with subsequent complete relief from pain (**b**)

5.1.9 Summary: Experiences in Own Patient Population

In the period from 2002 to 2019, the author surgically treated 138 pediatric or adolescent patients with talocalcaneal coalition. Figure 5.44 shows a summary of the patients operated until 2014 (Hamel et al. 2016). Isolated coalition resection or primary fusion was effective in about 87% of the cases, whereas combined resection and deformity correction was successful in about 77%.

In retrospect, regarding the own patient base, it seems advisable to limit resections to the really promising cases in view of the generally favorable results after fusion (cf. Fig. 5.45). The concept of simultaneous coalition treatment and malalignment correction has proved very successful; in cases where arthrodesis is required secondarily after resection, this is after deformity correction technically less complex in the sense of a pure in situ fusion.

The Author's Experience with Talocalcaneal Coalition Treatment

- Often long periods of time until diagnosis is made
- Coalition resection in younger children with small coalition is justified even without severe pain
- Simultaneous coalition resection and deformity correction advisable
- Critical differential indication between resection and fusion in patients at the end of growth and later
- Secondary fusion in patients with persisting pain after resection without longer delay (9–15 months)
- Restricted indication for secondary resection procedures

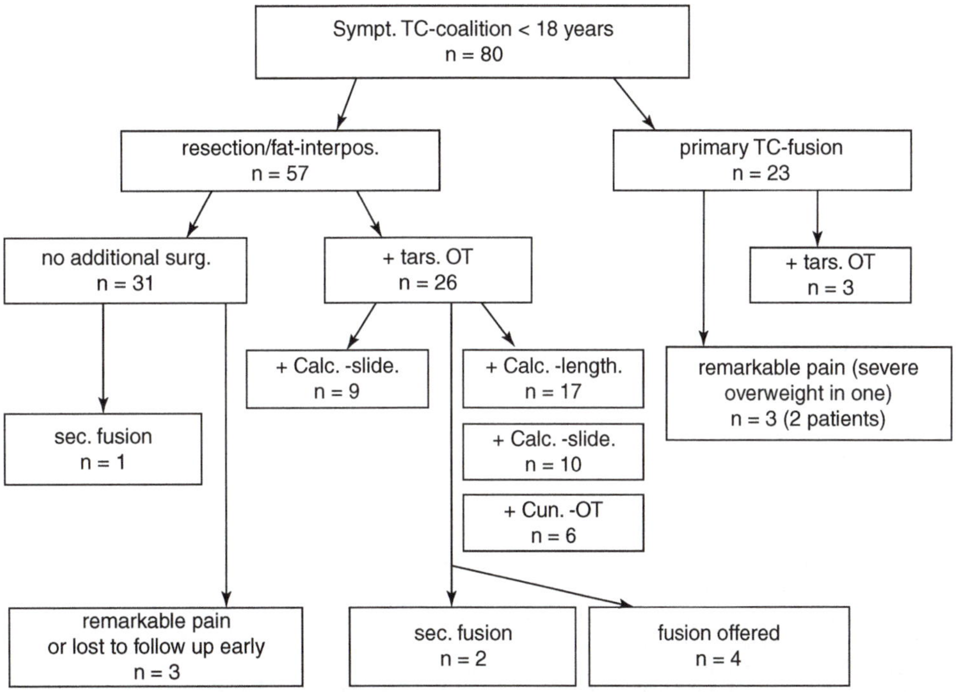

Fig. 5.44 Treatment paths of 80 surgically treated pediatric and adolescent patients with talocalcaneal coalition including the unfavorable results (from Hamel et al. 2016)

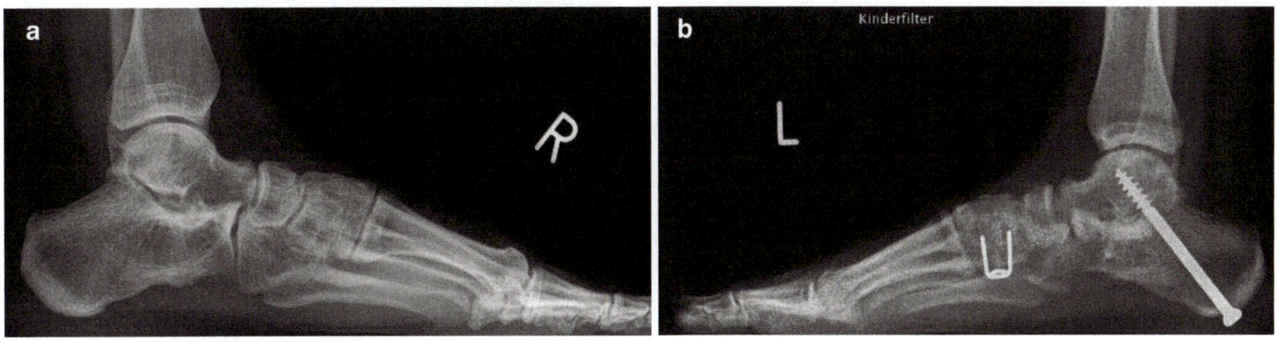

Fig. 5.45 18-Year-old female patient, who underwent a coalition resection with tarsal osteotomies at the age of 12 and 14 years (first on the right (**a**), then on the left (**b**)) in the presence of a pronounced rigid planovalgus deformity, with the difference that on the left side it was combined with a talocalcaneal fusion. The patient is largely satisfied with both sides, but when closely questioned, she sees slight functional advantages on the left side where a fusion was performed

5.2 Calcaneonavicular Coalition

The calcaneonavicular coalition is observed with about the same frequency as the talocalcaneal form and accounts for about 55% of the coalition surgeries in the author's practice. It presents significantly fewer questions about the treatment indication, and the surgical results are overall better than with the talocalcaneal coalition.

5.2.1 Therapeutically Relevant Pathomorphology and Pathophysiology

In the talocalcaneal-navicular joint complex, the osteoligamentous chain of calcaneus, cuboid, and navicular is closely linked to each other and moves opposite the talus. These first three bones, which move in almost the same direction, are interconnected by joints or ligaments. The ligamentum bifurcatum between the anterior calcaneal process and the lateral navicular pole, which always keeps these two skeletal elements in close spatial relationship during inversion and eversion, plays a special role here. If increasing rigidity occurs in this calcaneonavicular transition region due to the formation of a coalition which solidifies by progressive ossification as the patient grows older, it results in unphysiological forced movements. This has an impact especially at the talonavicular joint and often leads to arthritis in the long term. The complete or incomplete bone bridge (Fig. 5.47), interrupted by a gap, often extends far to the lower surface of the navicular bone (Fig. 5.48b) and can be more than 2.5 cm deep.

5.2.2 Clinic

The calcaneonavicular coalition often becomes symptomatic at the age of 9–12 years. Pain is expressed during sports or everyday activities above the calcaneonavicular transition region or diffusely in the entire hindfoot area. A peroneal spasm is also observed—somewhat less frequently than in the case of talocalcaneal coalition—and passive forced inversion is usually indicated as painful and is clearly limited. Malpositions are less frequent in the calcaneonavicular coalition than in the talocalcaneal form; if they occur, they are usually planovalgus deformities, rarely inversion malpositions.

5.2.3 Imaging

In most cases the standard X-rays are already sufficient for the diagnosis. In the lateral projection, the "anteater sign" (Fig. 5.46) is typical, an anterior process of the calcaneus extended far to the distal side. A "talar beak" (traction osteophyte at the head of the talus) is observed less frequently (Fig. 5.60a). A 45° oblique projection is required for a more precise representation of the coalition (Fig. 5.47). Cross-sectional imaging procedures such as MRI are diagnostically only useful if there is a suspicion of accompanying pathology (Figs. 5.49 and 5.50) or in individual cases as preparation for surgery (e.g., exclusion of an additional talocalcaneal coalition, Fig. 5.48). An anterolateral subtalar reshaping as in the talocalcaneal form (Sect. 5.1.3) can also be observed (Fig. 5.46).

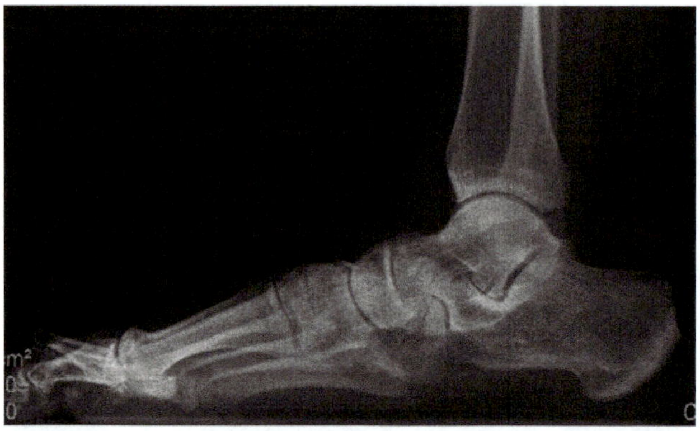

Fig. 5.46 Calcaneonavicular coalition, already clearly visible in the lateral X-ray projection. Typical is the so-called anteater sign, meaning an anterior calcaneal process that extends far distally. Note the marked cortical thickening of the calcaneal neck

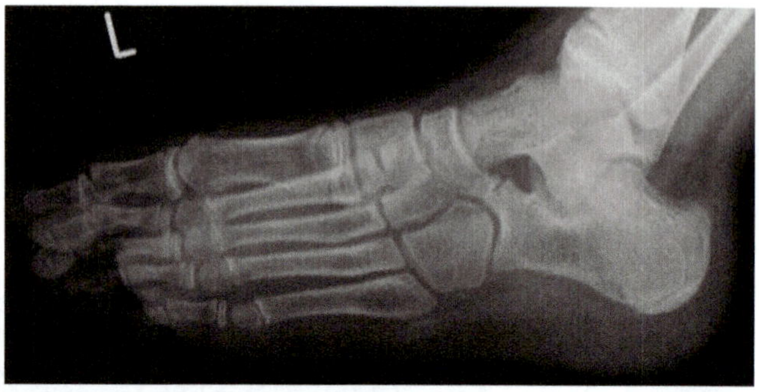

Fig. 5.47 In the 45° oblique view, the calcaneonavicular coalition can be seen well. In this case an incomplete bone bridge is clearly visible

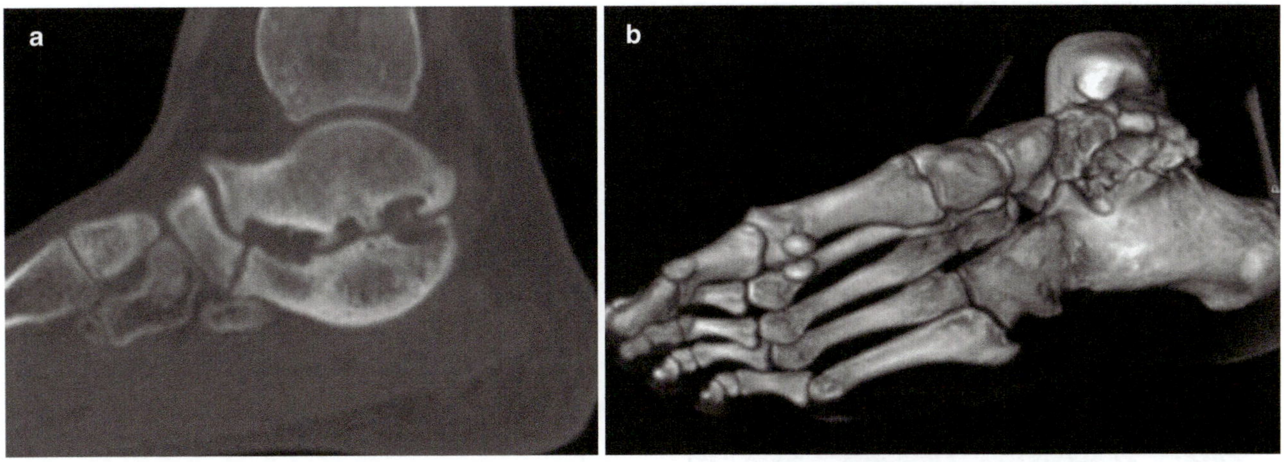

Fig. 5.48 Adolescent patient with calcaneonavicular and talocalcaneal coalition in CT (**a**) and three-dimensional reconstruction (**b**). The calcaneonavicular coalescence extends to the depth below the talonavicular joint

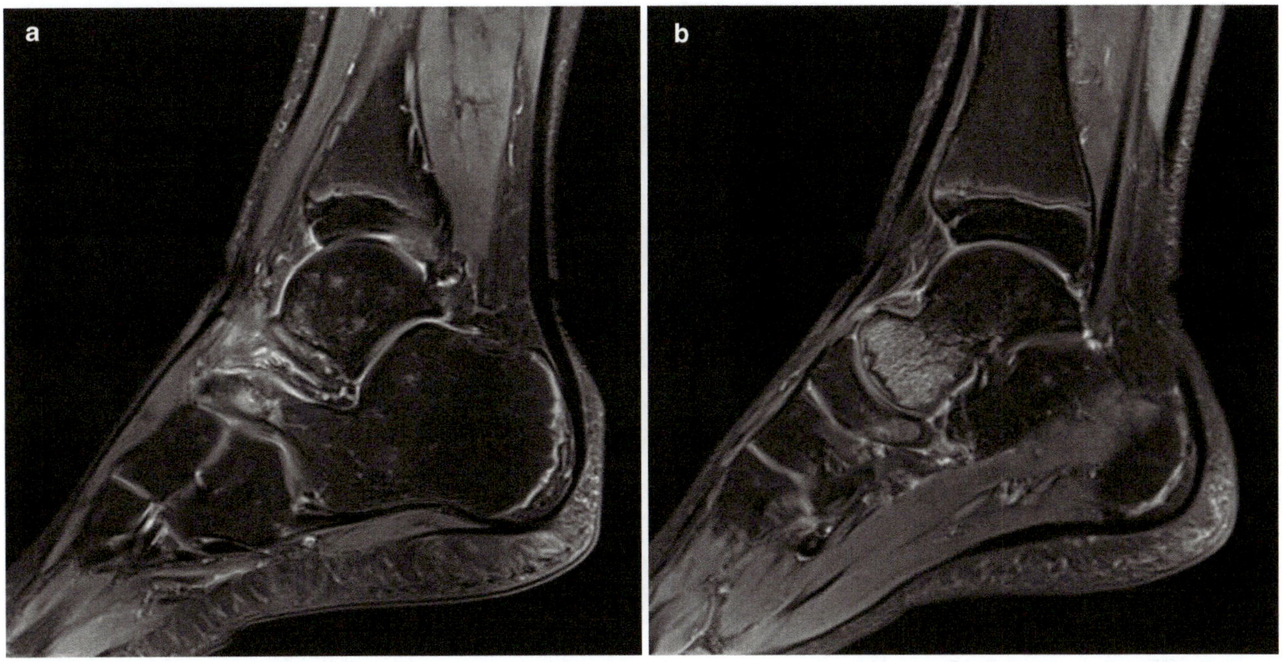

Fig. 5.49 11-Year-old girl with symptomatic, activated calcaneonavicular coalition (**a**) and additional clear bone bruise of the talar head with subchondral fracture line (**b**) in MRI

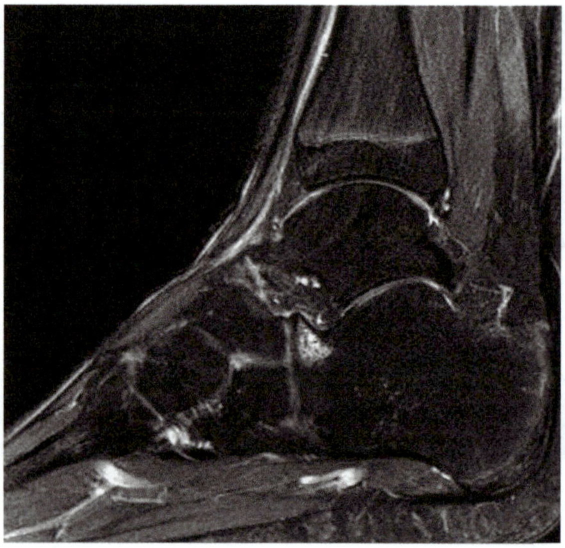

Fig. 5.50 Activation of the bony parts close to the coalition in symptomatic calcaneonavicular coalition in a 12-year-old boy in the MRI

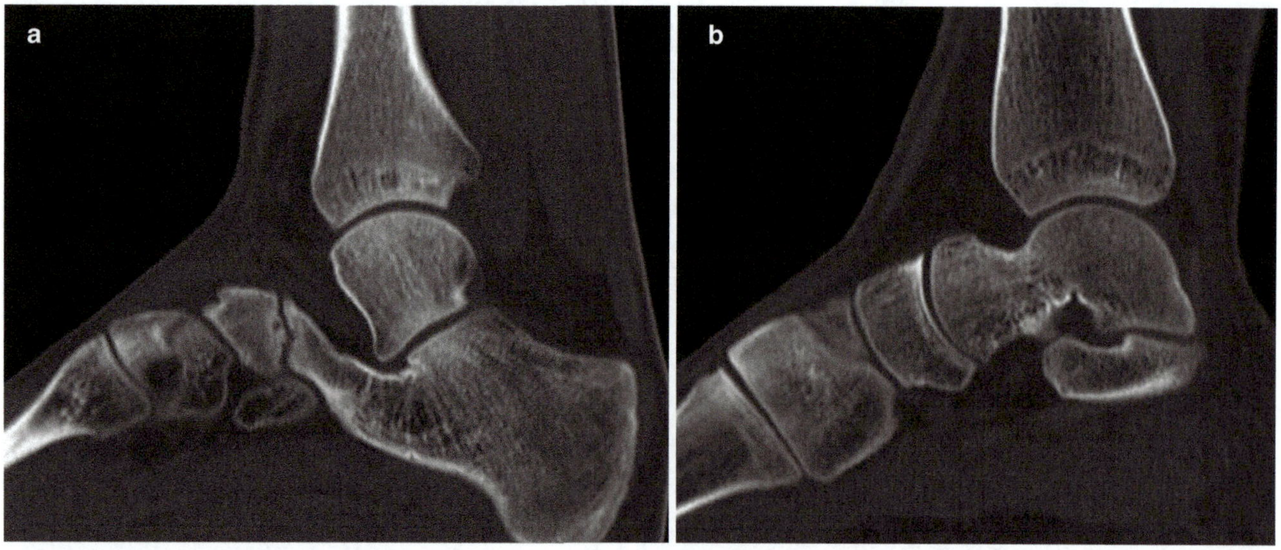

Fig. 5.51 CT sagittal section of a 15-year-old female patient with calcaneonavicular coalition (**a**). The distinct joint space narrowing of the talonavicular joint in its plantar part in the sense of a beginning arthritis is clearly visible (**b**)

5.2.4 Indication for Surgical Treatment

The surgical treatment of calcaneonavicular coalition in pediatric patients consists of the resection of the bone bridge with soft tissue interposition and—in some cases—additional correction of a planovalgus deformity. A primary fusion procedure is rarely considered in children and adolescents but may be necessary later in the case of more severe degenerative changes in the talonavicular joint.

The results of surgical resections in childhood and early adolescence are favorable in most of the cases, so that the indication can be generously given even without complaints. However, this does not represent the opinion of most of the authors in literature. The probability of later complaints or the development of arthritic changes (Fig. 5.51), due to the significantly disturbed tarsal mechanics as a result of the coalition, clearly outweighs the risks of resection. Nevertheless, especially in children with few complaints, possible complications such as—rarely—residual symptoms, skin nerve injury, or neuroma formation or even dystrophy must be pointed out during the informative discussion with the parents.

5.2.5 Coalition Resection with Muscle Interposition

Technique

The procedure is performed in the supine position with slightly raised ipsilateral buttocks. An oblique skin incision above the calcaneonavicular transition region exposes the origin of the extensor-digitorum-brevis muscle, which is detached and looped in an L-shaped manner (Fig. 5.52a). Here, both branches of the sural nerve and dorsally the branches of the superficial peroneal nerve must be spared (Fig. 5.53).

Below the detached muscle origin, the calcaneonavicular transition region with the coalition is exposed. Here, Kirschner wires can be used in the navicular for soft tissue retraction (Figs. 5.52b and 5.53b). In the cranial-proximal wound angle, parts of the lateral talar head are exposed; the calcaneocuboid joint is opened sparingly in the plantar distal region.

The resection of the coalition is performed—if necessary after K-wire marking, with image intensifier control—using narrow oscillating saws, various chisels, narrow Luer forceps, and, if necessary, also a bone burr in such a way that a resection gap of 8–10 mm is created (Fig. 5.52c). The direction of the resection is inclined by about 45° to medioplantar; the depth of the resection can be up to 2.5 cm until the talonavicular capsule (spring ligament) becomes visible at this depth. At the navicular, the resection should be approximately in the extension of the lateral neck of the talus; at the anterior process of the calcaneus, smaller parts of the calcaneocuboid joint surface often have to be included into the resection area (Fig. 5.54). The cancellous resection surfaces are covered with

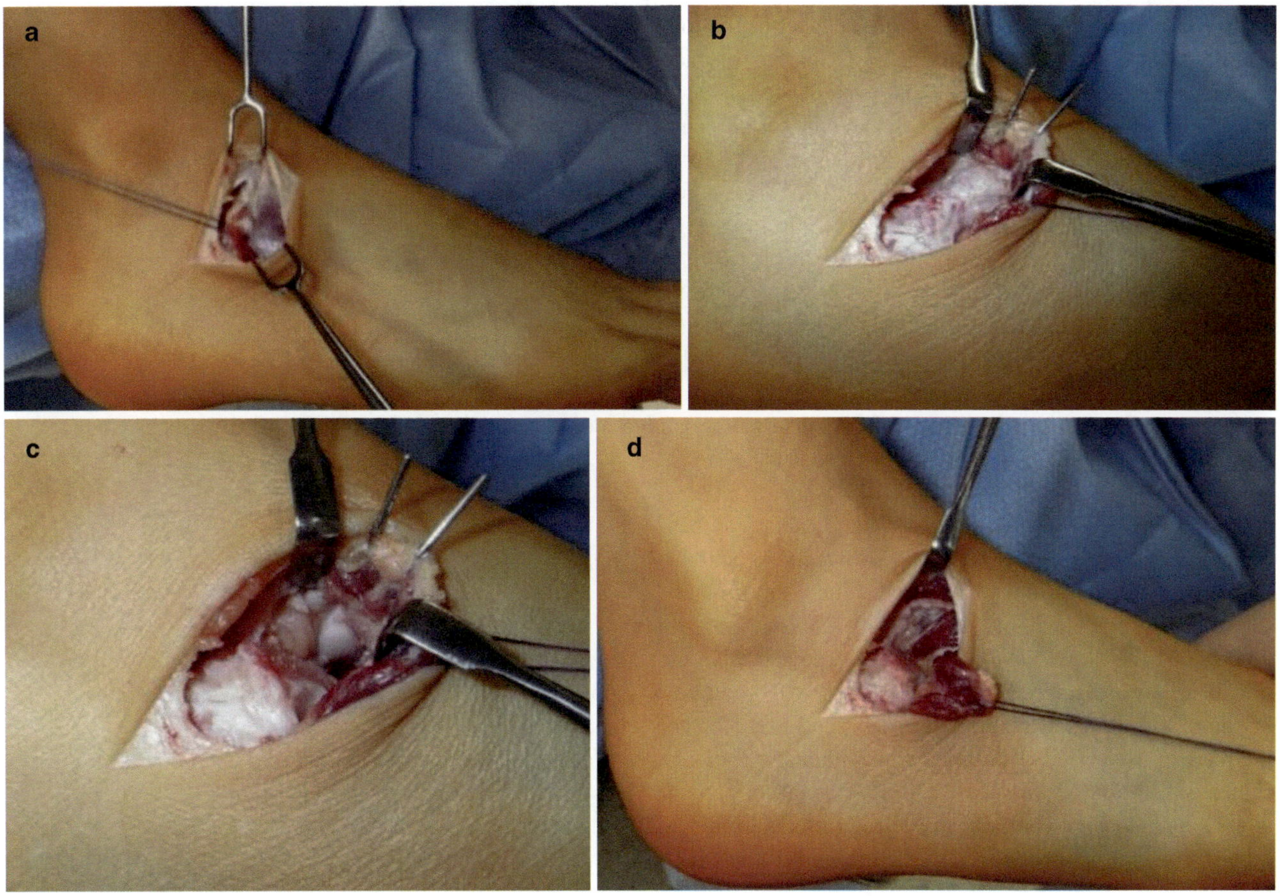

Fig. 5.52 Resection of the calcaneonavicular coalition: The extensor-digitorum-brevis origin is detached in an L-shape (**a**), and the underlying calcaneonavicular transition region is exposed. K-wires anchored in the navicular serve for soft tissue retraction (**b**). After resection, both the talonavicular joint (**c**) and the calcaneocuboid joint are visible. A split medial half of the M. extensor digitorum brevis origin is interposed into the resection gap (**d**), the attachment sutures are pulled out of the skin medioplantarly and knotted over a compress, and the lateral parts of the muscle (**d**) are refixed at the site of the original insertion to cover the soft tissue (see text)

bone wax. In rare cases with a far plantar location, it may be necessary to create a second, medioplantar access (see Fig. 5.62).

The detached extensor-digitorum-brevis origin is split into two approximately equal halves, and the dorsomedial half is pulled into the resection gap after sufficient mobilization, using an eyelet wire as a tool (Fig. 5.52d). The resorbable pullout sutures are finally knotted under slight tension in the medioplantar tarsal region above the skin and a swab (caution, danger of pressure sore!). The muscle interponate created in this way often does not fill the entire resection gap right down to the depth but reliably prevents a reossification at the coalition site. The lateral-plantar muscle parts are fixed in the soft-tissue in the area of the sinus tarsi to cover the situs. According to the literature, the entire extensor-digitorum-brevis origin may be interposed. Alternatively, a free fat tissue graft is also used. Without interposition, regeneration of the bony bridging may occur (see Fig. 5.55).

Postoperatively, the patient is immobilized for 3 weeks in a lower leg cast and kept non-weight-bearing, in order to ensure healing of the relocated muscle part. After removal of the swab and the pull-out sutures, the patient can be mobilized and weight-bearing is possible. Physiotherapeutically, inversion should be trained in particular, for which there was usually a clear restriction preoperatively.

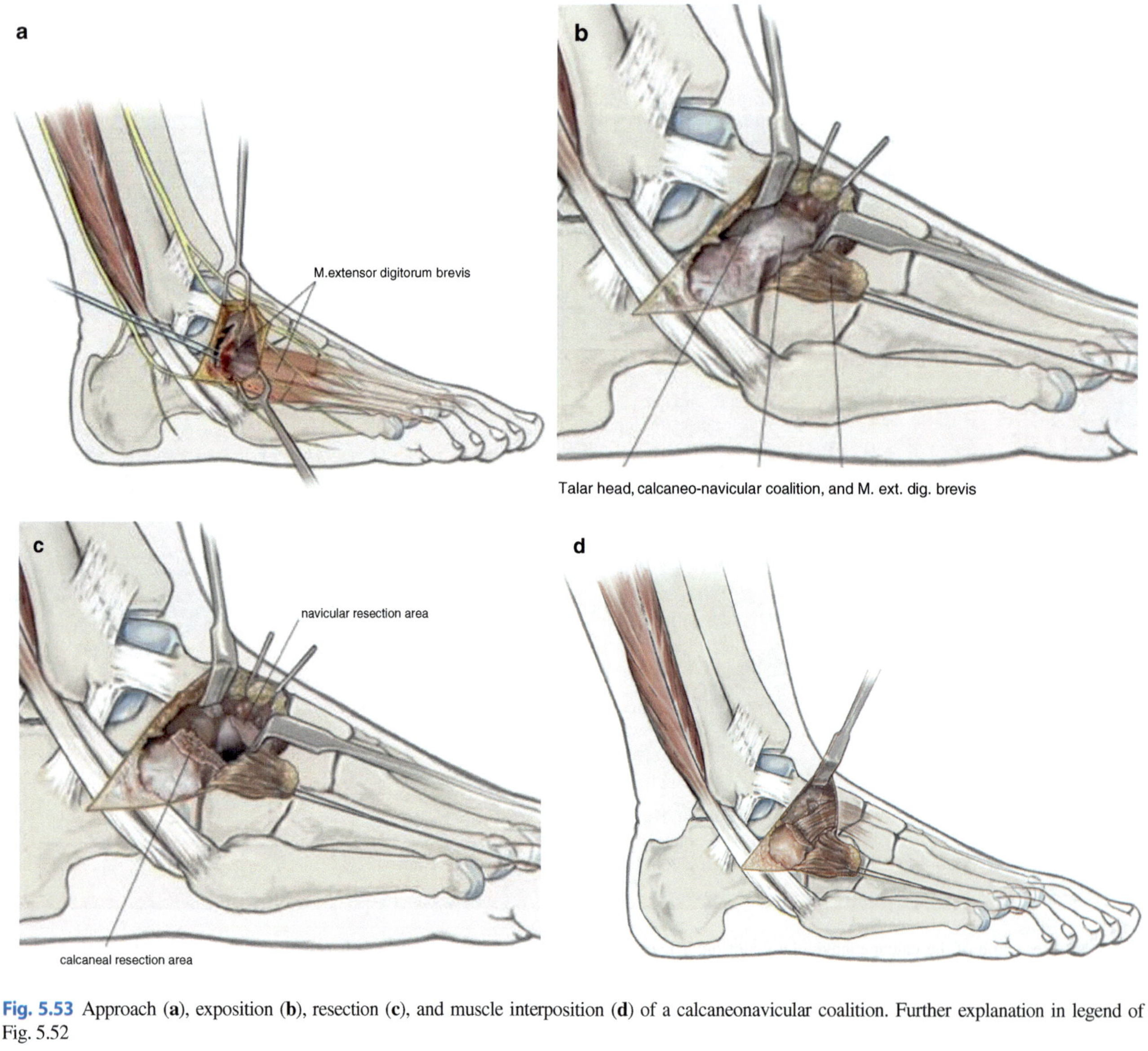

Fig. 5.53 Approach (**a**), exposition (**b**), resection (**c**), and muscle interposition (**d**) of a calcaneonavicular coalition. Further explanation in legend of Fig. 5.52

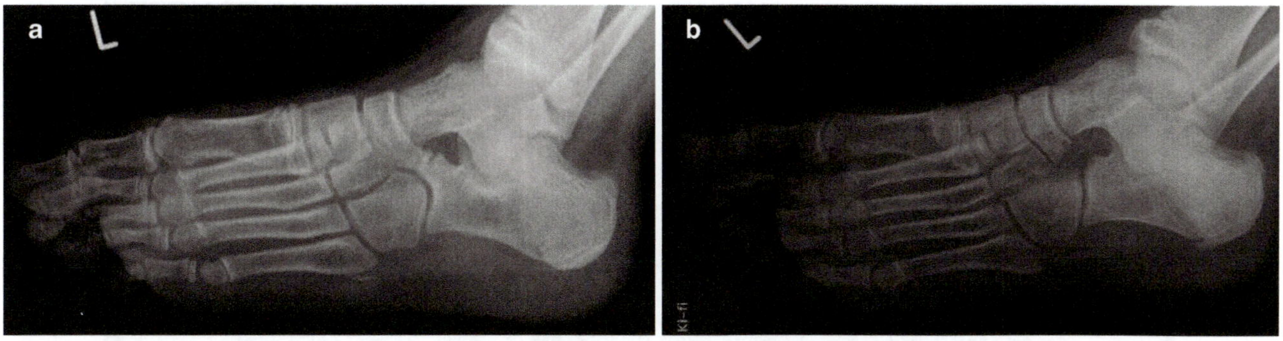

Fig. 5.54 Oblique X-ray projection before (**a**) and after (**b**) resection of the calcaneonavicular coalition in an 11-year-old patient. The resection surfaces at the navicular are approximately in line with the lateral-plantar talar neck-head contour, at the calcaneus with the medial-dorsal cuboid contour

5.2.6 Results

The results of older literature are summarized in a review by Lemley et al. (2006). Good clinical results of resection were observed in about 70–100% of cases, but with several cases of reossification, especially when no soft tissue interposition was used (see Fig. 5.55). Long-term studies report mostly good results (Inglis et al. 1986; Gonzales and Kumar 1990).

In the largest retrospective study in recent years, Mubarak et al. (2009) report on 96 cases in an 8-year period. They used a free fat interposition instead of muscle interposition with distally stemmed extensor-digitorum-brevis material, which according to their investigations is only able to fill about 64% of the resulting bone gap. 87% of their patients were fit to exercise at their previous level after 1 year with 5% reossification with the need for a new procedure.

In the author's patient group without systematic follow-up consisting of about 120 resections over a 15-year period, no cases of reossification have been reported so far. As a rule, the mobility of the hindfoot was postoperatively significantly improved, and few patients had minor residual symptoms; in two cases longer courses were observed due to postoperative dystrophy. A renewed intervention was only necessary in a 15-year-old patient, who already showed clear degenerative changes in the talonavicular joint at the time of resection (Fig. 5.56). Thus, the own results are more favorable than those reported in the literature; the disadvantages of interposition of extensor-digitorum-brevis muscles as described by Mubarak et al. (2009) cannot be traced when using the technique described above.

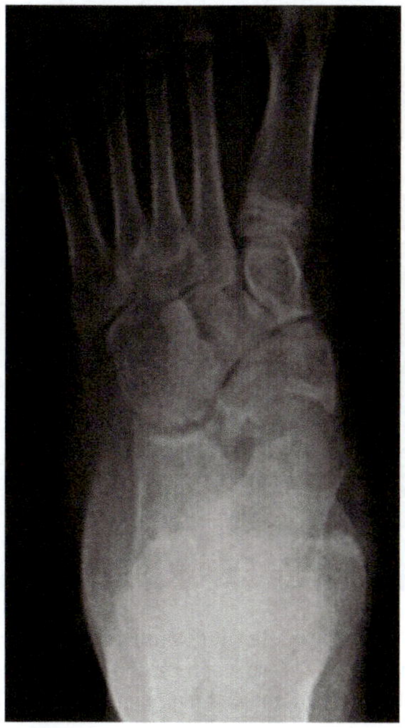

Fig. 5.55 12 Months after an externally performed resection of a calcaneonavicular coalition at the age of 13 years. Clinically distinct peroneal spasm, radiologically regenerated coalition and a severe narrowing of the talonavicular joint space

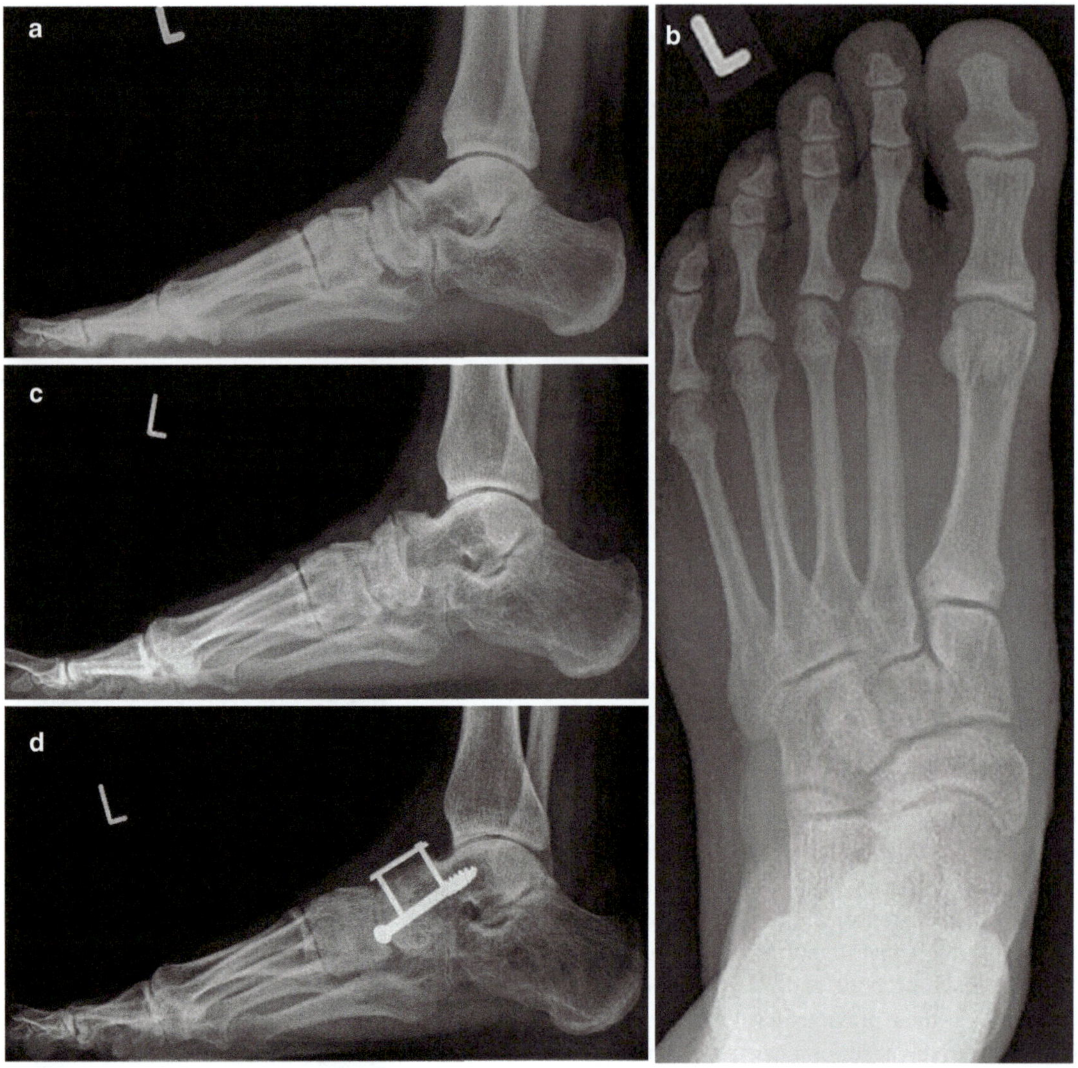

Fig. 5.56 15-Year-old patient with painful calcaneonavicular coalition and peroneal spasm (**a**, **b**). The resection and botulinum toxin treatment of the peroneal spasm did not lead to a pain-free result but to a rapidly progressive increase in the already pre-existing degenerative changes, so that 7 months after the initial intervention (**c**) a talonavicular fusion was performed (**d**)

5.2.7 Resection with Alignment Correction

Malpositions associated with calcaneonavicular coalition are less frequent than in the talocalcaneal form. If they do occur, they are also usually planovalgus deformities. Rarely and rather in cases with ossicles embedded into the coalition area, these are inversion malpositions (Fig. 5.61). In younger children and less severe planovalgus deformities, a spontaneous straightening of the foot after resection of the coalition can be expected without this being predictable. In more pronounced cases, an arthroereisis (Figs. 4.29 and 5.57) and/or osteotomies can be performed simultaneously (Figs. 5.58, 5.59, and 5.60). The indication criteria are similar to those for non-rigid planovalgus deformities (Chap. 4).

If there is only a hindfoot valgus component, the hindfoot statics can be normalized with a calcaneus sliding osteotomy (Fig. 5.58). However, the abductus component often predominates, and the navicular bone appears to be held laterally by the coalition. In this case a dosed calcaneal lengthening osteotomy can be performed from the same approach of the resection (Fig. 5.59). If the planovalgus deformity is pronounced in the three planes of space, a tarsal triple osteotomy (Hamel et al. 2014) can be used to correct it (Fig. 5.60). If hypermobility is pronounced, however, the resection of the coalition leads to further destabilization, and an arthrodesis is primarily preferable (see Fig. 4.51).

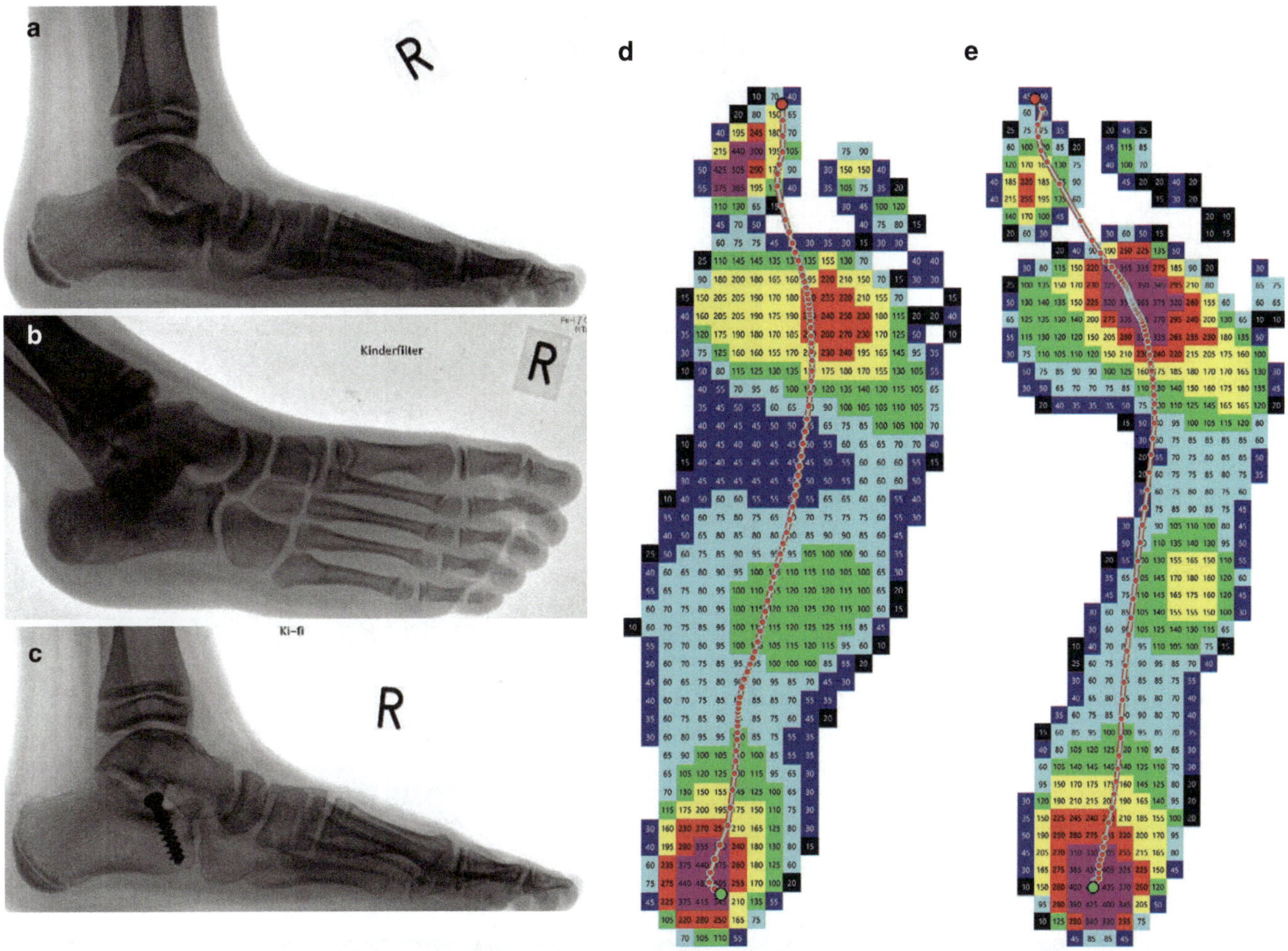

Fig. 5.57 11-Year-old patient with incomplete calcaneonavicular coalition and planovalgus deformity (**a**, **b**, **d**). 1 Year after resection of the coalition and calcaneostop arthroereisis good realignment of the foot (**c**) and clearly normalized pressure distribution (**e**)

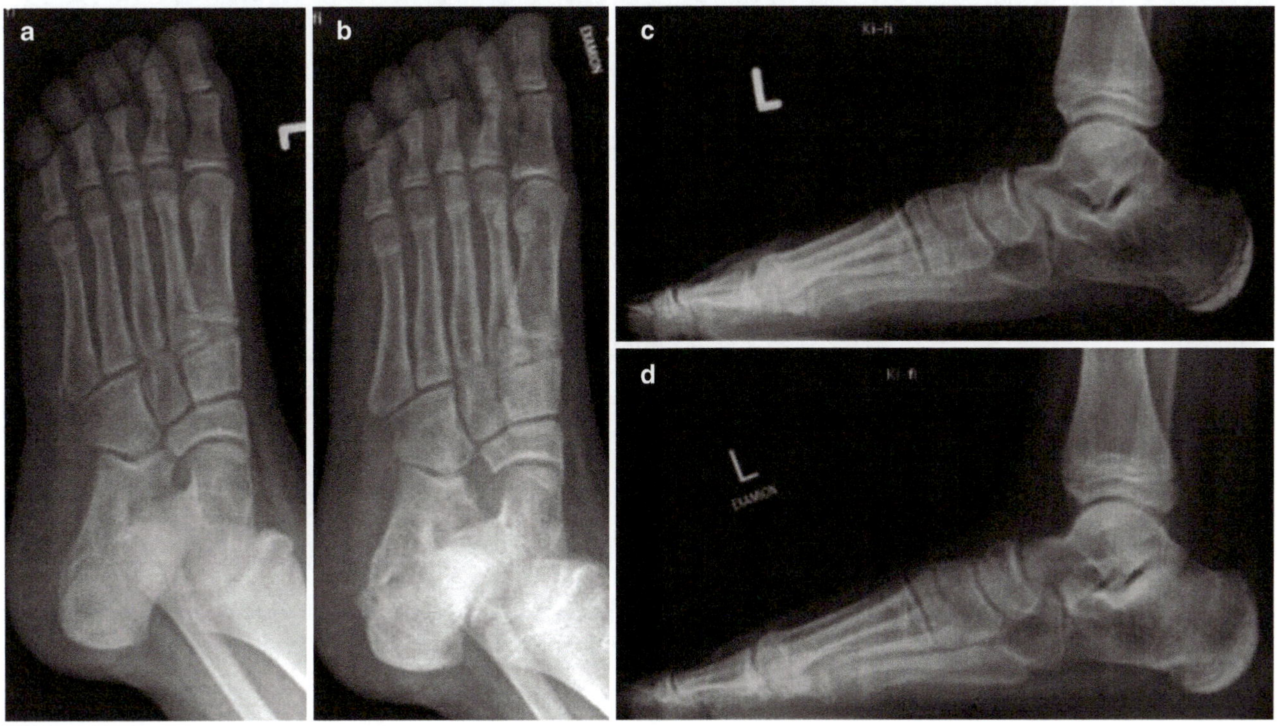

Fig. 5.58 12-Year-old patient before (**a**, **c**) and after (**b**, **d**) resection of a calcaneonavicular coalition with simultaneous calcaneal sliding osteotomy because of distinct hindfoot valgus. Postoperatively clinically completely free tarsal mobility

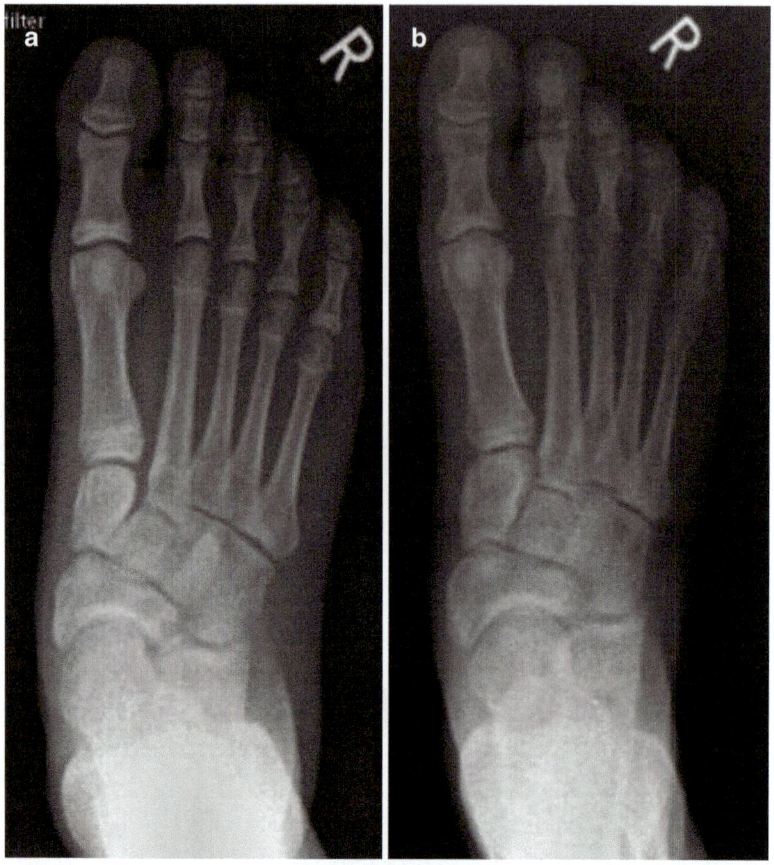

Fig. 5.59 15-Year-old patient before (**a**) and after (**b**) resection of a calcaneonavicular coalition with simultaneous calcaneal lengthening osteotomy in order to correct distinct abductus deformity in the transverse plane

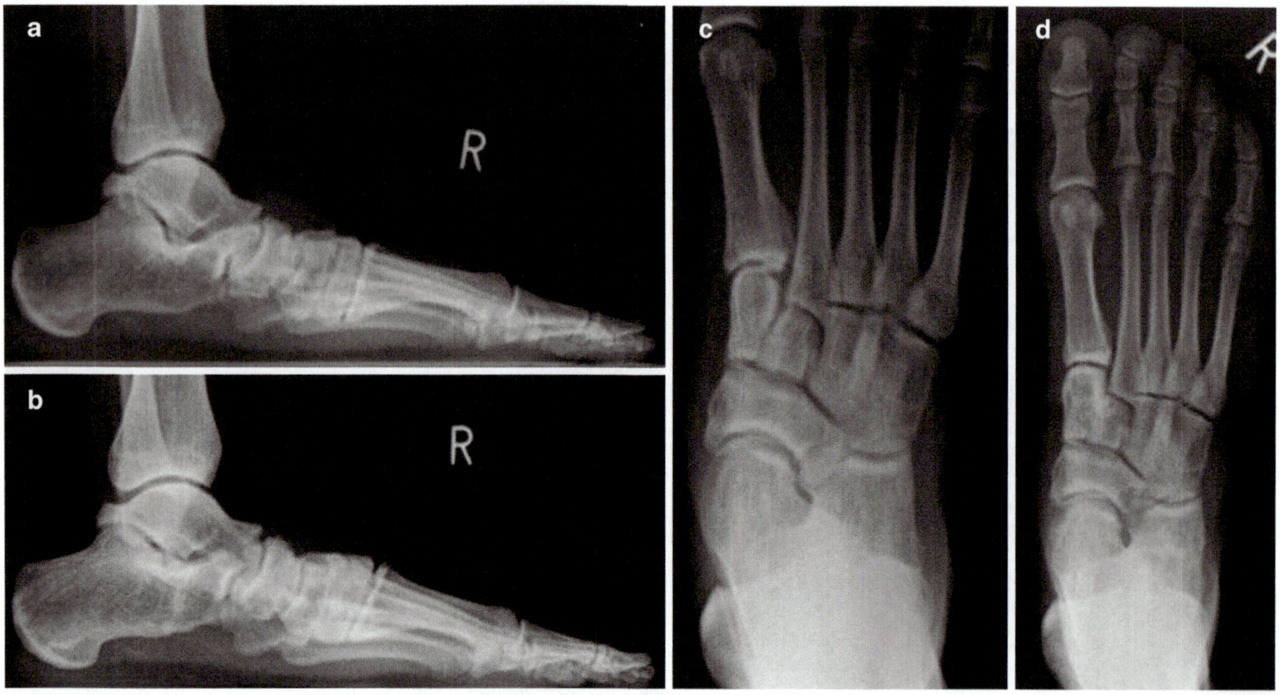

Fig. 5.60 18-Year-old patient with rigid planovalgus deformity in all three planes with calcaneonavicular coalition (**a**, **c**). In addition to resection of the coalition, a tarsal triple osteotomy with gastrocnemius lengthening was performed (**b**, **d**)

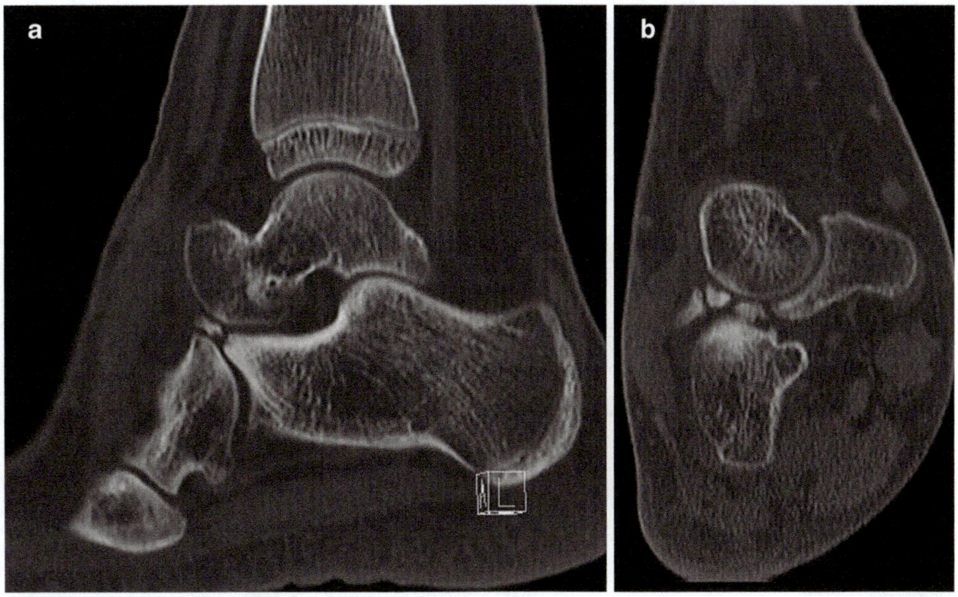

Fig. 5.61 In an 11-year-old girl (**a**, **b**). The patient showed increasing clubfoot posture. This was apparently a pain evasion phenomenon with embedded ossicles in the ligamentum bifurcatum, which immediately regressed after resection

5.3 Atypical Coalitions

Tarsal coalitions may be observed also at the plantar aspect of the calcaneonavicular region (Figs. 5.62 and 5.63), naviculo-cuboidal (Fig. 5.64), at the naviculo-cuneiforme joint line (Fig. 5.65), or at the tarsometatarsal region (Fig. 5.66). These are all rare conditions, and diagnosis as well as appropriate treatment sometimes may cause problems. Three-dimensional imaging like MRI, CT, and DVT is necessary in most of the cases.

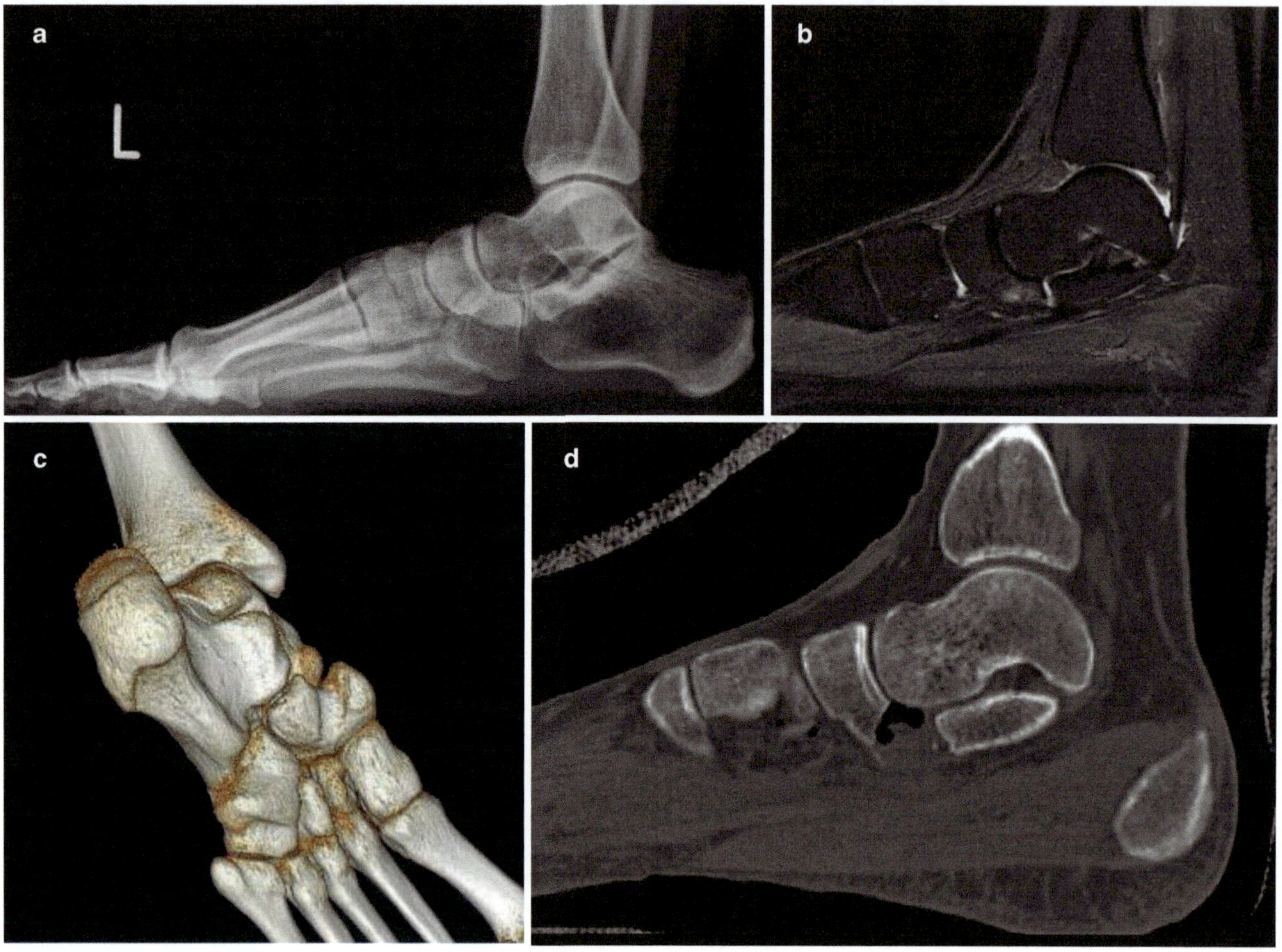

Fig. 5.62 15-Year-old female patient with calcaneonavicular coalition localized atypically at the plantar aspect below the talonavicular joint (**a**–**c**). Plantar excessive bone was removed from the os naviculare as can be seen in a postoperative CT scan (**d**)

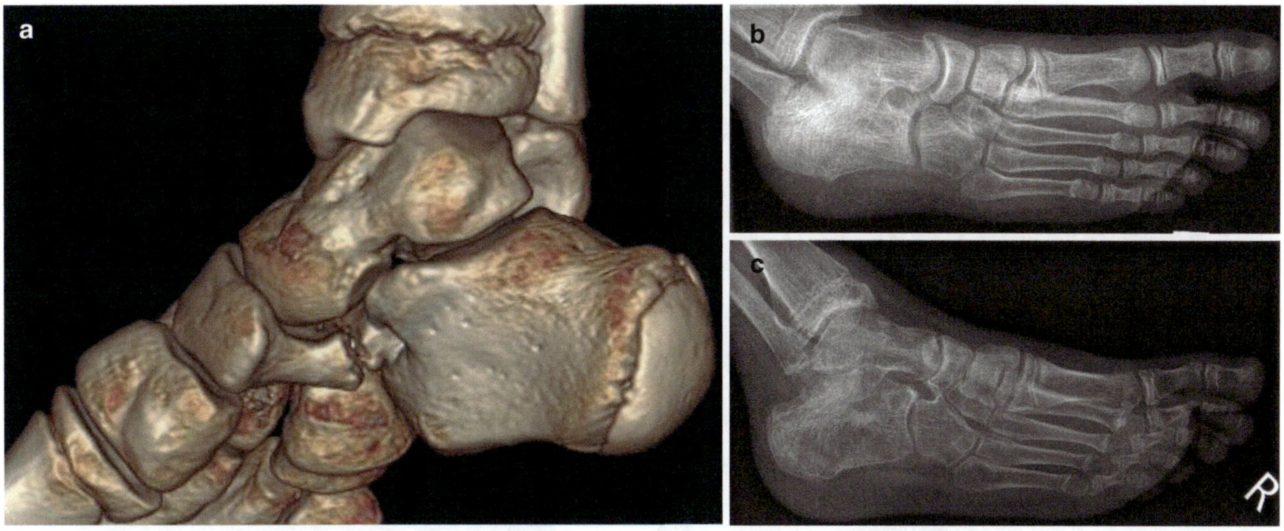

Fig. 5.63 This atypical calcaneonavicular coalition in a 10-year-old patient was located far plantar. The bifurcate ligament was preserved. CT scan (**a**) and oblique X-ray view pre- (**b**) and postoperatively (**c**). Resection in this case only was possible by two approaches (dorsolateral and medioplantar)

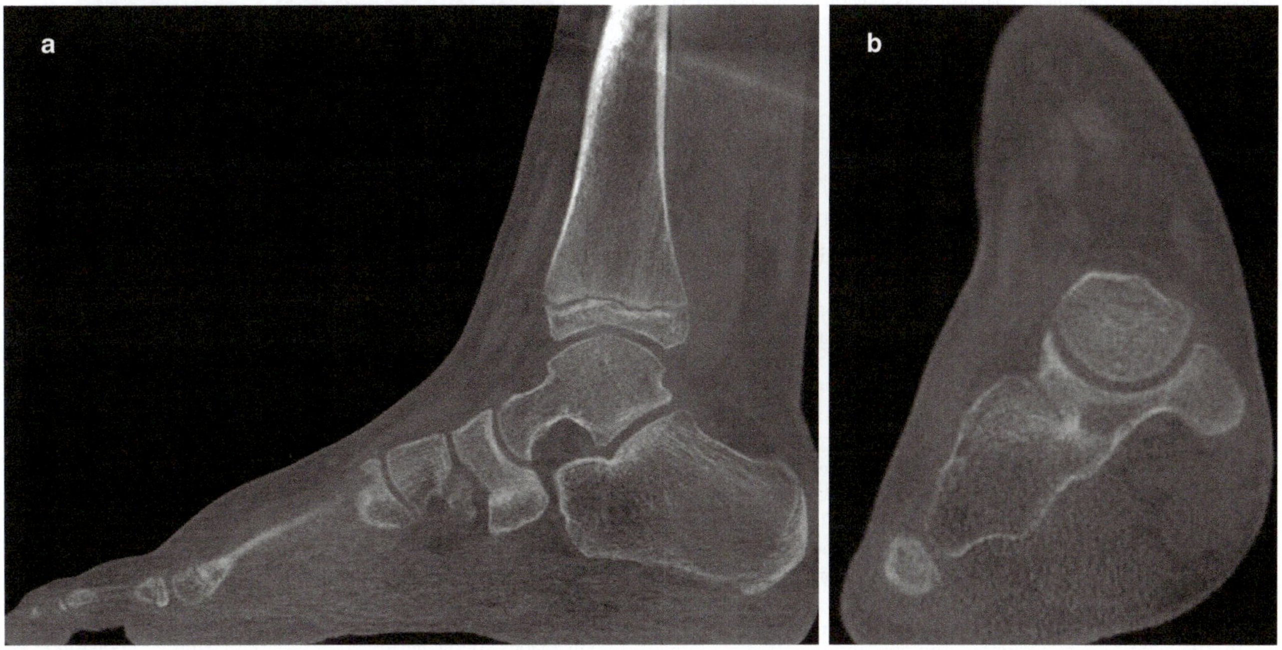

Fig. 5.64 Painful complete naviculo-cuneiforme coalition in an 11-year-old boy in sagittal weight-bearing (**a**) and frontal plane DVT (**b**)

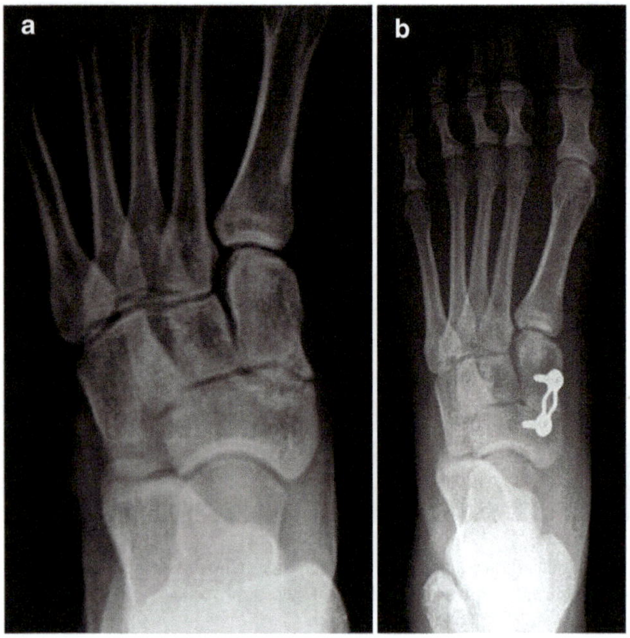

Fig. 5.65 Painful incomplete coalition in the plantar region of the medial naviculo-cuneiforme joint in an 18-year-old female patient (**a**), treated by interpositional fusion (**b**)

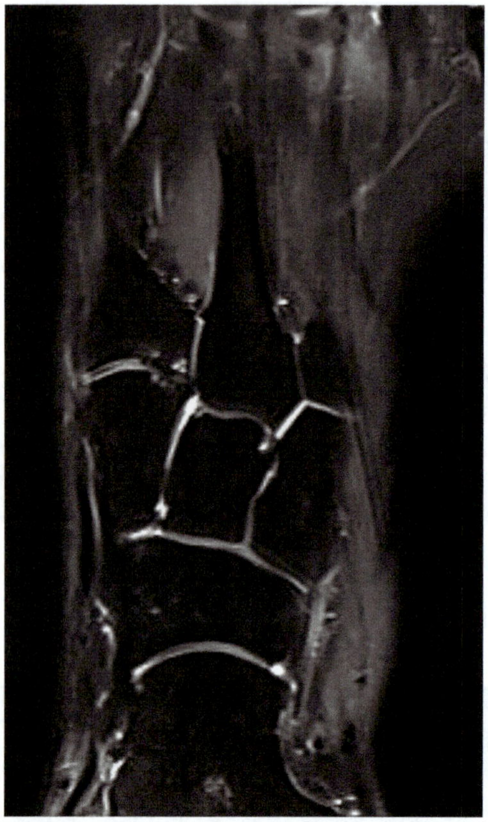

Fig. 5.66 MRI in an 18-year-old patient with localized coalition of the first tarsometatarsal joint

References

Blitz NM (2010) Pediatric & adolescent flatfoot reconstruction in combination with middle facet talocalcaneal coalition resection. Clin Podiatr Med Surg 27:119–133

Cass AD, Camasta CA (2010) A review of tarsal coalition and pes planovalgus: clinical examination, diagnostic imaging and surgical planning. J Foot Ankle Surg 49:274–293

Cowell HR, Elener V (1983) Rigid painful flatfoot secondary to tarsal coalition. Clin Orthop 177:54–60

Downey MS, DeWaters AM (2013) Tarsal coalition. In: Southerland JT et al (eds) Mc Glamry's comprehensive textbook of foot surgery, 4th edition, vol 1. Wolters Kluwer, Lippincott, Williams & Wilkins, Philadelphia

El Rassi G, Riddle EC, Kumar SJ (2005) Arthrofibrosis involving the middle facet of the talocalcaneal joint in children and adolescents. J Bone Joint Surg 87-A:2227–2231

Gantsoudes GD, Roocroft JH, Mubarak SJ (2012) Treatment of talocalcaneal coalitions. J Pediatr Orthop 32:301–307

Giannini S, Ceccarelli F, Vannini F et al (2003) Operative treatment of flatfoot with talocalcaneal coalition. Clin Orthop 411:178–187

Gonzales P, Kumar SJ (1990) Calcaneonavicular coalition treated by resection and interposition of the extensor digitorum brevis muscle. J Bone Joint Surg 72-A:71–77

Hamel J, Kinast C (2006) Der TMT-Index zur radiologischen Quantifizierung von Planovalgus-Deformitäten. FussSprungg 4:221–226

Hamel J (2008) Die dorsomediale Coalitio talocalcanearis—Präsentation von 7 operativ-resezierend behandelten Fällen im zweiten Lebensjahrzehnt. Fuss Sprunggelenk 6:207–213

Hamel J (2009) Die Resektion der talokalkanearen Coalitio im Kindes- und Adoleszentenalter ohne und mit Stellungskorrektur. Oper Orthop Traumatol 21:180–192

Hamel J (2012) 3–6-Jahres Ergebnisse nach Resektion einer talocalcanearen Coalitio kombiniert mit Calcaneus-Verlängerung im Kindes- und Jugendlichen-Alter. Fuss Sprunggelenk 10:175–183

Hamel J (2013) Diagnostik und Therapie der Koalitionen und Synostosen bei Kindern und Jugendlichen. Orthopade 42:442–448

Hamel J, Nell M, Kalpen A (2014) Das Konzept der Tarsalen Triple-Osteotomie (TTO) zur 3-DKorrektur schwerer Pes planovalgus-Deformitäten—erste radiologisch-pedographische Ergebnisse im Adoleszentenalter. Fuss Sprunggelenk 12:160–169

Hamel J, Nell M, Rist C (2016) Operative Behandlung der Coalitio talocalcanearis—Erfahrungen aus 80 Fällen kindlich-jugendlicher Patienten. Orthopade 45:1058–1065

Hetsroni I, Nyska M, Mann G, Rozenfeld G, Ayalon M (2008) Subtalar kinematics following resection of tarsal coalition. Foot Ankle Int 29:1088–1094

Inglis G, Buxton RA, Macnicol MF (1986) Symptomatic clacaneonavicular bars. The results 20 years after surgical excision. J Bone Joint Surg 68-B:128–131

Kawashima T, Uhthoff HK (1990) Prenatal development around the sustentaculum tali and its relation to talocalcaneal coalitions. J Pediatr Orthop 10:238–243

Kernbach KJ, Blitz NM (2010) A critical evaluation of subtalar joint arthrosis associated with middle facet talocacaneal coalition in 21 surgically managed patients: a retrospective CT-review. Clin Podiatr Med Surg 27:135–143

Kernbach KJ, Blitz NM, Rush SM (2008) Bilateral single-stage middle facet talocalcaneal coalition resection combined with flatfoot reconstruction: a report of 3 cases and review of the literature.

Investigations involving middle facet coalitions—part 1. J Foot Ankle Surg 47:180–190

Khoshbin A, Law PW, Caspi L, Wright JG (2013) Long-term functional outcomes of resected tarsal coalitions. Foot Ankle Int 34:1370–1375

Lateur LM, Hoe LR, Ghillewe KV, Ryspeerdt SS, Baert AL, Dereymaeker GE (1994) Subtalar coalition: diagnosis with the C sign on lateral radiographs of the ankle. Radiology 193:847–851

Lemley F, Berlet G, Hill K, Philbin T, Isaac B, Lee T (2006) Current concepts review: tarsal coalition. Foot Ankle Int 27: 1163–1169

Lisella JM, Bellapianta JM, Manoli A (2011) Tarsal coalition resection with pes planovalgus hindfoot reconstruction. J Surg Orthop Adv 20:102–105

Luhmann SJ, Schoenecker PL (1998) Symptomatic talocalcaneal coalition resection: indications and results. J Pediatr Orthop 18:748–754

Martus JE, Femino JE, Caird MS, Hughes RE, Browne RH, Farley FA (2008) Accessory anterolateral facet of the pediatric talus. J Bone Joint Surg 90-A:2452–2459

Masquijo JJ, Vazquez I, Allende V, Lanfranchi L, Torres-Gomez A, Dobbs MB (2017) Surgical reconstruction for talocalcaneal coalitions with severe hindfoot valgus deformity. J Pediatr Orthop 37:293–297

McCormack TJ, Olney B, Asher M (1997) Talocalcaneal coalition resection: a 10-year follow up. J Pediatr Orthop 17:13–15

Mosca VS (2014) Principles and management of pediatric foot and ankle deformities and malformations. Wolters Kluwer, Philadelphia

Mosca VC (2015) Subtalar coalition in pediatrics. Foot Ankle Clin 20:265–281

Mosca VS, Bevan WR (2012) Talocalcaneal tarsal coalitions and the calcaneal lengthening osteotomy: the role of deformity correction. J Bone Joint Surg 94-A:1584–1594

Mosier KM, Asher MA (1984) Tarsal coalition and peroneal spastic flatfoot. J Bone Joint Surg 66-A:976–983

Mubarak SJ, Patel PN, Upasani VV, Moor MA, Wenger DR (2009) Calcaneonavicular coalition—treatment by excision and fat graft. J Pediatr Orthop 29:418–426

Niki H, Aoki H, Hirano T, Akiyama Y, Fujiya H (2015) Peroneal spastic flatfoot in adolescents with accessory talar facet impingement: a preliminary report. J Pediatr Orthop 24-B:354–361

Rozansky A, Varley E, Moor M, Wenger DR, Mubarak SJ (2010) A radiologic classification of talocalcaneal coalitions based on 3D reconstruction. J Child Orthop 4:129–135

Vossen JA, Abbassi M, Qian Y, Hayes CW, Haar PJ, Hoover KB (2020) Correlation between the accessory anterolateral talar facet, bone marrow edema, and tarsal coalitions. Skeletal Radiology 49: 699–705

Wilde PH, Torode IP, Dickens DR, Cole WG (1994) Resection for symptomatic talocalcaneal coalition. J Bone Joint Surg 76-B:797–801

Neurogenic Deformities (Except Cavovarus Deformity)

6

Contents

Neurogenically induced deformities on the basis of spastic or flaccid paralysis and syndromal diseases in childhood and adolescence are extremely diverse. The basic principles of frequently indicated surgical treatment in the area of the lower leg and foot will be presented. Using the example of the neurogenic cavovarus deformity, this will be explained in more detail in Chap. 7.

Recommended Literature

- Döderlein L et al. (1999–2004) Fußdeformitäten, 4-volume work in German language (Der Klumpfuß, Der Knickplattfuß, Der Hohlfuß, Der Spitzfuß—Der Hackenfuß), Springer-Verlag, Heidelberg. *Lexical work with intensive consideration of neurogenic foot deformities, functional-anatomical aspects and history of orthopaedics*
- Tachdjian MO (1985) The child's foot. WB Saunders Company, Philadelphia. *Detailed description of neuromuscular deformities*
- Graham H (2010) Cerebral palsy. In: The child's foot and ankle (Hrsg.: Mc Carthy JJ, Drennan JC) Wolters Kluver Lippincott Williams and Wilkins, Philadelphia. *Good overview of foot and ankle problems in cerebral palsy in growing age*
- Perry J, Burnfield JM (2010) Gait analysis—normal and pathological function, Second edition, SLACK Incorporated. *Extensive presentation of gait analysis findings*

6.1 The Neuromotorically Affected Juvenile Patient

The neuromotorically handicapped pediatric or adolescent patient with a deformity in the lower leg-foot area requires a special approach, which differs significantly from dealing with localized problems. The following principles apply in particular for all neurogenic deformities:

J. Hamel, *Foot and Ankle Surgery in Children and Adolescents*, https://doi.org/10.1007/978-3-030-58108-4_6

- The overall neuromotor prognosis with formulation of a realistic treatment goal guides the indication.
- The team character of all therapeutic professional groups working with the child is of particular importance (e.g., physiotherapist, occupational therapist, orthopedic technician, in-patient rehabilitation facility, social pediatric center, psychologist).
- At a younger age, all orthotic and conservative treatment measures (e.g., serial casting, night splinting, botulinum toxin) should be exhausted first (Hamel 2000).
- Surgical interventions should generally be planned not before 6–8 years of age at the earliest with rare exceptions.
- Even more than with other deformities, an overall view of the complete lower extremity or the locomotor system as a whole is required. Often the surgical treatment has to start on several levels ("multi-level-surgery") and thus goes beyond the topic to be discussed here.
- The procedures of instrumental gait analysis are valuable in the context of diagnostics, documentation, and evaluation of results. The functional state of the neuromotorically impaired foot is documented especially by means of pedography; reference is made to the literature on differentiated instrumental gait analysis in the gait laboratory (Perry and Burnfield 2010).
- The long-term results of surgical interventions are often rather disappointing compared to the short-term corrections that can be achieved (cf. Chang et al. 2002).

Precise knowledge of the regular muscular activity during the stance and swing phase of gait is the most important:

Main Muscle Activity in the Five Phases of Gait

Heel contact	M. tibialis anterior
Shock absorption	M. tibialis posterior
Mid stance	Mm. soleus, tibialis posterior, peronei
Late stance	Mm. tibialis posterior, gastrocnemius, FHL, FDL
Swing phase	Mm. tibialis anterior, peronei, EHL, EDL

Of particular importance in neuromotor disorders is the distinction between disease-related muscular *dysfunction* and *compensation mechanisms*. The latter represent meaningful reactions of the locomotor organs to the actual functional disorder and are therefore never the primary approach of therapeutic efforts. It can be extremely difficult to differentiate between these mechanisms.

Typical Muscular Compensation Mechanisms (Clinical Examples)

Weakness of the calf muscles	Increased use of the long toe flexors (overcorrected clubfoot)
Tarsal hypermobility	Increased use of the long toe flexors (severe planovalgus def.)
Weakness of anterior tibial muscle	Extensor substitution (EHL, EDL) (cavovarus def.)
Weakness of ankle dorsiflexion (drop foot)	Increased hip and knee flexion in swing phase (peroneus paresis)
Weakness of the Mm. peronei	Extensor-digitorum-longus hyperactivity (cavovarus def.)
Weakness of the peroneus brevis muscle	Peroneus-longus hyperactivity (cavovarus def.)
Complete failure of the plantar flexors	Anterior tibial hyperactivity with heel push off (MMC)

6.2 Principles of Surgical Correction

The available surgical corrective measures must always be carried out in the following order: Soft tissue releases on contracted joint capsules and muscle-tendon units for the greatest possible correction of deformities, bony corrections, and arthrodeses to complete the correction and to provide sufficient stabilization and finally tendon transfers to optimize muscular balance. Physiotherapy and orthotic care are often required in addition to the surgical part of treatment. The approach and principles of correction will be explained using a particularly severe adolescent case of equinovarus deformity with hemispasticity as an example.

Case Study Equinovarus 1

A female patient, 17 years old at the time of surgery, was born in the 33rd week of pregnancy and developed hemispasticity due to perinatal brain damage. She and her family could not decide in childhood and adolescence to undergo the actually indicated surgical intervention and introduced herself with the most severe equinovarus deformity on the right side and marked instability with a tendency to twist and repeated ankle sprains (Fig. 6.1).

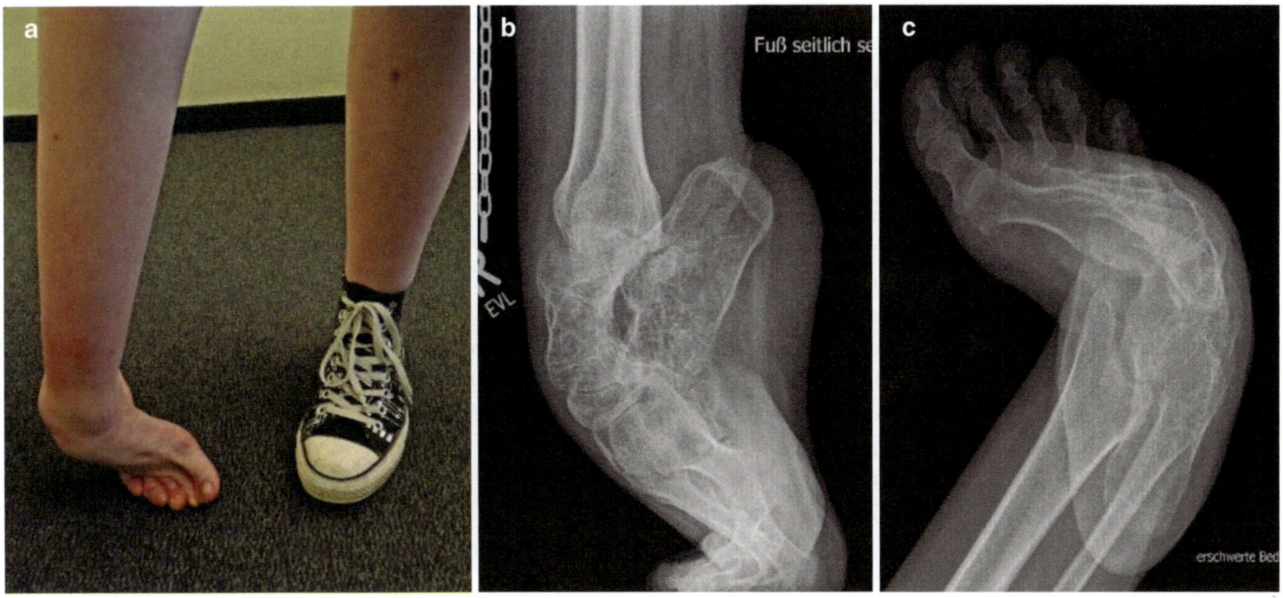

Fig. 6.1 Severe equinovarus deformity (**a**) in a 17-year-old female patient with hemispasticity (see text) and major skeletal malalignment (**b**, **c**)

6.2.1 Muscle-Tendon Lengthenings and Soft Tissue Release

Lengthening of muscle-tendon units has two main effects: A contract deformity can thereby be corrected and the affected muscle will be weakened. As a rule, the former effect in most cases is therapeutically desired; the latter usually represents an undesirable accompanying effect.

This will be illustrated using the example of muscular equinus contracture (Sect. 6.3.1) but applies in a similar way in general for any other muscular contracture:

- *In cases of shortened calf muscles which cannot be stretched conservatively (e.g. also using physiotherapy, dynamic braces, serial plaster cast treatment, botulinum toxin), very different surgical lengthening techniques can be considered (Sect. 6.3.1). In most cases, the aim is to achieve functionally usable mobility of the upper ankle joint, even with an extended knee joint, beyond about 10° of dorsal extension.*
- *In many cases only or predominantly the gastrocnemius part of the M. triceps surae is shortened. This can be determined by the translation test (comparison of the maximum dorsal extension of the ankle in knee flexion and knee extension). Intramuscular lengthening of only the gastrocnemius portion is a good solution in these cases, which allows about 10°–15° improvement in mobility and only causes a slight weakening and thus nearly no danger of overcorrection (Fig. 6.3a, b).*
- *If there are pronounced equinus deformity contractures and the soleus part of the calf muscles is also shortened, a percutaneous or open Achilles tendon lengthening can be considered (Fig. 6.3c, d). In these cases, however, the gastrocnemius part is often considerably more shortened than the soleus part, so that combinations of intramuscular lengthening of the gastrocnemius muscle with moderate lengthening of the Achilles tendon might also be an option. Each Achilles tendon lengthening should be performed in a measured manner to avoid overcorrection. The goal is a heel-to-toe gait with full load transfer of the heel in the early stance phase while maintaining a powerful forefoot plantar flection in the push-off phase of gait (Fig. 6.5).*
- *The risk of overcorrection depends on the type of disease. It is particularly high, for example, in spastic diplegia and less pronounced in spastic hemiplegia. The leg length (equinus foot compensation in shortened lower extremity) and the muscle status (caution with Achilles tendon lengthening in case of existing quadriceps weakness) should also be taken into account.*

Case Study Equinovarus 2

In the case of the 17-year-old female patient with hemispasticity, an open, Z-shaped Achilles tendon lengthening of about 4 cm was performed with lengthening also of the long flexor tendons of the toes as well as soft tissue releases of the plantar fascia and talonavicular joint. The dorsal upper ankle joint capsule could be released by forceful manipulation.

6.2.2 Bony Corrective Procedures

As with non-neurogenic deformities, corrective osteotomies can usually be carried out in childhood in order to preserve the joints, or corrective fusion can be performed in adolescence. Joints should never be sacrificed without careful consideration and with respect to the "hierarchy" of the tarsal joints (see box). In neurogenic deformities, fusion might be appropriate in order to correct pronounced deformities (Fig. 6.1), to stabilize an otherwise unstable situation, or to compensate for major muscle disbalance in order to prevent relapse of deformity. This can also be the case when a favorable muscular balance cannot be achieved in the foreseeable future (example in Fig. 6.12) or important joint-stabilizing muscle-tendon units are used for transfers. In such cases, it may be necessary to sacrifice single joints according to the principle of "simplify motion."

"Hierarchy" of the Joints in Foot and Ankle Region

Functionally extremely important	Ankle joint, talonavicular joint, tarsometatarsal joints IV and V, metatarsophalageal joints II to V
Functionally of medium importance	Talocalcaneal joint, calcaneocuboid joint, metatarsophalangeal joint I
Low functional significance	Naviculocuneiform joints, tarsometatarsal joints I–III

The pronounced neurogenic hindfoot inversion can best be treated in the Chopart line by corrective fusion (Sect. 6.3.2), in severe cases by triple arthrodesis. Eversion malpositions usually require the inclusion of the talocalcaneal joint (Sect. 6.3.3). As a rule: If the preserved range of motion of the peritalar complex – even after soft tissue release - does not include the neutral position, fusion of in neutral position should be considered. Arthrodeses are rarely performed before the age of about 10 years. Additional osteotomies are often necessary.

Case Study Equinovarus 3

In the example of the 17-year-old female patient with hemispasticity, only a triple arthrodesis according to Lambrinudi (Sect. 7.9.3) seemed appropriate for three-dimensional correction (Fig. 6.2). The anterior-based subtalar wedge removal allowed at least a slight plantar flexion of the talus and could have been even more extensive. This is of particular importance in such cases, since severe cartilage degeneration in the anterior region of the trochlea tali must be assumed, because of longstanding missing contact of the joint surfaces.

6.2.3 Muscular Rebalancing by Tendon Transfers

All neurogenic deformities in the ankle and foot area are based on muscular imbalances as the main cause. Muscle function diagnostics is therefore of particular importance and must take the following questions into account:

- What is the strength level of the single muscle and its antagonists?
- What are the lever arm ratios with the existing deformity?
- Does the muscle react spastically?
- Can the muscle be used arbitrarily?
- In which gait phase is the muscle active (Sect. 6.1)?
- Are compensation phenomena present (Sect. 6.1)?

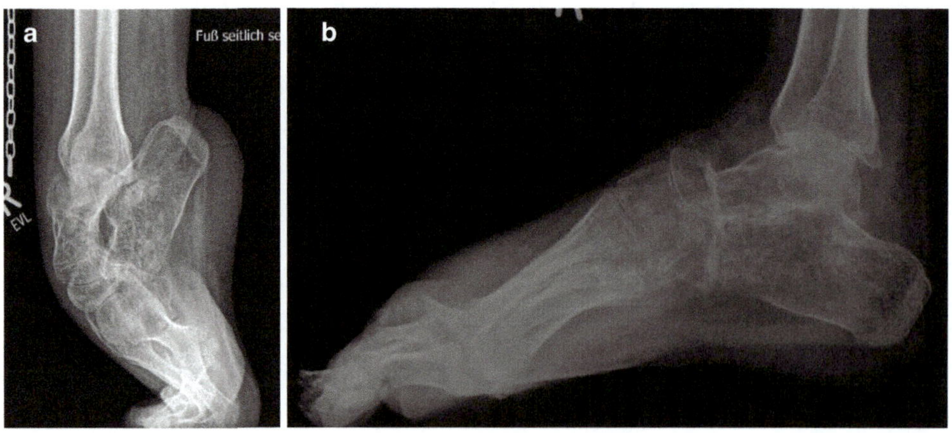

Fig. 6.2 Pre- (**a**) and postoperative image (**b**) after bony and soft tissue correction with triple arthrodesis in Lambrinudi technique in severe equinovarus deformity (see Fig. 6.1b)

The restoration or at least optimization of muscular balance with regard to the functional requirements through tendon transfers should be considered especially in the case of neurogenic deformities. The following basic rules apply:

- Tendon transfers are almost irreversible and must therefore be planned very carefully.
- Tendon transfers should only be indicated in cases of completely foreseeable muscular imbalance (e.g., rarely in early infancy).
- Possible further progression of the disease must be taken into consideration.
- Tendon transfers are preferable to lengthening with accompanying muscular weakening.
- Phasic transfers are less complicated than antiphasic transfers.
- A clearly deformity-promoting muscle should be transferred.
- Donor site and transfer morbidity should be considered.
- The effect of tendon transfers can often not be accurately predicted, and under- and overcorrections (see Fig. 6.12) are possible.
- Split-tendon transfers (see Sect. 6.3.2) are less susceptible to over- or undercorrections if the amount is well dosed (which in fact is not easy to accomplish), reduce the targeted controllability of the joints ("simplify motion"), but have the advantage over arthrodeses of maintaining at least passive mobility during the stance phase.

Case Study Equinovarus 4

In the case of the 17-year-old female patient with hemispasticity, the posterior tibial muscle was clearly shortened and overactive and thus highly conducive to deformity. However, this muscle could be controlled arbitrarily by the patient, so that a transfer was recommended. Since the anterior tibial and peroneal muscles were severely overstretched and insufficient, the posterior tibial tendon was transferred to the lateral midfoot (Sect. 7.11.2) to strengthen foot elevation and eversion or at least to create a tenodesis effect. In principle, an additional tendon shortening at the elongated muscle-tendon units could have also been considered (Rutz et al. 2011*).*

6.2.4 The Importance of Orthotics and Physiotherapy in the Context of Surgical Corrections

Expert peri- and postoperative physiotherapy on a neurophysiological basis is indispensable in the treatment of neurogenic deformities. Technical orthopedics as well plays a major role in the overall concept of neuro-orthopedic clinical manifestations. In connection with corrections in the lower leg-foot area, two indication areas are of particular importance:

- After surgical corrections, the result often has to be orthotically protected for longer periods of time in the sense of recurrence prophylaxis, to avoid overstretching of transferred muscle-tendon units or to support the foot mechanically (e.g., with insoles). In spastic paralysis, orthoses have a tonus-reducing effect.
- Often the aim of surgical intervention is to make indispensable bracing easier or even possible at all, e.g., in the case of paralysis of extensor weakness with drop foot (Fig. 6.17) or calcaneus foot deformity with severe calf muscle insufficiency (Fig. 6.18).

Case Study Equinovarus 5

In the case of the 17-year-old female patient with hemispasticity, a rigid ankle foot orthosis was worn for 6 months as well as a lower leg night brace. This was intended to further adjust the length of the overstretched extensor and evertor musculature and prevent overstretching of the transferred posterior tibial muscle. After the bone had healed, intensive physiotherapeutic treatment and gait training were carried out over several months.

6.3 Examples of Neuro-Orthopedic Corrections

Only the most common problems and procedures can be addressed. Since the cavovarus deformities constitute an independent entity group with specific questions, a separate chapter is devoted to them (Chap. 7).

6.3.1 Equinus Deformity

The aim is to achieve a sufficient but dosed lengthening of the muscle-tendon unit of the calf muscles (see Sect. 6.2.1), which permits the functionally required dorsal extension in the upper ankle joint (at least about 10°) with the least possible weakening of the plantar flexion. Surgical therapy is only indicated, if conservative treatment including physiotherapy, botulinum toxin application, or serial casting is not promising. From the large number of procedures described (Döderlein et al. 2004), four important techniques for lengthening the calf muscles—in the order of their correction potential—are presented here (Fig. 6.3).

1. ***Intramuscular gastrocnemius recession according to Baumann (Fig. 6.3a):***

   *Gastrocnemius lengthening according to Baumann (*Baumann and Koch 1989; *Herzenberg et al.* 2007*) is a frequently indicated procedure in childhood and adolescence not only in neurogenic conditions. The procedure is performed in a supine position with the patient's heel elevated on the instrument table and the calf muscles sagging freely. A longitudinal incision of about 4 cm length is made dorsomedially at the proximal one-third limit of the lower leg, sparing the saphenous vein and saphenous nerve in the epifascial subcutaneous tissue (Fig. 6.4a). After the longitudinal incision of the muscle fascia, the surgeon's finger can palpate the layer between the soleus and gastrocnemius muscles and the aponeurosis of the gastrocnemius muscle is visualized up to its lateral limit with very long Langenbeck hooks (Fig. 6.4b). The calf muscles are pretensioned by dorsal extension of the ankle joint. With a long knife, the aponeurosis above the muscular part of the gastrocnemius muscle is dissected once transversely on the distal side and further proximally a second time only on the medial side. Afterwards, the dorsal extension in the ankle joint can usually be extended significantly by about 10°–15° with the knee joint stretched and the gastrocnemius muscle fibers visibly stretched below the aponeurotical cut. If necessary, the soleus aponeurosis can also be notched in the same way.*

2. ***Gastroc-Slide (Fig. 6.3b):***

   The medial edge of the gastrocnemius aponeurosis is located via a dorsomedial longitudinal incision at the distal one-third limit of the lower leg. Above the junction of this aponeurosis with the soleus muscle to constitute the Achilles tendon, both muscle-tendon units are separated bluntly from each other and the gastrocnemius aponeurosis is completely severed from medial to lateral. Here, the laterally running sural nerve is to be particularly protected.

3. ***Percutaneous Achilles tendon lengthening (Fig. 6.3c):***

   Via three stab incisions at a distance of about 2–3 cm, the medial, lateral, and again medial half of the tendon is tenotomized from the middle of the tendon starting dis-

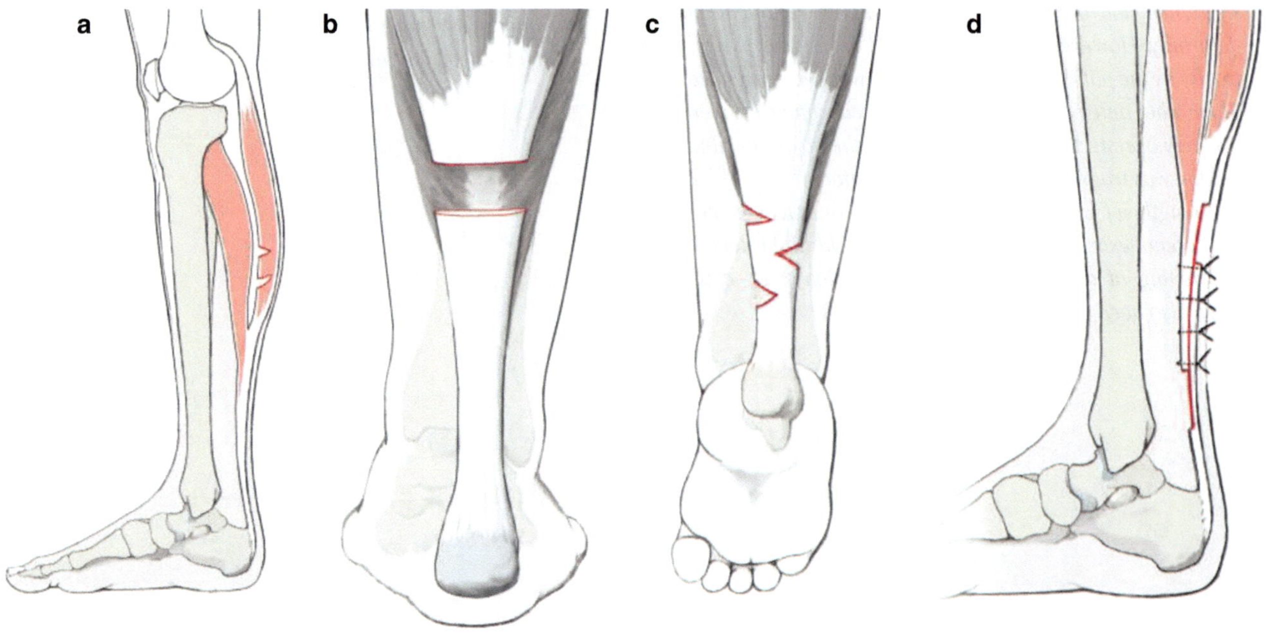

Fig. 6.3 Examples of lengthening techniques on the calf muscle-tendon unit: Intramuscular lengthening of the gastrocnemius part of the calf according to Baumann (**a**), complete severing of the gastrocnemius aponeurosis (Gastroc-slide) (**b**), percutaneous hemisection of the Achilles tendon (**c**) and Z-shaped Achilles tendon lengthening (**d**)

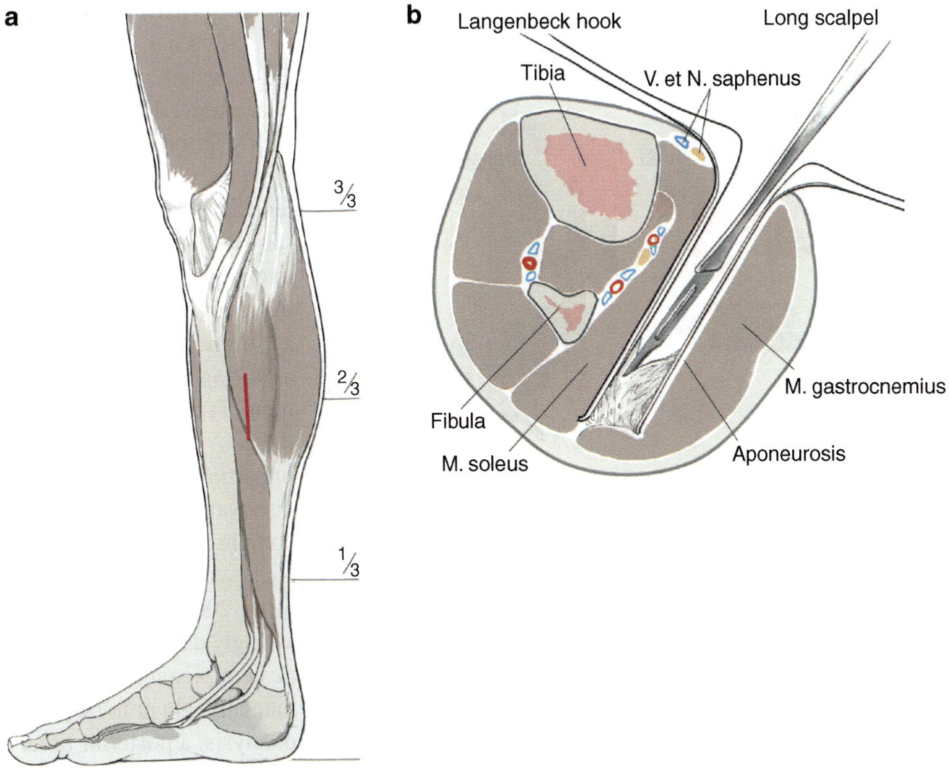

Fig. 6.4 The aponeurotic intramuscular lengthening of the gastrocnemius muscle according to Baumann and Koch (1989) is performed through an incision at the proximal dorsomedial one-third limit of the lower leg (**a**). The gliding layer between the gastrocnemius and soleus muscles is identified, and both muscles are separated bluntly to the lateral extent (**b**). Long, narrow Langenbeck hooks are required for this. Using a scalpel with a long handle, the gastrocnemius aponeurosis is dissected in two levels so that it can be expanded on the preserved muscular portion

tally, with the assistant tensioning the tendon. The subsequent mobilization (stretching) is performed very carefully to avoid a complete rupture of the tendon. Severe equinus deformities should not be treated by this procedure, because the expectable increase of dorsal extension is limited and complete rupture with severe loss of strength might occur.

4. ***Open Achilles tendon lengthening technique (Fig. 6.4d):***
   The access is made slightly curved medial to the Achilles tendon, whereby the access length is chosen according to the planned amount of lengthening. The tenotomy is performed frontally, leaving the dorsal tendon portion distally. Both tendon ends are reinforced medially and laterally with resorbable suture material. Suturing is usually performed at the end of the entire procedure and special attention is paid to the dosage: In neutral position of the foot, the sutured tendon should still have a slight tension. The tenotomy can also be performed in the sagittal plane, leaving either the medial (everted hindfoot) or the lateral (inverted hindfoot) tendon insertion at the calcaneal attachment preserved.

According to investigations by Herzenberg et al. (2007), the dorsal extension can be increased by about 10° by a single recession of the gastrocnemius aponeurosis (Baumann procedure) and by about another 5° through a second recession at another level. The effect of the Gastroc-slide is a gain of about 15° in dorsal extension. The percutaneous Achilles tendon lengthening is a very time-saving procedure, but it is only recommended for slight shortening of the calf muscles, since an unintentional complete severing of the tendon is associated with considerable functional disadvantages. With the open technique of the Z-shaped Achilles tendon lengthening, unlimited correction is possible, but overcorrection should be carefully avoided.

The success of calf muscle lengthening can be documented by clinical gait observation, gait analysis, but also pedographically. The aim is a strong and neither accelerated nor prolonged heel load, indicating a sufficient extension of the calf muscle/Achilles tendon unit, an anterograde course of the gait line, and a strong forefoot imprint in the late stance phase of walking (Fig. 6.5b) as an expression of the preserved calf muscle force.

Failure to lengthen the shortened calf muscle for a longer period of time during growth can have considerable disadvantages in the development of the upper ankle joint. The anterior parts of the trochlea tali cannot develop a physiologically formed hyaline joint cartilage due to the lack of formative movement stimuli (Döderlein et al. 2004), and this can lead to premature arthrosis after delayed calf muscle lengthening. The joint shape can also limit the desired effect of lengthening (Fig. 6.6).

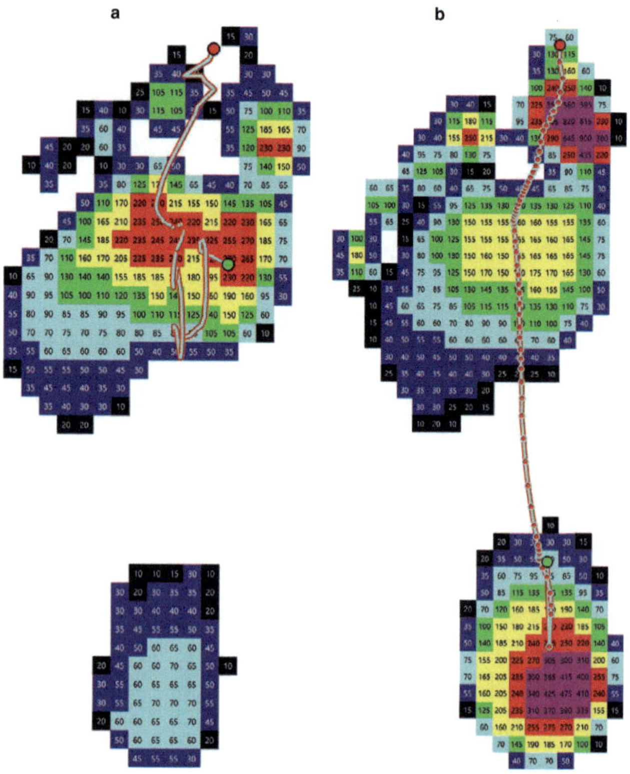

Fig. 6.5 9-Year-old boy with hemispasticity of the left side before (**a**) and 14 months after lengthening of the Achilles tendon (**b**). A heel-forefoot gait could be achieved again, recognizable by the COPP-line beginning in the heel area and running anterograde to the forefoot, as well as a physiological load on the heel with preserved forefoot load. The extensive imprint of the big toe can be interpreted as compensation for the still existing slight postoperative weakness of the calf muscle

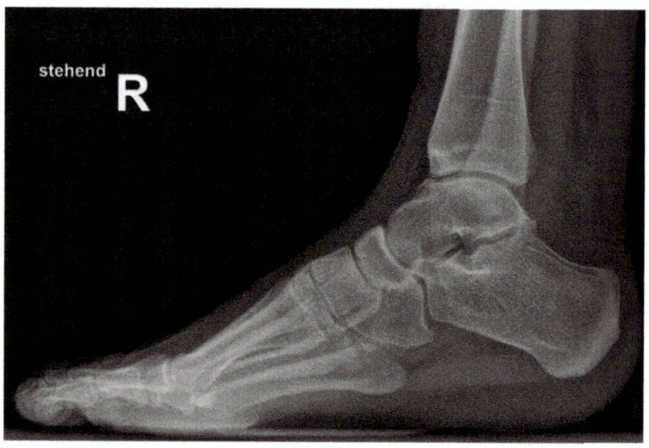

Fig. 6.6 Adolescent female patient with diplegic form of cerebral palsy. A calf muscle lengthening bilaterally was performed with delay at the age of 10 years, so that the anterior trochlea tali could not develop physiologically. In addition, there is a slight cavus component ("forefoot equinus"). It is obvious that calf muscle lengthening would not solve the problem. In addition to an osseous correction in the anterior tarsal region, a notch plasty of the talus (see Fig. 1.67) might be considered to compensate for the remaining equinus component

6.3.2 Neurogenic Equinovarus Deformity

Besides calf muscle shortening, the neurogenic clubfoot is characterized by a predominance of the invertor muscles over evertors. This leads to inversion of the hindfoot complex, overload of the lateral metatarsus and instability with a tendency to twist (Fig. 6.1). In addition to frequently necessary calf muscle lengthening, it must be decided preoperatively which muscle mainly contributes to the deformity. The overactivity of the posterior tibial muscle causes in particular a "stance phase varus," that of the anterior tibial muscle more a "swing phase varus." However, mixed patterns are common. Typical tendon transfers are split tendon transfers of the abovementioned muscles (see Fig. 6.10). The advantage of partial transfers is the lower risk of overcorrection, and the disadvantage is that the muscular control of the subtalar complex is deteriorated and the achieved distribution of muscle power to the two tendon halves is not always ideal (Piazza et al. 2003). The long-term results of tendon transfers are strongly dependent on the type of disease; for example, spastic hemiplegia can be expected to have more favorable results than diplegia or tetraspasticity (Chang et al. 2002). In spastic paralysis, a posterior tibial transfer to the dorsum of the foot (see Sect. 7.11.2) is only advisable, if the muscle can be controlled arbitrarily (like the case in Fig. 6.1).

Technique of the Split Transfer of the Tendons of the Anterior and Posterior Tibial Muscles

The proximal half of the anterior tibial tendon is detached at its insertion at the os cuneiforme mediale and separated as far as possible proximally from the distal half of the tendon. The split tendon half is pulled out through a supramalleolar incision, whereby a tunneling clamp can be helpful. At a third incision at the insertion of the peroneus brevis tendon, one half of this tendon is split off preserving its distal attachment, and the anterior tibial tendon half to be relocated is transferred thereto subcutaneously using a tunneling clamp. Both tendon halves are then sutured together under controlled tension with non-resorbable sutures. The anterior tibial tendon half, which is now inserted laterally, should have slightly more tension than the medial half. This can be easily checked by observing both tendon halves in the supramalleolar incision.

At the posterior tibial muscle, either an intramuscular lengthening to weaken the muscle or a split transfer to the lateral side can be considered. For this purpose, the cranial half of the posterior tibial tendon is detached directly at the insertion at the os naviculare and separated from the plantar half as far as possible proximally. This half of the tendon is pulled out through a dorsome-

dial incision on the distal lower leg, further split off proximally and transferred with a tunneling clamp into a third incision above the peroneal tendons retromalleolar, woven into the peroneus brevis in Pulvertaft-technique and fixed by sutures. Also a more distal coupling in the inframalleolar region is possible. The transfer can be combined with a more proximal intramuscular lengthening of the posterior tibial muscle.

In principle, the bony deformity can be corrected with soft tissue release and sliding osteotomy of the tuber calcanei in valgus direction in milder cases; however, in most cases a corrective fusion in the Chopart line is recommended for older children and adolescents. Thereby, the hindfoot varus deformity is also corrected in not too severe cases; otherwise a calcaneal osteotomy can be added.

Surgical Technique of Chopart Arthrodesis and Isolated Calcaneocuboid Fusion

Chopart correction arthrodesis is performed from two incisions (Hamel and Becker 1997). The talonavicular joint is exposed broadly from a dorsal incision over the distal course of the anterior tibial tendon, distracted with a spreader. The cartilage is removed, and the subchondral bone surface is prepared. The resection can be performed in a wedge-shaped manner according to the deformity (Fig. 6.7a). For the osteosynthesis, K-wires, compression screws, and claw-plates are considered depending on the age of the patient (Fig. 6.7b). The calcaneocuboid joint is exposed and resected through an oblique incision along the split lines of the

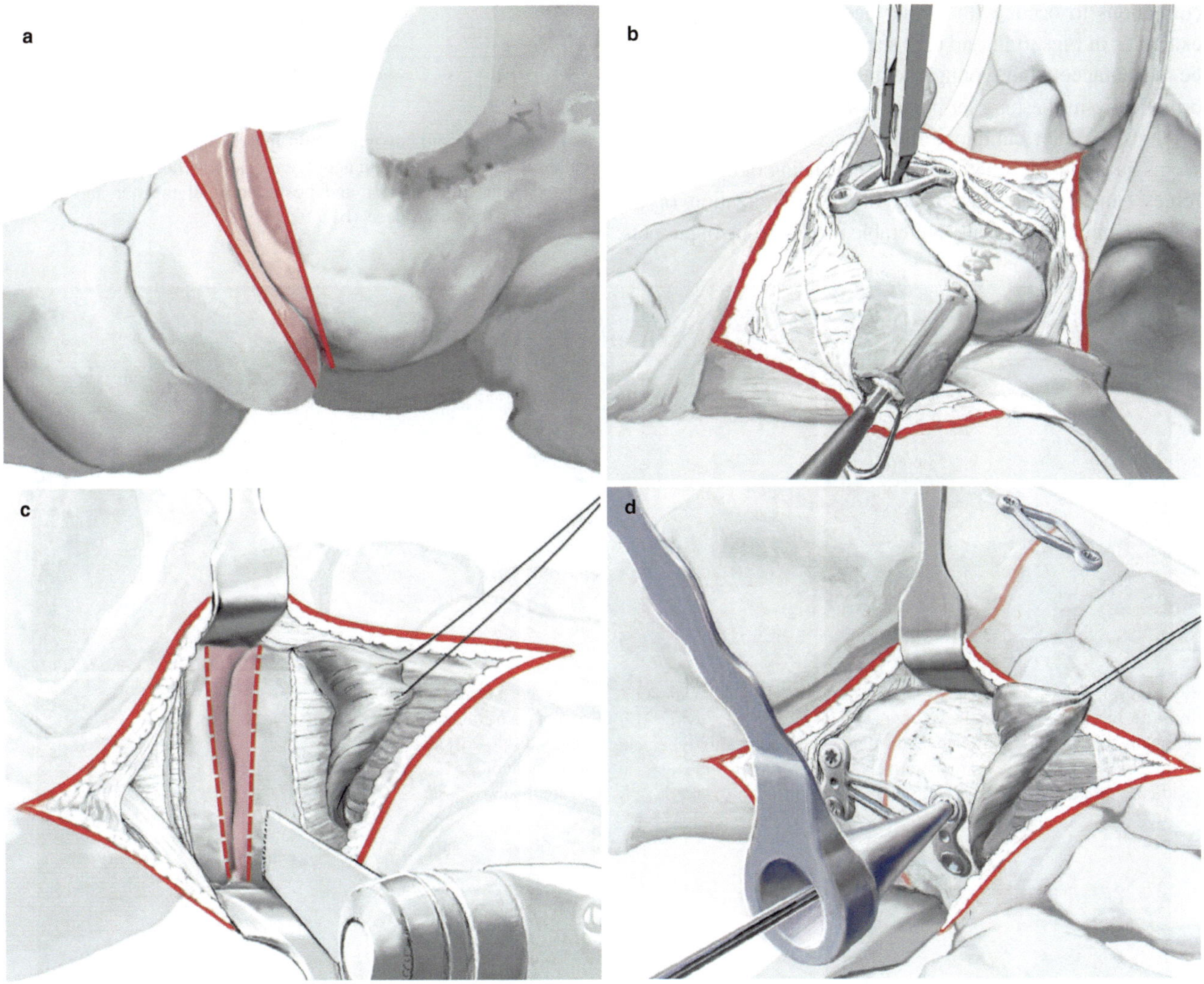

Fig. 6.7 Chopart arthrodesis via two incisions. The talonavicular joint is exposed by a dorsal incision and resected with appropriate wedge removal (**a**) and stabilized with screw and claw-plate (**b**). The calcaneocuboid joint is resected after temporary detachment of the extensor digitorum brevis origin (**c**) and fixed with a claw-plate (**d**) (from Hamel and Zwipp 2016)

skin and after L-shaped detachment of the extensor-digitorum-brevis origin (Fig. 6.7c). Depending on age and foot size, the fixation here is performed with K-wires, staples, screws, or claw-plates (Fig. 6.7d) in the desired position. In less severely deformed cases, the talonavicular joint can be left intact, and a resection arthrodesis of the calcaneocuboid joint with a shortening effect on the lateral tarsus is sufficient for correction (Fig. 6.8). In isolated calcaneocuboid fusion, the peritalar complex remains subtle in contrast to Chopart fusion, so that secondary deformity might occur.

The examples in Figs. 6.8, 6.9, 6.10, 6.11, and 6.12 demonstrate how a permanent orthograde alignment and stability can be achieved by a combined bony and soft tissue approach. However, especially when such corrections are carried out during the growth phase, it is not uncommon for over- and under-corrections to occur with further need for correction, as the examples in Figs. 6.11 and 6.12 show. In principle, it seems to be advantageous in younger children to initially stabilize orthotically in the long term and to schedule corrective interventions for later childhood or adolescence if possible. If it seems questionable whether a sole rebalancing of the muscular forces can be promising, an additional stabilization of the Chopart joint line is usually preferable for this group of patients.

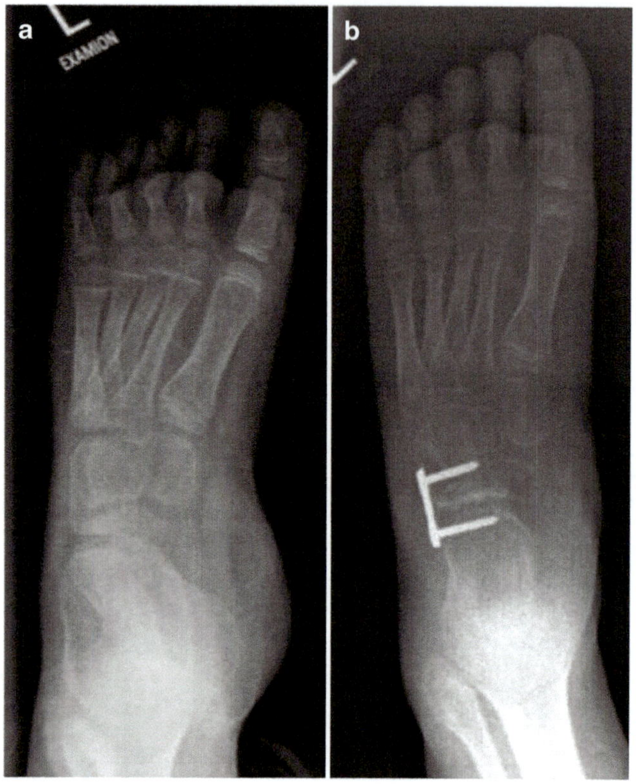

Fig. 6.8 9-Year-old boy with syndromal disease and mental and physical disability. The semirigid neurogenic clubfoot deformity (**a**) was stabilized with split anterior and posterior tibial transfer and isolated calcaneocuboid arthrodesis (**b**)

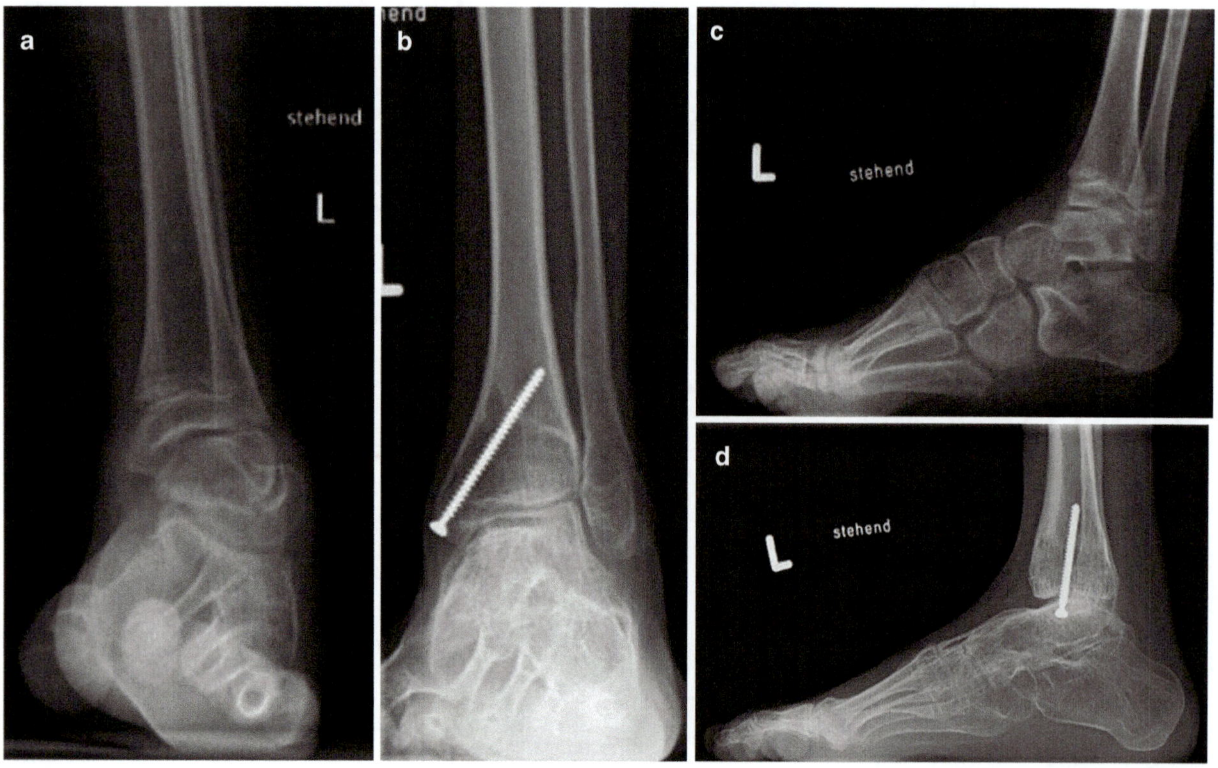

Fig. 6.9 11-Year-old patient with spinal muscle atrophy and severe neurogenic clubfoot deformity (**a**, **c**). An Achilles tendon lengthening with plantar fascia release was combined with a transfer of the posterior tibial tendon to the dorsum of the foot and the peroneus longus tendon to the peroneus brevis tendon (Sect. 7.11.1). For stabilization, the Chopart joint was fused, and a supramalleolar internal rotating osteotomy was additionally performed (**b**, **d**)

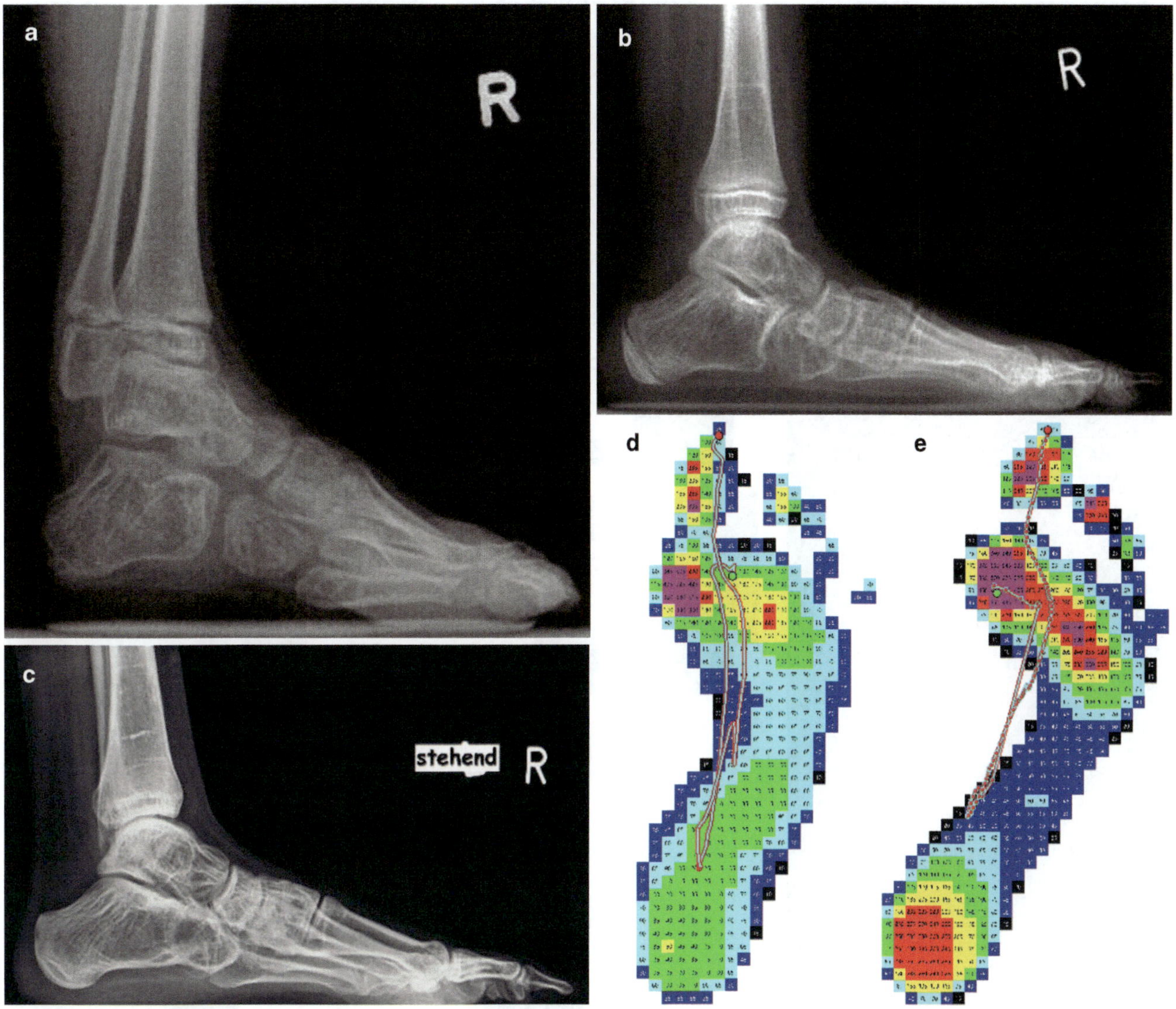

Fig. 6.10 Neurogenic clubfoot of a patient at the age of 9 years and peripheral neuropathy after chemotherapy treatment for leukemia (**a**, **d**). The peroneal musculature showed a complete loss. In addition to soft tissue release procedures medial and plantar, split anterior and posterior tibial tendon transfer was performed in combination with a Lichtblau resection arthroplasty at the lateral tarsus (**b**). A spontaneous ankylosis was observed after 8 years (**c**). Pedographically, 8 years postoperatively, a clearly normalized load pattern was found although with a persistent toe to heel gait (**e**). A dynamic orthosis to support weak dorsal extension should be considered here

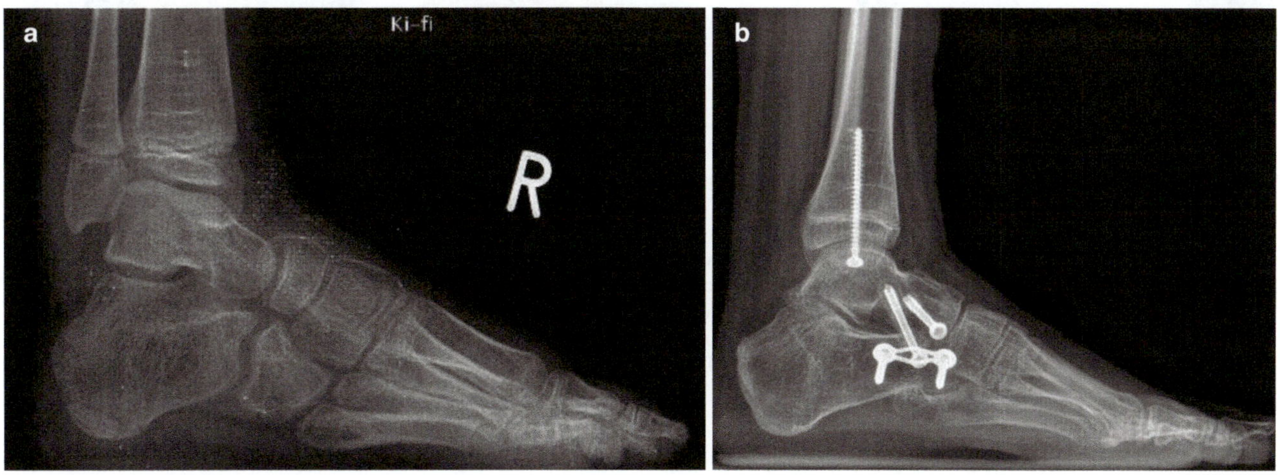

Fig. 6.11 12-Year-old patient with Curschmann-Steinert myopathy and neurogenic clubfoot deformity (**a**). An anterior tibial tendon transfer to the lateral cuneiform in combination with a split transfer of the posterior tibial tendon and a calcaneocuboid arthrodesis led to an overcorrection in the further course probably due to excessive tension of the transferred posterior tibial tendon part, which required an extension to Chopart arthrodesis with hemiepiphysiodesis at the distal tibia as a second operation with good alignment and function after 2.5 years (**b**)

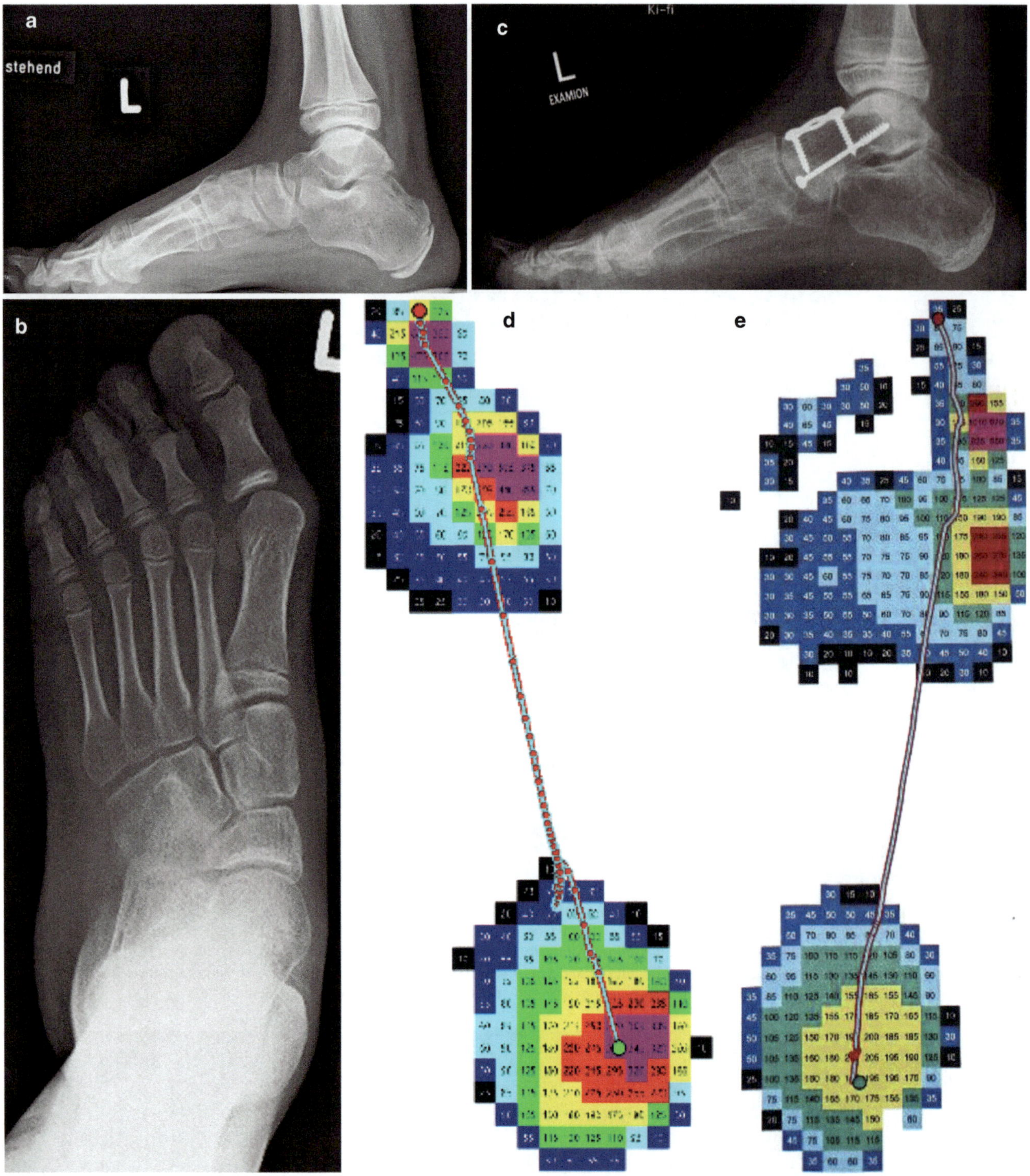

Fig. 6.12 11-Year-old patient with hemispasticity, externally overcorrected 1.5 years earlier by posterior tibial tendon transfer and (excessive) calf muscle lengthening. A progressive planovalgus deformity developed (**a**, **b**) with severe functional impairment, extreme loss of strength of the calf muscles, and an extreme pathological load pattern (**d**). By shortening the Achilles tendon with reinforcement by flexor-hallucis-longus transfer to the tuber calcanei, transfer of the anterior tibial tendon back to medial side, and stabilization of the tarsus by corrective talonavicular arthrodesis (**c**), a significant increase in strength and an overall functional improvement could be achieved. Already 6 months postoperatively (**e**), a normalized load pattern was observed

6.3.3 Neurogenic Equino-Planovalgus Deformity

In the neurogenic equino-planovalgus deformity, there is an increased activity of the evertors, especially of M. peroneus brevis. Calf muscle shortening or overactivity plays an important role in connection with the ground reaction forces. Inability of the talocalcaneal-navicular complex to adopt its stabil form, destabilization of the midfoot and forefoot abduction ("lever arm disease") will add to functional deterioration especially in the push-off-phase of gait.

Surgical correction usually includes a dosed calf muscle lengthening and stabilization of the talocalcaneal-navicular joint complex by arthroereisis, osteotomy, or arthrodesis. With arthroereisis, only preliminary results are available in cases of basic neuromotor diseases. Osteotomies (calcaneus lengthening osteotomy, TTO; see Sect. 4.11) can be used in principle as for flexible planovalgus deformities of non-neuromotor patients (Zeifang et al. 2006; Ettl et al. 2009). Here, talocalcaneal arthrodeses will be described, which can be combined with tarsal osteotomies. Good results were also described with talonavicular arthrodesis (de Coulon et al. 2011). Dussa et al. (2017) describe a Chopart arthrodesis with complete removal of the navicular bone to shorten the medial column in older children and adolescent patients. In some cases, a lengthening of the tendon of the peroneus brevis muscle and a rerouting of the anterior tibial tendon attachment (Fig. 4.14) should also be considered (Hamel et al. 1994). The Grice extra-articular arthrodesis is partly replaced today by an arthroereisis in combination with a transfer of the peroneus brevis tendon to the posterior tibial tendon attachment (Dr. A. Krebs, Wien-Speising, personal communication). Pure soft tissue surgery is not sufficient. In this deformity, the foot development and function of children with good walking capacity can be significantly improved by surgical intervention at an early school age, so that it is not advisable to wait until the end of the growth period. Patients who are unable to walk (e.g., tetraspasticity) have significantly worse results after surgical correction (Hamel et al. 1994; Ettl et al. 2009). According to the rule: "Fusion of a joint is treatment of the neighbouring joints," the capacity of the ankle joint for alignment changes of the talus in the sagittal plane should be taken into account (Figs. 6.15 and 6.16).

Technique of Extra-Articular Grice Arthrodesis and the "Princess Margret Rose Technique"

The extra-articular talocalcaneal corrective arthrodesis according to Grice (1952) is performed via an oblique skin access to the sinus tarsus. After removal of the soft tissue from the sinus tarsi, grooves are made cranially at the corpus-collum-transition of the talus and caudally at the calcaneus. From the facies anteromedialis of the proximal tibia (distal to the growth plate), an elongated corticospongious graft is harvested and cut into two halves, which are put together with their spongious surfaces like a sandwich. This double layer graft is precisely fitted into the prepared grooves in the corrected position and approximately as an extension of the tibial longitudinal axis, so that it prevents the talocalcaneal joint from eversion (Figs. 6.13 and 6.14); temporary stabilization with K-wires talocalcaneal is advisable. The disadvantage of the technique, which can be performed from about the age of 7 years and does not cause any growth disturbances of the tarsal skeleton, is the need for at least 6 weeks of weight relief until the bony incorporation of the graft. A combination with soft tissue stabilization medially is possible (Hamel et al. 1994). Varus overcorrection should be avoided.

An alternative for somewhat older children is the "Princess Margret Rose Technique" (Denneyson and Fulford 1976), in which cancellous bone material is impacted into the sinus tarsi area after removal of soft tissue and roughening of the surrounding bone, but without resection of the joint surfaces. A talocalcaneal screw osteosynthesis is performed for stabilization (Fig. 6.15). From about the age of 11–12, conventional fusion by resection of the joint surfaces is also possible.

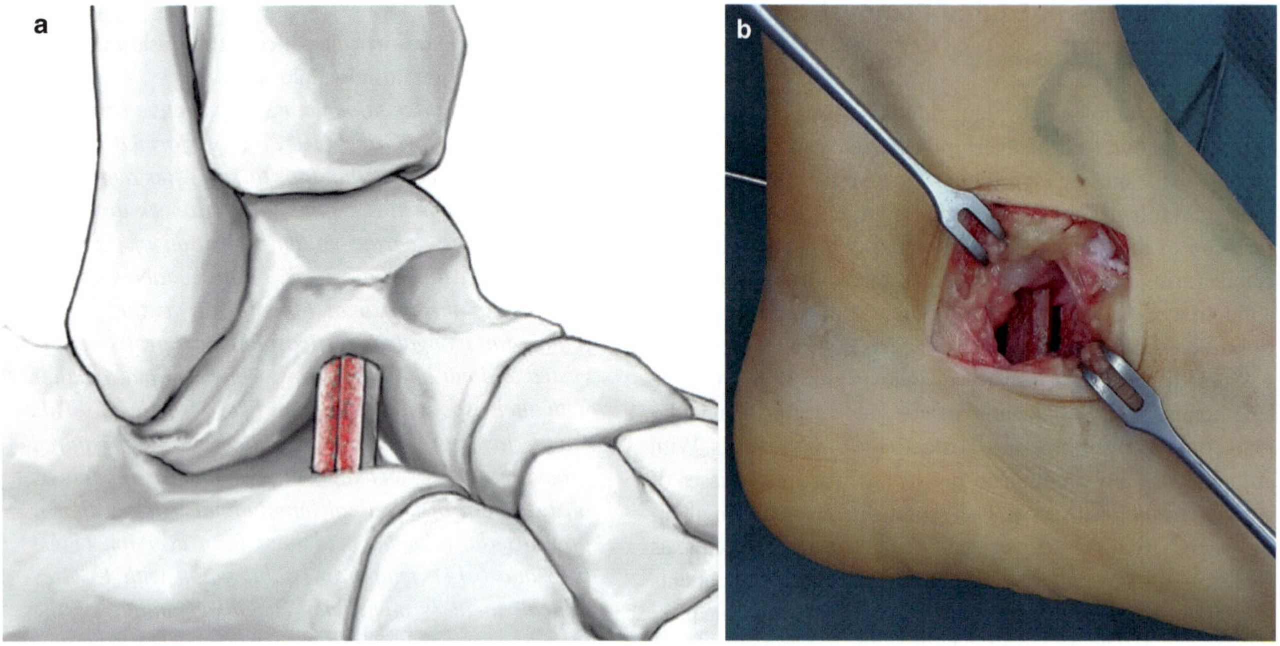

Fig. 6.13 Extra-articular graft arthrodesis according to Grice. A sandwich-like doubled tibial graft is anchored in the sinus tarsi and prevents excessive eversion (**a**, **b**)

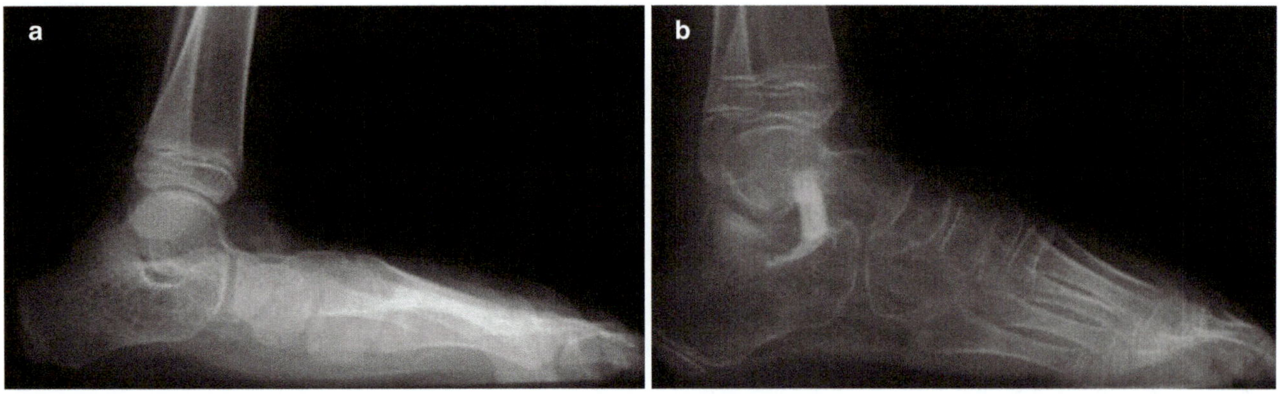

Fig. 6.14 8-Year-old girl with equino-planovalgus deformity in severe spastic diplegia (**a**). By means of dosed calf muscle lengthening and Grice arthrodesis, a complete straightening of the foot could be achieved (**b**). The graft has healed in on the talar and calcaneal side

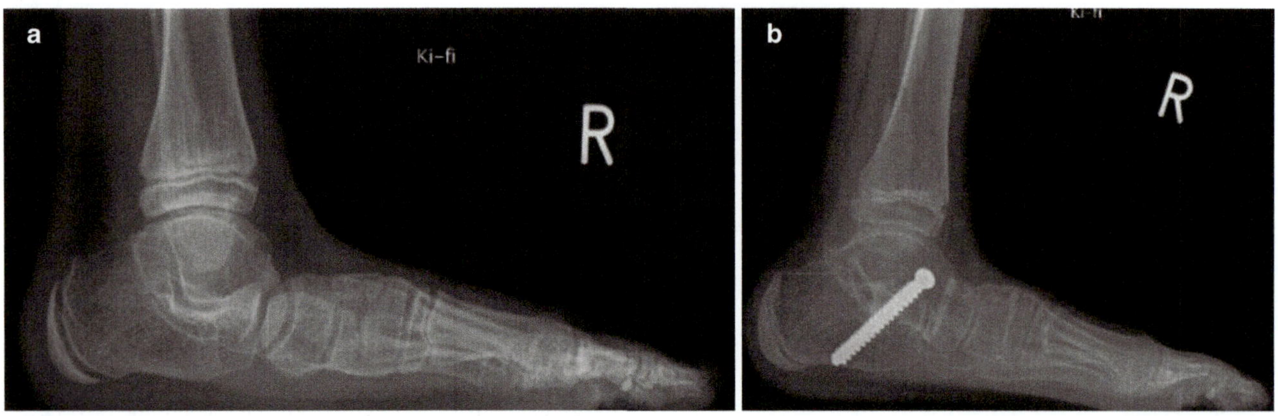

Fig. 6.15 12-Year-old girl with syndromal underlying disease and completely fixed subtalar joint in arthrogryposis (**a**). The severe equino-planovalgus deformity was straightened by tarsal arthrodeses with soft tissue surgery, whereby a complete correction of the talar inclination was deliberately omitted in order to avoid an early degeneration of the ventral parts of the upper ankle joint (**b**)

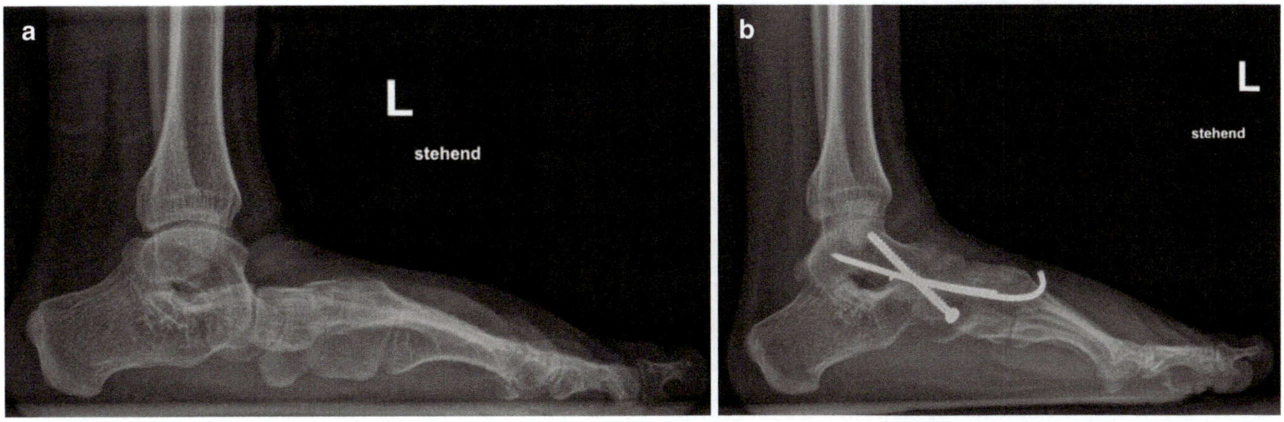

Fig. 6.16 Adolescent patient with neurogenic planovalgus deformity and severely plantar-flexed talus (**a**), externally treated by complete correction at the talonavicular joint and adverse effect on the ankle joint alignment (**b**)

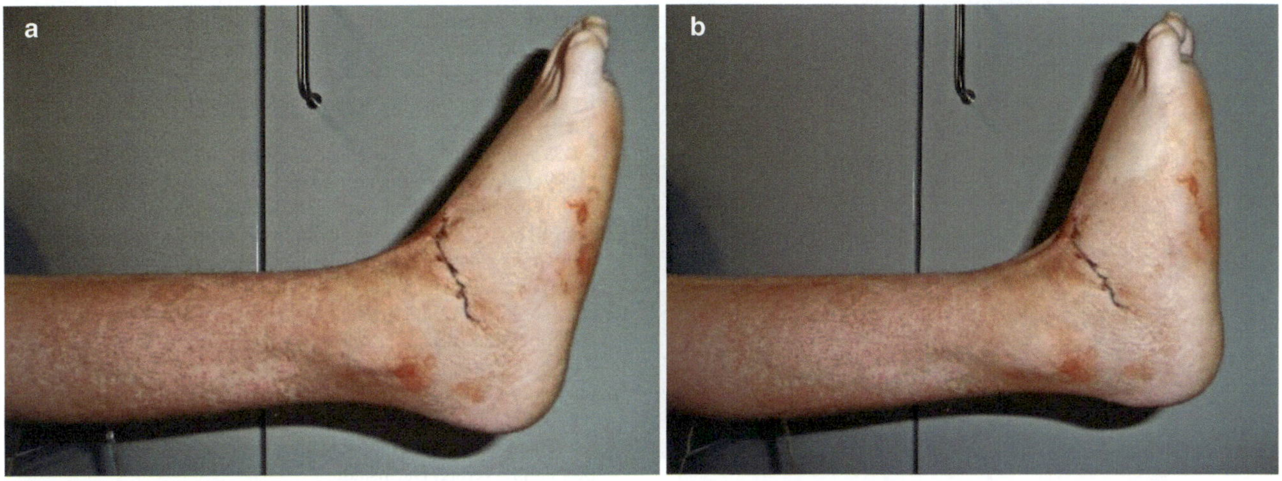

Fig. 6.17 11-Year-old girl with neurogenic clubfoot deformity due to peroneal paresis after removal of a vascularized fibular graft. 10 weeks after calcaneocuboid arthrodesis and transfer of the posterior tibial muscle to the dorsum of the foot, an active dorsal extension is possible again to a limited extent (**b**) in addition to the plantar flexion (**a**), the tensed tendon is visible after subcutaneous relocation

6.3.4 Flaccid Lower Leg Muscle: (Partial) Paralysis

In the case of flaccid (partial) paralysis of the lower leg muscles, a combined surgical and orthotic procedure is often necessary. For orthotic treatment, a stable neutral position of the foot should be aimed for. Deformities and pronounced instabilities of the hindfoot complex should be corrected by arthrodesis (e.g., Grice arthrodesis for deformities with tarsal eversion, Chopart arthrodesis for inversion malpositioning). Improvement of the disturbed muscular balance is also useful, even if this does not make orthotic fitting unnecessary, but facilitates orthotic support (Fig. 6.17). For example, the support of a weak active ankle extension with a foot lifting orthosis is much easier to achieve than in cases without any active function. A calcaneus foot deformity (Fig. 6.18) can be better treated orthotically after transfer of anterior tendons to the tuber calcanei. It should therefore be examined whether a tendon transfer can improve active control or whether the deficiency can be compensated for by bony stabilization. The following measures, for example, can be considered:

Examples of Typical Corrections for Flaccid Paralysis of the Lower Leg

Drop foot	Transfer of long toe extensors, M. tibialis post., M. peroneus long.
Posterior tibial muscle failure	Talonavicular- or Chopart Arthrodesis (FDL-transfer)
Peroneal muscle failure	Transfer of the anterior tibial tendon to the midline of the foot
Calf muscle failure	Surgically not compensable! Nevertheless posterior transfer of anterior tibial tendon sometimes useful
Flail toes	MTPJ-fusion at the first ray. Alternatively, extensor tendon tenodesis to prevent disturbing drop toes and to preserve passive mobility for late stance phase

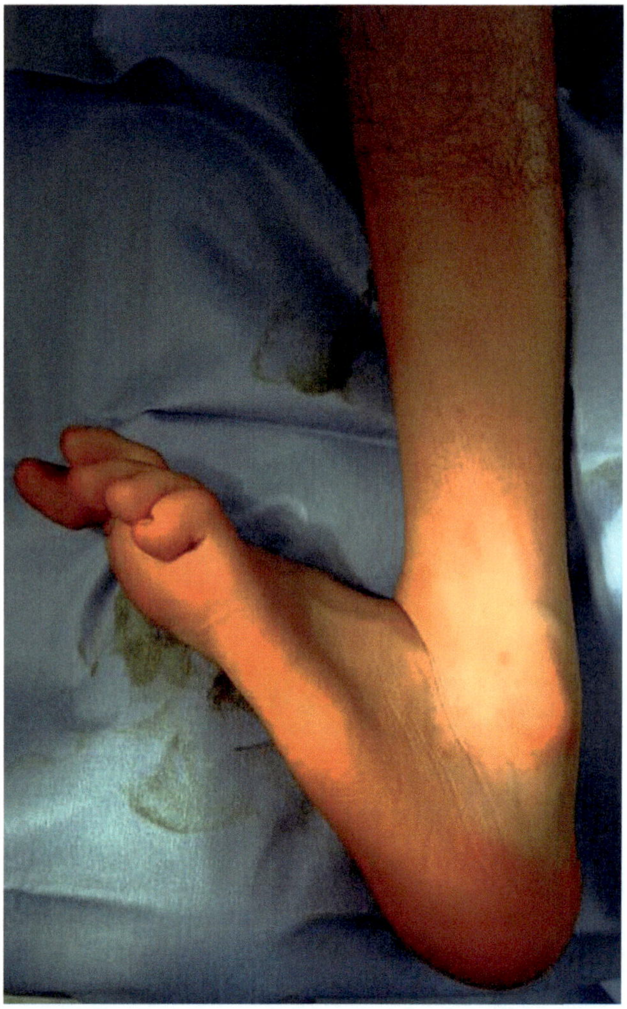

Fig. 6.18 In this patient with meningomyelocele and S1 paralysis level with severe calcaneus foot due to complete failure of the calf muscles, a significant improvement of the muscular balance could be achieved by transfer of the anterior tibial muscle to the calcaneal tuber, thus facilitating the use of a lower leg orthosis

As a foot lifter replacement in the event of failure of the anterior muscle group, e.g., in peroneal paresis, a transfer of the posterior tibial muscle through the interosseous membrane to the dorsum of the foot (see Sect. 7.11.2, Fig. 6.17) or the relocation of the tendon of the long peroneal muscle around the fibula to the anterior side of the foot can be considered. To compensate for the donor site morbidity, a transfer of the flexor-digitorum-longus tendon or a Chopart arthrodesis should be added in the first case, in the second case a coupling of the peroneus brevis tendon to the distal peroneus-longus tendon stump.

In severe calcaneus foot, e.g., in meningomyelocele with deep-lumbar or sacral paralysis (Fig. 6.18), a transfer of anterior muscle-tendon units through the interosseous membrane to the tuber calcanei usually does not nearly compensate for the loss of calf muscles, but it can contribute to undisturbed foot development and better orthotic fitting (Park et al. 2008).

References

Baumann JU, Koch HG (1989) Ventrale aponeurotische Verlängerung des M. gastrocnemius. Oper Orthop Traumatol 1:254–258

Chang CH, Albarracin JP, Lipton GE, Miller F (2002) Long-term follow-up of surgery for equinovarus foot deformity in children with cerebral palsy. J Pediatr Orthop 22:792–799

de Coulon G, Turcot K, Canavese F, Dayer R, Kaelin A, Ceroni D (2011) Talonavicular arthrodesis for the treatment of neurological flat foot deformity in pediatric patients: clinical and radiographic evaluation of 29 feet. J Pediatr Orthop 31:557–563

Denneyson WG, Fulford GE (1976) Subtalar arthrodesis by cancellous grafts and metallic internal fixation. J Bone Joint Surg 58-B:507–510

Döderlein L, Wenz W, Schneider U (2004) Der Spitzfuß—Der Hackenfuß. Springer-Verlag, Berlin, Heidelberg, New York

Dussa CU, Döderlein L, Forst R, Böhm H, Fujak A (2017) Management of severe equinovalgus in patients with cerebral palsy by naviculectomy in combination with midfoot arthrodesis. Foot Ankle Int 38:1011–1019

Ettl V, Wollmerstedt N, Kirschner S, Morrison R, Pasold E, Raab P (2009) Calcaneal lengthening for planovalgus deformity in children with cerebral palsy. Foot Ankle Int 30:398–404

Graham KH (2010) Cerebral palsy. In: Mc Carthy JJ, Drennan JC (eds) The Child's foot and ankle. Wolters Kluwer, Lippincott Williams and Wilkins, Philadelphia

Grice DS (1952) An extra-articular arthrodesis of the subastragalar joint for correction of paralytic flat feet in children. J Bone Joint Surg 34-A:927–940

Hamel J (2000) In: Venbrocks R (ed) Fußdeformitäten im Rahmen neuroorthopädischer Krankheitsbilder—Diagnostik und konservative Therapie. Neuroorthopädie und Rheumaorthopädie des Kindes. Steinkopff-Verlag, Darmstadt

Hamel J, Becker W (1997) Die Korrekturarthrodese des Chopart-Gelenkes bei neurogenen Fußdeformitäten. Oper Orthop Traumatol 9:109–119

Hamel J, Kissling C, Heimkes B, Stotz S (1994) A combined bony and soft-tissue tarsal stabilization procedure (Grice-Schede) for hindfoot valgus in children with cerebral palsy. Arch Orthop Trauma Surg 113:237–243

Hamel J, Zwipp H (2016) Sprunggelenk und Rückfuß – Meistertechniken in der operativen Orthopädie und Unfallchirurgie. Springer-Verlag Berlin, Heidelberg

Herzenberg JE, Lamm BM, Corwin C, Sekel J (2007) Isolated recession of the gastrocnemius muscle: The Baumann procedure. Foot Ankle Int 28:1154–1159

Park KB, Park HW, Joo SY, Kin HW (2008) Surgical treatment of calcaneal deformity in a select group of patients with myelomenigocele. J Bone Joint Surg 90-A:2149–2159

Perry J, Burnfield JM (2010) Gait analysis – normal and pathological function. Thorofare: SLACK incorporated

Piazza SJ, Adamson RL, Moran MF, Sanders JO, Sharkey NA (2003) Effects of tensioning errors in split transfers of tibialis anterior and posterior tendons. J Bone Joint Surg 85-A:858–865

Rutz E, Baker R, Tirosh O et al (2011) Tibialis anterior tendon shortening in combination with Achilles tendond lengthening in spastic equinus in cerebral palsy. Gait Posture 33:152–157

Tachdjian MO (1985) The child's foot. WB Saunders Company, Philadelphia

Zeifang F, Breusch SJ, Döderlein L (2006) Evans calcaneal lengthening procedure for spastic flexible flatfoot in 32 patients (46 feet) with a follow up of 3 to 9 years. Foot Ankle Int 27:500–507

Cavovarus Deformities

7

Contents

The very broad spectrum of cavovarus deformities includes on the one hand the less severe forms of the "high arched" foot type ("idiopathic cavovarus foot"), whose muscular imbalances usually remain below the neurophysiological detection limit. These cases require foot surgery advice, e.g., due to metatarsalgia, peroneal tendon degeneration, metatarsal V stress fracture, or symptoms of ankle instability in adulthood. On the other side of the spectrum, there

J. Hamel, *Foot and Ankle Surgery in Children and Adolescents*, https://doi.org/10.1007/978-3-030-58108-4_7

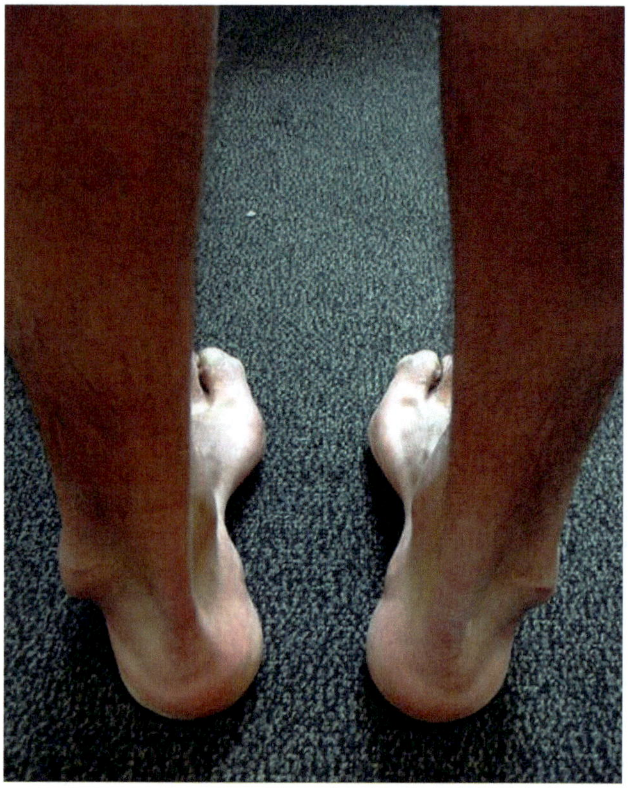

Fig. 7.1 Bilateral cavovarus deformity in a young patient with hereditary sensomotoric neuropathy (HSMN)

are progressive deformities in the presence of a clear muscle imbalance, due to an underlying neurologic disease.

Characteristic and eponymous for the cavovarus deformities are the hindfoot varus component and the increased medial longitudinal arch (Fig. 7.1). In contrast to the neurogenic clubfoot, there is no hindfoot equinus component, and the medial foot ray shows an overload—except in late cases—as does the lateral foot rim. All the basic principles described in Sects. 6.1 and 6.2 for the evaluation of neuromotor deformities in the lower leg-foot region apply also for cavovarus deformities. The phenomena of muscular imbalance and the principles of correction will be described in greater detail for this group of diseases.

Recommended Literature

- *Döderlein L et al. (*2000*)* Der Hohlfuß. *Extensive, lexical work with a broad presentation also of the history (in German)*
- *Tachdjian MO (*1985*)* The child's foot
- *Smith TF et al. (*1992*)* Pes cavus. In: Comprehensive textbook of foot surgery, 2. Ed. (Ed.: Mc Glamry et al.), *not included in later editions*
- *Coleman SS (*1983*)* Complex foot deformities in children. *Very detailed description of the indications for the child*

7.1 Therapeutically Relevant Aspects of Etiology and Pathogenesis

Cavovarus deformities are in most cases foot deformities that develop during childhood or adolescence and can be caused by various neurogenic diseases. Often the underlying disease belongs to different subgroups of hereditary sensomotoric neuropathy (HSMN), M. Charcot-Marie-Tooth (CMT). Common to the cavovarus deformities is a pathogenetic muscular imbalance. This can be clinically obvious but is often only detectable by subtle muscle strength testing. Typical is an early—at least relative—weakness of peroneus brevis muscle, anterior tibial muscle, and the short foot muscles. Due to this weakness of individual muscles—which varies greatly from case to case—compensatory processes (cf. Sect. 6.1) and ground reaction forces, progressive deformities of various types and characteristics frequently occur during the growth age and also thereafter. Some of these biomechanical relationships, which are important for understanding the pathogenesis, will be explained in more detail below, since they also have direct therapeutic significance.

7.1.1 Phenomena of Muscle Dynamics

The paralysis-related weakness of a muscle causes compensation mechanisms and results in a relative predominance of antagonists. Important examples are:

- ***Peroneal dysfunction***

  The weakness of the M. peroneus brevis and thus of the active eversion results in compensatory hyperactivity of the—initially less weakened—long peroneal muscle, which simultaneously is a strong plantar flexor of the medial ray (Fig. 7.2).
- ***Anterior tibial/long peroneal muscle antagonism***

  The weakness of the anterior tibial muscle in combination with overactivity of the long peroneal muscle (see above) leads to increased plantar flexion of the medial ray (Fig. 7.3).
- ***Posterior tibial/peroneus brevis antagonism***

  Normal activity of the posterior tibial muscle leads to a hindfoot inversion when the peroneus brevis muscle is weak at the same time.
- ***Extensor substitution***

  The weakness of the anterior tibial muscle is compensated by overactivity of the long toe extensor muscles; this favors claw toe formation and reinforces the cavus component by tensioning the plantar fascia.

7.1.2 Muscle Mechanical Factors

Purely muscle-mechanical conditions and interactions are also involved in the progression of the cavovarus deformation. Some examples are:

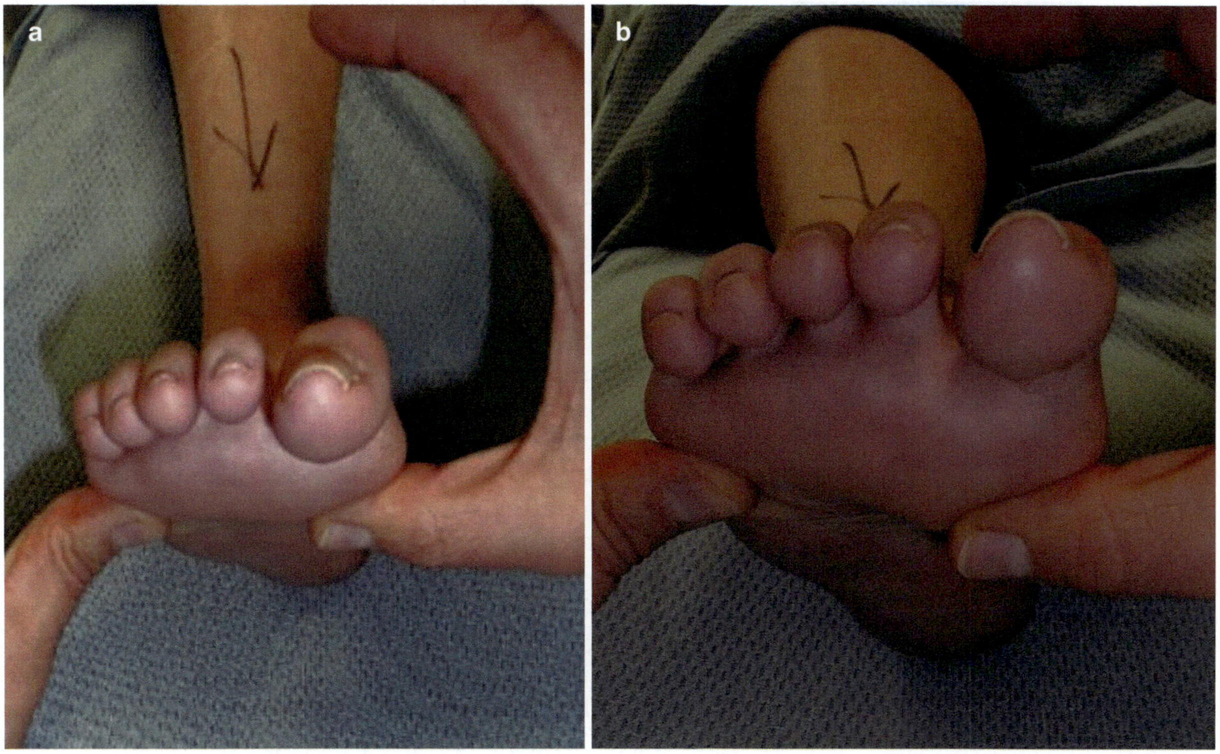

Fig. 7.2 Muscle testing of the M. peroneus longus activity level: from a neutral foot position (**a**), the patient is asked to plantarflex. With active plantar flexion of the foot, in the presence of peroneal dysfunction, an increased plantar flexion of the medial metatarsal ray occurs due to the overactivity of the M. peroneus longus (**b**)

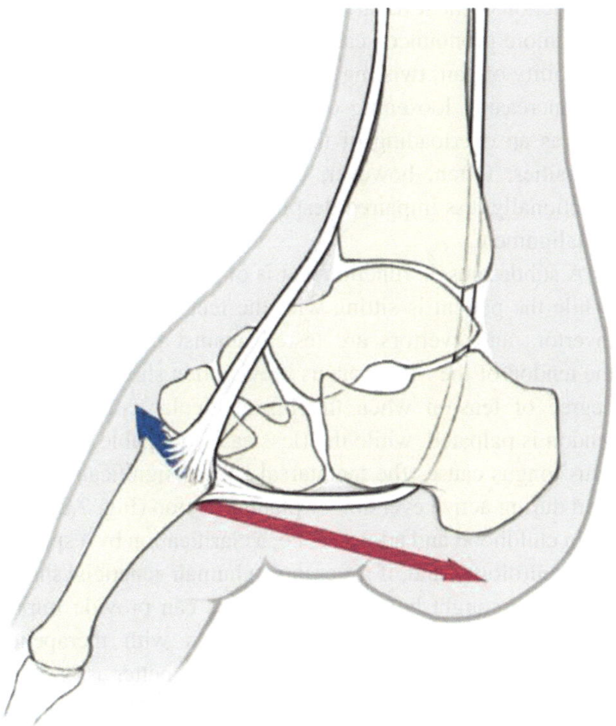

Fig. 7.3 Assuming equal force development of the anterior tibial muscle and the long peroneal muscle, the balance of forces in relation to the dorsal extension or plantar flexion of the medial ray—represented by the two arrows—is already shifted strongly in favor of the long peroneal muscle and the plantar flexion by the initial position in spontaneous posture

- With increasing cavus deformity, the leverage ratio becomes even more unfavorable for the—weakened—anterior tibial muscles (Fig. 7.3), while it becomes more favorable for the—already overactive—long peroneal muscles ("peroneal overdrive," Manoli and Graham 2005).
- With increasingly hyperextended initial position of the metatarsophalangeal joints, the extending torque of the long toe extensors on these joints increases further.
- The plantar fascia also plays an important role: due to claw toe deformity, it comes under increased tension ("windlass mechanism") and thus reinforces the cavus component and the hindfoot inversion.

7.1.3 Couplings Caused by Tarsal Mechanics

The interactions of the three deformity components (mid-forefoot pronation, hindfoot inversion, and supramalleolar outward rotation), which are based on tarsal mechanics, continue to favor the development of the cavovarus deformity: mid-forefoot pronation and hindfoot inversion are mutually dependent and reinforce each other; a lowering of the medial foot ray causes an inversion of the hindfoot complex ("forefoot-driven hindfoot varus," "tripod effect"), and a hindfoot inversion of the tarsal joints results in an (over) active M. peroneus longus favoring the plantarflexion of the medial ray.

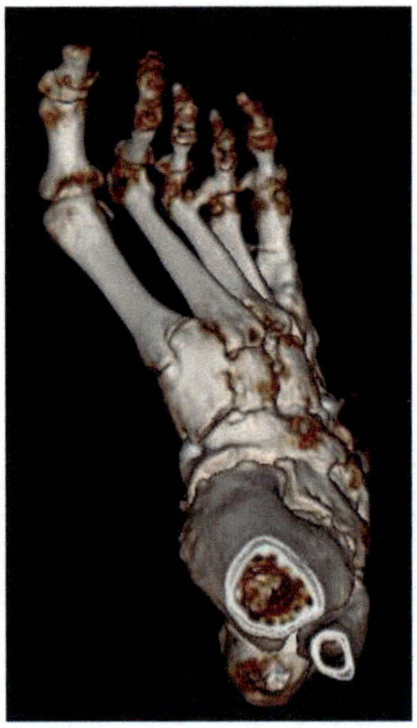

Fig. 7.4 3-D CT reconstruction of a cavovarus deformity. The pronounced external rotation of the malleolar region in combination with inversion of the talocalcaneal-navicular complex is clearly visible. This is accompanied by a medialization of the tuber calcanei

Due to the cardanic property of the hindfoot joints, inversion of the peritalar complex leads to increased outward rotation of the lower leg. This is supported by the influence of the posterior tibial muscle and the lack of its antagonist [Hansen 2008]. The outward rotation of the lower leg vice versa increases hindfoot varus deformity by shifting the tuber calcanei towards medial (see Figs. 7.4 and 7.30).

Malposition Components of the Cavovarus Deformity

- Mid-forefoot pronation
- Hindfoot inversion
- Supramalleolar outward rotation

7.2 Clinical Examination

Characteristics of the cavovarus deformities are clinically the increased longitudinal arching of the foot (cavus component), which particularly affects the medial foot ray (mid-forefoot pronation) and a varus malposition of the heel when viewed from behind. However, cases are also observed in which the cavus component is predominant compared to the hindfoot inversion (Fig. 7.23a). The Coleman block test (Coleman and Chesnut 1977) allows an examination of the proportion of forefoot-related hindfoot deformity and the flexibility of the hindfoot joints: If the medial ray is allowed to plantarflex when the other parts of the sole are positioned on a piece of wood of appropriate height, the hindfoot becomes partially or completely straightened by reducing the tarsal inversion (Fig. 7.5). The hindfoot varus deformity when viewed from behind is composed of the inversion of the talocalcaneal-navicular complex and the medialization of the heel by supramalleolar outward rotation. Basically, the cavovarus deformity is always rather rigid for tarsal-mechanical reasons, since the hindfoot complex is exclusively in its stable "rigid-lever" mode during the stance phase of gait and cannot adopt the flexible "mobile adaptor" mode even during heel contact and in the early stance phase.

In the forefoot area, a tendency towards claw-toe development with hyperextension of the metatarsophalangeal joints and flexion of the proximal and distal interphalangeal joints is usually dominant. In gait analysis, the increased activation of the long toe extensors (extensor substitution) is particularly noticeable. A similar excessive recruition of the long toe extensors can be observed in active dorsal extension of the foot.

The lower leg outward rotation is best estimated in knee flexion (Fig. 1.75). The angle of the intermalleolar axis in relation to the knee motion axis in most cavovarus cases is above the normal level of about 20°–25° outward rotation. The range of motion of hip rotation in extended position of the hip joint should also be checked; it is not uncommon to see an outward rotation contracture, which adds to the lower leg outward rotation and can be unmasked by foot correction and thus become clinically relevant. An excessive outward rotation of the foot in relation to the direction of gait causes a reduction of the lever arm in late stance phase and push off.

In more pronounced cases, patients report a tendency for instability of gait, twisting the ankle, frequent ankle sprains, and increasing loosening of the lateral ankle ligaments as well as an overloading of the lateral foot ray with painful callosities. Often, however, the affected persons are still functionally less impaired despite the advanced stage of the malalignment.

A subtle muscle function test is of particular importance: While the patient is sitting with the feet hanging down the invertors and evertors are tested against resistance, here, the tendon of the M. peroneus brevis often shows a reduced degree of tension when the inframalleolar course of the tendon is palpated, while the (less easily palpable) M. peroneus longus causes the metatarsal I to be significantly lowered during active eversion or plantar flexion (Fig. 7.2).

In childhood and adolescence, a clarification by a specialized neurologist and, if necessary, a human geneticist should always be sought before surgery. This can provide important differential diagnostic information with therapeutic consequences (e.g., "tethered cord") and a better assessment of the progression to be expected. From our own experience, however, we must warn against prolonged and costly "endless diagnostics," which allows the optimal time for a correction to pass by unused.

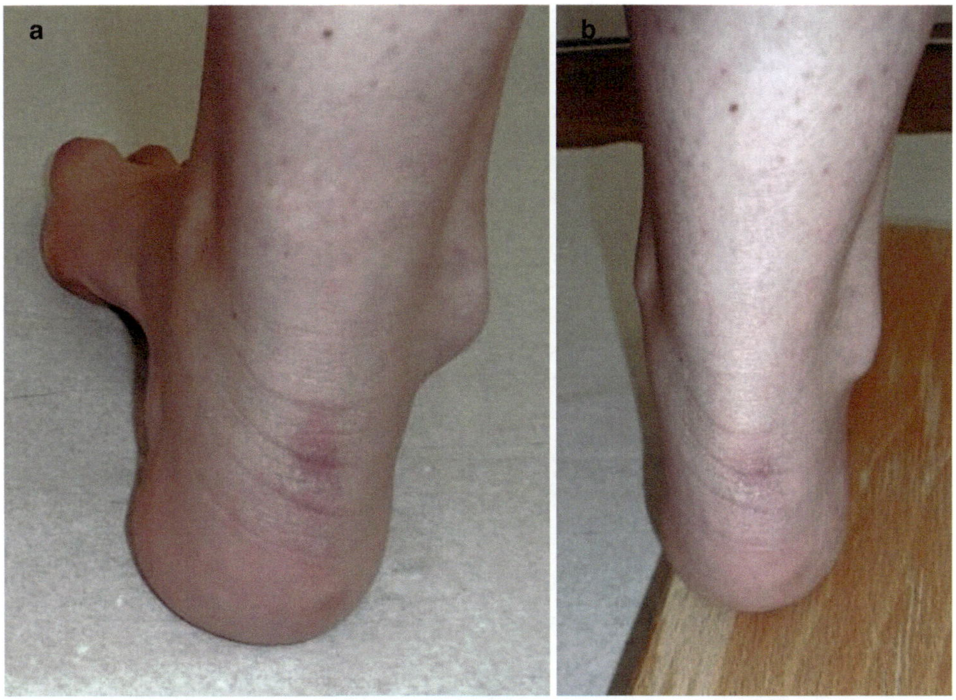

Fig. 7.5 In the Coleman block test, the hindfoot varus malposition (**a**) is eliminated by plantarflexing the medial pronated ray, if the hindfoot joints are flexible (**b**)

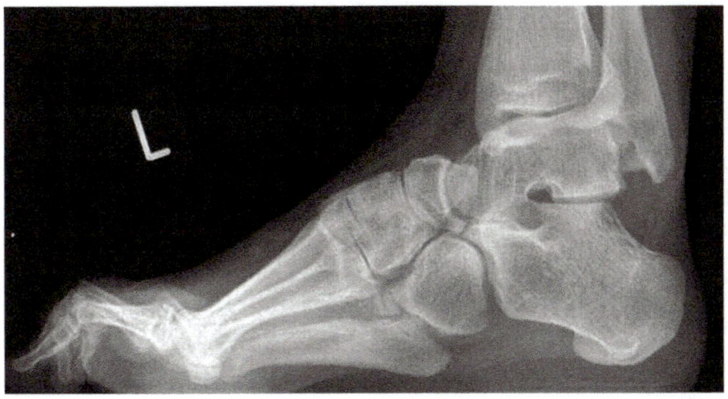

Fig. 7.6 Cavovarus deformity in the lateral projection without compensation of the lower leg outward rotation. In such an imaging technique, the medial cavus component, for example, cannot be detected in its true extent (cf. d'Astorg et al. 2016), whereas the hindfoot inversion is depicted excessively

7.3 Radiological Imaging

For radiological diagnostics, it should be taken into account that three coupled lower leg-foot segments (see Sect. 7.1.3) must be depicted: the pronated midfoot-forefoot segment, the inverted hindfoot complex, and the outward rotated lower leg-talus segment. The following characteristics can be observed (Figs. 7.6, 7.7, and 7.8):

- **Mid-forefoot pronation or medial cavus** component evaluated in the lateral projection: divergence of the metatarsal bones, lack of overlap between the navicular and cuboid, increased talus-metatarsal I angle ("Meary's angle," normally <0°), calcaneal pitch angle, normally <25°, calcaneus metatarsal I angle ("Hibbs' angle," normally >150°).

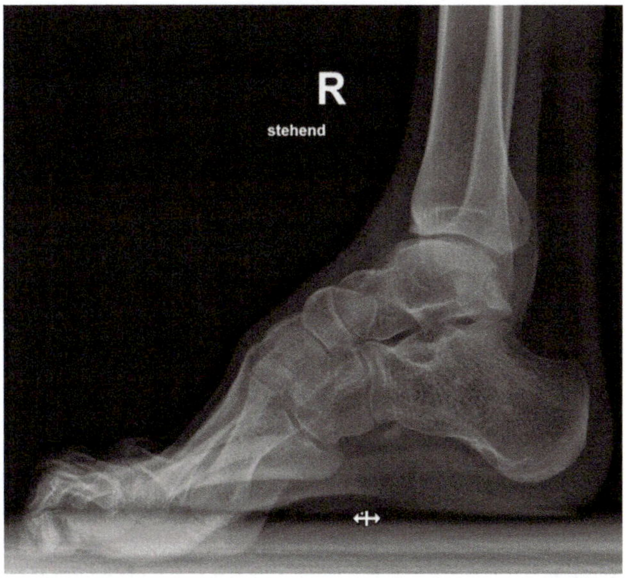

Fig. 7.7 "Hindfoot-centered" lateral X-ray projection of a cavovarus deformity with compensation of the mid-forefoot pronation through allowing the medial ray to plantarflex and the lower leg outward rotation through inward rotation of the foot. This allows the evaluation of the real positional relationships at the ankle and peritalar joints to be assessed in the furthest possible correction position. However, the extent of the mid-forefoot pronation with divergence of the metatarsalia and pathologically increased talus-metatarsal-I angle is shown excessively

- **Inversion of the talocalcaneal-navicular joint complex** evaluated in the lateral projection: parallel alignment of talus and calcaneus, horizontal position of the posterior facet of the subtalar joint; medialized position of the navicular in relation to the talar head in the dorsoplantar image.

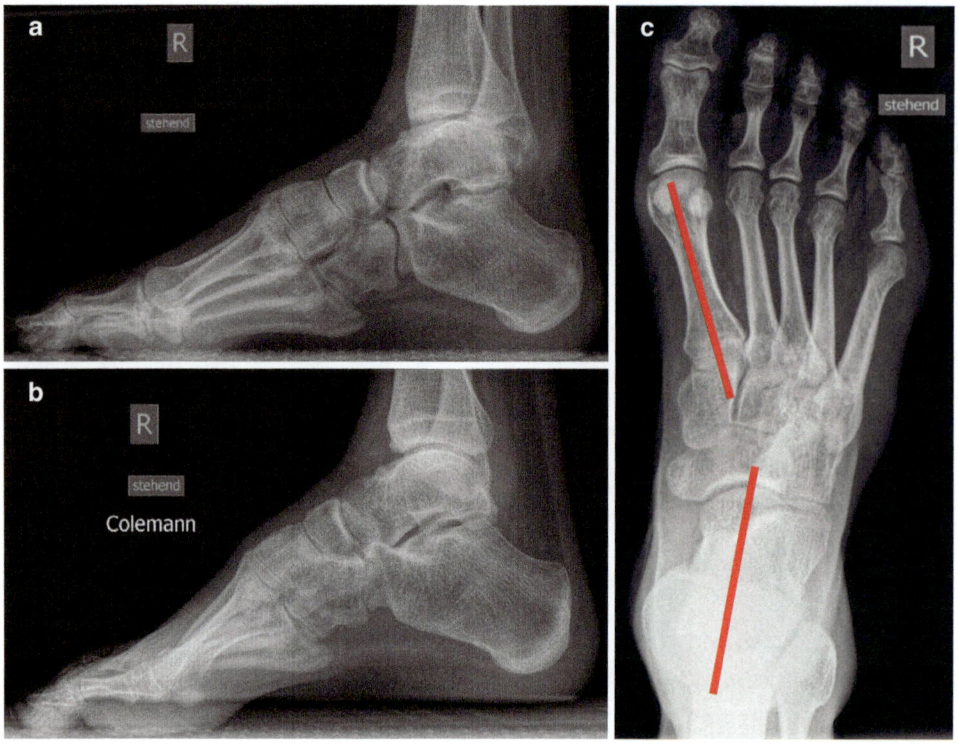

Fig. 7.8 Moderately pronounced cavovarus deformity of an 18-year-old patient, in uncorrected position (**a**) and with compensation of the outward rotation of the lower leg "hindfoot-centered," as well as recorded with the Coleman block test on the same day (**b**). The divergence of the metatarsalia, the clearly positive talometatarsal I angle (approx. +20°), and the conditions at the anterior tibiotalar joint are shown much better in the hindfoot-centered recording technique. This allows more precise planning, for instance, of the necessary cavus correction and the elevation at the medial ray. The rotational correction for the hindfoot-centered lateral view (**b**) is derived from the talometatarsal I angle in the dorsoplantar projection with Coleman block test (**c**)

- **Supramalleolar outward rotation** (dorsal positioning of the lateral malleolus, double contour of the trochlea tali and increased visibility of the ("open") sinus tarsi in the lateral projection, lack of visibility of the medial and lateral compartment in the ankle ap projection).

The described phenomena can be seen at a glance in the lateral X-ray image of the cavovarus foot in the common mid-forefoot-centered X-ray adjustment technique. If a lateral X-ray image is taken with the length axis of the foot parallel to the X-ray cassette, the extent of the malpositioning of the abovementioned segments is shown in a distorted way that does not do justice to the depiction of the actual deformity (Fig. 7.6): The mid-forefoot pronation with the pronounced plantar flexion of the medial ray, readable, e.g., at the talus-metatarsal-I angle, appears much less pronounced than it really is; the conditions at the tibiotalar joint with a tendency to anterior impingement cannot be assessed because of the supramalleolar outward rotation and the talocalcaneal-navicular complex is not shown in the furthest corrected position and also outwardly rotated with a wide "open" sinus tarsi.

It is not possible to show all deformity components of the three-dimensional deformity in one two-dimensional projection. However, each of the lower leg-foot segments mentioned above can be isolated by means of specific adjustment techniques and thus be presented more precisely for the planning of an intervention. The "hindfoot-centered" adjustment has proven itself in practice (Hamel et al. 2020): A plantar flexion of the medial ray as in the Coleman block test (Sect. 7.2) allows an assessment of the hindfoot contracture independent of the influence of midfoot-forefoot pronation. Thus the talocalcaneal-navicular complex is positioned in the furthest possible correction position. Compensation of supramalleolar outward rotation by inward rotation of the foot allows a more precise assessment of the hindfoot position and the conditions at the upper ankle joint (Fig. 7.7). The difference of an uncorrected lateral view and a hindfoot-centered projection is shown in Fig. 7.8.

Also in the ankle ap projection, the lower leg outward rotation should be compensated for in order to obtain an exact representation of the tibiotalar joint. This image is not taken using the Coleman block test to document the extent of tibiotalar tilting and instability (Fig. 7.29c). If the ankle joint does not open laterally, this does not, however, exclude a higher degree of anterolateral instability, which often only becomes radiologically (and clinically) apparent after subtalar arthrodesis. The Saltzman image is generally used to document the hindfoot varus component; however, this imaging technique is highly dependent on the selected rotational position of the foot, so that it has proven less suitable for the author. In the cavovarus foot, the hindfoot varus component is a combination of inversion of the talocalcaneal-navicular complex and the easily underestimated supramalleolar outward rotation and is therefore clinically more easily detected than radiologically.

Three-dimensional CT reconstructions (Fig. 7.4) and in particular DVT in a weight-bearing position and in combination with the Coleman block test allow an even more precise analysis of the malposition components for surgical planning. In special cases, the MRI can be used to diagnose the lower leg muscles and damage of the peroneal tendons.

Recommended X-Ray Imaging Technique for Cavovarus Deformities (Hamel et al. 2020)

- Dorsoplantar image with plantarflexion of the medial ray (Coleman block test), determination of the TMT-I angle (Fig. 7.8c), to which 10° are added. This is the "rotation angle."
- Lateral image in "hindfoot-centered" projection with compensation of the supramalleolar rotation by inward rotation of the foot according to the "rotation angle" previously determined from the dorsoplantar image and with plantarflexion of the medial ray (Coleman block test).
- Ankle joint ap projection with compensation of supramalleolar rotation (see above) without plantarflexion of the medial ray also show tibiotalar instability (Fig. 7.29c).
- (Saltzman projection).

7.4 Pedography

Pedography (cf. Sect. 1.4.3) is particularly suitable for depicting and documenting the extent of the cavovarus deformity, the resulting functional disorder, the progression of the disease, and the results of surgical corrections from a functional point of view. Five phenomena particularly characteristic for this group of diseases could be identified from the peak pressure recording (Hamel 2016a) (Fig. 7.9).

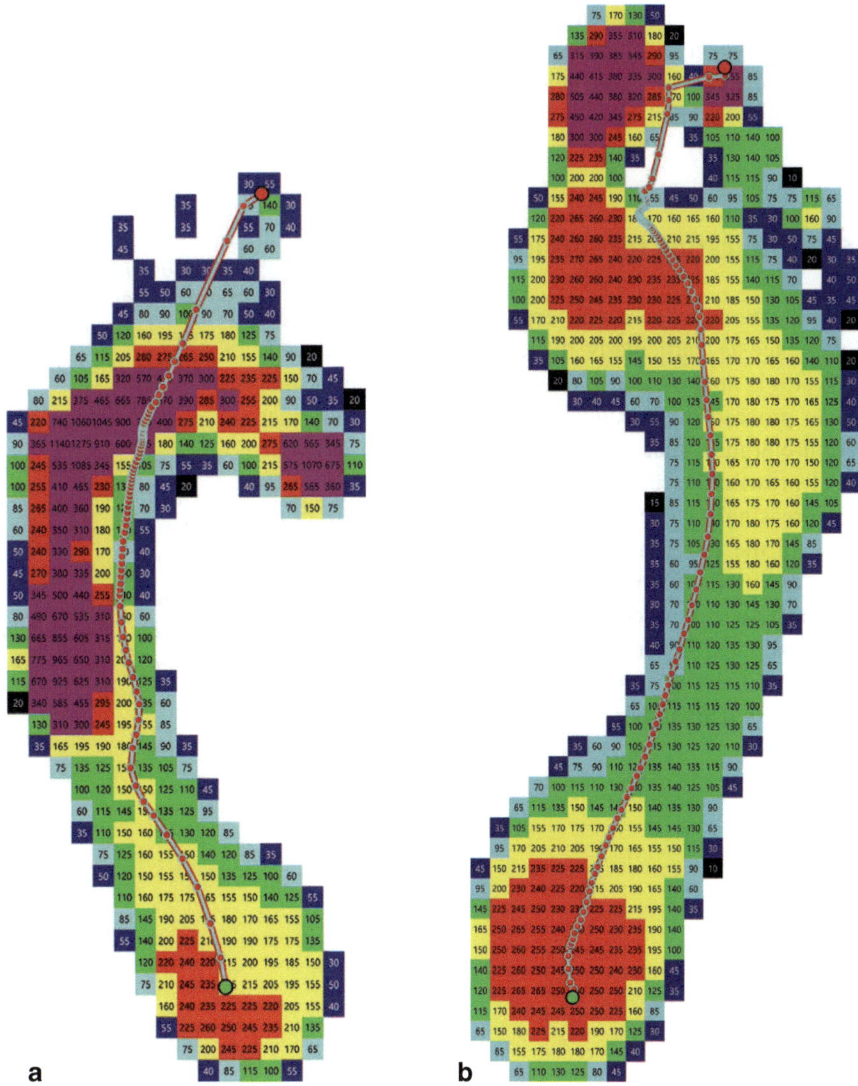

Fig. 7.9 Pedographic image of an advanced cavovarus deformity (**a**) compared to the healthy opposite side (**b**). All characteristics mentioned in the text can be seen

Pedographic Characteristics of the Cavovarus Deformity

- Reduction and shortening of the load-bearing area (increased indentation).
- Absence of medial convexity of the center of pressure line at initial heel contact as an expression of missing eversion and shock absorption at the beginning of the stance phase of gait.
- Overloading of the lateral foot ray especially the metatarsal V base.
- High pressure on the metatarsal V and I head, the latter caused by the activity of the M. peroneus longus (after the rupture of its tendon, however, the pressure on the metatarsal I head rapidly decreases).
- Progressive loss of the toe imprint.

Through suitable corrections, the loaded plantar area can often be significantly increased and the locally achieved peak pressure in the forefoot area can thus be effectively reduced (Fig. 7.29). The postoperative load distribution of the metatarsalia provides information as to whether it has been successful to relieve the metatarsal I in a dosed and non-excessive manner by elevation of the medial ray and peroneus longus transfer (Fig. 7.18). The toe imprint shows whether the toes have been reintegrated at least as tactile organs (Figs. 7.15 and 7.22) and thus extend the loaded sole surface (Fig. 7.29).

7.5 Indication for Surgical Correction

The indication for surgical correction in childhood and adolescence is particularly difficult for several reasons, and it still is not possible to present a consistent algorithm how to proceed therapeutically. While some of the older literature argued, that one should basically wait until the end of growth, the recommendation for earlier correction has increasingly gained acceptance (e.g., Döderlein et al. 2000). In the last years, new concepts have been added to this discussion. A new aspect is the presentation of an apparently successful conservative approach with 6 weeks of redression in lower leg walking casts and subsequent night splinting with at least a suspensive effect (d'Astorg et al. 2016). The authors describe that surgery could be at least postponed thereby and was frequently definitive without necessity for revision. However, compliance for long-time splinting seems to be a problem. For patients in the growing age, Sanpera et al. (2018) published first results of a concept of guided growth with hemiepiphysiodesis at the first metatarsal bone to correct or at least prevent deterioration of plantar flexion in combination with plantar fascia release.

One important prerequisite for the decisive process is close observation of the course to detect any deterioration. Pedographic follow-up analysis (Hamel 2016c and 2017) is particularly suitable for monitoring the course of the condition and helpful in determining the timing of surgery (Fig. 7.10). Rough algorithms on how to proceed and what decisions have to be made are given in Figs. 7.36 and 7.37.

When determining the indication for surgical intervention, the question of "whether" to proceed invasively is less important than "when" and "how" to correct. The arguments for and against a surgical intervention already in the growth age have to be carefully weighed against each other in each individual case ("when?"):

Arguments Against Early Correction

- *The progression of the paralysis and thus the deformity is often not yet definitively foreseeable, even if the underlying disease could be precisely classified (which is not always possible).*
- *The patients are often functionally little impaired in the earlier stages and therefore difficult to convince of a major procedure with probably prolonged healing time.*
- *Some of the necessary procedures (e.g., fusions and tendon transfers) are irreversible but may subsequently prove inadequate or insufficient in the further course of the disease.*

Arguments for Early Correction

- *In many cases it is possible to intervene very effectively in the pathogenetic process (e.g., by eliminating peroneal dysfunction, see above) and thus prevent further progression.*
- *An increasing deformation is associated with secondary damage and makes a later intervention more difficult (e.g., fusion instead of joint sparing surgery).*

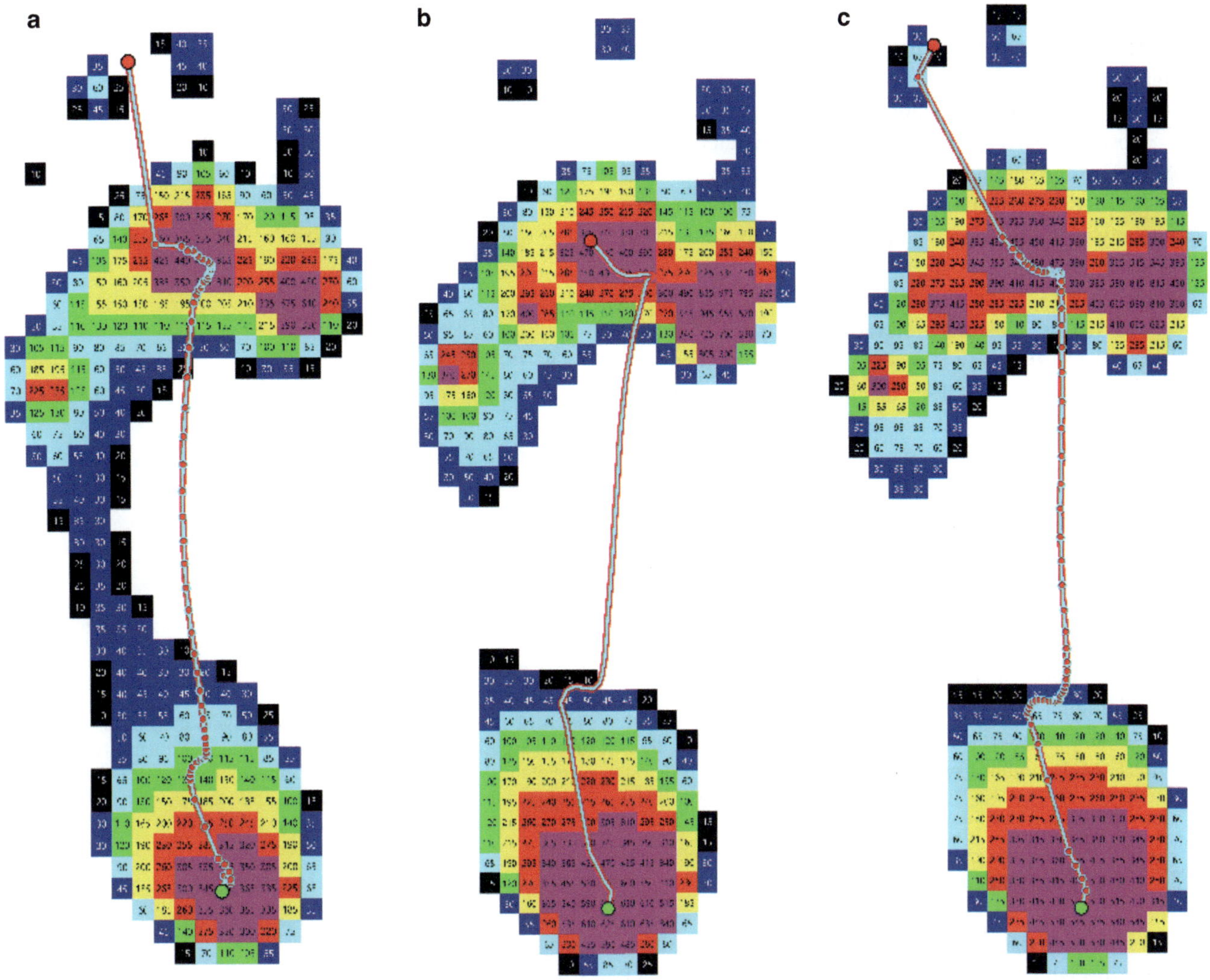

Fig. 7.10 Pedographic recording of peak pressure in juvenile cavovarus deformity due to HSMN at the age of 12 (**a**), 14 (**b**), and 15 years of age (**c**). The progression of the dysfunction can be seen in the relative reduction of the load-bearing surface and the increasing overload of metatarsals I and V. The sharp bend of the COPP-line (Center of Pressure Progression) at the begin of midstance is typical

7.6 Principles of Correction

An operative correction of the cavovarus deformity includes the following components in different combinations ("how?"):

- *Soft tissue release (plantar fascia release, lengthening of the shortened posterior tibial tendon, and release of the soft tissue structures in the medial tarsal area, in some cases also a calf muscle lengthening).*
- *Joint-preserving correction or realigning fusion of midfoot pronation and hindfoot inversion, in severe cases correction of supramalleolar outward rotation.*
- *Elimination of muscular imbalance (peroneus longus to brevis transfer, posterior and anterior tibial tendon transfer, rerouting of the long toe extensors and flexors).*
- *Forefoot corrections.*

In some cases, the individual steps to be performed are determined only intraoperatively in detail. Preoperatively, however, the procedure should be planned in its basic features, e.g., whether in pronounced cases a complete correction of the hindfoot complex should be performed with additional compensation of the supramalleolar outward rotation or whether a compromise in the positioning of the talocalcaneal-navicular complex should be aimed for; from the muscle function testing, it should be derived how to proceed with the tendons of posterior and anterior tibial muscles and whether an active eversion of the peroneal muscle group is still present or can be restored. In the following, the most important procedures are presented and typical procedure combinations are explained using twelve application examples.

Typical Intervention Combinations in Cavovarus Deformity

- Pure soft tissue correction (quite rarely indicated, mostly in early schoolchild age, mostly later secondary correction required; see Fig. 7.13).
- Soft tissue correction + elevation of the medial ray (only if the hindfoot complex is still fully mobile when testing with the Coleman block test; see Fig. 7.15).
- Soft tissue correction + elevation of the medial ray + sliding osteotomy of the calcaneus (if partial contracture of the hindfoot complex is not too pronounced; see Fig. 7.18).
- Soft tissue correction + elevation of the medial ray + Chopart arthrodesis (in case of pronounced hindfoot contracture or expected progression; see Fig. 7.22).
- Soft tissue correction + elevation of the medial ray + Lambrinudi arthrodesis (in case of pronounced horizontal position of the talus and anterior upper ankle impingement; see Fig. 7.28).
- Additional supramalleolar rotation (Fig. 7.31).
- Isolated cavus correction in the anterior tarsus (in case of dominant cavus component (Fig. 7.21)).

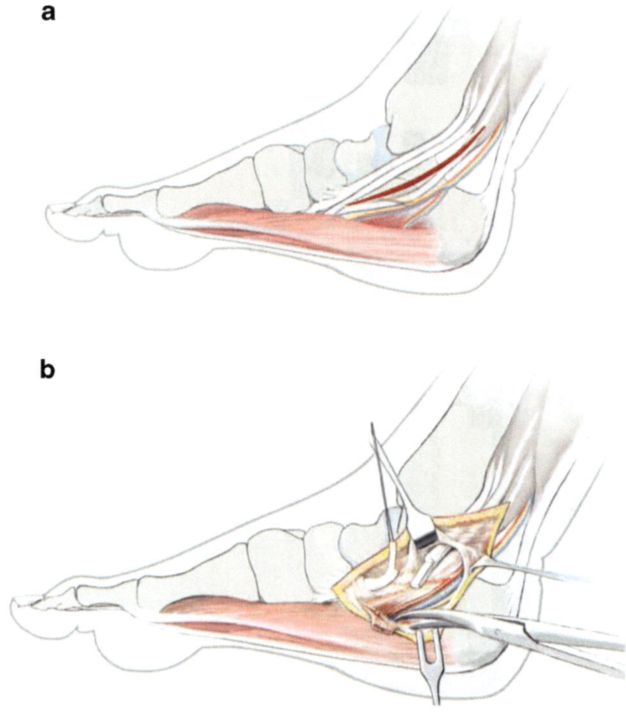

Fig. 7.12 Extended medioplantar release with dorsomedial approach (**a**) and exposition of the medioplantar soft tissue structures (**b**), detachment of the three origins of the abductor hallucis muscle (Mosca 2014), incision of the medial talonavicular capsule (not shown), and Z-shaped lengthening of the posterior tibial tendon

7.7 Soft Tissue Surgery

A predominantly soft tissue procedure in practice can be considered especially for the younger age group (see Figs. 7.11 and 7.12) and can be combined with a redressive plaster treatment.

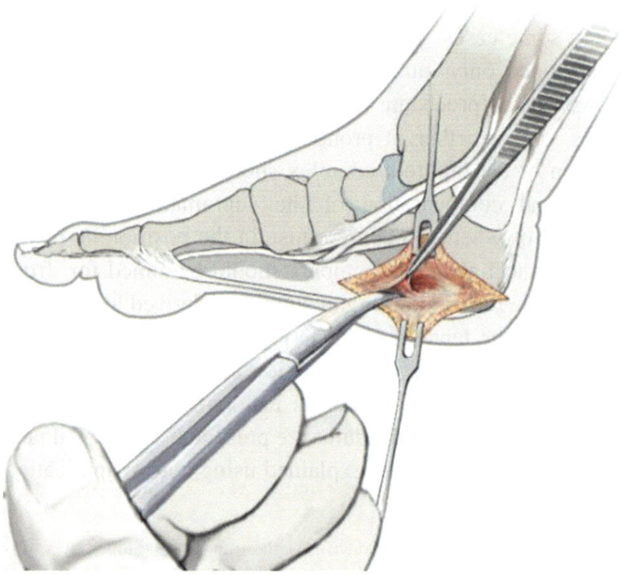

Fig. 7.11 Plantar fascia release from a medial access. The skin incision can be limited to 3–4 cm; also percutaneous procedures and pricking with cannulas are possible

7.7.1 Plantar Release (Steindler)

Technique

A longitudinal incision of about 3–4 cm length is made at the medial edge of the palpable plantar fascia and thus slightly medial to the loaded sole surface. The plantar fascia is located with a raspatory and isolated and separated from the short foot muscles (Fig. 7.11). The plantar fascia is cut completely close to its calcaneal origin with a scalpel or strong scissors until it can be expanded manually with visible distance of the cut ends. The original procedure according to Steindler (1920) additionally includes a detachment of parts of the short foot muscles from their origin at the calcaneus. Alternatively, percutaneous release of the markedly tensioned parts of the plantar fascia via a stab incision is also possible.

It should be noted that the plantar fascia is the most important passive plantar flexor of the metatarsophalangeal joints in the late stance phase via the "windlass" mechanism (tension of the plantar fascia through dorsal extension of the metatarsophalangeal joints) and thus counteracts claw toe development. Whether this is of therapeutic relevance and the plantar fascia release thus can be counterproductive is difficult to assess. The plantar fascia release is generally recommended in the literature as a primary corrective measure in children and adolescents. Further stretching of the plantar soft tissue structures is possible with follow-up treatment with postoperative redressive plaster casts (Coleman 1983).

7.7.2 Medioplantar Soft Tissue Release

If there is already an inversion contracture of the talocalcaneal-navicular complex, which can also be detected in the Coleman block test, an extended medioplantar soft tissue release should be considered (Coleman 1983; Mosca 2014), as is similarly the case with surgical clubfoot correction (Fig. 7.12).

Technique

For the medioplantar release, a curved skin incision is made below the medial malleolus (Fig. 7.12a), the neurovascular bundle is exposed proximally behind the medial malleolus, and first the laciniate ligament above the tarsal canal is severed until the entry of the neurovascular structures into the abductor hallucis muscles is identified (Fig. 7.12b). The abductor hallucis muscle is detached close to its origin and the plantar fascia is severed as described above. The short foot musculature can also be somewhat detached from its origin at the medioplantar calcaneal surface. Further cranially, the course of the posterior tibial tendon is displayed close to its insertion point. Depending on the planning, the tendon is extended in a Z-shaped manner or detached and looped for transfer. Depending on the extent of the contracture, the strong talonavicular capsule is pricked multiple times or completely cut through. The medial capsule of the subtalar joint may also be included in the release. Figure 7.13 shows an example of a predominantly soft tissue cavovarus correction in early school children age.

7.7.3 Lengthening of the Calf Muscles

A shortening of the calf muscles is not usually present in cavovarus deformities, so that a lengthening of the calf muscles is usually not useful; however, in the case of pronounced weakness of the foot extensors or as part of a transfer of the posterior tibial tendon, a slight intentional weakening of the gastrocnemius portion of the calf muscles to improve the balance of forces can still be useful in individual cases. Since the calf muscles can also weaken with progressive paralysis, intramuscular release according to Baumann (Fig. 6.3a) or dosed percutaneous lengthening of the Achilles tendon should be preferred, and a Z-shaped lengthening of the Achilles tendon should be avoided in most cases.

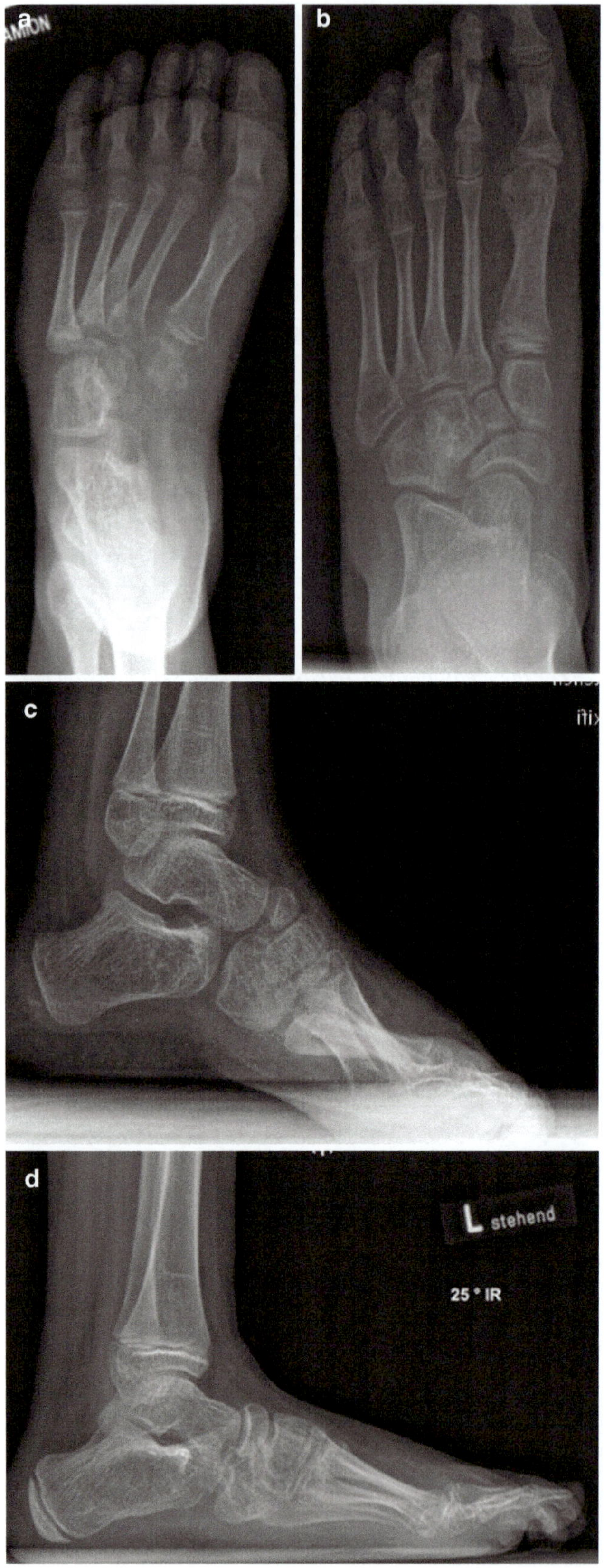

Fig. 7.13 Example 1, predominantly soft tissue correction in younger age. 8-Year-old boy with known HSMN and progressive cavovarus deformity, increasing tendency of twisting in status after externally performed plantar release and peroneus longus transfer with insufficient effect. Preoperatively still distinct cavovarus adductus deformity (**a**, **c**), note the significantly increased talometatarsal I angle in the lateral, nearly hindfoot-centered image (**c**). Medioplantar soft tissue release with lengthening of posterior tibial and Achilles tendon (percutaneous), cuboid osteotomy, split anterior tibial tendon transfer to the peroneus brevis insertion. Postoperative redressive plaster casts in order to further stretch the plantar soft tissue structures, which is still promising at this age. An ankle foot orthosis with passive foot lifting function was applied afterwards. 2 Years postoperatively significant correction (**b**, **d**). Further measures such as fusions did not yet seem justified due to the young age of the patient

7.8 Joint-Preserving Bony Tarsometatarsal Correction

If the extent of the deformity and the expected progression is not too pronounced, especially in childhood and adolescence, correction is possible without fusion. Shock absorption properties of the hindfoot complex can thereby be preserved. In most cases, the following individual bony corrections—in addition to the soft tissue measures—should be considered:

- Correction of mid-forefoot pronation by elevating osteotomy of the proximal first metatarsal bone or at the lesser tarsus.
- Correction of the hindfoot varus by calcaneal osteotomy.

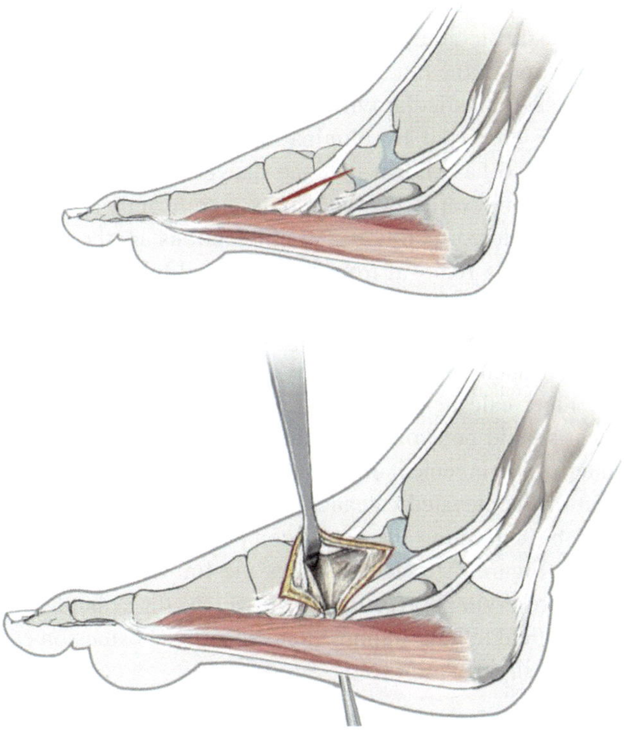

Fig. 7.14 Dorsal-based wedge removal from the medial cuneiform for elevation of the plantar-flexed medial ray. Careful protection of the anterior tibial tendon insertion is important

7.8.1 Correction of the Mid-Forefoot Pronation

Elevation of the plantar flexed medial ray by wedge resection from the metatarsal I base, taking into account the possibly still open growth plate, is necessary in most cases. However, it must not be overdosed, especially if soft tissue procedures such as the peroneus longus to brevis transfer and/or a Jones transfer (Sect. 7.12) are added, as otherwise it can result in a troublesome "dorsal bunion" in the sense of an overcorrection (see Sect. 1.6.3). In cases of more pronounced mid-forefoot pronation, a correction by wedge removal at the level of the cuneiformia is possible as an alternative (Fig. 7.18), which can also include the second and third ray. Mosca (2014) and the French group of Wicart and Seringe (2006), on the other hand, recommend an additive open-wedge osteotomy of the cuneiform bones to avoid shortening the medial ray; however, this requires an effective plantar soft tissue release either in combination or as a preceding procedure with subsequent redressive plaster treatment beforehand.

Technique

The metatarsal I base is exposed from a dorsal approach and an oblique osteotomy is performed from distal-dorsal to proximal-plantar, respecting a possibly still open growth plate and otherwise the first tarsometatarsal I joint. After removal of a dorsal open wedge while preserving the plantar cortex and elevation of the medial ray, the osteotomy can be fixed with a double-threaded screw (Fig. 7.15). Alternatively, a dorsal-based wedge removal can be performed at the medial cuneiform from the extensor side or from a medial approach while preserving the anterior tibial tendon insertion (Fig. 7.14) and can be fixed with a K-wire.

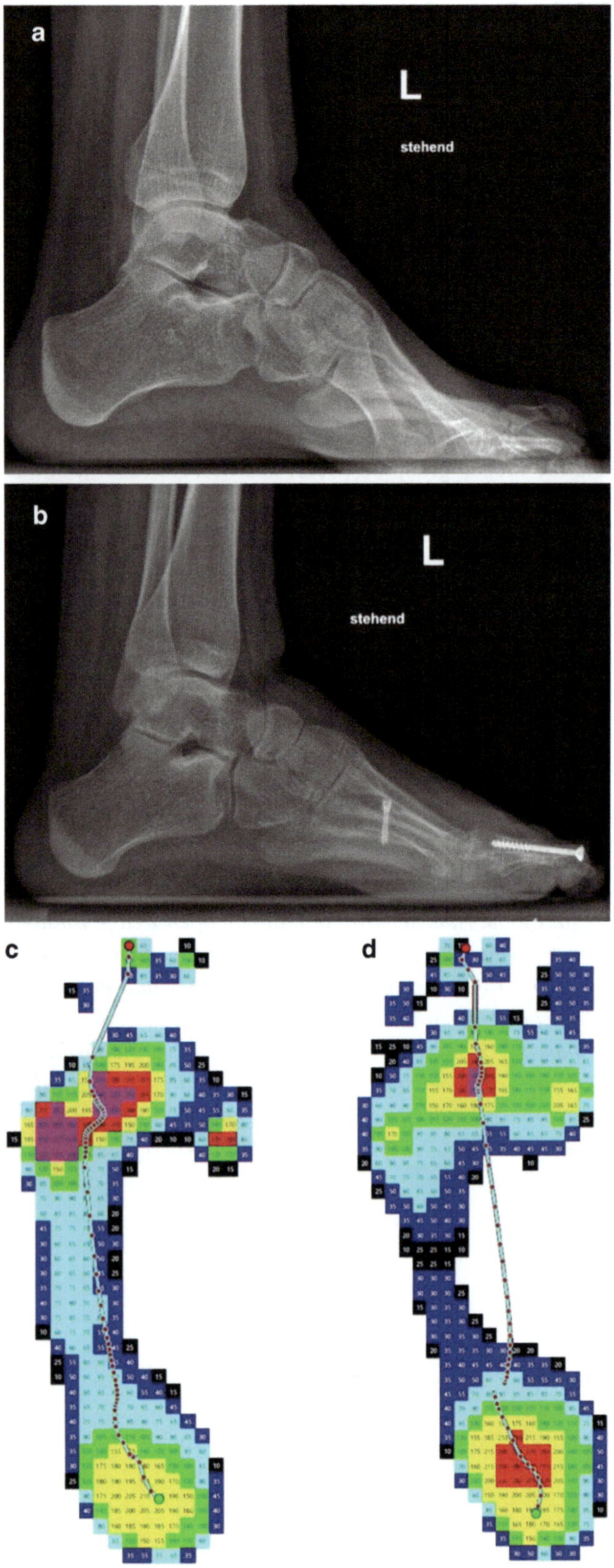

Fig. 7.15 Example 2, 13-year-old female patient with HSMN before (**a**, **c**) and 7 months after (**b**, **d**) joint-preserving surgery (soft tissue release of plantar fascia, talonavicular joint and posterior tibial tendon, peroneus longus to brevis transfer, rerouting of flexor hallucis longus tendon and extensor digitorum longus tendon, elevating osteotomy of the first ray and toe fusions). Especially improvement of toe function is already visible at this early postoperative examination (**d**)

7.8.2 Correction of the Hindfoot Varus Deformity

The elevation at the medial ray has a significant correction effect on the (flexible) hindfoot varus component, which is considered sufficient by some authors in less pronounced cases (Ward et al. 2008). The need for an additional calcaneal osteotomy to correct the hindfoot varus component is usually assessed using the Coleman block test (Fig. 7.5). However, it should be considered here that an alignment to the neutral position of the hindfoot axis is not sufficient for this test, but a relative measure of eversion to inversion in a ratio of 1:2 should be aimed for in order to allow the talocalcaneal-navicular complex to work in its mid-position. In consequence, slight hindfoot valgus should be observed in the Coleman block test to decide against calcaneal osteotomy. It should also be noted that a larger proportion of the hindfoot varus position is predetermined by the supramalleolar outward rotation (Fig. 7.4) and can only be corrected by eliminating the latter (Fig. 7.30). Experience has shown that the danger of overcorrecting the hindfoot varus component is significantly less than that of undercorrecting it. Possible options are the lateral-based wedge removal from the calcaneal tubercle (Dwyer osteotomy), open or percutaneous lateralizing osteotomy or multidimensional correcting open osteotomies, such as the Calcaneus-Scarf osteotomy (Fig. 7.16). Shortening of the tuber calcanei as well as elevation of the tuber fragment should be avoided, as this may adversely affect the anterior impingement of the ankle joint. Instead, the reduction of the elevated calcaneal pitch angle should be realized by correcting the cavus component (Figs. 7.16 and 7.21). Figure 7.17 demonstrates the limits of the purely joint-preserving corrections with which, for example, the anterior ankle joint impingement and dorsal extension can only be slightly improved.

Technique of Calcaneus-Scarf Osteotomy

A clear valgus effect on the hindfoot can be achieved by three-dimensional Scarf osteotomy (Figs. 7.16 and 7.18) (Hamel 2015). After visualization of the lateral calcaneal wall, a Z-shaped osteotomy is performed using a saw gauge from forefoot surgery. The tuber fragment is shifted laterally, slightly inward rotated in the transverse plane, and a slight rotation is achieved in the frontal plane as well by bony wedge removal from the horizontal part of the osteotomy. A prophylactic splitting of the tarsal tunnel is recommended, as otherwise the tibial nerve may develop symptoms of entrapment.

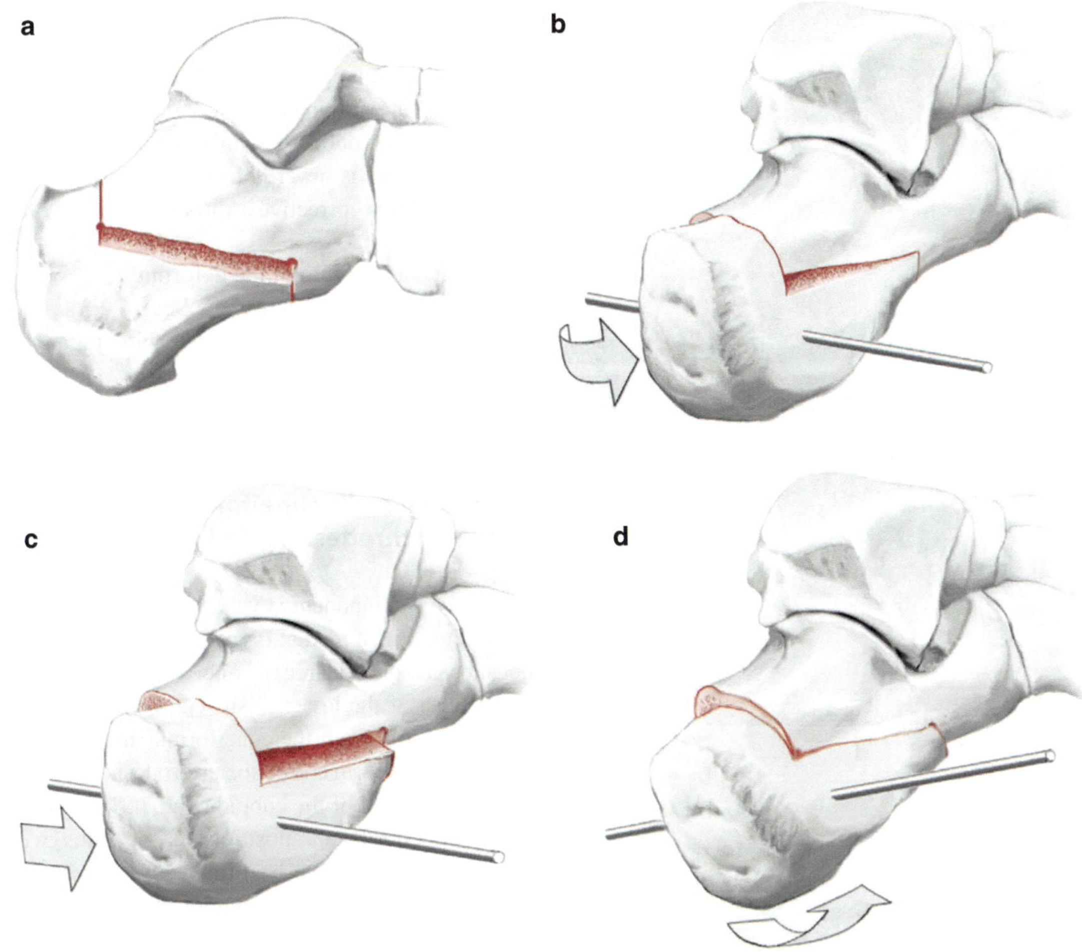

Fig. 7.16 Three-dimensional Calcaneus-Scarf osteotomy for correction of the hindfoot varus deformity: lateral displacement and rotation of the tuber fragment in the transverse plane and lateral wedge removal for additional correction in the frontal plane

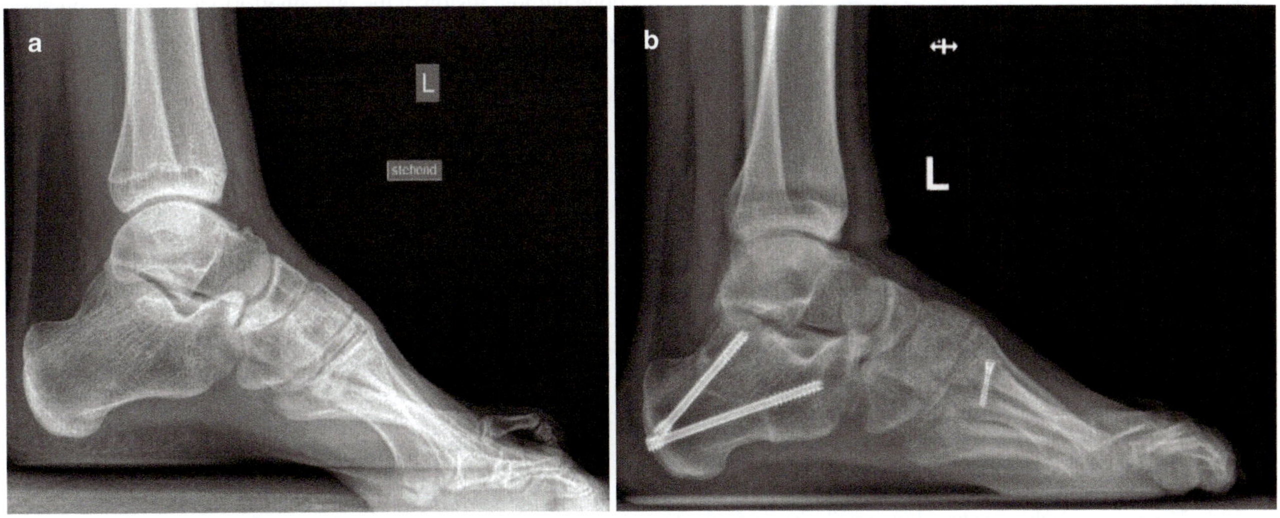

Fig. 7.17 Example 4, 16-year-old male patient before (**a**) and after (**b**) joint-preserving correction including Calcaneus-Scarf osteotomy with good tarsometatarsal alignment but still signs of mild anterior ankle impingement (**b**)

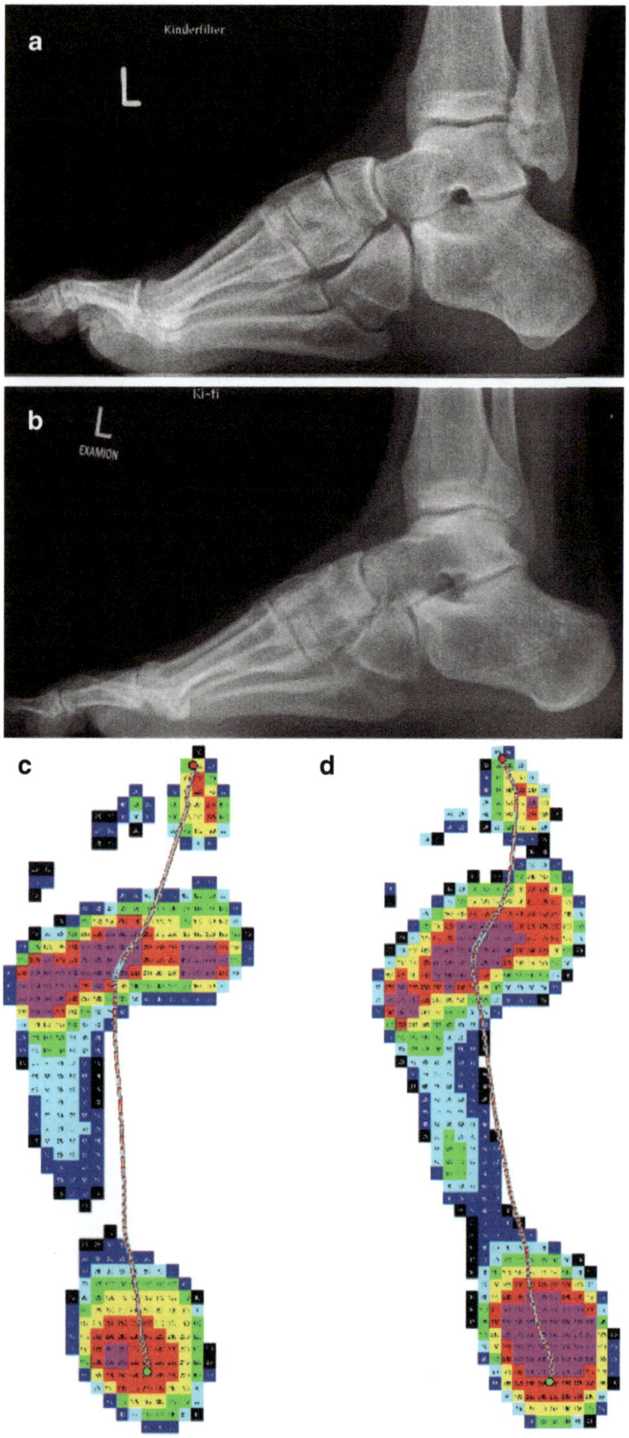

Fig. 7.18 Example 3, (largely) joint-preserving correction in a 15-year-old patient with HSMN and cavovarus deformity. Before (**a, c**) and after Calcaneus-Scarf osteotomy, naviculo-cuneiform 1–3 correction arthrodesis (see below), peroneus longus tendon transfer, and split posterior tibial tendon transfer. 1 Year postoperatively good alignment correction (**b**) and function but still significantly reduced toe involvement (**d**). The preoperatively pronounced supramalleolar outward rotation in the (not hindfoot-centered) lateral image (**a**) is clearly reduced postoperatively (**b**)

7.9 Tarsal (Partial) Arthrodesis

Particularly with a given progression, (partial) fusion is recommended already in later childhood and adolescence, as it prevents further deformation. However, a rebalancing of the muscular forces is nevertheless indispensable. The joints to be included in a corrective arthrodesis depend on:

- Extent and location of the deformity.
- "Hierarchy" of the joints (see Sect. 6.2.3)
- Necessity of stabilization also with regard to possible progression.

7.9.1 Naviculo-cuneiform Correction Arthrodesis (Cole Procedure)

If the cavus component is very pronounced and in particular not limited to the medial ray, and the peritalar complex does not show a higher degree of contracted deformity, a correction at the level of the lesser tarsus can be considered, either by wedge removal from the cuneiformia and the cuboid or as a naviculo-cuneiform correction arthrodesis without (Fig. 7.18) or with inclusion of the cuboid (Fig. 7.21) (Cole 1940). This allows the horizontal position of the talus with anterior ankle impingement to be effectively corrected. With this procedure, the pure cavus component can be well addressed without affecting functionally important joints. Even minor cavovarus deformities can be corrected with the Cole procedure in combination with other measures (Fig. 7.21) (Simon et al. 2019). For very severe cavus correction Mubarak and Dimeglio (2011) recommended the excision of the navicular bone without fusion of the talocuneiform joint in combination with closed-wedge osteotomy of the cuboid bone.

Technique Naviculo-Cuneiform Correction Arthrodesis (Cole Procedure)

The naviculo-cuneiform joint line is displayed subperiostally via a dorsal longitudinal incision while sparing the soft tissues as much as possible (Fig. 7.19). The planned wedge removal is marked with two K-wires with control in the lateral image intensifier projection. The arthrodesis runs laterally into the cuboid without affecting either the calcaneocuboid joint or the functionally particularly important fifth tarsometatarsal joint (Fig. 7.20). This is checked in the image intensifier prior to the osteotomy. The arthrodesis can be fixed with Kirschner wires and bone clamps or a claw plate and heals quickly in the cast. Alternatively, an anterolateral approach with temporary detachment of the extensor digitorum brevis origin is also possible.

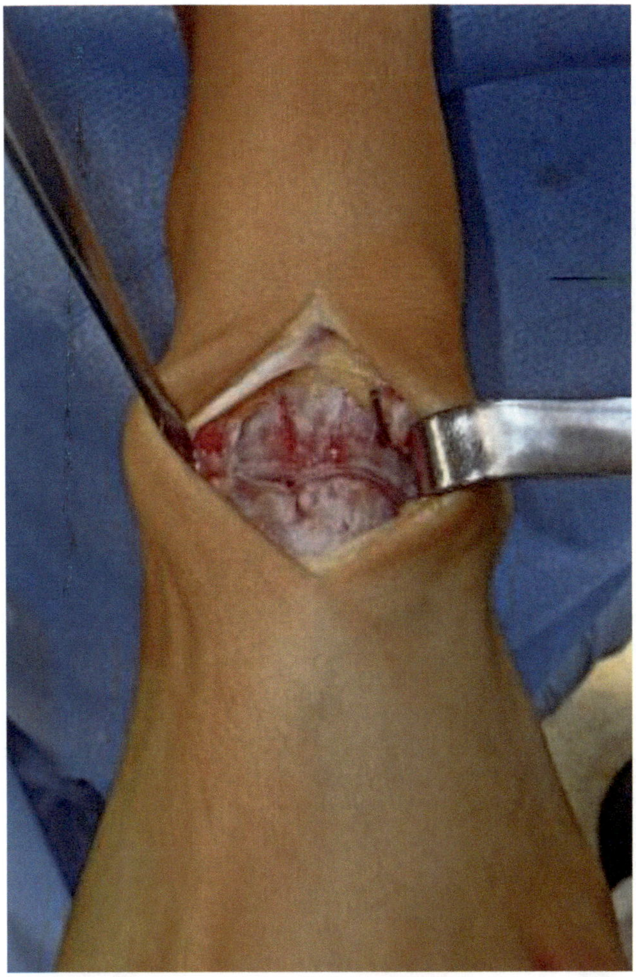

Fig. 7.19 Intraoperative site after subperiostal exposure of the NC joint line to perform a naviculo- cuneiform correction arthrodesis with cuboid osteotomy (Cole procedure) to correct the cavus component and mid-forefoot pronation

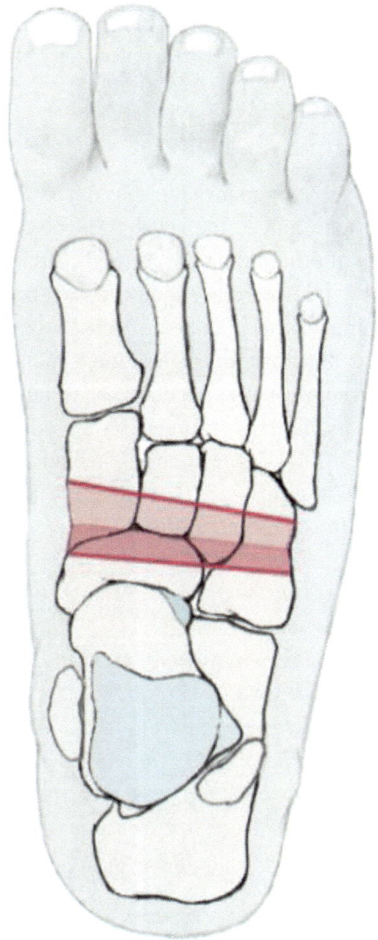

Fig. 7.20 Naviculo-cuneiform correction arthrodesis with dorsal-based wedge removal to correct the cavus deformity. More appropriate is a wedge resection that runs not straight from medial to lateral but angled with the apex in the center of the foot and the legs of the angle orientated slightly in proximal direction

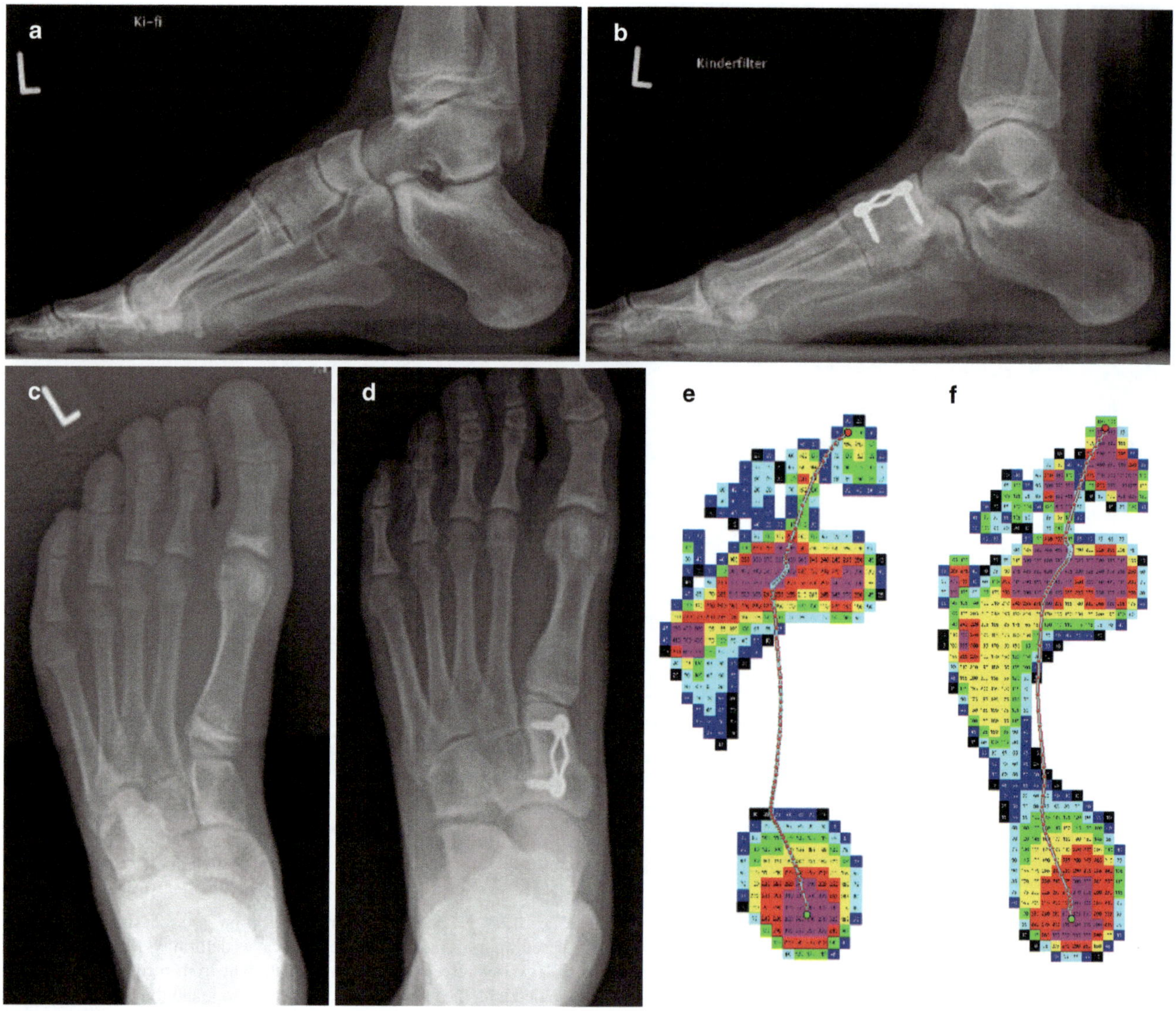

Fig. 7.21 Example 5, 13-year-old patient with cavovarus deformity, before (**a**, **c**, **e**) and 1 year after naviculo-cuneiform-1–3 correction arthrodesis and cuboid osteotomy (Cole procedure), additionally plantar fascia release, peroneus longus to brevis transfer and elevating metatarsal-I-base wedge resection (b, d, f). Note in particular the reduction of the preoperatively distinct anterior impingement in the ankle joint due to the changed talar position (**b**) and the normalized load distribution (**f**)

7.9.2 Chopart Realignment Fusion

If there is an inversion of the talocalcaneal-navicular complex that cannot be sufficiently corrected by soft tissue release and/or if progression is probable due to considerable muscular imbalance, a three-dimensional correction and permanent stabilization can be achieved with Chopart arthrodesis from the age of about 10 years on, although with almost complete loss of function of the hindfoot joints (Fig. 7.22). For the technique, see Sect. 6.3.2. By removing appropriate bone wedges, a correction of the cavus component is possible in cases that are not extremely deformed. An isolated calcaneocuboid arthrodesis while preserving the talonavicular joint is also possible in some cases (Fig. 7.23).

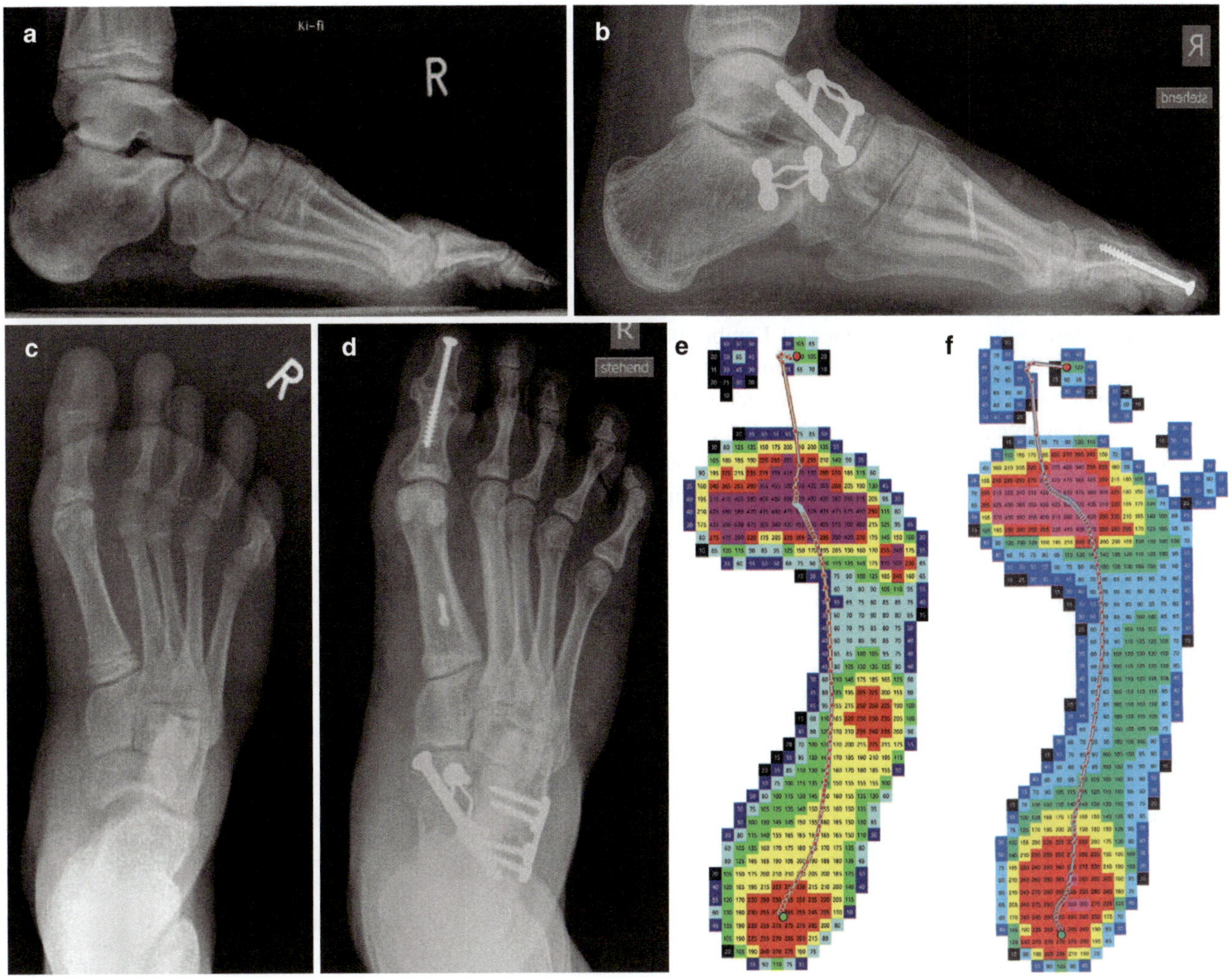

Fig. 7.22 Example 6, 13-year-old patient with suspected HSMN and cavovarus deformity. Before (**a**, **c**, **e**) and 18 months after (**b**, **d**) Chopart correction arthrodesis, elevating metatarsal osteotomy, minimally invasive IP/PIP arthrodesis and rerouting of the extensor digitorum longus tendons. Pedography 28 months postop. (**f**) Shows especially the well restored toe function compared to the preoperative state

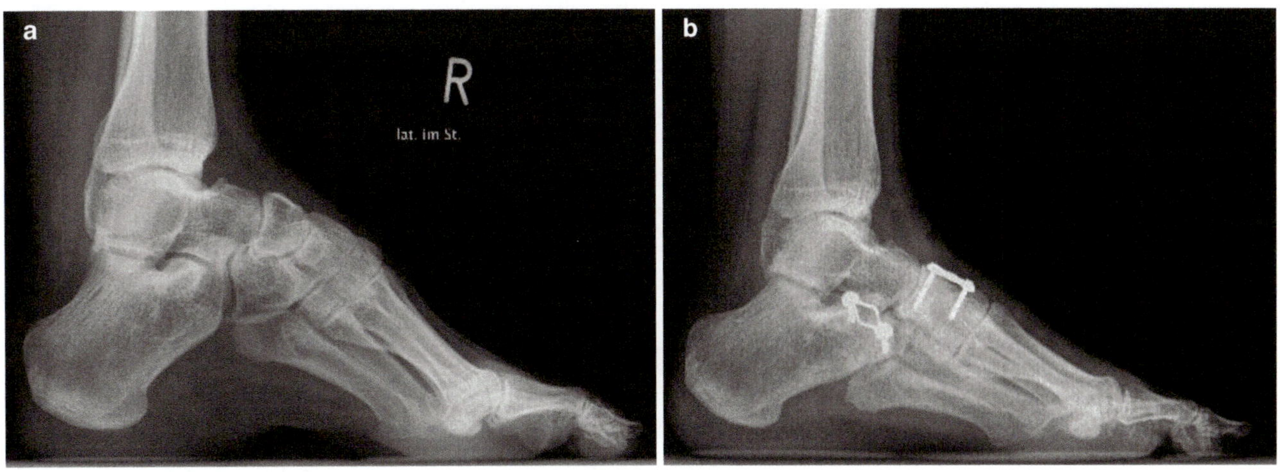

Fig. 7.23 Example 7, severe "idiopathic" cavus foot without evidence of a proven underlying disease. Pronounced cavus component without peritalar inversion. In this case a calcaneocuboid arthrodesis was combined with a naviculo-cuneiform correction arthrodesis while preserving the talonavicular joint. The significantly improved calcaneal pitch angle and the correction of the preoperatively nearly horizontally positioned talus with anterior upper ankle joint impingement (**a**) are visible postoperatively (**b**)

7.9.3 Lambrinudi Arthrodesis

Triple arthrodesis is still considered the gold standard for treating severe hindfoot deformity with muscular imbalance. Saltzman et al. (1999) found a high proportion of residual deformities and secondary degenerative changes in the neighboring joints in an extensive long-term follow-up; nevertheless, there was a high degree of subjective satisfaction among patients even in the long-term course. The modification according to Lambrinudi (1927) is suitable for cavovarus deformities. The advantage of Lambrinudi's arthrodesis over Chopart arthrodesis is that, in contrast to Chopart arthrodesis, an even more extensive correction of the hindfoot varus can be carried out and using anterior wedge removal from the subtalar joint (Fig. 7.25), in particular a significantly higher flexion of the talus and thus better function of the upper ankle joint can be achieved in severe cases (Fig. 7.28). Especially in cases of considerable weakness of the extensors and in connection with the posterior tibial tendon transfer to the dorsum of the foot, the upper ankle joint should be brought into the best possible working position without anterior impingement situation (Hamel 2016b). For the Lambrinudi modification technique, see Sect. 1.7.2 and Fig. 7.25. Approaching from anterolateral (Fig. 7.24), the talar blood supply should be carefully preserved medially to prevent talar necrosis. For stabilization, talocalcaneal screw osteosynthesis in combination with talocuboidal claw-plate fixation has proven particularly effective (Figs. 7.26 and 7.27). Cavus components of considerable extent can also be completely corrected with Lambrinudi arthrodesis (Fig. 7.28). Marked functional improvement in terms of stability and load distribution can be achieved (Fig. 7.29).

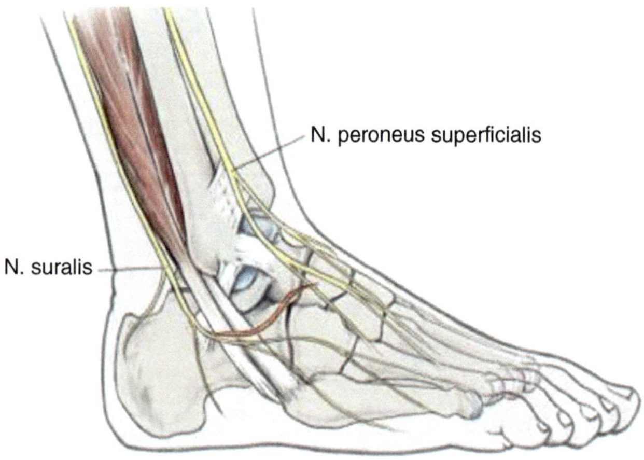

Fig. 7.24 Approach to the peritalar complex for Lambrinudi arthrodesis with S-shaped incision above the muscle belly of M. extensor digitorum brevis. N. suralis and N. peroneus superficialis should be preserved carefully

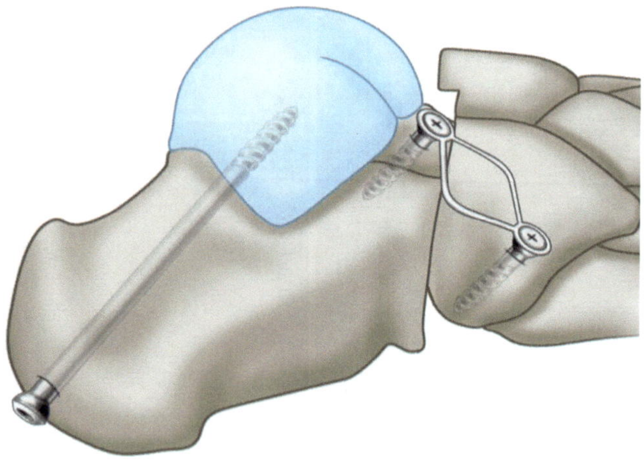

Fig. 7.26 Talocuboidal stabilization with a claw plate. Sufficient stability at Chopart joint line is achieved by talocuboidal fixation with a claw plate. In most cases there is hardly any bone contact talonavicular and additional percutaneous K-wire-fixation is sufficient

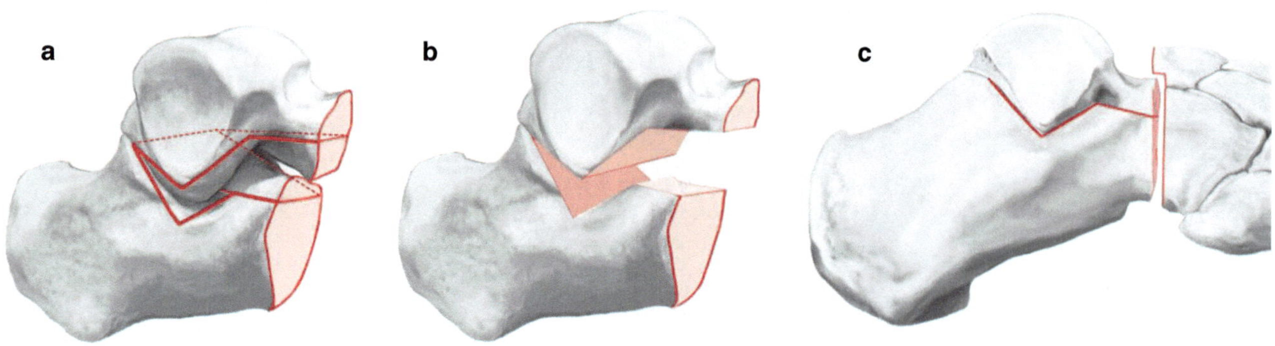

Fig. 7.25 Principle of Lambrinudi arthrodesis with removal of a ventral based bone wedge (**a**, **b**) from the subtalar joint for flexion of the preoperatively horizontally adjusted talus (**c**)

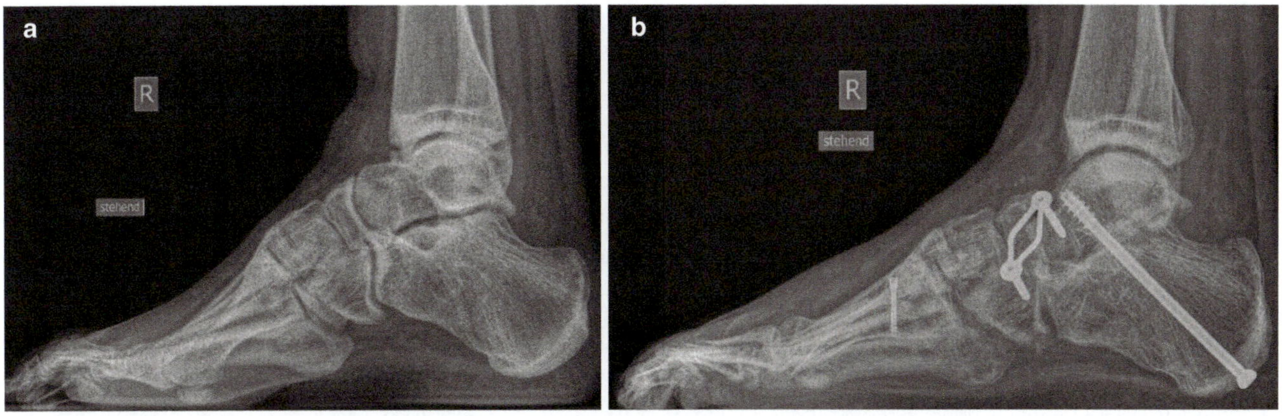

Fig. 7.27 Example 8, pre- (**a**) and postoperative (**b**) lateral X-ray projection of a cavovarus foot correction with Lambrinudi arthrodesis, stabilized with compression screw and claw plate osteosynthesis

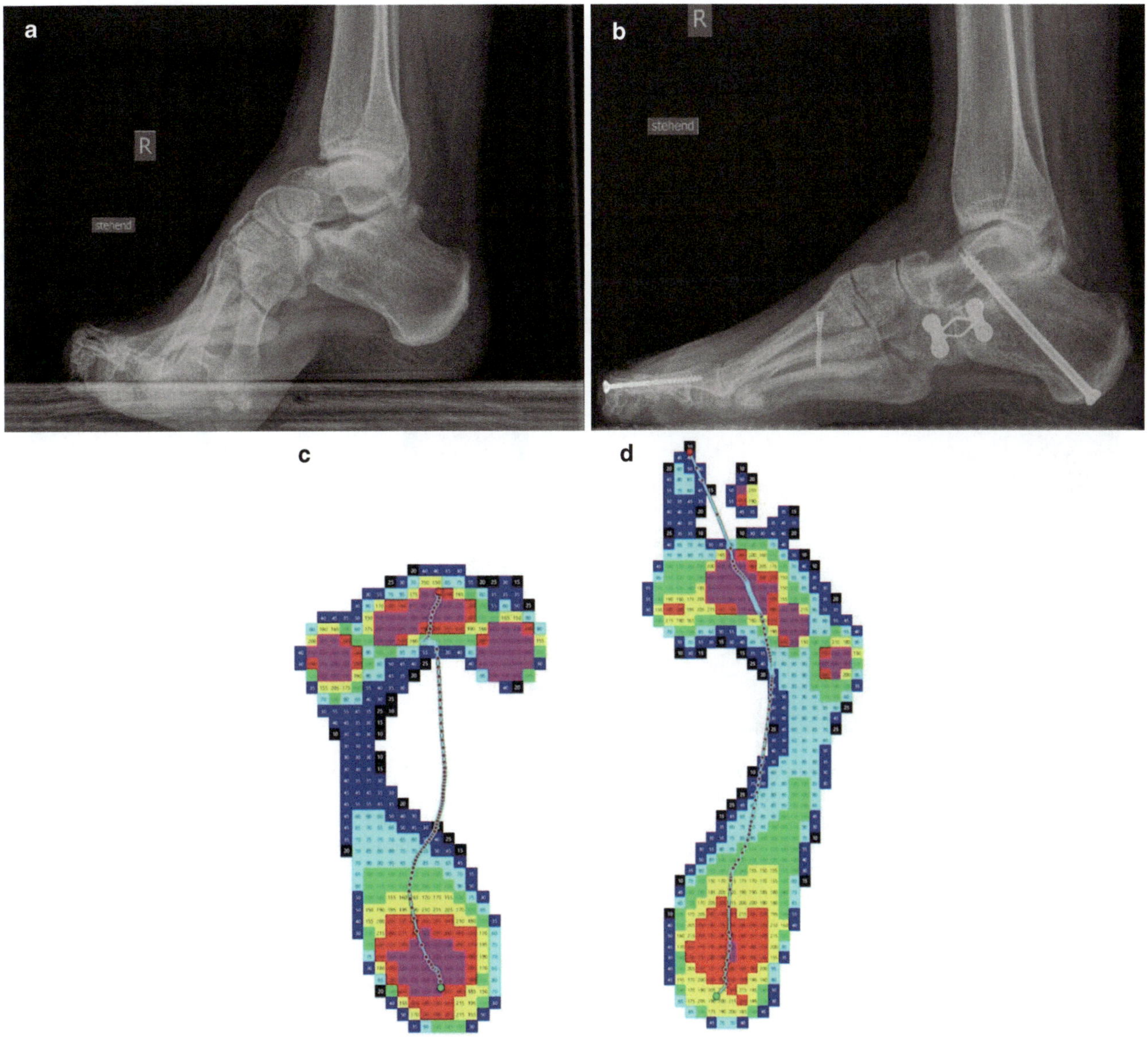

Fig. 7.28 Example 9, severe cavovarus deformity with extreme cavus component (**a**) and realignment with Lambrinudi arthrodesis, transfer of the long peroneal and the posterior tibial tendon and forefoot correction (**b**). The range of motion of the ankle joint has been improved significantly. The pedographic result 18 months postoperatively (**d**) shows clear improvement in comparison to the similarly affected contralateral side (**c**)

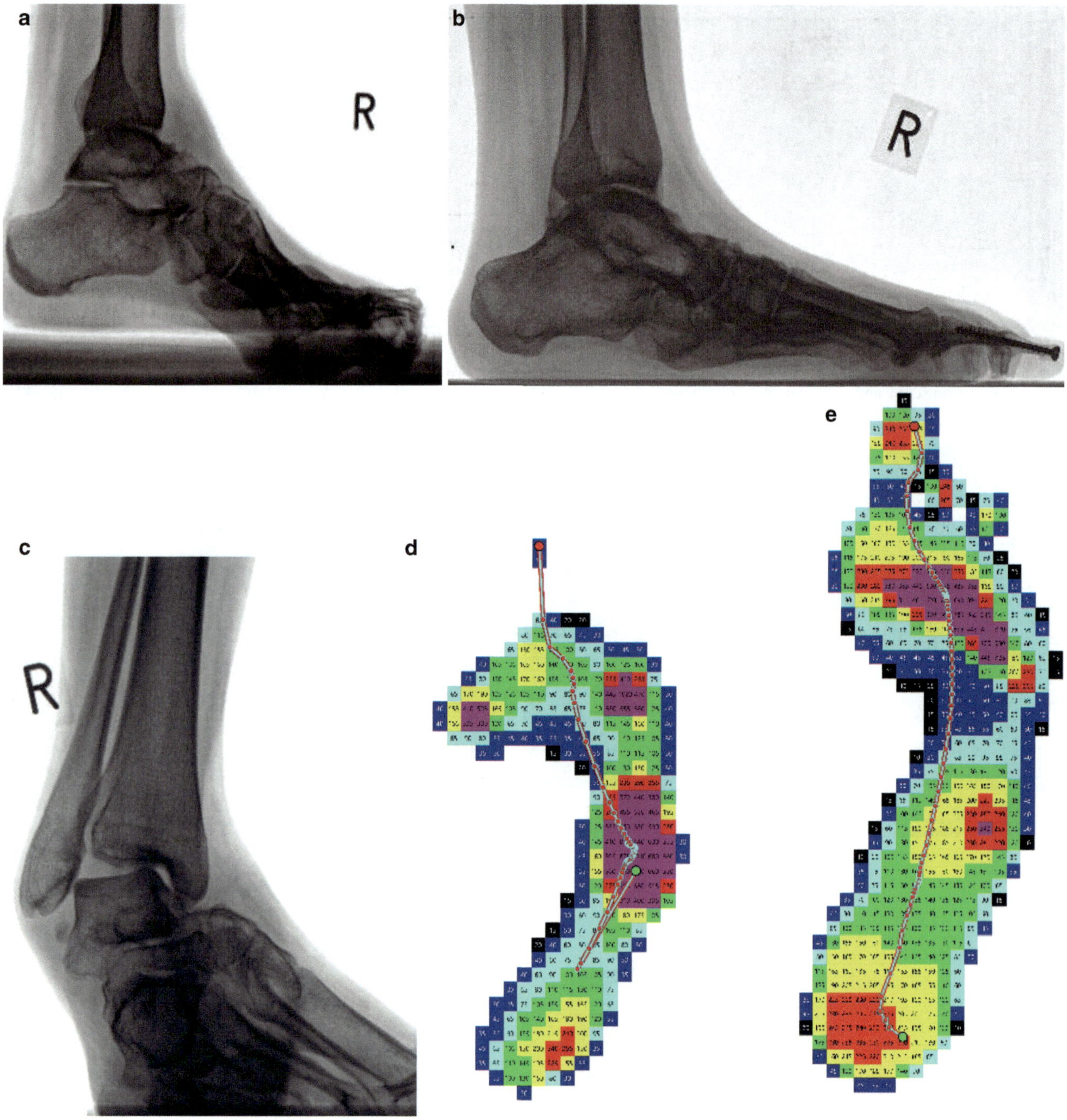

Fig. 7.29 Example 10, 17-year-old female patient with known HSMN and cavovarus deformity (**a**, **c**, **d**). After Lambrinudi arthrodesis, peroneus longus and posterior tibial transfer, significant alignment correction (**b**), and functional improvement (**e**). Ligamentous ankle stabilization was not performed despite considerable instability (**c**). Pedography pre- (**d**) and 3 years postoperatively (**e**), increase of the loaded area by 70%. An even more extensive pronatory realignment of the anterior tarsus in the Chopart line would have avoided the persistent pressure peak over the metatarsal V base (**e**)

7.10 Supramalleolar Corrections and Ankle Joint Degeneration

The conditions at the tibiotalar joint must be taken into special consideration with every correction, since this joint has a particular influence on the late overall prognosis. The following phenomena must be considered:

7.10.1 Supramalleolar Outward Rotation Malposition

If this is not corrected, either the foot correction will have to remain incomplete with a persisting hindfoot varus or the outward rotation previously compensated for by the foot malposition will be unmasked, with a clear outward rotation of the foot in relation to the direction of gait (foot opening angle), especially in the presence of the frequently observed outward hip rotation contracture. A supramalleolar internal rotating osteotomy (Fig. 7.31) is recommended even in milder cases (Hansen 2010). In addition to correcting the overall alignment of the foot, it causes a lateralization of the tuber calcanei and thus contributes significantly to the correction of the hindfoot varus (Fig. 7.30).

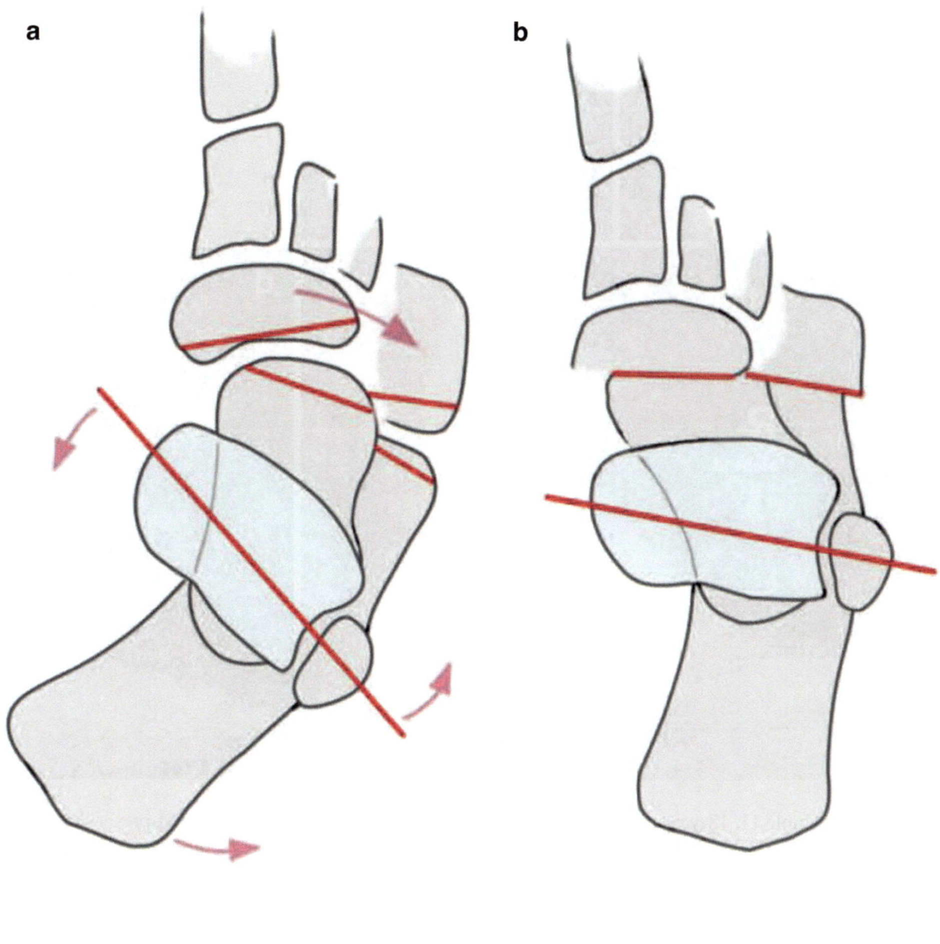

Fig. 7.30 Before and after a supramalleolar inward rotation osteotomy. The preoperatively distinct outward rotated malleolar axis (**a**) was corrected by more than 20° (**b**) in combination with a corrective Chopart arthrodesis. As a result, the tuber calcanei (**a**), which is positioned far medially, is clearly lateralized (**b**) with an unchanged foot opening angle. An additional sliding osteotomy of the calcaneus should be added as a rule, but with rigid supramalleolar outward rotation; this alone would not be able to eliminate the hindfoot varus component

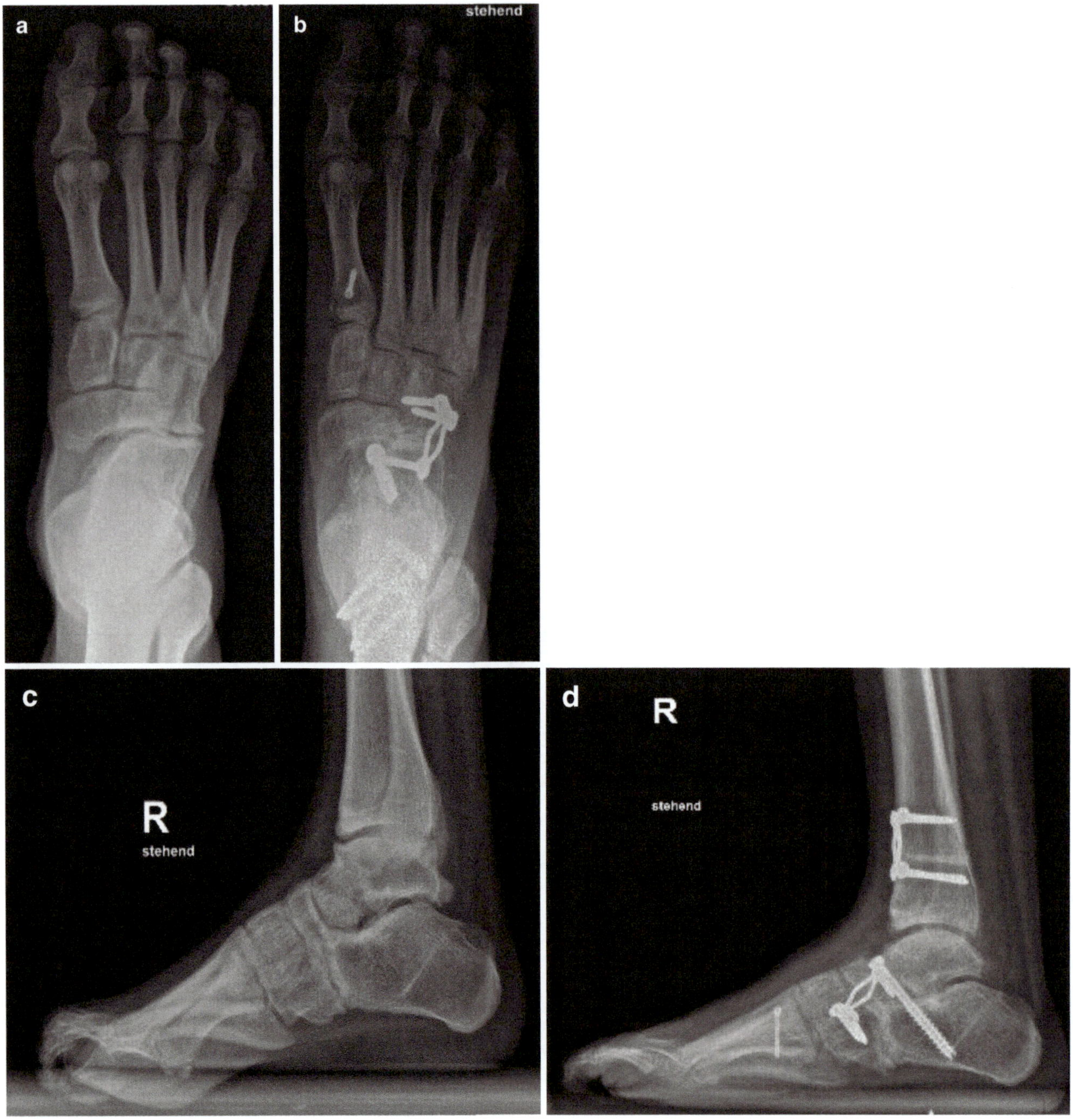

Fig. 7.31 Example 11, 18-year-old patient with persisting cavovarus deformity after joint-preserving correction years before (**a**, **c**). Tarsal realignment with Lambrinudi arthrodesis was combined with an inward rotation at the supramalleolar level of about 25° (**b**, **d**)

7.10.2 Anterior Impingement Due to Horizontal Position of the Talus

Particularly in a pronounced cavus component, the dorsal extension of the upper ankle joint is thereby limited and can be significantly improved by cavus correction (Fig. 7.21) and in pronounced cases most effectively by a Lambrinudi modification of the triple arthrodesis (Fig. 7.32), which improves the function of the weakened dorsal extensors and the efficiency of a posterior tibial transfer. In extreme cases, a strong flexion of the talus due to the resulting posterior impingement can deliberately limit the plantar flexion in such a way that in the swing phase the foot drops only slightly if the foot extensors are very weak. This effect also significantly facilitates the use of a dynamic ankle foot orthosis with foot lifting function.

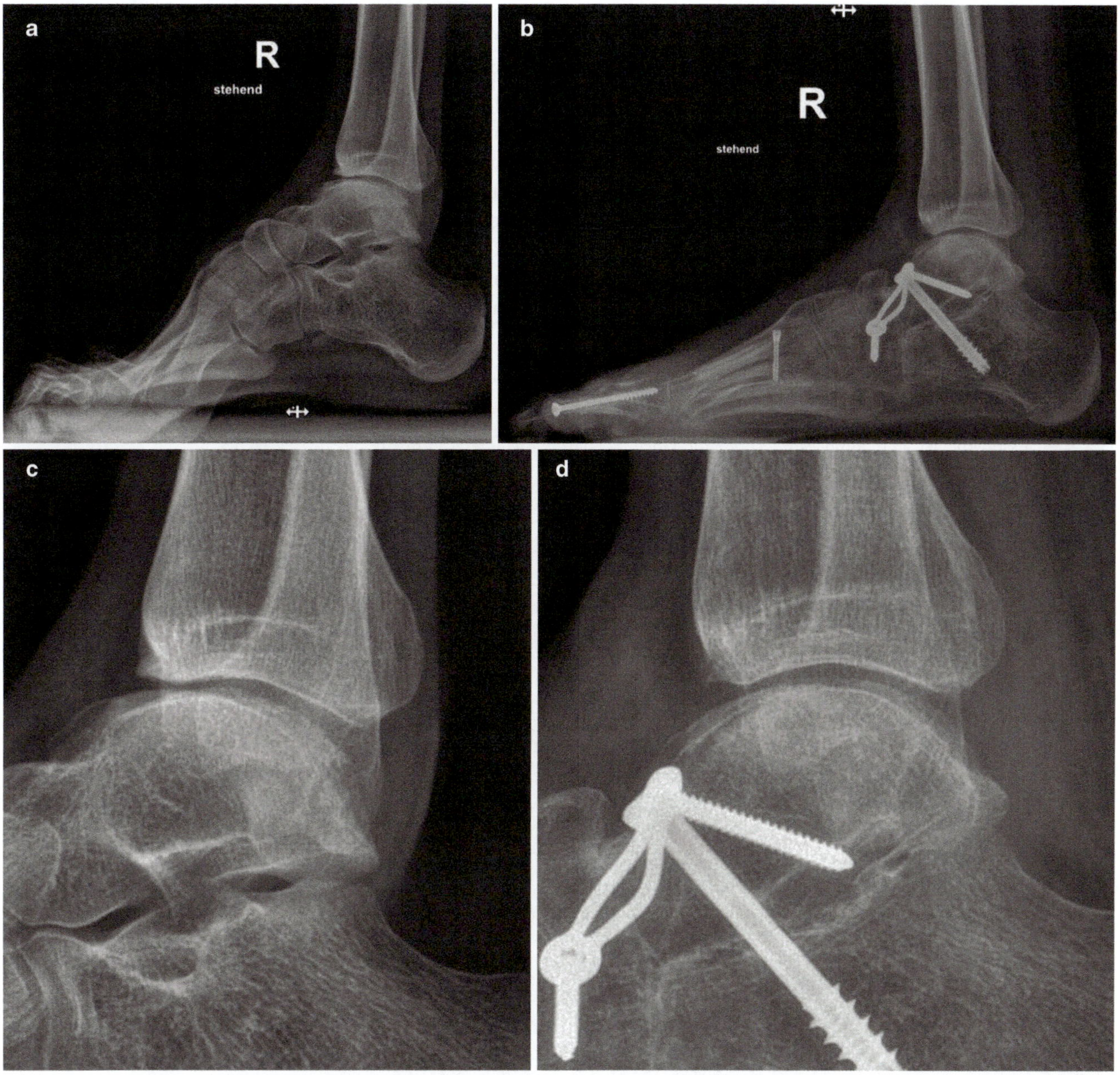

Fig. 7.32 Example 12, anterior dislocation with signs of initial degenerative arthritis at the tibiotalar joint (**a**, **c**) was improved by tarsometatarsal realignment including Lambrinudi arthrodesis (**b**, **d**)

7.10.3 Anterolateral Ankle Joint Instability

Instability of the upper ankle joint can be largely compensated by complete foot correction and peroneus longus transfer for these patients with limited functional needs (Fig. 7.29). If this is not the case, ligament reconstructive measures can also be considered, e.g., if the loss of strength of the peroneus brevis muscle is already advanced, the transfer of the distally stemmed peroneus brevis tendon to the ventral fibula region using the very effective Orthner technique (2011).

7.11 Elimination of Muscular Imbalance

Muscular imbalance (cf. Sect. 7.1.1) is the pathogenetically most significant factor in the development of cavovarus deformities and thus also decisive for the risk of recurrent malposition. Nevertheless, the importance of correcting muscular imbalance in particular is viewed very differently in the literature: Wicart and Seringe (2006), for example, do not recommend any tendon transfer within the context of combined interventions, Mosca (2014) considers the peroneus longus tendon transfer, which is common in adult correction, to be indispensable in childhood as well and advises against the posterior tibial tendon transfer, while Kumar et al. (2010) recommend the latter as a standard intervention and again do not mention the peroneus longus transfer. Döderlein et al. (2000) consider the posterior tibial tendon transfer onto the dorsum of the foot to be less effective in most cases and relocate the tendon to the Achilles tendon instead.

According to the author's experience, the deformity-promoting peroneus longus and posterior tibial muscles should generally also be addressed in most cases. However, the therapist should be aware that tendon transfers in particular are irreversible interventions—in contrast to osteotomies, for example—and their effect can hardly be reduced or increased by a follow-up intervention.

7.11.1 Peroneus Longus Transfer

The weakness of the peroneus brevis muscle with compensatory hyperactivity of the peroneus longus muscle, which is usually affected much later in the paralysis pattern ("peroneal dysfunction" Sect. 7.1.1), will in many cases suggest a transfer of the peroneus longus tendon to the peroneus brevis tendon. The plantarizing effect of the peroneus longus muscle on the medial ray of the foot as a deforming force can thus be reduced, with a strengthening effect on the active eversion. This can be modified according to Manoli and Graham (2005) (Fig. 7.33) in such a way, that the plantar course of the tendon is preserved in the sense of a tenodesis in order to avoid overcorrection with development of a dorsal bunion (especially with additional bony elevation on the medial tarsometatarsal ray and Jones transfer).

Technique: Transfer of the Peroneus Longus Tendon to the Peroneus Brevis Tendon

The technique of Manoli and Graham (2005) has proven to be effective for the peroneus longus to brevis transfer. The peroneus longus tendon is split longitudinally in the inframalleolar course, and the cranial half of the tendon is severed. Both split tendon halves are woven into the peroneus brevis tendon with the Pulvertaft technique and slight tension, using non-resorbable suture material (Fig. 7.33). This corresponds functionally to a complete shift of the peroneus longus action onto the peroneus brevis insertion while maintaining a plantar peroneus longus portion as tenodesis to avoid excessive elevation of the medial ray. If the tendon coupling is technically insufficient however, the peroneus longus effect on the first ray might not be completely eliminated.

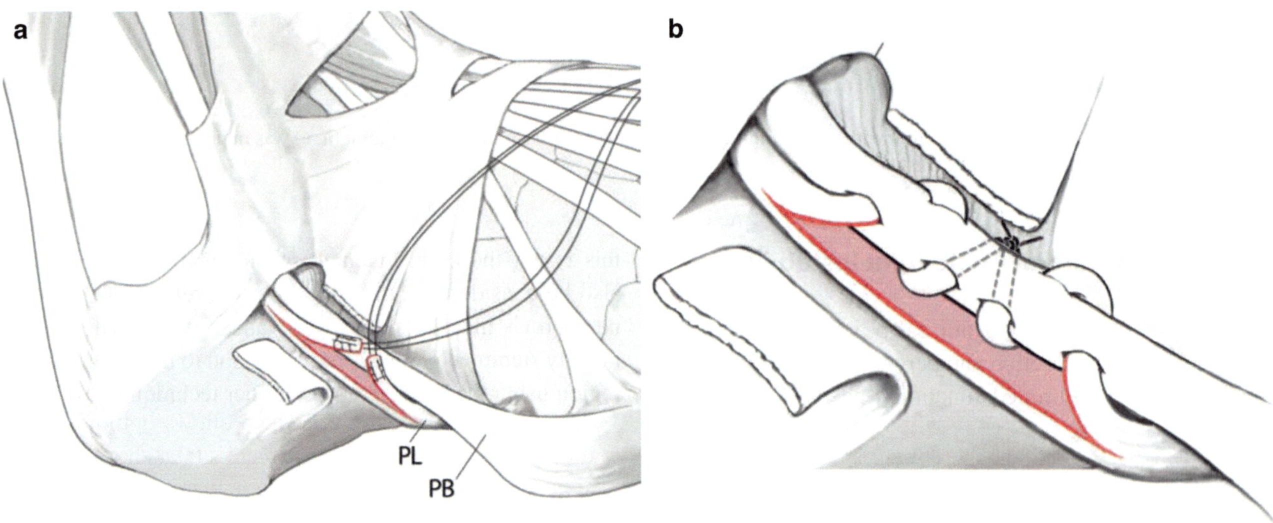

Fig. 7.33 Peroneus longus transfer in the modification according to Manoli and Graham (2005) with preservation of a plantar portion as tenodesis (**a**, **b**). The tendon of the M. peroneus longus (PL) is coupled with that of the M. peroneus brevis (PB) by a non-resorbable suture

7.11.2 Posterior Tibial (and Anterior Tibial) Tendon Transfer

Due to the weakness of the peroneus brevis muscle, the posterior tibial muscle loses its most important antagonist and thus becomes a deforming force that promotes the inversion of the talocalcaneal-navicular complex. Therefore, a weakening of the muscle by tendon lengthening or transfer of its terminal tendon is often necessary. The eversion can also be supported by a (split) transfer of the anterior tibial tendon, as is common in neurogenic clubfoot deformity (see Sect. 6.3.2); however, in cavovarus deformities in the context of progressive neurogenic disease, this muscle is usually affected early in the progressive paralysis process. Therefore anterior tibial tendon transfer is not the procedure of first choice.

For the posterior tibial tendon transfer, either a split transfer to the peroneus brevis tendon is suitable (Sect. 6.3.2) (then, however, under consideration of symmetrical tension and possibly combined with intramuscular lengthening further proximally to weaken the remaining tendon branch) or usually a transfer through the interosseous membrane to the dorsum of the foot (Hamel 2016c). A transfer to the tuber calcanei is also advocated by some surgeons. As a rule, a complete posterior tibial tendon transfer is combined with a hindfoot arthrodesis, so that the muscular control of the subtalar complex is no longer of great importance.

The posterior tibial tendon transfer to the dorsum of the foot completely eliminates its deformity-promoting effect on the talocalcaneal-navicular complex, generally without the risk of planovalgus deformation. However, this is an antiphasic transfer, and often only a tenodesis effect can be expected. In the literature this transfer is evaluated differently (cf. Kumar et al. 2010; Mosca 2014). In the follow-up treatment, an orthotic fitting with a foot-lifting effect and night splinting should be provided for several months. According to the author's experience, the functional effect of the transfer is particularly dependent on whether the upper ankle joint is additionally adjusted—for example, by Lambrinudi arthrodesis—to a physiological range of motion with sufficient dorsal extensibility.

Technique: Anterior Transfer of Tibialis Posterior Tendon (Fig. 7.34)

The posterior tibial tendon is completely detached at its insertion at the navicular bone and, after slight thinning, is neatly looped with strong, non-resorbable suture distally. After mobilization it can be pulled out through a supramalleolar dorsomedial incision. A third anterolateral incision exposes the membrana interossea to the lateral side of the tibia, where a window of about 1 cm wide and about 4–5 cm long is created. Directly behind it, the peroneal artery must be carefully protected. Using a curved clamp, the end of the tendon is moved extraperiostally around the distal tibia from the aforementioned incision to the anterior compartment. From there, it is guided above or below the retinaculum extensorum to the dorsum of the foot, where it is anchored at the end of the procedure under tension in a slightly extended position of the ankle joint using a biotenodesis screw. The subcutaneous transfer above the retinaculum seems to ensure a slightly better strength development due to the more direct course; however, the tendon can protrude slightly under the skin here (Fig. 6.17).

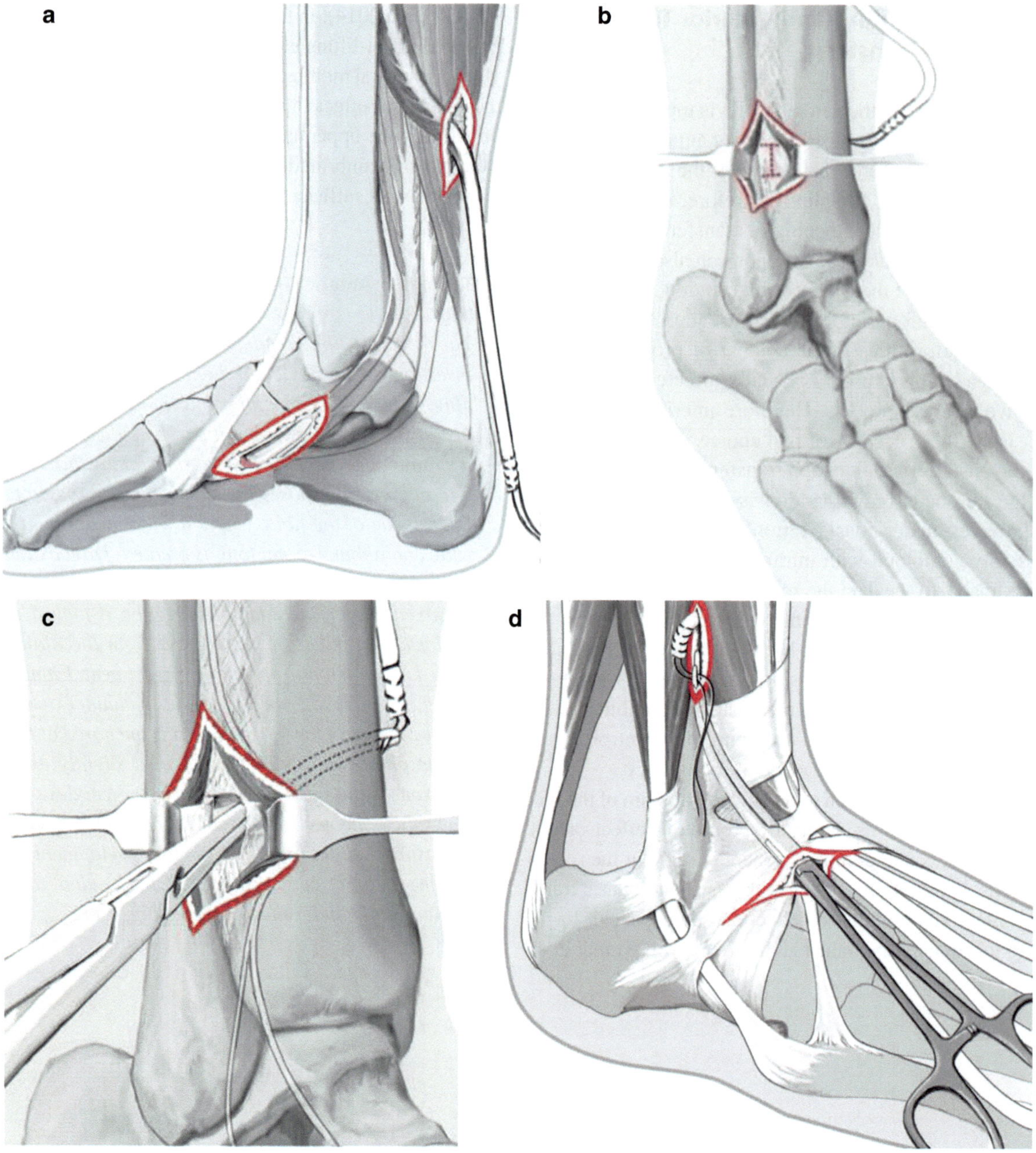

Fig. 7.34 Posterior tibial tendon transfer to the dorsum of the foot. After detachment of the tendon at its insertion point and mobilization into a second dorsomedial incision (**a**), a window is created in the interosseous membrane (**b**), and the tendon is guided anteriorly (**c**). It is transferred above (**d**) or below the retinaculum extensorum to the dorsum of the foot, where it is fixed in the lateral os cuneiforme through a drill hole, the loop threads are led out to plantar, the tendon is tensioned and fixed with an interference screw

7.12 Claw Toes

In addition to the weakness of the short foot muscles including the flexor hallucis brevis muscle, which is clinically difficult to assess, predominantly the long extensor and flexor muscles are pathogenetically involved in the development of claw toes in progressive cavovarus deformity (Fig. 7.35a). The overactivity of the long extensors (extensor substitution) leads to hyperextension of the metatarsophalangeal joints.

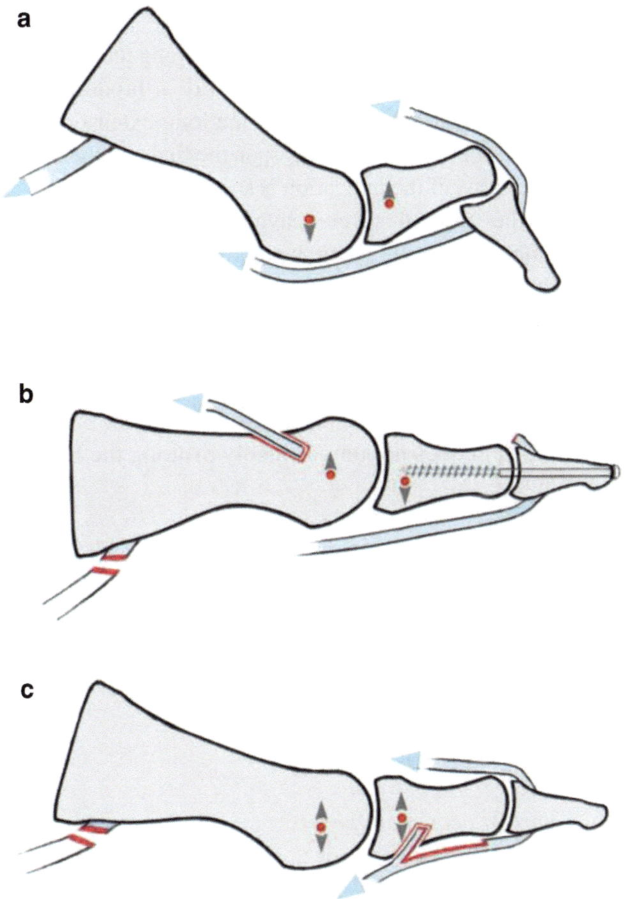

Fig. 7.35 Muscular imbalance in the development of the claw toe deformity at the first ray (**a**): Overactivity of the peroneus longus muscle and the extensor hallucis longus muscle (extensor substitution) leads to plantarization of the medial ray and hyperextension in the metatarsophalangeal joint of the big toe, which is reinforced by the flexor hallucis longus muscle inserting at the distal phalanx (in case of weakness of the flexor hallucis brevis muscle). Peroneus longus transfer in combination with a relocation of the extensor hallucis longus tendon and interphalangeal arthrodesis (Jones procedure) (**b**) can lead to an excessive effect with development of a dorsal bunion. On the other hand, a relocation of the flexor hallucis longus tendon back to the proximal phalangeal base is suitable for muscular rebalancing without loss of active dorsal extension (**c**) in cases that are not too pronounced. In case of simultaneous IP fusion, the flexor tendon rerouting should be complete. If the IP joint is preserved, split transfer is preferred with tenodesis of the distal stump to stabilize the interphalangeal joint against hyperextension

The main effect of the long toe extensors acts on the metatarsophalangeal joint. The long flexors have a flexing effect on the proximal and distal interphalangeal joints and thus indirectly also support the hyperextension of the metatarsophalangeal joints.

Functional results can be evaluated best by pedographic examination. Treatment examples are presented in Figs. 7.15, 7.22, and 7.29. Three principles of correction can be applied alternatively or in combination, but tendon lengthening of the extensor tendons does not appear to be advisable:

– ***PIP- (or IP-) Arthrodesis***

Technique

Open resection of the proximal interphalangeal joint or the interphalangeal joint of the big toe via a U-shaped or S-shaped access with temporary tenotomy of the extensor tendon and K-wire fixation (screw osteosynthesis at the IP joint). Minimally invasive arthrodesis with resection of the cartilaginous joint surfaces is also possible.

Advantage: Increases the flexing effect of the long flexors on the metatarsophalangeal joint.

Disadvantage: Does not eliminate the troublesome extensor substitution unless it is reduced by other measures and may lead to hyperextension of the straightened toe or relapse of flexion contracture with pseudarthrotic healing.

– ***Rerouting of the long flexors back to the proximal phalangeal base (also in combination with PIP/IP fusion)***

Technique

Via two plantar accesses, the long flexor tendon is detached distally at the lesser toes, drawn out at the proximal phalangeal level, split longitudinally and directed dorsally, where it is sutured in the extensor tendon hood. Fixation via a drill hole in the base of the proximal phalanx is recommended for the first ray (Kadel et al. 2005) (Fig. 7.35c).

Advantage: Significantly increases the flexing effect of the long flexors on the metatarsophalangeal joint.

Disadvantage: In cases of very pronounced extensor substitution, not sufficiently effective, especially on the first ray. If necessary, a percutaneous tenotomy of the extensor tendon at the level of the proximal joints should be added.

– ***Relocation of the long toe extensors back to the midfoot (Jones 1916, Hibbs 1919)***

Technique

The long extensor tendons are detached at the level of the distal metatarsus, and either sutured to the peroneus tertius tendon (if present) or a bony fixation on the tarsometatarsal region is performed. It is sufficient for the effect to fix two end tendons of the extensor digitorum longus muscle. The distal tendon stumps are sutured to the extensor digitorum brevis tendons. At the first ray, the extensor hallucis longus tendon is relocated to the metatarsal I neck, usually in conjunction with suturing the distal tendon stump to the extensor hallucis brevis tendon and arthrodesis of the interphalangeal joint (Jones procedure) (Fig. 7.35b). Mosca (2014) always adds a percutaneous tenotomy of the long flexor tendon at the level of the proximal flexor crease. Alternatively the extensor hallucis longus tendon can be transferred to the lateral tarsal region to reinforce eversion.

Advantage: Very effective, complete elimination of the extensor substitution.

Disadvantages: On the first ray danger of "hanging" big toe and dorsal bunion development (Breusch et al. 2000). In HSMN, a progressive weakening of the long toe extensors is also to be expected in the further course of the disease. The procedure should therefore only be indicated in particularly severe cases, when flexor transfer (see above) does not seem sufficient.

Author's Recommendation for the Treatment of Claw Toes in Cavovarus Deformities

In mild cases, initially only cavovarus correction, at the most IP/PIP arthrodeses.

In moderate cases: Relocation of the long toe flexors (Fig. 7.35c) in combination with IP/PIP arthrodeses.

In severe cases: Rerouting of the long extensors of the lesser toes is unproblematic; on the first ray, there is no alternative if the indication is stringent (Fig. 7.35b).

In the case of severe cavovarus deformities, a two-stage procedure can be considered, in which the hind- and midfoot are corrected in the first step with bone and soft tissue procedures and about 6 weeks later supramalleolar rotation, ankle ligament reconstruction, and forefoot corrections are added as needed. This has a favorable effect on the dosage and does not unreasonably prolong the healing phase.

7.13 Algorithm

The algorithms given in Figs. 7.36 and 7.37 are meant to summarize, how to proceed in "early" and "late" corrections. Some important diagnostic tools and observations that should be evaluated preoperatively and are useful for decision making during surgery are mentioned on the right side of the algorithms.

7.14 Results

The results for less severe underlying disease and progression are extremely favorable, especially for the so-called "idiopathic" cavus feet. In contrast, there are only limited long-term results after joint-preserving surgery in severe neurogenic underlying disease. Ward et al. (2008) found favorable long-term results after metatarsal I base osteotomy in

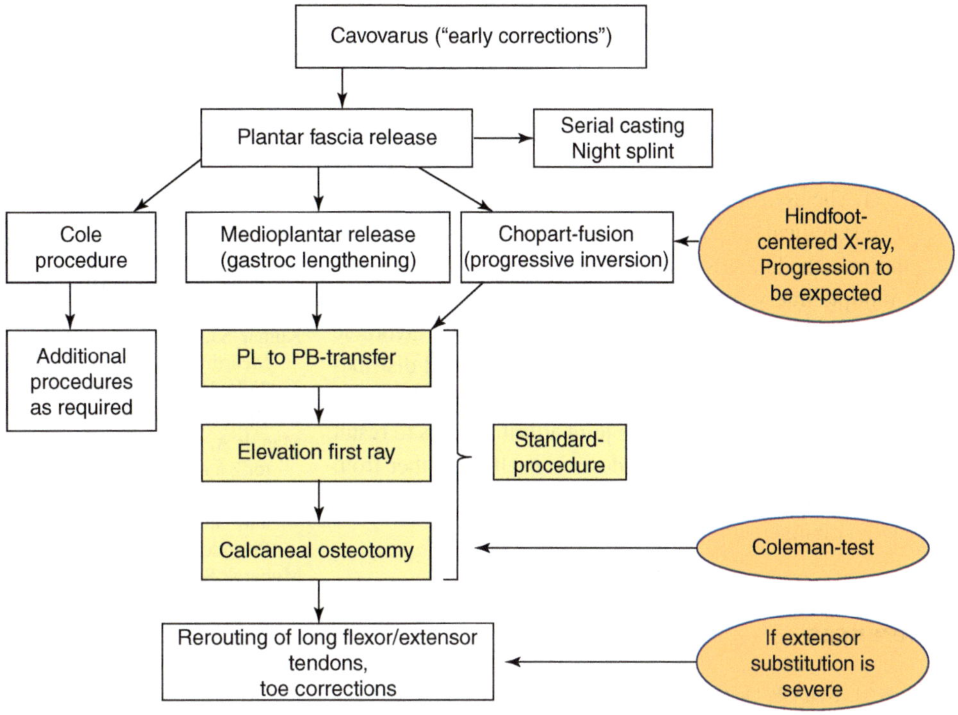

Fig. 7.36 Algorithm for "early correction" of a cavovarus deformity of minor severity, often possible in late childhood and adolescence as a rough template on how to proceed and what decisions have to be made (right side)

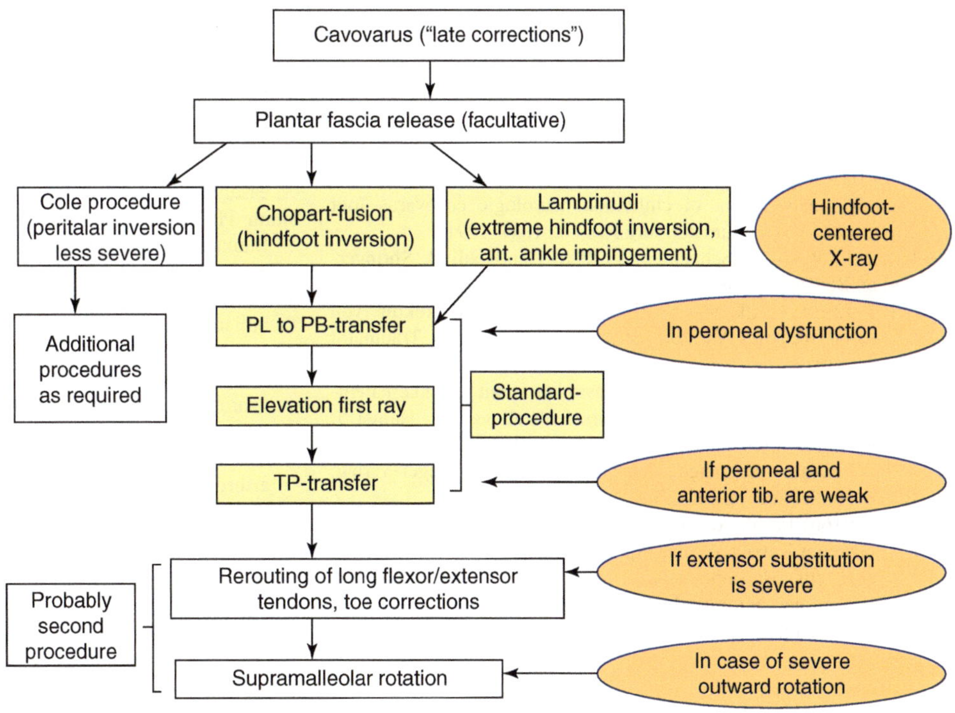

Fig. 7.37 Algorithm for "late correction" in more severe and rigid neurogenic cavovarus deformities as a rough template on how to proceed and what decisions have to be made (right side)

combination with tendon transfers in 41 treated feet of adolescent patients with Charcot-Marie-Tooth disease after an average of 26.1 years. However, frequent recurrence of hindfoot varus was observed, but only eight follow-up operations and no need for secondary triple arthrodesis. The medium-term results of Wicart and Seringe (2006) showed satisfactory results in 63.9% after tarsal osteotomies with soft tissue correction. Secondary triple arthrodesis was required in 33% of the 36 cases. The same group reported good or fair long-term results after Cole procedure in 81% of the 26 cases after 6.2 years in the mean (Simon et al. 2019).

Since the reported long-term results after triple arthrodesis are not favorable (Wetmore and Drennan 1989), a timely joint-preserving correction in adolescence seems to be entirely advisable. However, a considerable follow-up surgery rate must be expected. The assessment of the further course (family anamnesis, neurological clarification, monitoring of the course) and the optimal scheduling with avoidance of undercorrections and thus multiple interventions are decisive. If a triple arthrodesis is necessary, the exact positioning with regard to a favorable range of motion of the upper ankle joint and a good distribution of the remaining muscle forces will determine the long-term prognosis. Progressive ankle joint arthritis seems to result less from the fact of tarsal arthrodesis in itself but rather from incomplete correction, persisting muscular disbalance, or anterior ankle impingement (cf., e.g., Fig. 7.32a, c).

References

Breusch SJ, Wenz W, Döderlein L (2000) Function after correction of a clawed great toe by a modified Robert Jones transfer. J Bone Joint Surg 82-B:250–254

Cole WH (1940) The treatment of claw-foot. J Bone Joint Surg 22-A:895–908

Coleman SS (1983) Complex foot deformities in children. Lea & Febiger, Philadelphia

Coleman SS, Chesnut WJ (1977) A simple test for hindfoot flexibility in the cavovarus foot. Clin Orthop 123:60–62

d'Astorg H, Rampal V, Seringe R, Glorion C, Wicart P (2016) Is non-operative management of childhood neurologic cavovarus foot effective? Orthop Traumatol Surg Res 102:1087–1091

Döderlein L, Wenz W, Schneider U (2000) Der Hohlfuß. Springer-Verlag, Berlin, Heidelberg

Hamel J (2015) Kalkaneus-Scarf-Osteotomie zur Korrektur von subtalaren Rückfuß Varusdeformitäten. Oper Orthop Traumatol 27:308–316

Hamel J (2016a) Peronäalsehnenrekonstruktion mit gelenkerhaltender Korrektur bei leichter Kavovarusfehlstellung. In: Hamel J, Zwipp H (eds) Meistertechniken in der operativen Orthopädie und Unfallchirurgie—Sprunggelenk und Rückfuß. Springer-Verlag, Berlin, Heidelberg, pp 235–246

Hamel J (2016b) Tarsale Arthrodesen mit Sehnentransfer zur Korrektur der schweren Kavovarus und Equinovarusdeformität. In: Hamel J, Zwipp H (eds) Meistertechniken in der operativen Orthopädie und Unfallchirurgie—Sprunggelenk und Rückfuß. Springer-Verlag, Berlin, Heidelberg, pp 247–258

Hamel J (2016c) Pedografie bei Cavovarus-Deformitäten. Orthopädie-Schuhtechnik, Sonderheft Pedografie, pp 54–56

Hamel J (2017) Korrekturen und Indikationen einer Pes-cavovarus-Deformität bei Kindern und Jugendlichen. Oper Orthop Traumatol 29:473–482

Hamel J, Hörterer H, Gottschalk O, Harrasser N, Walther M (2020) Die "Rückfuß-zentrierte Röntgentechnik" zur Erfassung von Cavovarus-Deformitäten—Vorschlag zur Optimierung der radiologischen Darstellung mit Behandlungsbeispielen. Der Orthopäde, zur Publikation angenommen

Hansen ST (2008) The cavovarus/supinated foot deformity and external tibial torsion: the role of the posterior tibial tendon. Foot Ankle Clin 13:325–328

Hansen ST (2010) Adult consequences of pediatric foot disorders. In: McCarthy JJ, Drennan JC (eds) Drennan's the child's foot and ankle, 2nd edn. Lippincott, Philadelphia, pp 526–530

Hibbs RA (1919) An operation for "Claw Foot". J Am Med Assoc 73:1583–1585

Jones R (1916) The soldier's foot and the treatment of common deformities of the foot. Part II. Claw foot. Br Med J 1:749–752

Kadel NJ, Donaldson-Fletcher EA, Hansen ST, Sangeorzan BJ (2005) Alternative to the modified Jones procedure: outcomes of the flexor hallucis longus (FHL) tendon transfer procedure for correction of clawed hallux. Foot Ankle Int 26:1021–1026

Kumar SJ, Kowtharapu DN, Rogers KJ (2010) Cavus deformity. In: Mcarthy JJ, Drennan JC (eds) Drennan's the child's foot and ankle, 2nd edn. Lippincott, Philadelphia, pp 174–187

Lambrinudi C (1927) New operation on drop-foot. Br J Surg 15:193

Manoli A, Graham B (2005) The subtle cavus foot, "the underpronator", a review. Foot Ankle Int 26:256–263

Mosca VS (2014) Principles and management of pediatric foot and ankle deformities and malformations. Wolter Kluwer, Philadelphia

Mubarak SJ, Dimeglio A (2011) Navicular excision and cuboid closing wedge for severe cavovarus foot deformities: a salvage procedure. J Pediatr Orthop 31:551–556

Orthner E (2011) OSG-Prothese bei Varusinstabilität—eine neue Möglichkeit der Korrektur. FussSprungg 9:96–101

Saltzman CL, Fehrle MJ, Cooper RR, Spencer EC, Ponseti IV (1999) Triple arthrodesis: twenty-five and forty-four-year average follow-up of the same patients. J Bone Joint Surg 81-A:1391–1402

Sanpera I, Frontera-Juan G, Sanpera-Iglesias J, Corominas-Fraces L (2018) Innovative treatment for pes cavovarus: a pilot study of 13 children. Acta Orthop 89:668–673

Simon AL, Seringe R, Badina A et al (2019) Long term results of the revisited Meary closing wedge tarsectomy for the treatment of the fixed cavo-varus foot in adolescent with Charcot-Marie-Tooth disease. Foot Ankle Surg 25:834–839

Smith TF, Pitts T, Green DR (1992) Pes cavus. In: McGlamry ED, Banks A, Downey MS (eds) Comprehensive textbook of foot surgery, vol 1, 2nd edn. Williams & Wilkins, Baltimore

Steindler A (1920) Stripping of the os calcis. J Orthop Surg 2:8–12

Tachdjian MO (1985) The child's foot. WB Saunders, Philadelphia

Ward CM, Dolan LA, Bennet DL, Morcuende JA, Cooper RR (2008) Long-term results of reconstruction for treatment of flexible cavovarus foot in Charcot-Marie-Thooth Disease. J Bone Joint Surg 90-A:2631–2642

Wetmore RS, Drennan JC (1989) Long-term results of triple arthrodesis in Charcot-Marie-Tooth Disease. J Bone Joint Surg 71-A:417–422

Wicart P, Seringe R (2006) Plantar opening-wedge osteotomy of cuneiform bones combined with selective plantar release and Dwyer osteotomy for pes cavovarus in children. J Pediatr Orthop 26:100–108

Supramalleolar Deformities

8

Contents

Growth disturbances and malpositions of the supramalleolar region are observed—with divergent genesis—either isolated or in the context of complex lower leg/foot deformities.

8.1 Physiological Growth Behavior of the Distal Lower Leg

The harmonious growth of the tibia and fibula is a prerequisite for the axial development of the supramalleolar region and the ankle joint, in which both skeletal elements are involved in joint formation. In infancy, a supramalleolar valgus is physiological.

The relative importance of the distal tibial and fibular growth plate for longitudinal growth at the age of the treatment examples presented here decreases continuously compared to the proximal physes from early school age (fibula) and from about 10 years of age (tibia). Nevertheless, the remaining average residual growth for the distal fibular growth plate is still quite considerable in the growth phases of schoolchild age and, for example, is still over 5 cm in boys at 10 years of age (girls over 3 cm) and over 2 cm (girls over 1 cm) at 12 years of age (Pritchett 1992). The residual growth on the tibia after surgery can easily be read on the Harris line retrospectively (e.g., Fig. 8.2c).

8.2 Clinical and Radiological Examination

When clinically assessing the hindfoot axis by inspection from behind, it must be taken into account that supramalleolar malalignments can be compensated by the subtalar joint. Supramalleolar varus deformity, for example, will not become clinically significant until the motion limit of compensatory eversion of the talocalcaneal navicular complex is reached. On palpation, the tip of the fibula is physiologically much lower than the tip of the medial malleolus, whereas in supramalleolar valgus conditions, the malleoli might appear at the same level.

Furthermore, the rotational profile of the lower extremity should be clinically examined. Physiologically, the malleolar axis shows about 20°–25° outward rotation relative to the knee joint motion axis (Fig. 1.75). This is checked in knee flexion by adjusting the knee joint motion axis relative to the intermalleolar axis. Inversion contractures of the hindfoot complex lead to supramalleolar outward rotation malposition (see Chap. 7). An inward rotated gait pattern, as is frequently observed in healthy children especially between the age of 3 and 8 years, can have its cause on three levels (apart from conditions following fractures of the long tubular bones that healed in malrotated position): Increased femoral neck anteversion, inward rotation of the lower leg, and in the

J. Hamel, *Foot and Ankle Surgery in Children and Adolescents*, https://doi.org/10.1007/978-3-030-58108-4_8

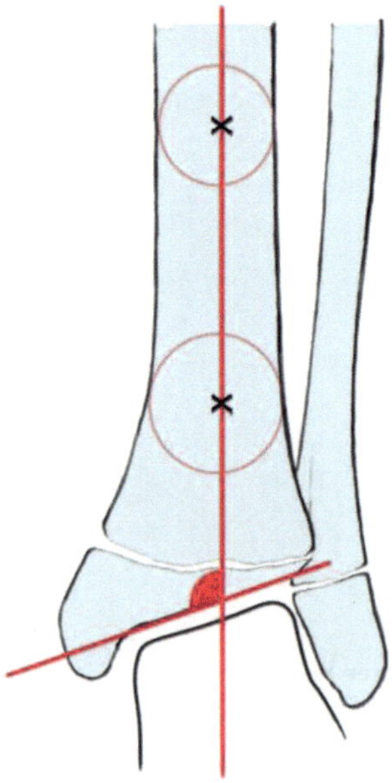

Fig. 8.1 Determination of the medial distal tibial angle (MDT angle) from the longitudinal axis of the tibia and the inclination of the tibial joint surface

subtalar region (skew foot condition, peritalar inversion as in clubfeet). Rotational malpositions of the lower leg usually show no spontaneous correction during the growth period.

A clinically observable hindfoot valgus deformity is in most cases localized in the subtalar complex; however, if a supramalleolar component is suspected, it should be excluded via an ankle joint ap X-ray in a weight-bearing position. In the ankle joint ap projection, the distal fibula growth plate is normally located approximately at the height of the tibiotalar joint space, in infants slightly higher (Dias 1985). The determination of the medial distal tibial angle (MDT angle) has proven to be useful for the quantitative assessment of supramalleolar deformities in the frontal plane (Fig. 8.1), which physiologically is approximately 90°, but is significantly higher in infants (Sect. 4.1). Davids et al. (2005) found mean values of 91.1° (SD = 3.75°) in children between 5 and 17 years of age. Knupp et al. (2005) found normal values of an average of 92.4° (SD = 3.1°) after the end of growth. A non-horizontal direction of central beam when the X-ray tube is tilted or directed further proximal (e.g., also for full leg radiographs) can represent false pathological angles.

8.3 The Supramalleolar Non-traumatic Valgus Deformity

While supramalleolar valgus deformities are observed in numerous underlying diseases, varus deformities are extremely rare except after growth plate injuries to the distal tibia (Sect. 8.4).

8.3.1 Pathogenesis

Supramalleolar valgus deformity may be the result of a lack of continuity (e.g., fibula defect, condition after fibula removal) or insufficient length development of the fibula (e.g., fibular hemimelia, neurofibromatosis). In other cases, osteonecrosis of the anterolateral tibial epiphysis (Nell et al. 2015) or tibiofibular coupling (e.g., synostosis or exostosis) may be the cause, apparently in conjunction with fibular shortening. The frequently observed valgus deformity in idiopathic clubfeet (especially in postoperative overcorrection (see Sect. 1.6.3) is not completely clear in its pathogenesis (Hamel 2015). The destabilization of the medial tarsometatarsal column probably seems to play an important role. Occasionally "idiopathic" cases are observed. Love et al. (1990) found a persistence of a physiological valgus adjusted supramalleolar region in early infancy in children with hindfoot valgus deformities.

Clinical Pictures with Supramalleolar Valgus Deformity (Selection)

Neurofibromatosis	(Fig. 8.9)
Multiple cartilaginous exostoses	(Figs. 8.6 and 8.7)
Condition after lower leg lengthening	(Fig. 8.4)
Fib. hemimelia/condition after fibula resection	
Cerebral palsy/MMC (ambulatory)	
Clubfoot (overcorrection) and talus verticalis	(Figs. 8.2 and 3.10)
Osteonecrosis of the anterolateral tibial epiphysis	(Figs. 8.3, 8.8, and 8.9)
"Idiopathic supramalleolar valgus"	
Ball and socket ankle joint	(Fig. 8.11)
Tibiofibular synostosis	(Fig. 8.18)

The supramalleolar valgus deformity can be compensated by inversion of the subtalar joint complex and thus become clinically masked. The shearing forces acting in the ankle joint can lead to a destabilization of the syndesmosis with a widened medial "clearspace" (medial malleolus - talus distance) (Figs. 8.4, 8.6, 8.9, 8.14, and 8.15).

8.3.2 Guided Growth by Hemiepiphysiodesis

By temporarily or definitively terminating the growth of the distal medial tibial growth plate, a directed longitudinal growth can be achieved with the aim of correcting the valgus deformity. A correction effect of approximately 0.6° per month has been observed (Rupprecht et al. 2015; Stevens et al. 2011). The use of clamps, eight-plates (Stevens et al. 2011), or a screw (Figs. 8.2 and 8.3) is alternatively possible.

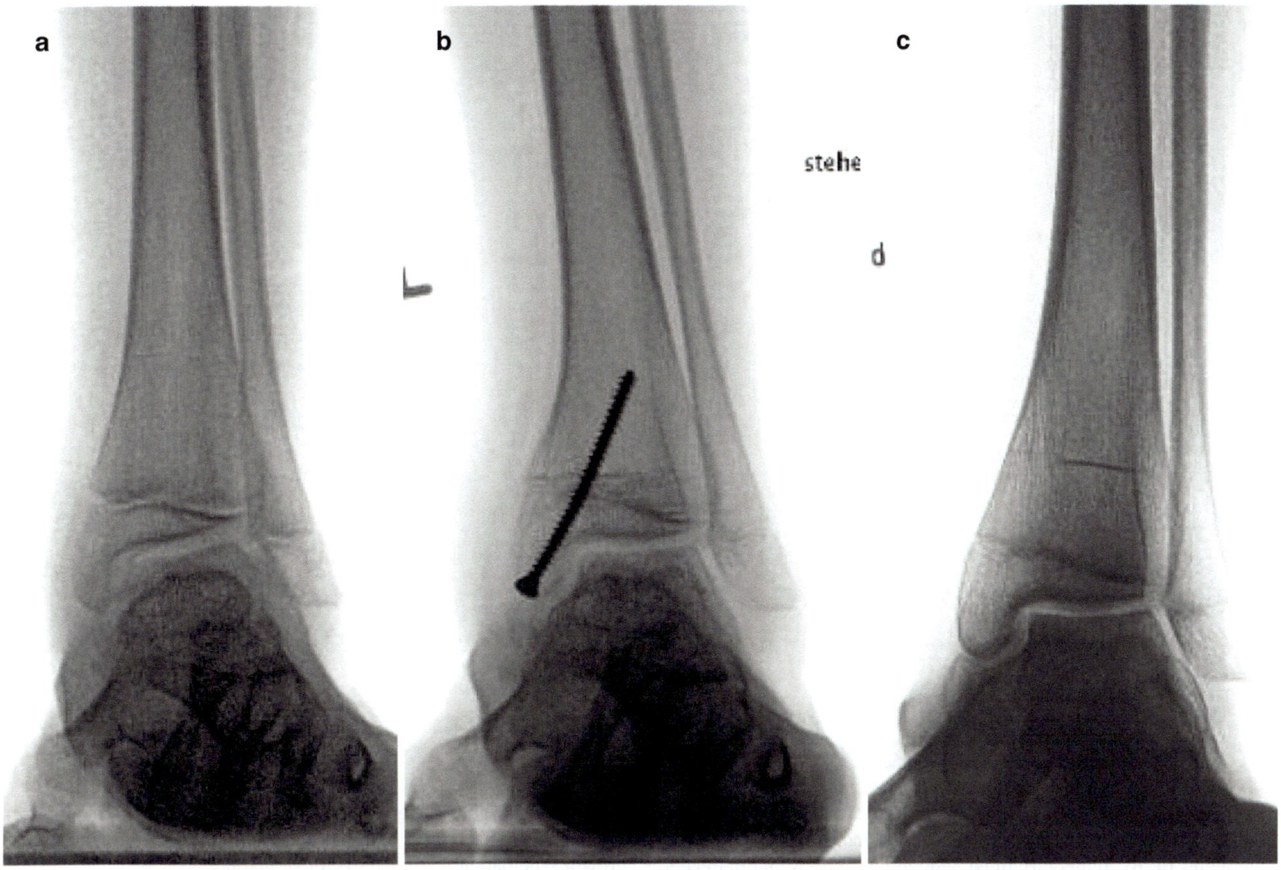

Fig. 8.2 11.5-Year-old boy, symptoms of overcorrection following externally surgically treated idiopathic clubfoot. A clear supramalleolar valgus deformity (**a**) could be corrected by medial hemiepiphysiodesis. The screw was left in place for 1.5 years (**b**). A stronger inclined placement of the screw with an even more medial intersection with the growth plate would have been superior. The considerable residual growth of the tibia until the end of the growth period is clearly visible by the Harris line (**c**)

By positioning more ventral or posterior, the effect is also active in the sagittal plane to a limited extent. The implant is retained during the temporary growth inhibition until a slight overcorrection is achieved. A certain loss of correction after metal removal must be expected ("rebound effect"). Figures 8.2 and 8.3 show two application examples. Further examples of temporary epiphyseodesis in idiopathic clubfoot can be found in Figs. 1.70, 1.79, 1.81, and 1.114. However, one basic problem of medial hemiepiphysiodesis is that the fibular side of the joint with the shortening of the fibula is not corrected at the same time and thus suboptimal bony conditions can remain in the lateral ankle joint compartment (see Figs. 1.114b and 8.18).

Technique of Hemiepiphyseodesis

A K-wire is placed in the distal tibia through a stab incision in the medial malleolus under image intensifier control in such a way, that it crosses the growth plate as far as possible medially and does not affect the upper ankle joint. A threaded small fragment cancellous screw (fully threaded) is applied over the guide wire. A steel screw should be used, a titanium screw may cause troubles during removal.

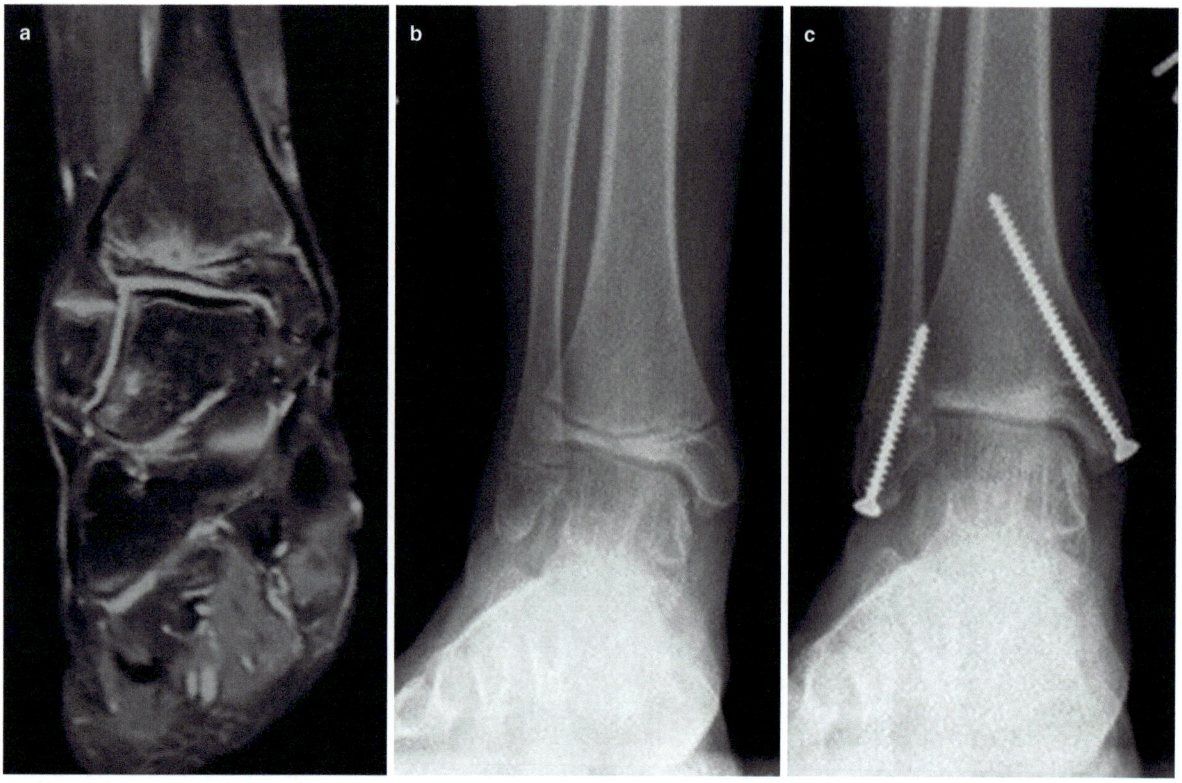

Fig. 8.3 13.2-Year-old boy, valgus deformity caused by osteonecrosis of the anterolateral tibial epiphysis with considerable load-dependent complaints (**a**, **b**). Temporary tibial hemiepiphysiodesis and fibula epiphysiodesis largely corrected the malposition within 13 months (**c**), although epiphysiodesis was performed only just before the end of growth. The patient was then free of symptoms

8.3.3 Supramalleolar Osteotomy in Valgus Deformity

If a purely growth-modifying measure is not sufficient due to limited residual growth or the extent of the deformity, or if a rotation is additionally required, a corrective osteotomy may be considered, possibly in combination with epiphysiodesis. This osteotomy can be performed with smaller correction angles using the closed-wedge or open-wedge technique (Fig. 8.15).

One problem of supramalleolar osteotomies with a more pronounced correction effect in the frontal plane is that the pivot point of the osteotomy to be selected should be located centrally and approximately at joint space height. However, both, open-wedge and closed-wedge osteotomies, will produce a considerable side to side offset because of the position of their respective pivot point in the area of the corticalis, which is to be preserved. This is demonstrated in Fig. 8.4b in the form of a planning sketch.

A simple closed or open-wedge osteotomy of the distal tibia is therefore only recommended if the amount of correction is limited. Otherwise, according to the laws of CORA (center of rotation of angulation) (Paley 2002), the technique according to Wiltse (1972) is preferable, with which excessive prominence of the medial malleolus and excessive shortening can be avoided in the varus osteotomy. As a rule, an additional fibula osteotomy with a varus effect and, if necessary, a lengthening effect, appears to be necessary. In effect, the correction of the Wiltse osteotomy corresponds to the dome-osteotomy described for adults with far distally located CORA.

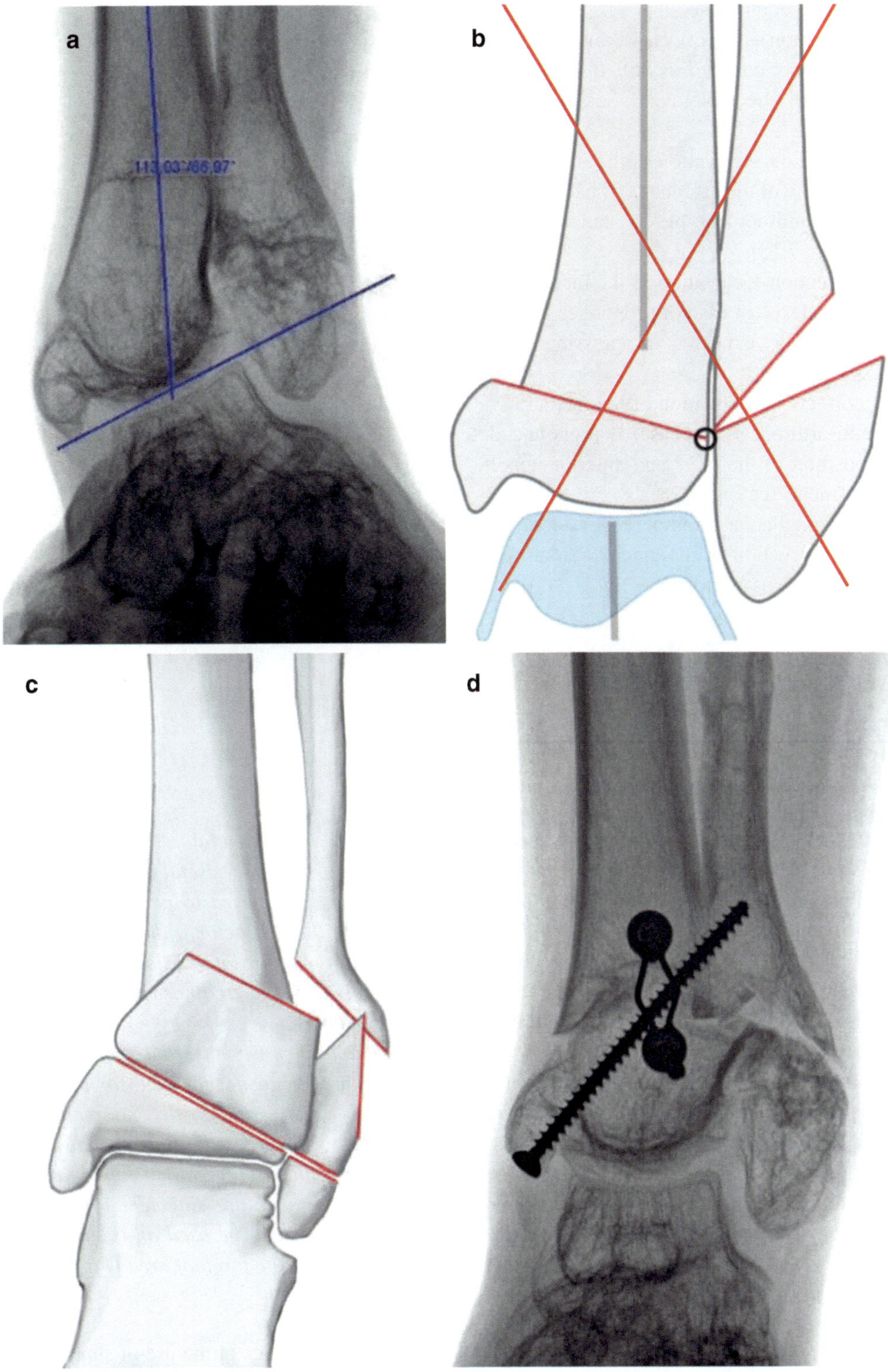

Fig. 8.4 10.5-Year-old girl with Ollier disease (enchondromatosis) and severe valgus malformation in condition after lengthening of the lower leg (**a**), MDT angle approx. 113°. The planning sketch for a closed-wedge osteotomy of the tibia (**b**) shows a pronounced medialization of the talus in relation to the tibia at a pivot point of the osteotomy in the lateral cortical tibia (circle drawn). As the planning sketch shows, this form of osteotomy increases the varus effect on the hindfoot alignment but results in a distinct prominence of the medial malleolus and is therefore less recommendable. In contrast, a correction using the Wiltse technique (Wiltse 1972) (**c**) results in good tibiotalar alignment (**c**, **d**)

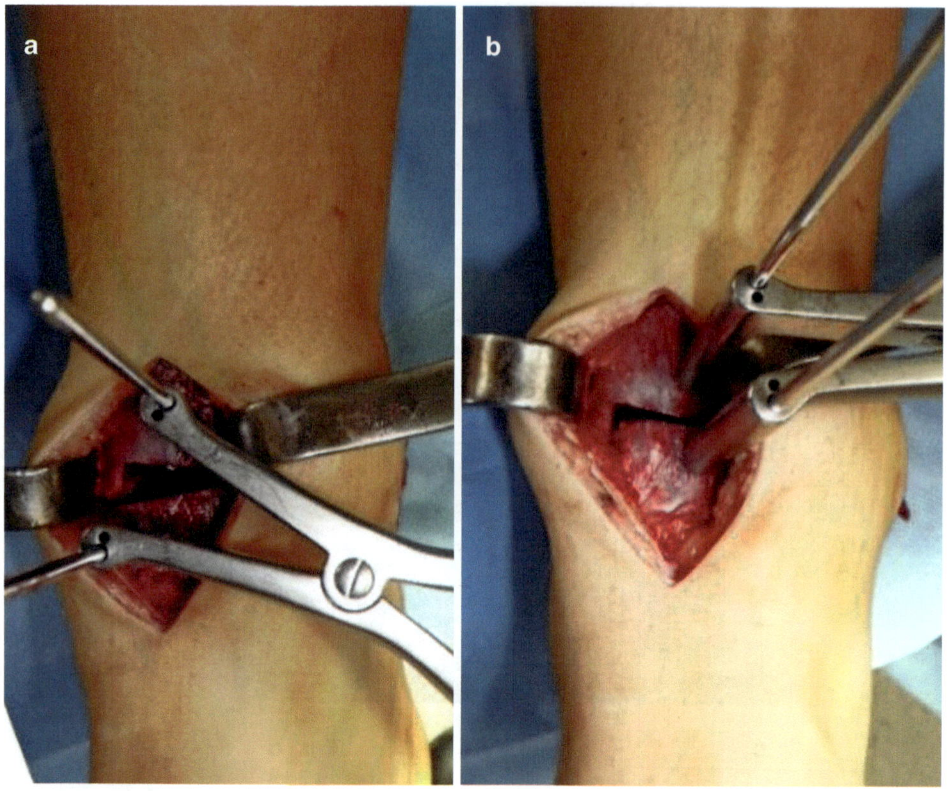

Fig. 8.5 Use of the Hintermann distractor for lateral displacement of the distal fragment in supramalleolar osteotomy with varus orientation effect. Two K-wires are placed asymmetrically in the two osteotomy partners (**a**). The required lateralization of the distal fragment can be achieved by rotating the distractor (in this case counterclockwise) (**b**). The groove made in the proximal fragment is clearly visible

Technique of the Supramalleolar Osteotomy with Varus Orientation Effect According to Wiltse

Prior to the procedure, a planning sketch is prepared, which shows in particular the extent of the required lateral displacement (Figs. 8.4b and 8.13b). The distal tibial base is exposed via an anterior longitudinal incision between the tibialis anterior and extensor hallucis longus tendon while sparing the superficial and deep neurovascular structures. Approximately 2.5 cm above the joint space, a transverse osteotomy is performed after marking with a K-wire under image intensifier. A tent-shaped step is sawn into the proximal osteotomy surface while preserving the medial corticalis, the lateral part of which corresponds to the planned correction angle. The fibula is osteotomized obliquely from lateral caudal to medial cranial through a separate longitudinal incision at approximately the same height as the tibia. If the fibula is significantly shortened, a lengthening here is advisable, which can be realized either in a Z-shaped manner or by interposition of a graft. Depending on the extent of the axial correction required, the distal fragment of the tibial osteotomy must now be moved laterally. The Hintermann distractor has proven very useful as a manipulation tool (Fig. 8.5). It can be used to perform the lateral offset by rotating the distractor with slight extension. The bony protrusion on the lateral side resulting from the lateral offset is removed, as otherwise a conflict with the fibula can occur.

Percutaneously inserted crossed Kirschner wires have proven to be effective for osteosynthesis (Fig. 8.7b), which can usually be removed after about 4 weeks. In older children and adolescents, screws and claw plates (Fig. 8.8) in combination with mandatory hard casts are sufficient for stabilization. Less bulky plates can be used on the fibula, as are otherwise used in the forefoot area (Figs. 8.6 and 8.7).

Further examples of the use of supramalleolar osteotomy with varus effect are shown in Figs. 8.6, 8.7, 8.8, 8.9, 8.10, and 8.11. In the case of supramalleolar valgus malformations with a need for correction, there are characteristic disease-specific additional features, which will be addressed in the context of the presented clinical examples:

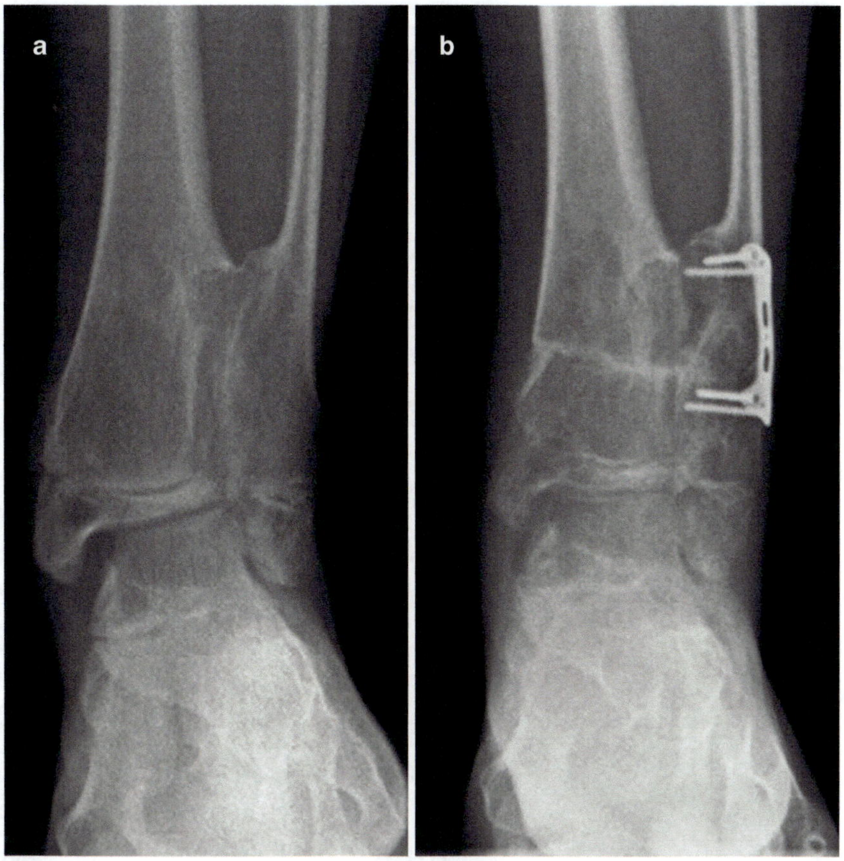

Fig. 8.6 14-Year-old patient with multiple cartilaginous exostoses and supramalleolar valgus deformity (**a**). The medial clear space (medial malleolus-talus distance) is significantly enlarged. After tibia and fibula osteotomy restored ankle alignment (**b**)

- In multiple cartilaginous exostoses, the exostoses usually originate from the fibula, which can cause the fibula to entangle with the tibia and must then be resected. In addition, the fibula is usually significantly shortened, so that lengthening is usually necessary (Figs. 8.6 and 8.7).
- In the case of osteonecrosis of the lateral tibial epiphysis, a (temporary) medial epiphysiodesis of the tibia (and possibly also of the fibula) should be considered in addition to axial correction (Fig. 8.8; see also Fig. 8.3). This rare entity was, apart from some case reports in patients without other concomitant diseases, explicitly described for the first time by the author's group with accompanying literature research (Nell et al. 2015).
- In cases of fibular continuity interruptions with cranial migration of the ankle-forming distal fibula components, the lateral counter-support for the talus must be restored, which may require tibiofibular synostosis (Fig. 8.10).
- The formation of a ball and socket ankle joint, as observed in tarsal synostoses involving the talonavicular joint (but not in coalitions) (Hamel et al. 1993), is usually associated with fibula shortening and supramalleolar valgus deformity. A distinct supramalleolar osteotomy with varus effect should be combined with a medial calcaneal osteotomy (Fig. 8.11), as the supramalleolar varus effect may be partially reduced by increased valgus of the talus due to the spherical joint geometry. Alternatively, a reorientating osteotomy of the synostosis itself is also possible.

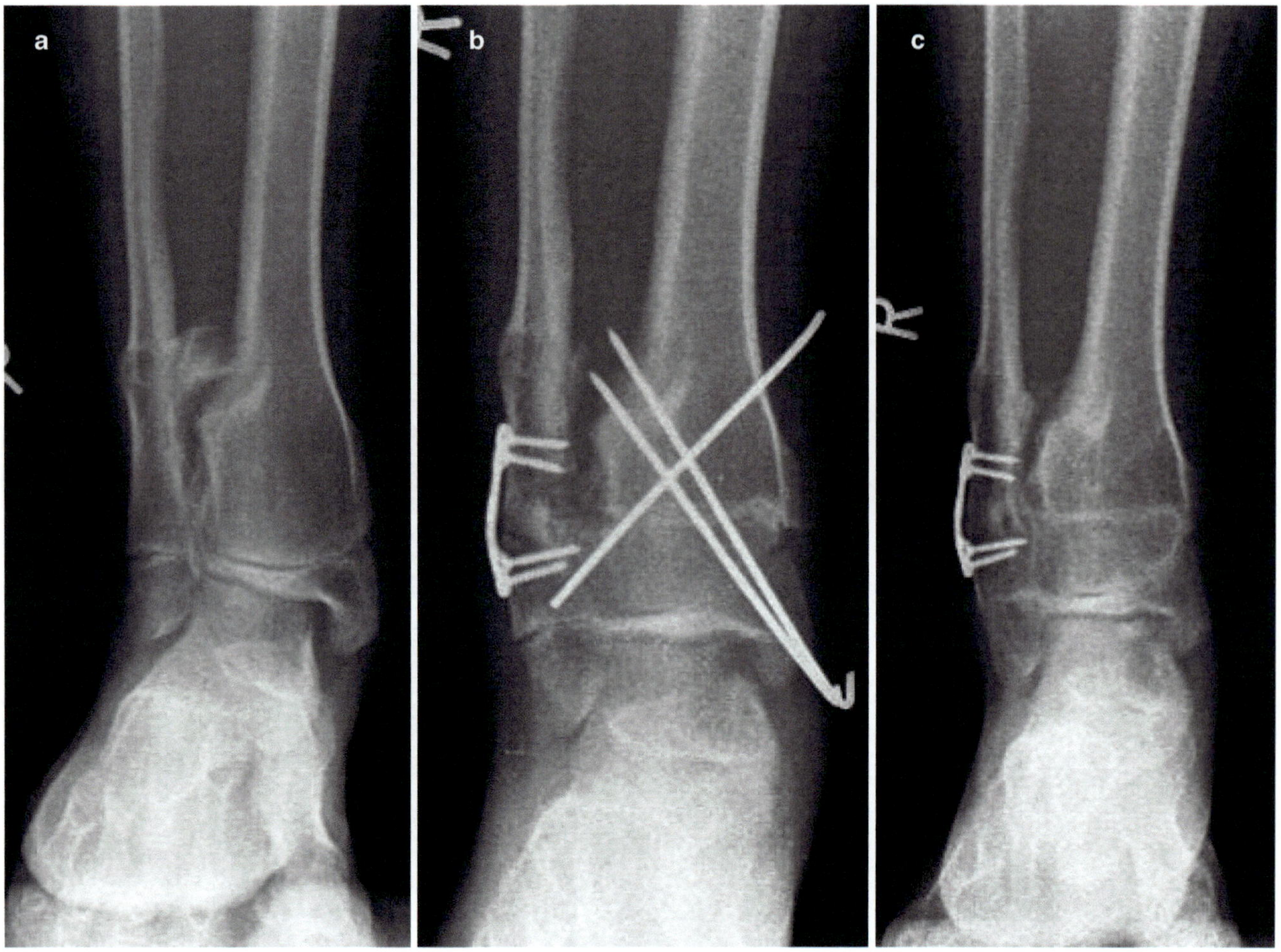

Fig. 8.7 14-Year-old patient with multiple cartilaginous exostoses and the typical valgus malformation (**a**). Supramalleolar tibial osteotomy with fibula lengthening osteotomy and resection of the fibula exostosis (**b**, **c**)

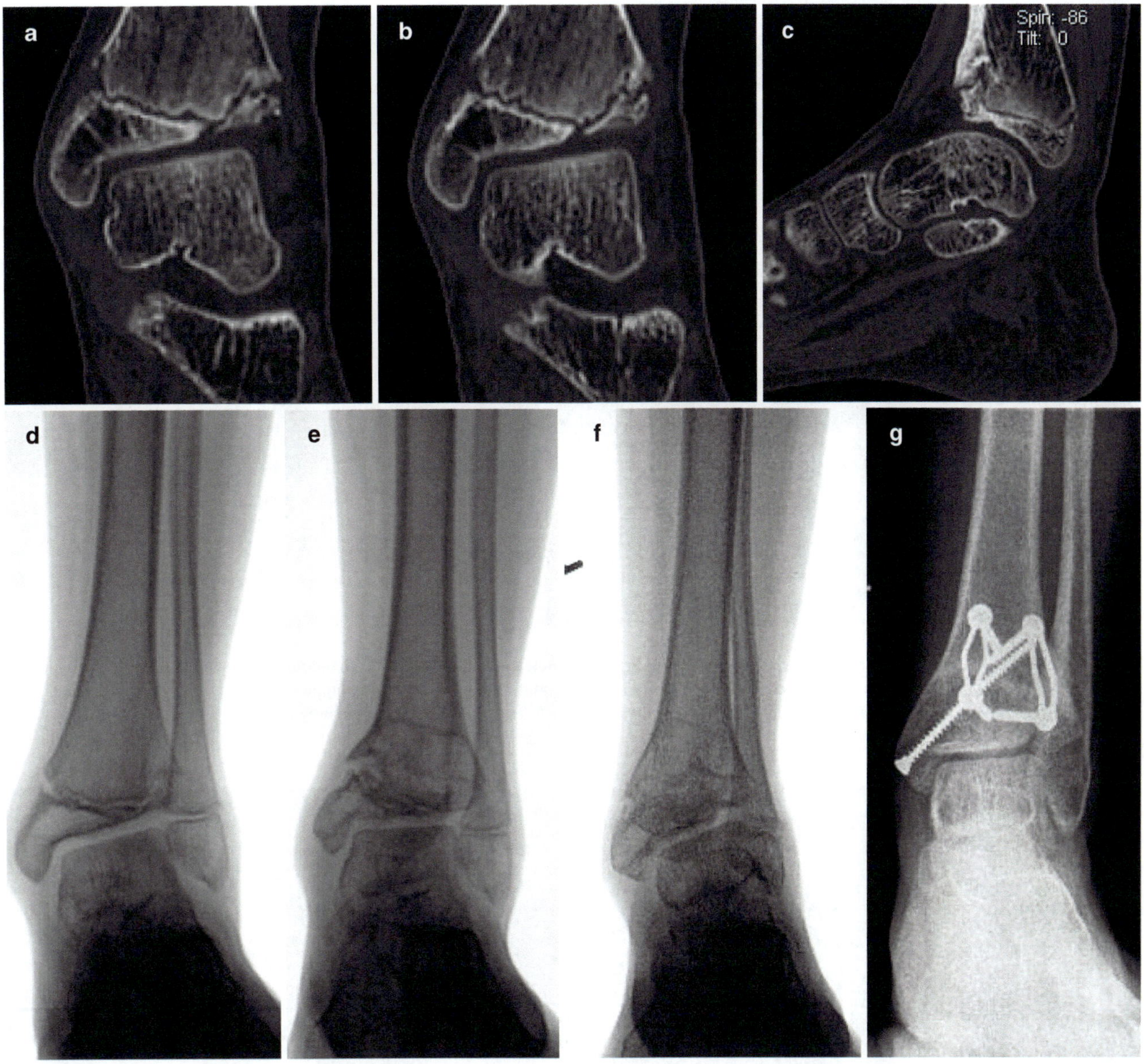

Fig. 8.8 10.8-Year-old boy with osteonecrosis of the anterolateral distal tibial epiphysis, supramalleolar valgus deformity with distinctly shortened fibula, possibly corresponding to a mild form of fibular hemimelia (**a**–**d**). After supramalleolar osteotomy and temporary epiphysiodesis, sufficient axial realignment at 12 years (**e**). However, the epiphysis has not recovered. Subsequently, a renewed valgus malformation occurred with formation of a bone bridge in the area of the lateral tibial growth plate (**f**). The need for a renewed osteotomy using the open-wedge technique and resection of the bone bridge (bar-resection) from the osteotomy area followed at 13.8 years (**g**)

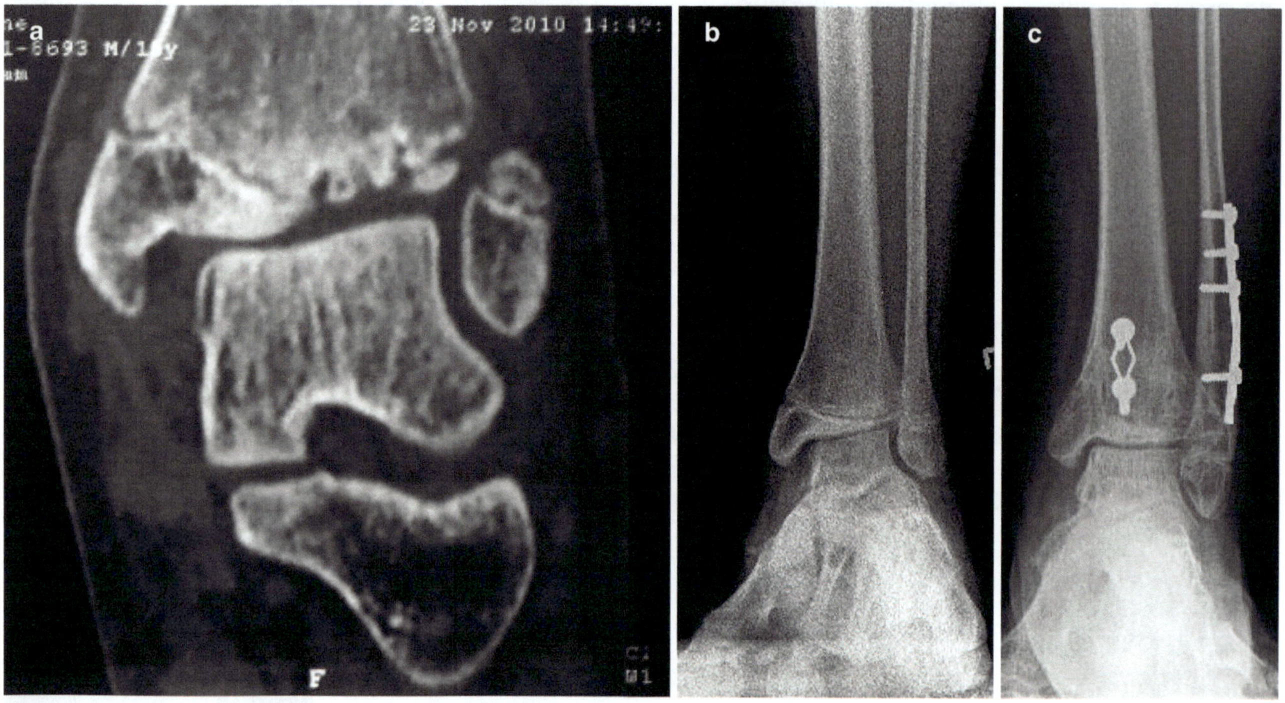

Fig. 8.9 15-Year-old boy with progressive symptoms since a few months. Radiologically clear signs of osteonecrosis of the anterolateral tibial epiphysis (**a**) with relative fibula shortening (**b**). The significantly increased talus to medial malleolus distance due to the lack of lateral counter support could be completely reduced by supramalleolar tibial osteotomy and fibula lengthening (**c**)

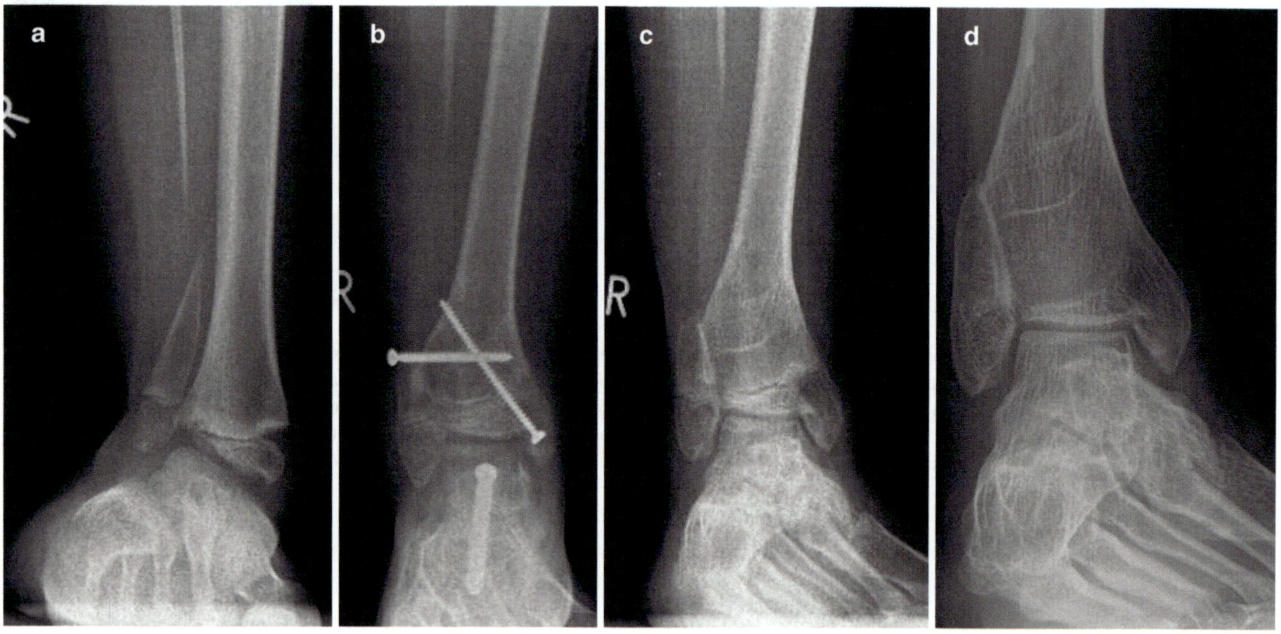

Fig. 8.10 8-Year-old boy with neurofibromatosis and fibula pseudarthrosis with atrophy of the fibular diaphysis (**a**). Stabilization of the ankle joint by tibiofibular synostosis with distalization of the distal fibula segment and supramalleolar tibial osteotomy with temporary hemiepiphysiodesis. Additionally a Grice arthrodesis was performed (**b**). Almost 3 years postoperatively (**c**) and after the end of growth stable conditions and good axial position (**d**)

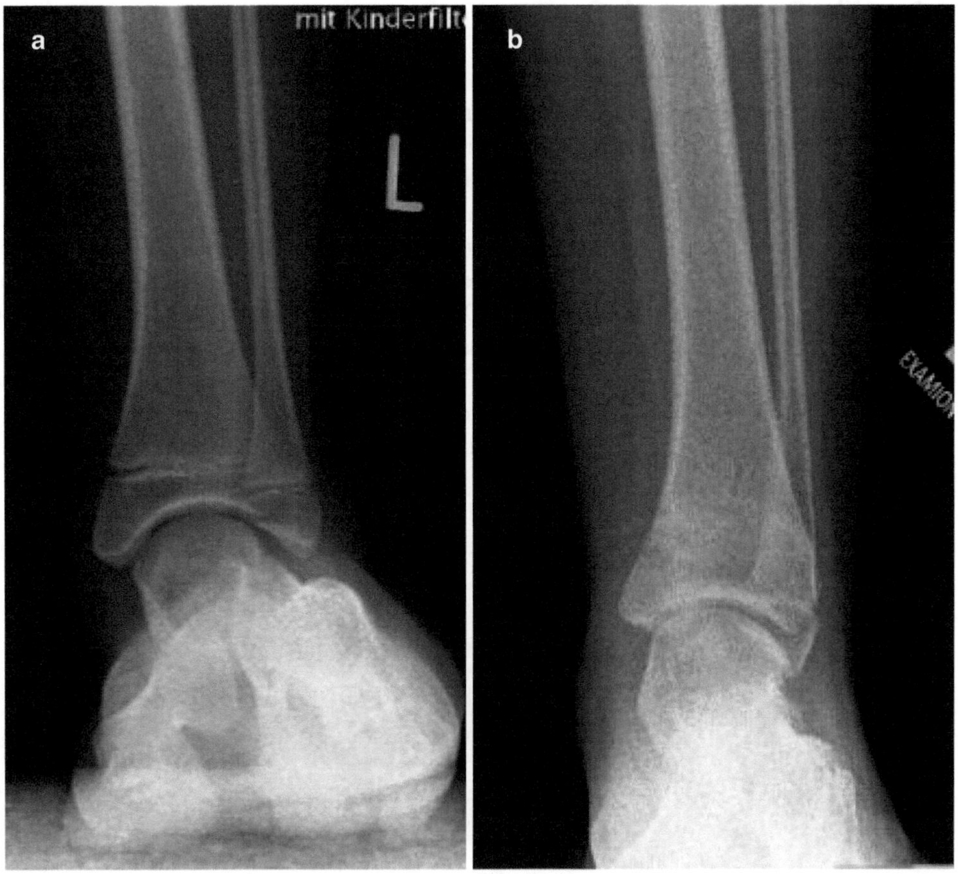

Fig. 8.11 12.5-Year-old girl with ball and socket ankle joint in fibular hemimelia, hindfoot synostoses, and a forefoot with four metatarsal rays (**a**). After supramalleolar osteotomy, calcaneus sliding osteotomy and plantarizing medial cuneiform osteotomy, sufficient foot realignment (**b**). Lower leg lengthening planned

8.4 The Post-traumatic Supramalleolar Deformity

Injury to the distal tibial or fibular growth plate can lead to premature growth plate closure and asymmetrical growth (Wachowsky et al. 2015). For a comprehensive overview, see Peterson (2007). First of all, CT scans should always be performed to determine whether removal of the bone bridge (bar resection) is promising (see Fig. 8.8) and whether this can prevent further growth disturbance (Wilkins 2000). If this is not the case, epiphysiodesis and/or osteotomies can be used for correction.

Injury to the medial tibial growth plate can result in supramalleolar varus malgrowth if growth of the lateral tibial joint and fibula is not reduced (Figs. 8.12 and 8.13). In less severe cases, an open-wedge or closed-wedge osteotomy (Fig. 8.12) of the tibia can be performed with fibula epiphysiodesis; in pronounced malalignment, the pivot point of the osteotomy must be shifted far distally, and the distal fragment must be shifted to medial in accordance with the procedure described in Sect. 8.3 in severe valgus deformity, to avoid unfavorable lateral displacement (Fig. 8.13).

If the fibula growth plate is injured, resulting in its premature closure, valgus malformation occurs and especially a lateral dislocation of the talus due to the lack of fibular support. In these cases, repositioning by fibular lengthening is necessary to prevent severe joint damage (Figs. 8.14 and 8.15). Ligamentous injuries of the syndesmosis are not observed in growing age.

Also in the sagittal plane, relevant malpositions requiring correction can occur due to premature closure of the joint. Figures 8.16 and 8.17 show two examples of correction osteotomies addressing sagittal plane deformity.

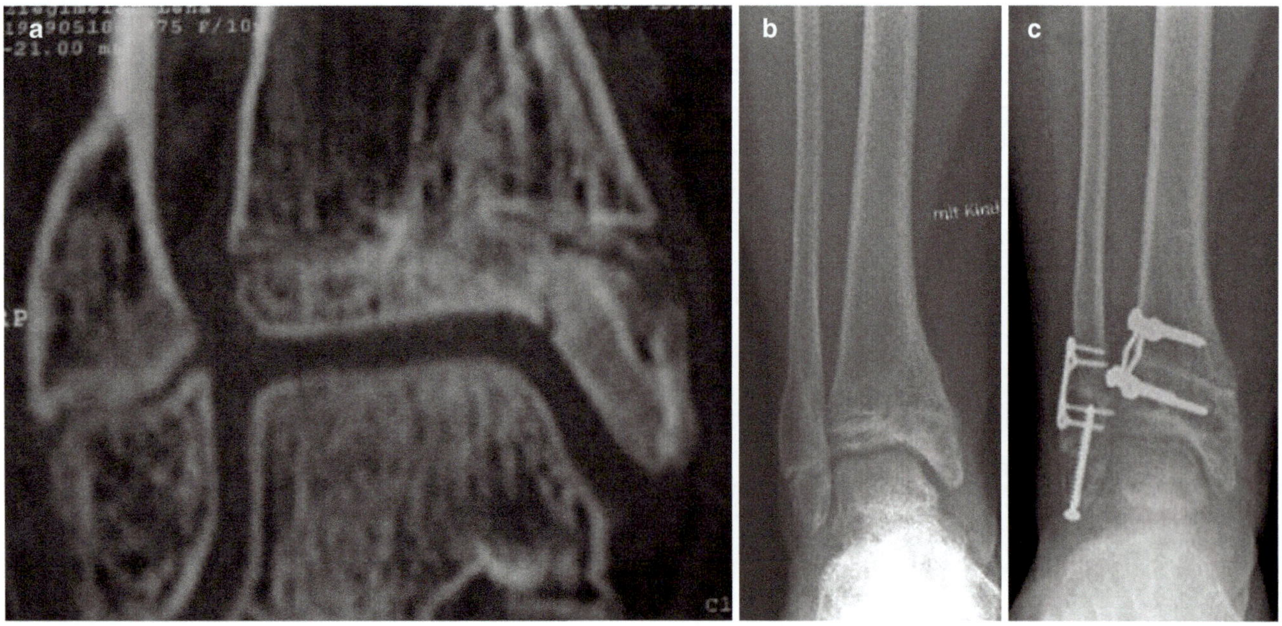

Fig. 8.12 12-Year-old female patient with condition after severe axial compression injury of both distal lower legs at the age of 10 years and extensive premature growth plate closure of the central-medial tibial growth plate portions (**a**) with undisturbed fibular growth (**b**). A bar resection did not appear promising. A supramalleolar tibial and fibular osteotomy with epiphysiodesis of the lateral tibial and fibular growth plates, further incorrect growth was prevented (**c**). Since the opposite side is also affected, a considerable difference in leg length was not to be expected

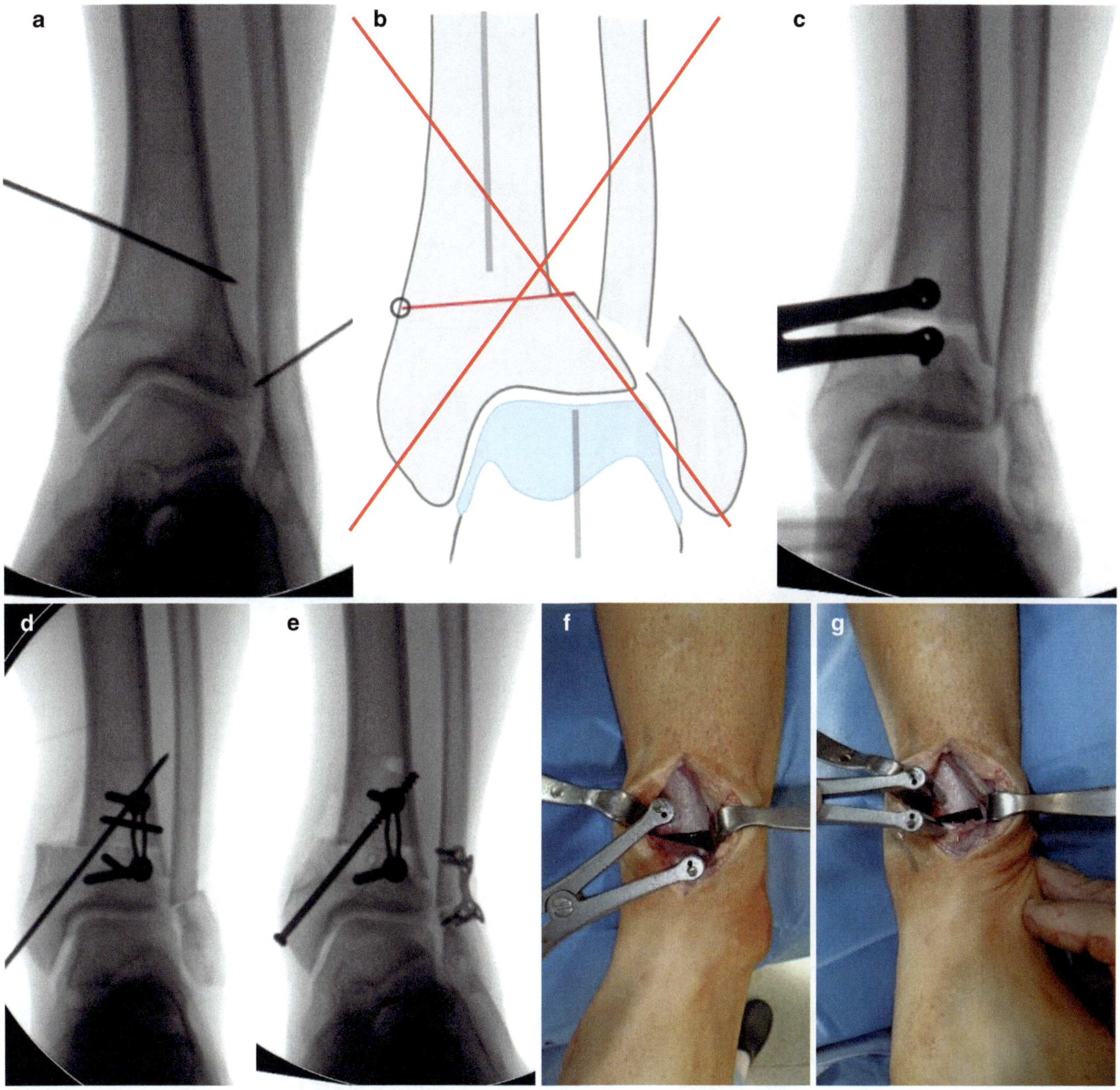

Fig. 8.13 Almost 14-year-old girl with a condition following meningococcal sepsis in early childhood (Waterhouse-Friderichsen syndrome), damage to the distal tibial growth plate, and severe varus malformation with undiminished fibula growth (**a**). If a closed-wedge osteotomy with a pivot point in the medial tibial corticalis would have been performed, a pronounced lateral dislocation of the ankle joint in relation to the tibial shaft with a clear prominence of the lateral malleolus would have been created (**b**). A distinct medial shift of the tibial base in relation to the tibial shaft (**c**–**e**) with the creation of a groove in the proximal fragment, using the Wiltse technique (Wiltse 1972), results in a sufficient realignment of the talus under the tibia (**d**). The bony excess medial to the distal fragment was removed (**e**). Manipulation to medialize the distal fragment is facilitated by the use of the Hintermann distractor, which in this case is rotated clockwise (**f**, **g**)

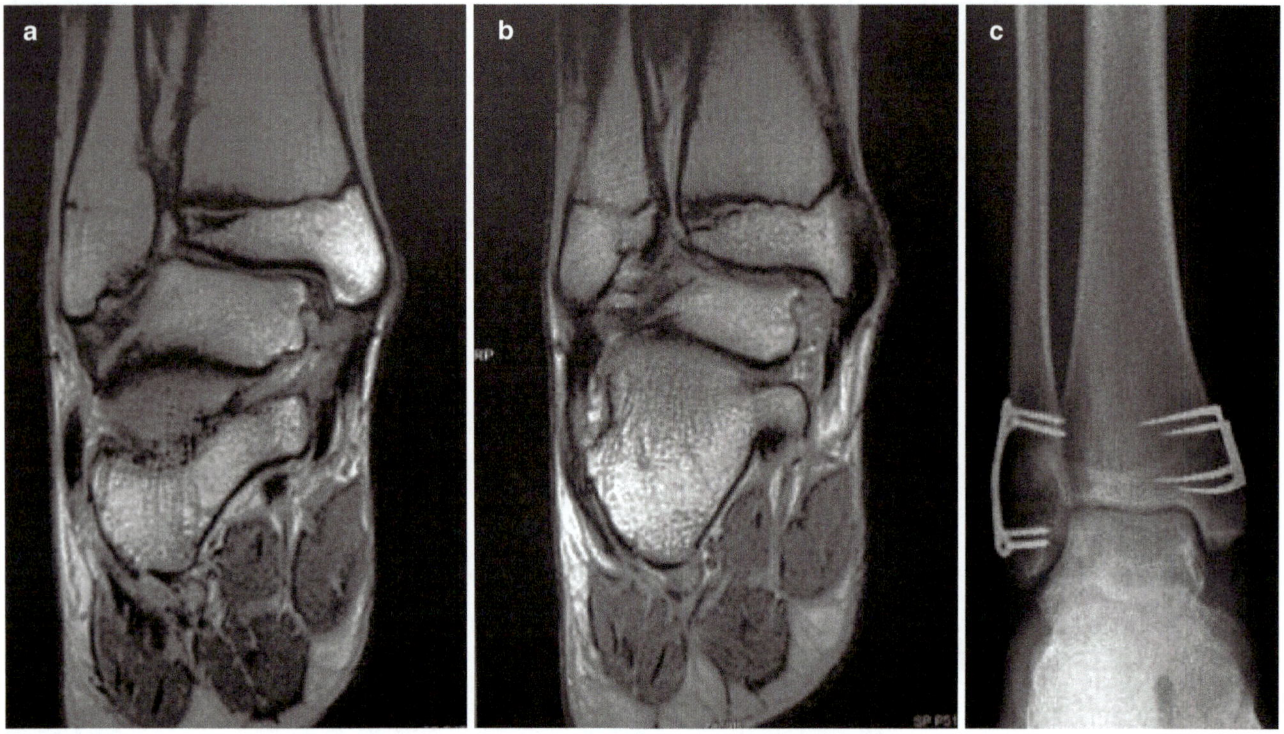

Fig. 8.14 15-Year-old female patient, status after severe ankle sprain about 12 months ago with premature closure of the fibular growth plate (**a**). This resulted in significant valgus malformation with increased medial clear-space (**b**). Due to fibular lengthening and definitive epiphysiodesis of the tibia complete realignment and sufficient stability at the ankle joint could be achieved (**c**)

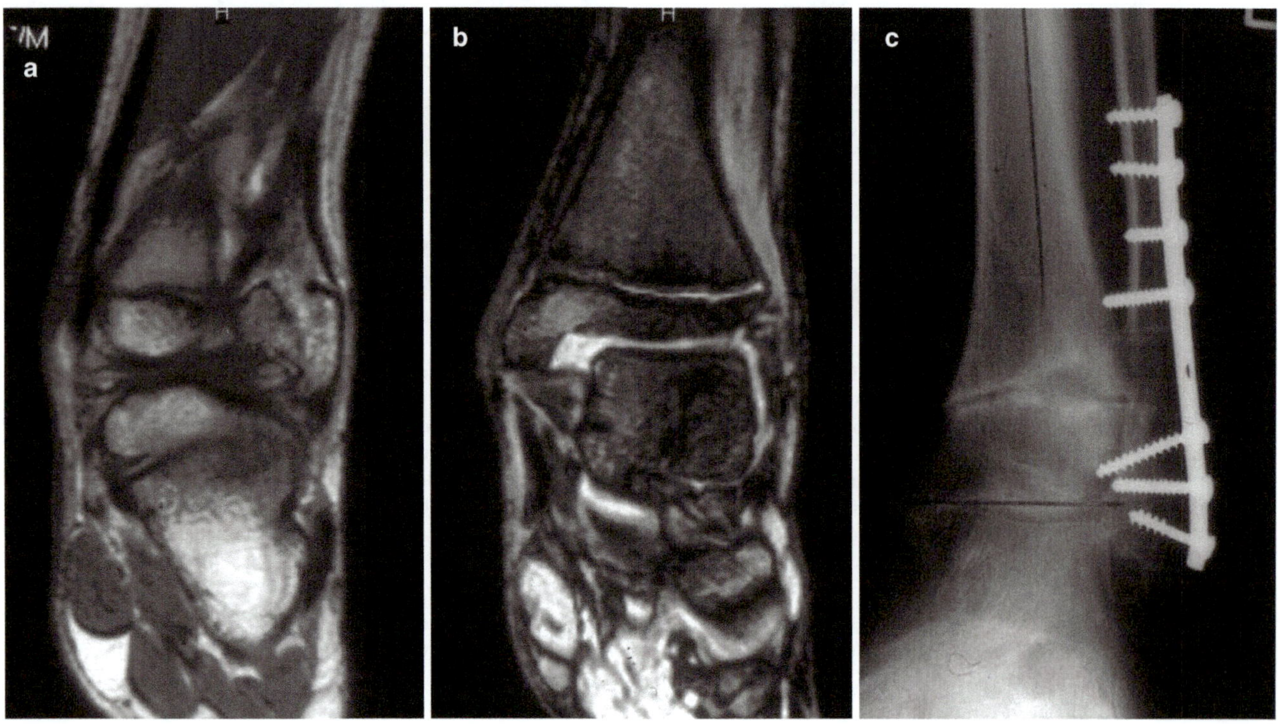

Fig. 8.15 14-Year-old boy with post-traumatic premature closure of the fibular growth plate (**a**) and distinct lateral shift of the talus due to the lack of fibular support (**b**). This could be corrected by open-wedge osteotomy (slightly overcorrecting) and fibular lengthening (**c**)

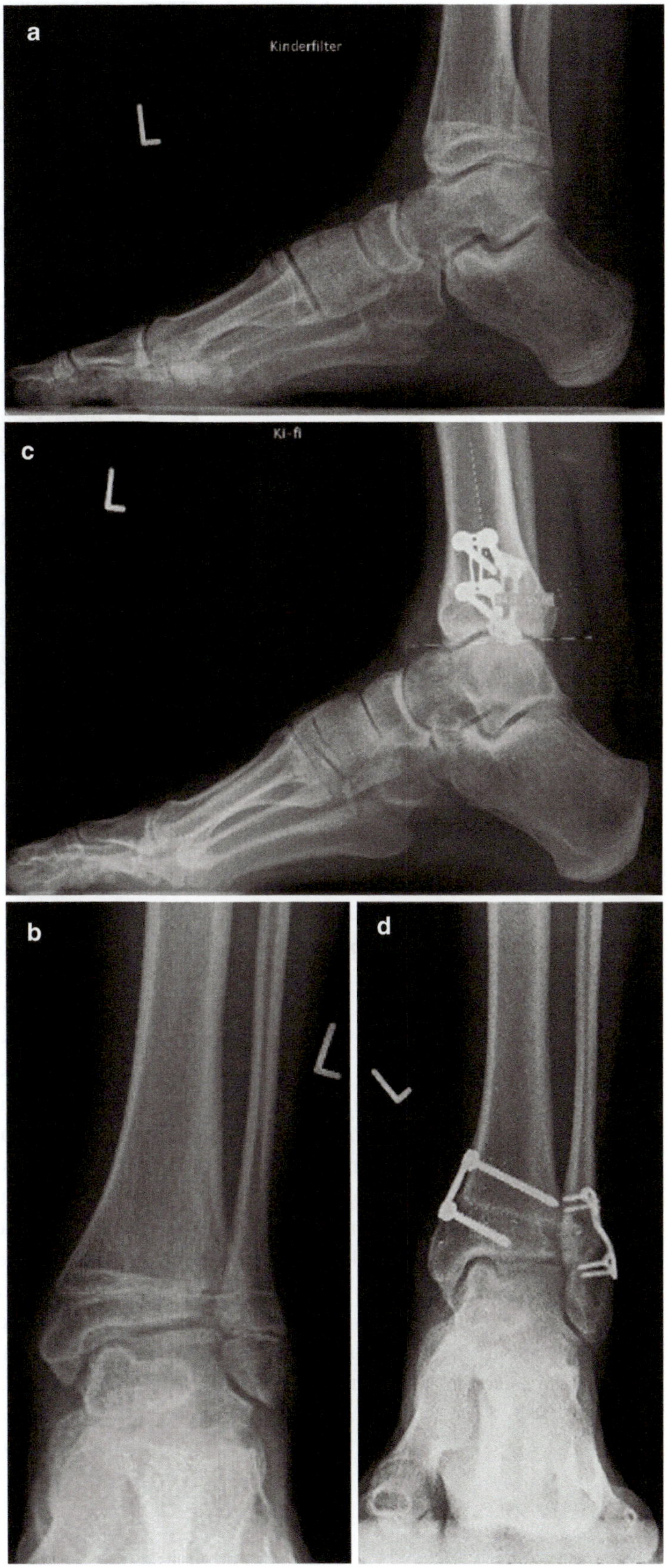

Fig. 8.16 16-Year-old patient with post-traumatic dorsolateral premature growth plate closure of the tibia. The flexion malposition of the distal tibia has resulted in a significant limitation of the dorsal extension of the ankle joint (**a**), aggravated by a moderate cavovarus foot component. In addition, there was a supramalleolar valgus deformity (**b**). This could be sufficiently corrected by a closed-wedge osteotomy with varus and extension effect at the tibia and additional mild open-wedge osteotomy of the fibula (**c**, **d**), so that a slight dorsal extension is possible again and the deformity is compensated in the frontal plane

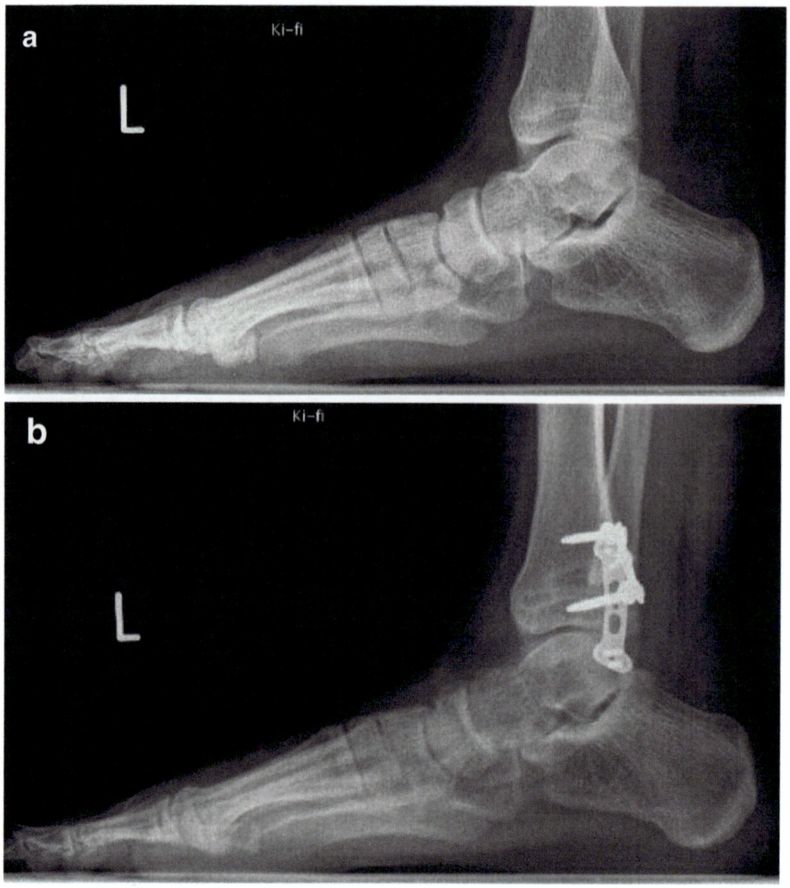

Fig. 8.17 15-Year-old patient with condition after premature growth plate closure at the distal tibia dorsolateral and thus reduced slope of the distal tibial joint surface (**a**). An open-wedge tibial osteotomy from a posterior approach with slight fibular lengthening was performed (**b**)

8.5 Supramalleolar Rotational Malpositions

Rotational malpositions at the level of the lower leg occur in connection with foot deformities or even independently. They can be compensated by the two joints of the lower extremity with motion capacity in the transverse plane (hip joint and subtalar joint complex). A spontaneous correction of rotatory malpositions in the course of growth cannot be assumed. Therefore, if the findings are clear, a surgical correction should be considered, which is technically rather less complex. If the need for correction is lower, the fibula can be left untreated, while if the need for correction is higher, the fibula should undergo osteotomy too, also to accommodate the rotation center of the osteotomy. The osteotomies of tibia and fibula should be performed at different levels to prevent synostosis. Depending on the age, screws, claw-plates, K-wires, and, for adolescent age, angle-stable plates have proven to be suitable for osteosyntheses. A known complication is the tibiofibular synostosis, which leads to a reduced distal migration of the fibula (Fig. 8.18) (Frick et al. 2001).

Supramalleolar inward rotating osteotomies are sometimes necessary, for example, in the correction of severe cavovarus deformities (see Chap. 7). In the idiopathic clubfoot, the constellation often consists of an internal rotation gait with a clinically rather externally rotated malleolar region. In this case, the causes of the inward rotational gait are usually located in the foot itself, so that outwardly rotating supramalleolar osteotomies are only very rarely indicated (see Sect. 1.6.2.6).

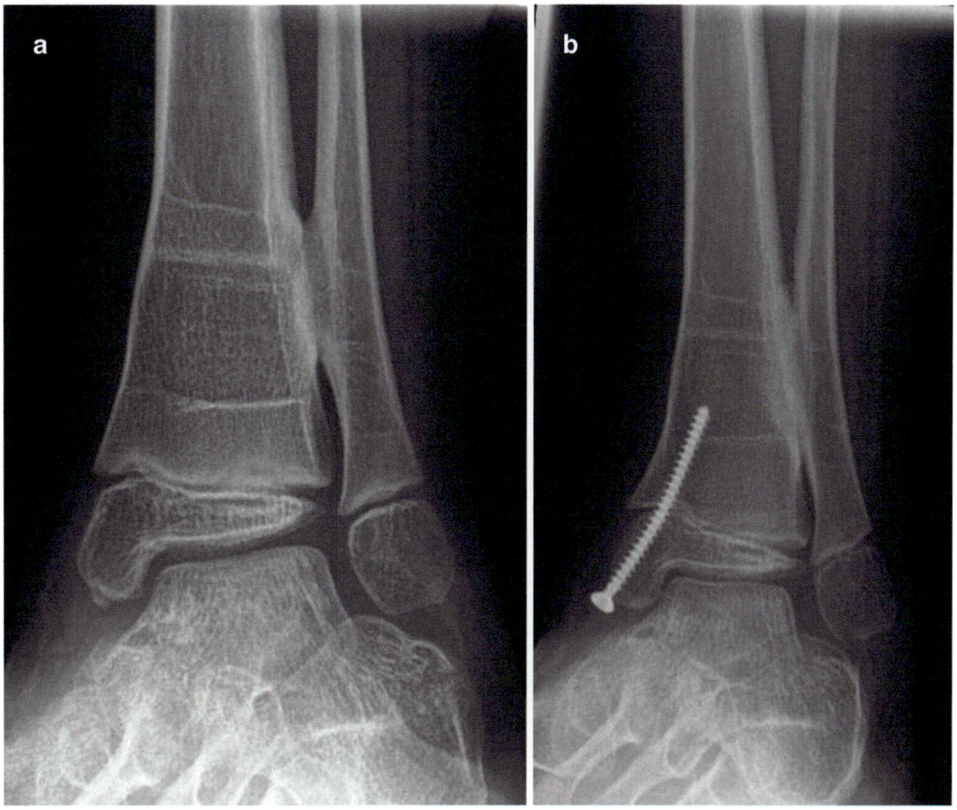

Fig. 8.18 Condition following supramalleolar rotational osteotomy with consecutive tibiofibular synostosis (**a**). Hemiepiphysiodesis can correct the tibial malposition but cannot adjust the fibular length and the position of the lateral malleolus (**b**)

References

Davids JR, Gibson W, Pugh LI (2005) Quantitative segmental analysis of weight-bearing radiographs of the foot and ankle for children—normal alignment. J Pediatr Orthop 25:769–776

Dias LS (1985) Valgus deformity of the ankle joint: pathogenesis of fibular shortening. J Pediatr Orthop 5:176–180

Frick SL, Shoemaker S, Mubarak SJ (2001) Altered fibular growth patterns after tibiofibular synostosis in children. J Bone Joint Surg 83-A:247–254

Hamel J (2015) Knöcherne Deformitäten des Oberen Sprunggelenkes beim operativ behandelten idiopathischen Klumpfuß. OUP 4:349–355

Hamel J, Müller G, Becker W (1993) Ein Fall von beidseitiger isolierter talonavicularer Synostose im Kindesalter—Beobachtungen zur Mechanik des Tarsus und der funktionellen Adaptation des Oberen Sprunggelenkes. Z Orthop 131:275–278

Knupp M, Ledermann H, Magerkurth O, Hintermann B (2005) The surgical tibiotalar angle: a radiologic study. Foot Ankle Int 26:713–716

Love SM, Ganey T, Ogden JA (1990) Postnatal epiphyseal development: the distal tibia and fibula. J Pediatr Orthop 10:298–305

Nell M, Rist C, Hamel J (2015) Supramalleoläre Valgus-Deformität bei partieller Nekrose der distalen Tibiaepiphyse. OUP 4:356–362

Paley D (2002) Principles of deformity correction. Springer-Verlag, Berlin

Peterson HA (2007) Epiphyseal growth plate fractures. Springer-Verlag, Berlin, Heidelberg

Pritchett JW (1992) Longitudinal growth and growth-plate activity in the lower extremity. Clin Orthop 275:274–279

Rupprecht M, Spiro AS, Breyer S, Vettorazzi E, Ridderbusch K, Stücker R (2015) Growth modulation with a medial malleolar screw for ankle valgus deformity. Acta Orthop 86:1–5

Stevens PM, Kennedy JM, Hung M (2011) Guided growth for ankle valgus. J Pediatr Orthop 31:878–883

Wachowsky M, Fernandez FF, Wirth T (2015) Vorzeitiger posttraumatischer Wachstumsfugenverschluss am distalen Unterschenkel. OUP 4:364–368

Wilkins KE (2000) Management of physeal arrest of the ankle and foot. In: Myerson M (ed) Foot and ankle disorders. W.B. Saunders Company, Philadelphia

Wiltse LL (1972) Valgus deformity of the ankle as a sequel to acquired or congenital anomalies of the fibula. J Bone Joint Surg 54-A:595–606

Osteochondral Lesion of the Talus

9

Contents

9.1 Clinical Presentation

Osteochondral lesions of the talus are observed with an age peak in the second decade of life. They are predominantly located in the area of the medial talar shoulder, less frequently laterally or centrally. They are sectorial aseptic necroses of the bone with secondary damage to the cartilage covering. However, lesions of the cartilage with inflow of synovial fluid may as well be the beginning of the pathogenetic chain. In some cases a connection with trauma can be assumed. The spontaneous healing tendency is rather favorable in adolescents, so that invasive treatment procedures are usually only considered in case of complaints or progression in later stages during the course of observation. Asymptomatic patients with MRI changes should only be observed.

In connection with the treatment of osteochondral talar lesions, the medial and anterolateral stability of the ankle joint should always be checked and, if necessary, treated by ligamentous reinforcement. In addition to the tightening of the anatomical ligament structures by reinsertion or the utilization of local soft tissue structures (e.g., the retinaculum inferius in the form of a Brostrom/Gould procedure), stabilization with the autologous semitendinosus tendon is most effective in particularly severe cases after closure of the growth plates (Hamel 2016).

9.2 Surgical Treatment Procedures

Three therapeutic options are generally considered in childhood and adolescence:

- **Arthroscopic procedures:** The diagnostic clarification often shows in childhood and adolescence that the cartilage is still intact in early stages. In later stages, the arthroscopic examination serves to test the stability of the dissected cartilage and can provide results that differ from those of the magnetic resonance tomogram. If the lesion is unstable, fixation with resorbable pins may be considered. Otherwise, reconstructive procedures should be preferred. Completely detached, smaller fragments can be removed arthroscopically with anterograde drilling of the defect. Predominantly good results have been described, but with a substantial proportion of therapy failures, for children and adolescent patients (Reilingh et al. 2014; Jurina et al. 2018). With the use of K-wire anchored distractors, arthroscopically osteochondral defects can often be inspected clearly and can be treated with similar precision as with open procedures when performed by an experienced surgeon. Also reconstructive surgery is possible arthroscopically (D'Ambrosi et al. 2017).
- **Retrograde bone drilling:** If the cartilage cover is intact, retrograde drilling from the sinus tarsi can be performed

J. Hamel, *Foot and Ankle Surgery in Children and Adolescents*, https://doi.org/10.1007/978-3-030-58108-4_9

under X-ray control and, if necessary, with the aid of targeting devices (Fig. 9.1), or it can even be filled with cancellous bone. This should have a positive effect on blood circulation and healing processes. The therapeutic value is difficult to assess, and there is hardly any meaningful information on this in the literature. Masquijo et al. (2016) report on six cases at the age of 11–15 years with good clinical results after 3 years, but radiologically incomplete healing in half of the cases. At least these procedures often have an analgetic effect.

– **Open reconstruction**: A larger defect can be treated directly via an arthrotomy with or without medial malleolar detachment. The competing methods are cartilage-bone replacement by *OATS cylinders* from the knee joint, and the principle of *autologous matrix-induced chondrogenesis (AMIC) with insertion of collagen membranes* (Walther et al. 2012; Wiewiorski et al. 2016; Gottschalk et al. 2017). Refixation of larger fragments can be attempted, but does not always lead to the desired healing (Fig. 9.8).

The open procedure with the use of collagen membranes will be described in more detail here, as it has proven to be particularly effective in adolescents. It is possible in the form shown here without or—after growth plate closure—with extended medial malleolar detachment and allows reconstruction under optimal visibility. The available literature mainly refers to the adult age: Good results with OATS plasty (Paul and Imhoff 2016) have been reported in young adults with, however, significant donor site morbidity in the knee joint (Paul et al. 2009). Good clinical results are now available for osteochondral lesions in young adults for the AMIC procedure (overview in Gottschalk et al. 2017), which only requires the harvesting of autologous cancellous bone chips.

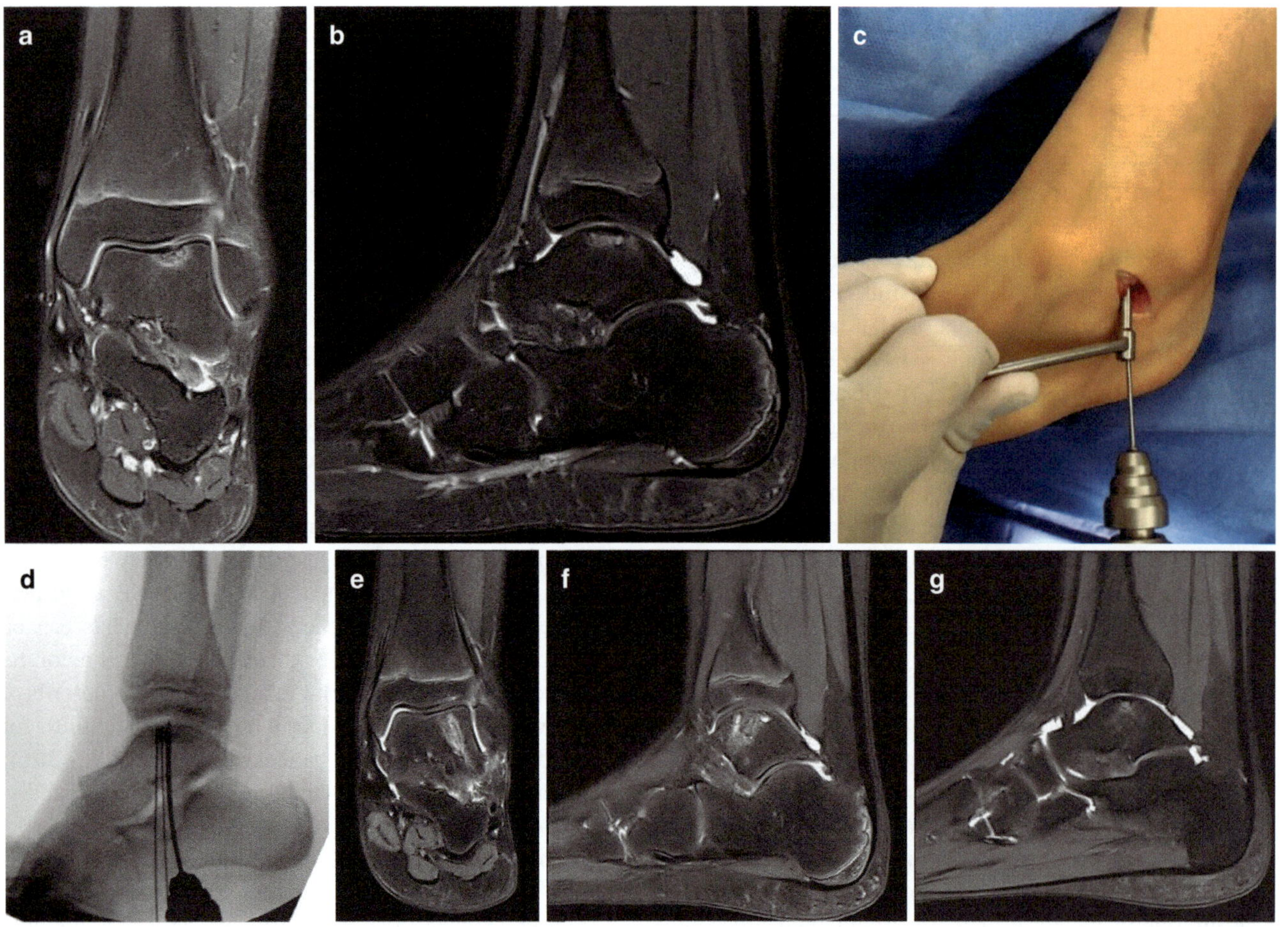

Fig. 9.1 11-Year-old girl with a history of significant complaints for several months, with centrally located osteochondral lesion (**a**, **b**). Retrograde drilling was performed from an access at the sinus tarsi under image intensifier control (**c**, **d**). Thin K-wires were placed in the affected area from the lateral processus tali and redrilled with a 1.8 mm drill. 6 Weeks postoperatively, the effect of drilling is visible in MRI (**e**, **f**). Nearly 2 years later, still ongoing healing of the subchondral bone could be observed (**g**)

9.3 Cancellous Bone Graft with Collagen Membrane

In pronounced cases of an osteochondral lesion in adolescents, careful debridement of the defect and filling with cancellous bone graft is an option that has opened up since the introduction of collagen membranes to cover the embedded cancellous bone.

Cancellous Bone Graft with AMIC Membrane *The extent of the osteochondral defect is determined by palpation of the cartilage. The affected cartilage area is resected with a scalpel or a sharp curette until stable cartilage margins are visible. The underlying bony defect is debrided with curettes and then with the high frequency bone burr up to the healthy cancellous tissue of the talus. In addition, very thin holes are drilled in a fan shaped manner (Fig. 9.6a). Cancellous bone is harvested from the calcaneus or the tibial osteotomy site and embedded in the defect. An AMIC membrane is precisely cut to size and applied to the defect with fibrin glue, so that it exactly matches the surrounding cartilage margins. After the fibrin glue has hardened, the joint is mobilized, and the stable position of the membrane is checked again. This membrane allows the cancellous bone and the mesenchymal cells infiltrated from the inside of the bone to be held in place, and a cartilage regenerate is formed.*

Access to the anterior parts of the medial talar shoulder can be gained by anteromedial arthrotomy (Fig. 9.2). By distraction with the K-wire anchored distractor, it is thus possible to gain access to the more posterior parts of the medial talar shoulder (Fig. 9.3). However, the more posterior located the necrotic process is, the more difficult a complete debridement becomes, including fan-shaped oriented drilling to open the sclerotic marginal structures of the lesion, and the reconstructive measures overall.

Alternatively, with already closed tibial growth plate, the medial compartment can be reached via an osteotomy of the medial malleolus at the level of the tibiotalar joint space. The disadvantage is that with this procedure, full visibility and orthograde instrumentation of the defect may be suboptimal and the osteosynthesis of the small medial malleolar fragment may present problems. These disadvantages can be eliminated by an "extended medial malleolar osteotomy," and reconstruction can be performed under direct view and at a 90° angle to the talar joint surface. It is also possible to work on central areas of the talus (Fig. 9.4). The author has had good experiences with the form of extended medial malleolar osteotomy shown here, which allows optimal access to the osteochondral defect of the medial talar shoulder. With technically exact performance, permanent damage to the joint surface by this intra-articular osteotomy can be safely avoided. In recent literature, the medial malleolar osteotomy is by some authors (Wiewiorski et al. 2016) recommended as a regular form of access, almost never necessary according to others (Gottschalk et al. 2017).

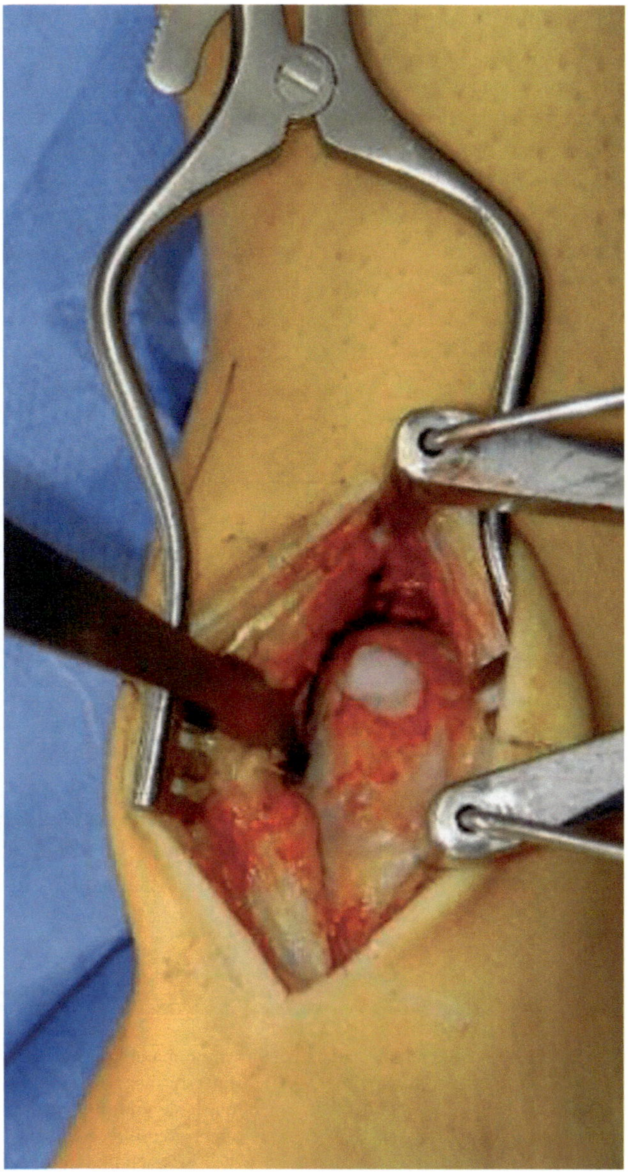

Fig. 9.2 Treatment of an anteromedially located osteochondral lesion with curettage, cancellous bone graft and AMIC membrane via an anteromedial arthrotomy using a K-wire anchored distractor. The image was provided by Dr. O. Gottschalk, Munich

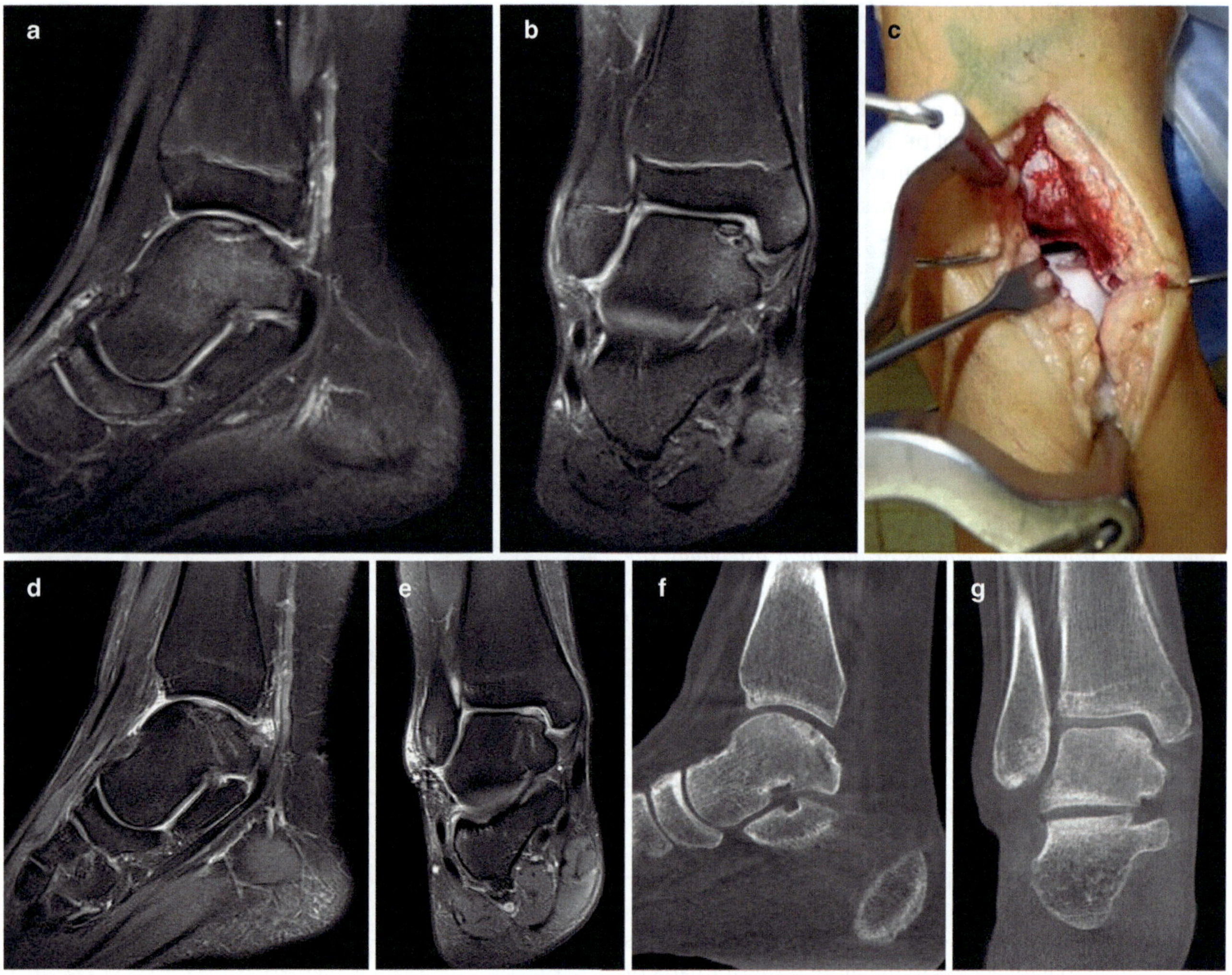

Fig. 9.3 13-Year-old female patient with a symptomatic osteochondral lesion, with still open growth plates (**a**, **b**), located further posterior than in the case of Fig. 9.1. Debridement, cancellous bone grafting and covering with an AMIC membrane (**c**). The defect could be adequately reached and treated by distraction with a K-wire-anchored spreader from the anterior side. In the MRI 7 months postoperatively, the inserted cancellous bone shows the beginning of healing and incorporation (**d**, **e**), the joint contour seems to be restored in the DVT 18 months postoperatively (**f**, **g**)

Technique of Extended Medial Malleolar Osteotomy

Through a curved incision, the medial malleolus is exposed up to about 5 cm proximal to its tip. After epiperiostal dissection in an anterior direction, the ankle joint is opened sparingly anteromedially, and the lesion at the medial edge of the talus is inspected, if it is partially visible. Posteriorly, the posterior tibial tendon must be identified in its gliding groove and protected throughout its further course. The V-shaped osteotomy is marked by incision into the periosteum. The preparation of the subsequent screw placement is done before the osteotomy, by drilling holes and determining the screw length. An image converter is used for this purpose. The proximal screw runs approximately horizontally, the distal one obliquely from the tip of the medial malleolus without penetrating the joint (Figs. 9.4 and 9.5). The osteotomy is started with the oscillating saw, using the thinnest possible saw blades. The osteotomy is completed with chisels that are as thin but also as wide as possible. It ends in the articular surface of the tibiotalar central compartment. The large medial malleolar fragment is mobilized, shifted distally, and kept aside for further surgery with K-wires, which are inserted into the non-cartilaginous medial parts of the talus or into the tibia (Fig. 9.6). This provides direct orthograde access to the entire medial edge of the talus. The osteosynthesis of the medial malleolar osteotomy is performed with two small fragment corticalis screws with continuous thread to avoid compression.

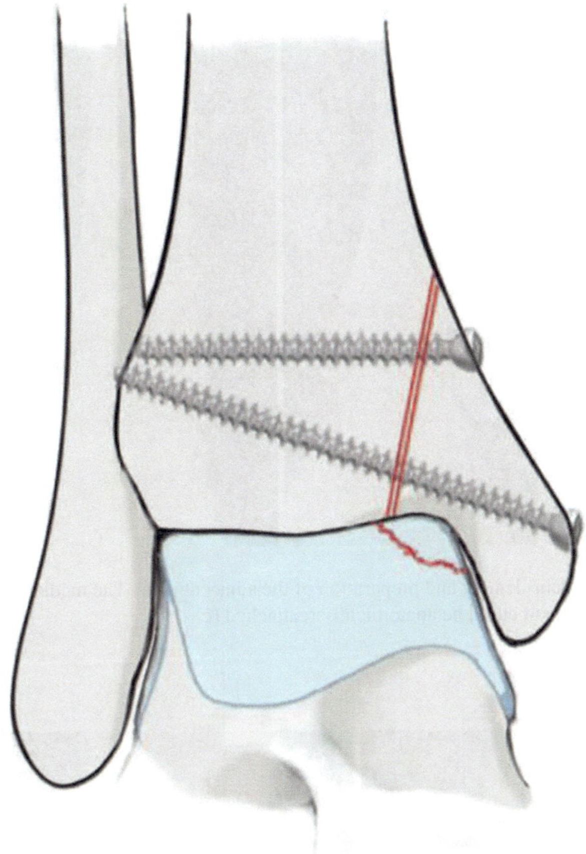

Fig. 9.4 Extended medial malleolar osteotomy as approach to the defect of the medial talar shoulder

9.4 Results

In the literature, there are hardly any reports on the application of reconstructive procedures in children and adolescents. Gottschalk et al. (2017) observed clinically favorable medium-term results in young adult patients. Wiewiorski et al. (2016) also report predominantly on middle-aged patients, who generally did not regain their pre-existing athletic level. Nevertheless, it may be assumed that the healing processes in adolescents are more favorable. According to the author's experience with a limited number of cases, the clinical results so far are favorable. Radiologically, a complete filling of the defect with completely congruent talar joint surface is not always to be expected. Postoperative incongruence after intra-articular tibial osteotomy has never been observed. Three exemplary courses of adolescent patients are presented (Figs. 9.7, 9.8, and 9.9).

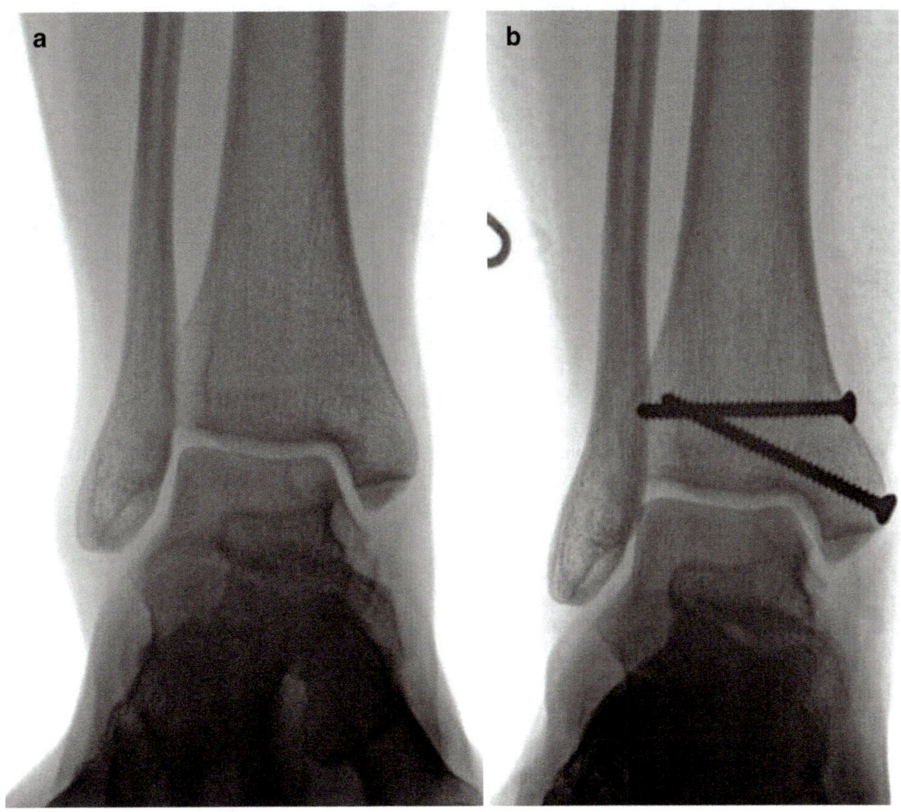

Fig. 9.5 Before (a) and after medial malleolar osteotomy (b) with osteosynthesis through two non-compressive small fragment cortical screws in an 18-year-old female patient

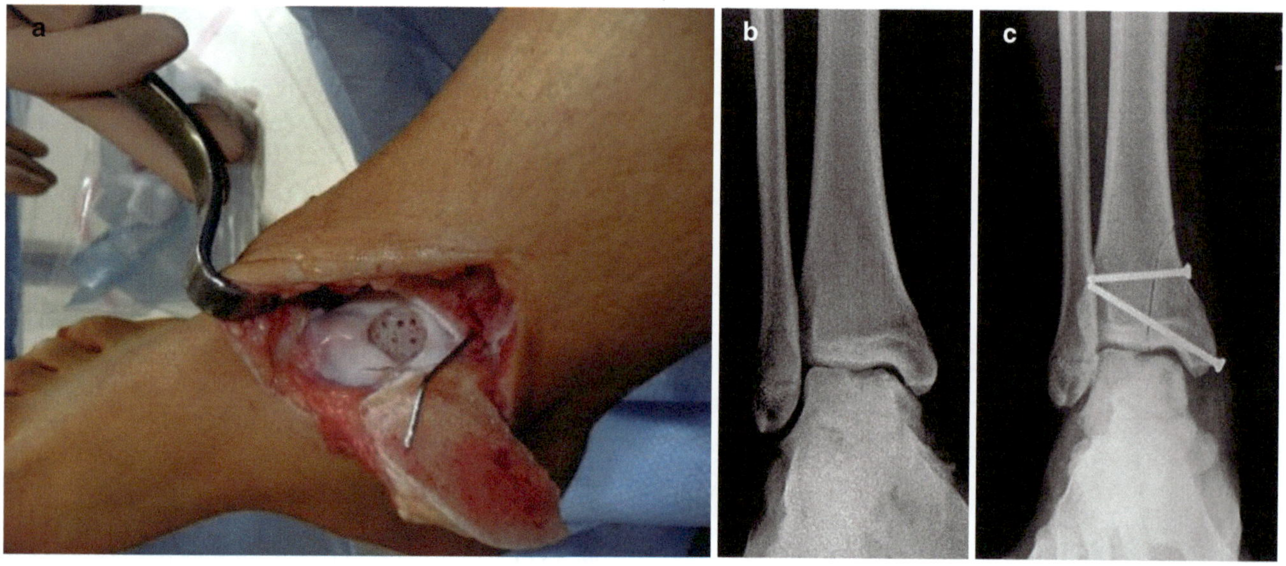

Fig. 9.6 18-Year-old female patient with large central osteochondral lesion of the talus (**a**, **b**). Temporary detachment of a large medial malleolar fragment allowed direct orthograde visualization of the defect (**a**) for debridement and preparation of the adjacent bone. The medial tibial fragment could be anatomically reattached (**c**)

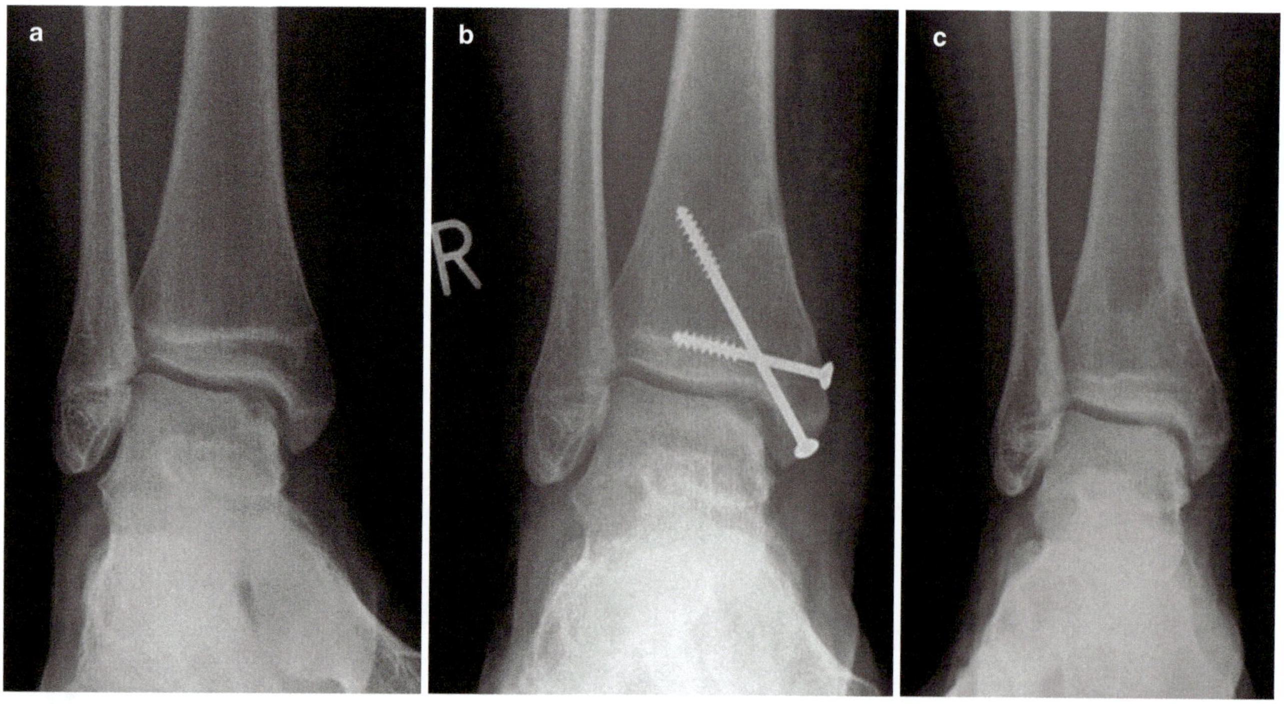

Fig. 9.7 15-Year-old patient with complaints since 3 years (**a**). A large osteochondral lesion of the medial edge of the talus was treated with cancellous bone graft and AMIC membrane covering after medial malleolar osteotomy (**b**). 5 years after the procedure, the patient is free of complaints. A smaller residual defect is still visible (**c**)

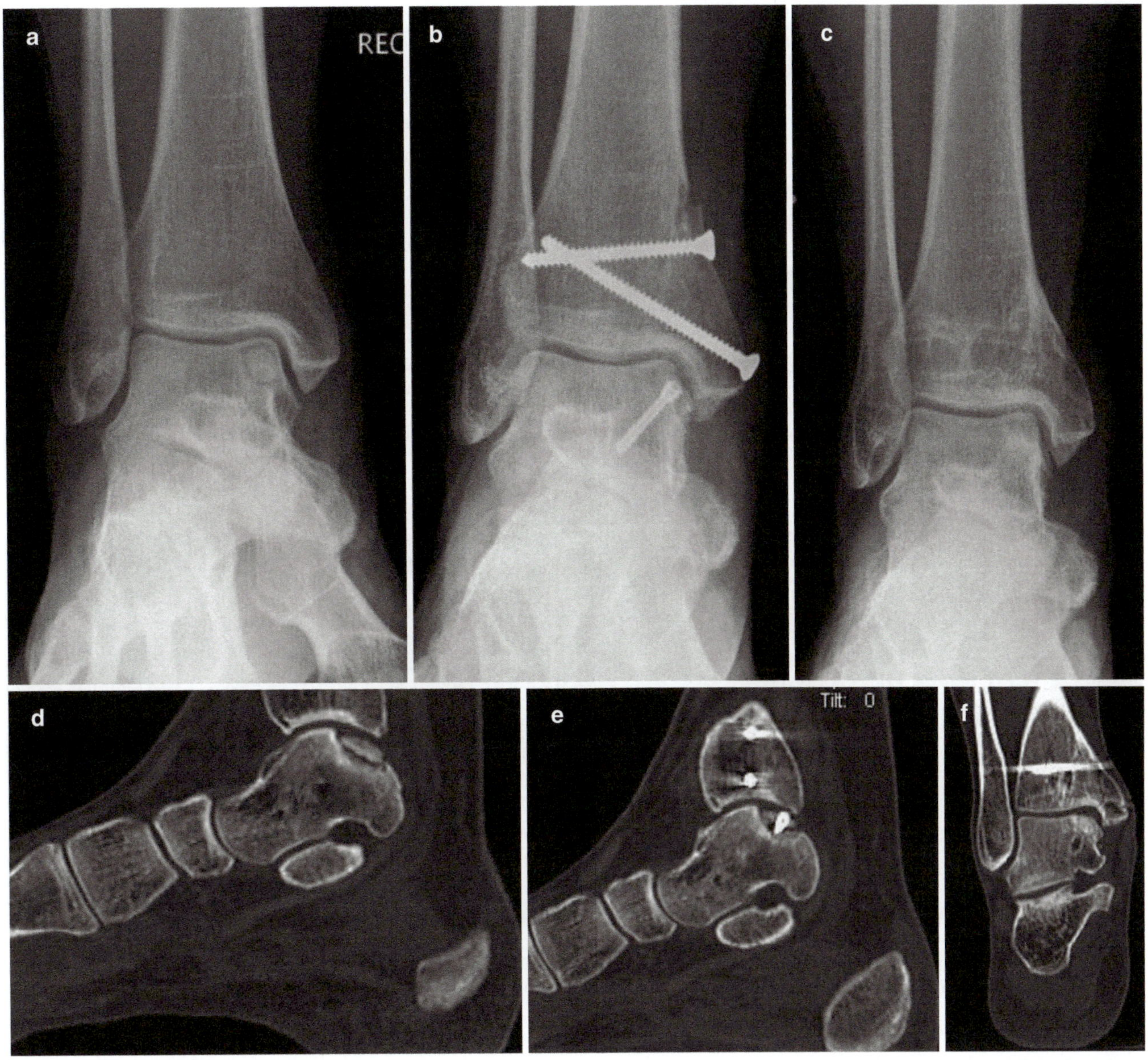

Fig. 9.8 18-Year-old female patient with large osteochondral fragment at the dorsomedial talus (**a**, **d**). Cancellous bone graft with refixation (**b**) resulted in incomplete healing with persisting symptoms (**e**). Therefore, 1 year later, cancellous bone graft with AMIC membrane covering was performed with good radiological and clinical results 3 years postoperatively (**c**, **f**)

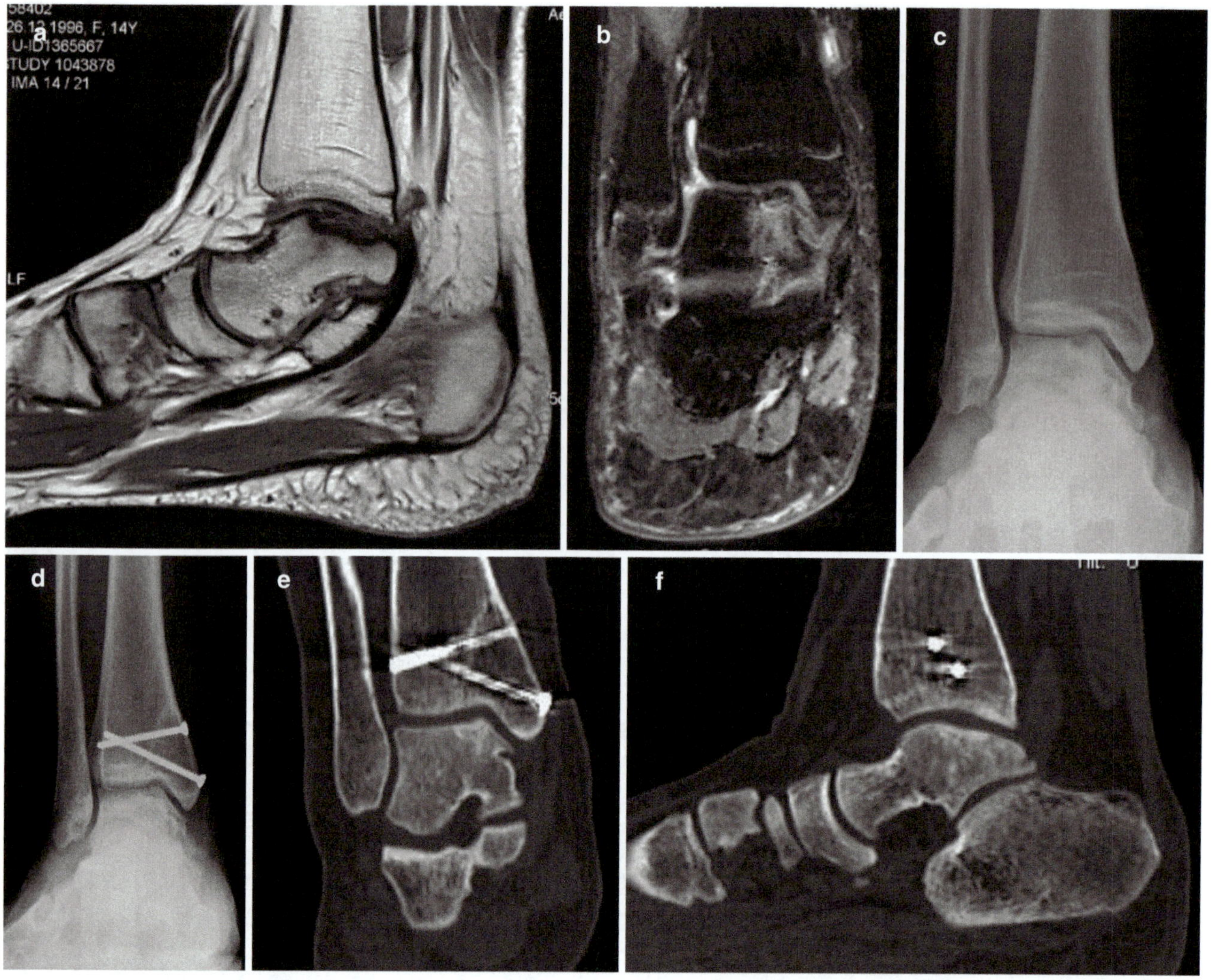

Fig. 9.9 18-Year-old female patient with large medial osteochondral talar lesion (**a**–**c**). One year after cancellous bone graft and covering with AMIC membrane, extensive filling of the defect, however, in CT incomplete congruence of the talar joint surface (**d**–**f**)

References

D'Ambrosi R, Maccario C, Ursino C et al (2017) Combining microfractures, autologous bone graft, and autologous matrix-induced chondrogenesis for the treatment of juvenile osteochondral talar lesions. Foot Ankle Int 38:485–495

Gottschalk O, Altenberger S, Baumbach S et al (2017) Functional medium-term results after autologous matrix-induced chondrogenesis for osteochondral lesions of the talus: a 5-year prospective cohort study. Foot Ankle Surg 56:930–936

Hamel J (2016) Anatomische Außenbandrekonstruktion mit freiem Sehnentransplantat bei schwerer Instabilität des oberen Sprunggelenkes. In: Hamel J, Zwipp H (eds) Sprunggelenk und Rückfuß. Springer-Verlag, Berlin, Heidelberg

Jurina A, Dimnjakovic D, Mustapic M, Smoljanovic T, Bojanic I (2018) Clinical and MRI Outcomes after surgical treatment of osteochondral lesions of the talus in skeletally immature children. J Pediatr Orthop 38:122–127

Masquijo JJ, Ferreyra A, Baroni E (2016) Arthroscopic retrograde drilling in juvenile osteochondritis dissecans of the talus. J Pediatr Orthop 36:589–593

Paul J, Imhoff AB (2016) Osteochondrale Läsion des Talus. In: Hamel J, Zwipp H (eds) Meistertechniken in der operativen Orthopädie und Unfallchirurgie—Sprunggelenk und Rückfuß. Springer-Verlag, Berlin, Heidelberg, pp 49–54

Paul J, Sagstetter A, Kriner M, Imhoff AB, Spang J, Hinterwimmer S (2009) Donor-site morbidity after osteochondral autologous transplantation for lesions of the talus. J Bone Joint Surg 91-A:1683–1688

Reilingh ML, Kerkhoffs GMMJ, Telkamp CJA, Struijs PAA, van Dijk CN (2014) Treatment of osteochondral defects of the talus in children. Knee Surg Sports Traumatol Arthrosc 22:2243–2249

Walther M, Becher C, Volkering C et al (2012) Therapie chondraler und osteochondraler Defekte am Talus durch Autologe Matrix Induzierte Chondrogenese. FussSprungg 10:121–129

Wiewiorski M, Werner L, Paul J, Anderson AE, Barg A, Valderrabano V (2016) Sports activity after reconstruction of osteochondral lesions of the talus with autologous spongiosa grafts and autologous matrix-induced chondrogenesis. Am J Sports Med 44(10):2651–2658

Middle-Forefoot Deformities in Children

10

Contents

The isolated mid-forefoot deformities in the growth age shall be described. Forefoot involvement in complex deformities, such as claw-toe problems in cavovarus deformities (Sect. 7.12) and dorsal bunion as an overcorrection phenomenon in idiopathic clubfoot and also skew foot deformity (Chap. 2), is dealt with in the corresponding chapters.

10.1 Typical Deformities of the First Ray in Growth Age

10.1.1 Juvenile Hallux-Valgus-Syndrome

Already at an early school age—primarily in girls—a combined malposition of the first ray is often observed, which is very similar to the adult form in most aspects and frequently the precursor of a typical hallux valgus in adult age. Etiologically, a genetic disposition, as well as the constitutional type of the connective tissue (especially, e.g., Marfan syndrome, Trisomy 21), are apparently important here; the role of constricting footwear already in childhood is not conclusively clarified. A radiomorphological feature of the juvenile form is in some cases the altered contour of the metatarsal I joint surface with a lateral indentation (Fig. 10.4), the often clearly pathological distal joint surface angle (Fig. 10.6), and the usually absent or, compared to the adult form, low expression of the medial pseudoexostosis. The following aspects require special attention in indication and treatment of juvenile hallux valgus syndrome:

- The decentering of the metatarsophalangeal joint in growth age can contribute to an osseous maldevelopment of the joint partners (form follows function), e.g., to a lack of development of the plantar guide ridge of the metatarsal I head, or to a lack of cartilage development of the medial metatarsal I head (Fig. 10.1). Dys- and aplasia of the sesamoids are observed in the juvenile hallux valgus syndrome.
- Significant malpositioning can have a negative growth-directing effect on the neighboring toes.

J. Hamel, *Foot and Ankle Surgery in Children and Adolescents*, https://doi.org/10.1007/978-3-030-58108-4_10

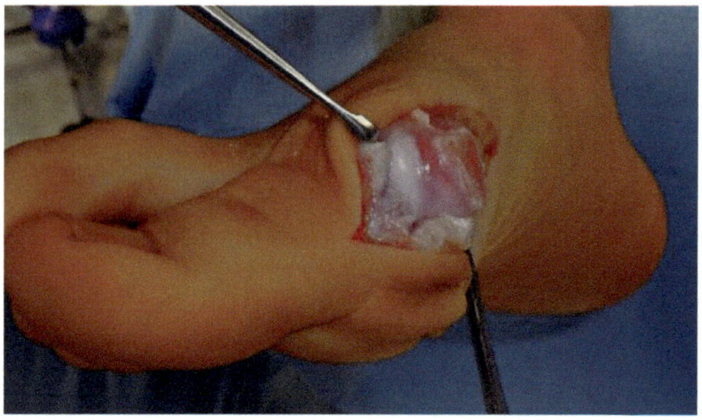

Fig. 10.1 Absence of cartilage cover of the medial metatarsal I head in juvenile hallux valgus. Due to the defective containment caused by the malalignment, the articular cartilage cannot develop

- All surgical measures must take into account the growth and development potential, especially in the area of the epiphyseal plates.

10.1.1.1 Indication for Surgery

As in adults, the indication boundaries are not sharply defined. In the literature, surgical interventions in the growth age are sometimes generally advised against—in the author's experience to some extent wrongly (Fuhrmann 2013; Ricco et al. 2014). However, the following aspects should be considered from the author's point of view in childhood:

- Slight deformities should not be surgically corrected in the growth age, among other reasons because of the increased risk of recurrence and overcorrection before the end of growth. However, in the case of pronounced deformities, correction can be carried out well before the end of growth.
- Caution with girls in the peripubertal age group. Here, inadequate expectations on the part of the child (and parents) and sometimes insufficient compliance often make follow-up treatment difficult.
- The use of redressive (night-) splints for growth modification and to avoid progression can be integrated into the treatment concept and delay a surgical intervention.

The overall constellation of the patient in childhood and adolescence must always be taken into consideration: In the case of a pronounced planovalgus deformity, an additional hindfoot correction is necessary (Fig. 10.8), since otherwise an increased risk of recurrence must be expected. Especially in the case of hallux valgus of the juvenile patient with cerebral palsy, an isolated forefoot correction is rarely advisable, since disorders and deformities of the entire lower extremity are usually present (see Chap. 6). In the case of generalized hypermobility, permanent correction results of non-fusing interventions are not to be expected and surgical treatment is better scheduled for later in life.

10.1.1.2 Standard Surgical Technique

As a standard procedure, the author considers a combination of Scarf osteotomy of the metatarsal I (Fuhrmann 2013), common in adult foot surgery, with a distal soft tissue intervention and an osteotomy with varus effect to the phalangeal base, carefully preserving the growth plate (Fig. 10.2). With the Scarf osteotomy, a wide shift for reduction of the usually significantly increased intermetatarsal I–II angle is possible without worsening the joint surface angle and without disturbing the proximal metatarsal I growth plate. A distal metatarsal I osteotomy (Fig. 10.7) is also possible, or a metatarsal I double osteotomy, in which—taking the growth plate into account—an angulation in the area of the metatarsal I base is combined with a correction of the distal articular surface angle by distal osteotomy.

Technique Scarf Osteotomy with Soft Tissue Correction and Phalangeal Osteotomy

From a medial longitudinal incision, the metatarsophalangeal joint capsule is exposed in an epicapsular fashion and opened dorsotibially lengthwise. A pseudoexostosis is usually not developed, but the medial side of the metatarsal I head is trimmed with the oscillating saw to induce a stable capsular scar fixation. An intra-articular and occasionally pain-causing meniscoid can often be detected and should be resected, corresponding to a rupture of the deep layer of the medial collateral ligament. In mild cases, lateral release can be performed transarticularly as a horizontal splitting of the sesamoidal ligament complex; in more pronounced cases, a separate approach is advisable, with which the adductor-hallucis tendon can also be detached from the phalangeal base under visual control. A transfer to the metatarsal I (McBride 1967) should be considered at best in the case of neurogenic hallux valgus in the context of cerebral palsy. A Scarf osteotomy is performed using a target K-wire and a saw gauge. As a rule, this does not have to extend beyond the proximal one-third limit of the metatarsal I and thus does not affect the proximally located growth plate. After sufficient mobilization, the distal-plantar fragment can be shifted medially, whereby a correction of the distal articular surface angle can also be achieved by slight rotation in the transverse plane. Fixation is performed with threaded K-wires (Fig. 10.3), resorbable screws (Fig. 10.4) or double threaded screws.

The metatarsal I head is repositioned onto the sesamoid bone plate by means of medial capsuloplasty with Vicryl-0 sutures placed in a pulley-like manner. Afterwards, it is particularly important to make sure that a complete correction of the joint is achieved without signs of overcorrection. Since there is usually still a residual valgus of the toe after this, it is fully corrected distal to the phalangeal growth plate by tibial-based wedge removal. In this case, percutaneous K-wire stabilization for about 3 weeks is usually sufficient (Fig. 10.5).

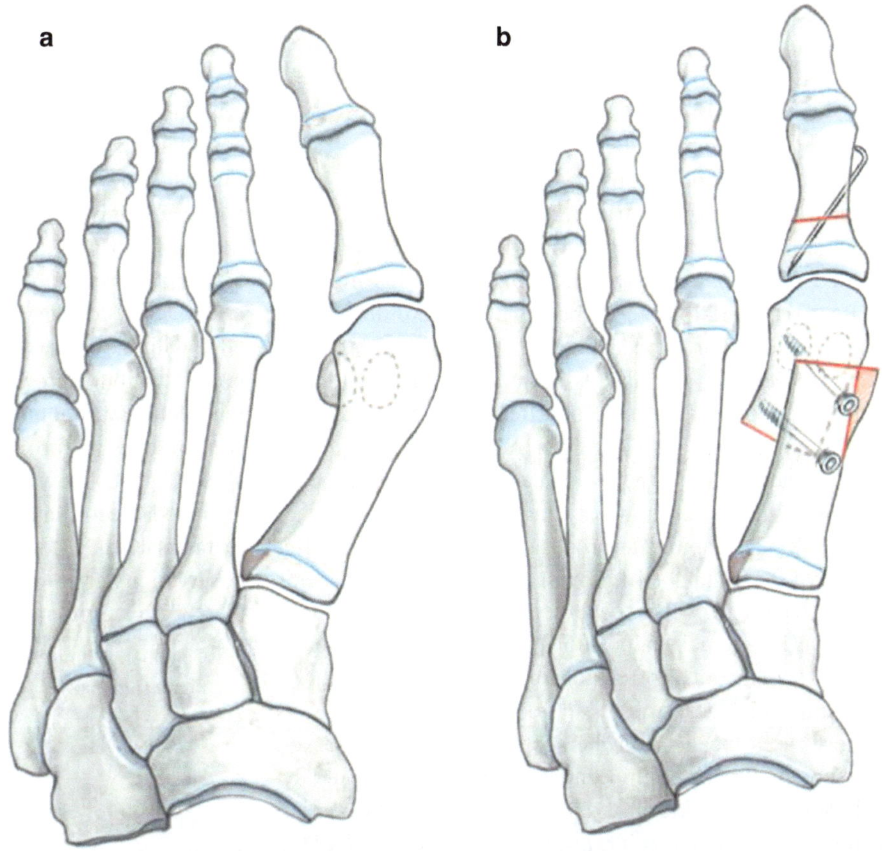

Fig. 10.2 Correction of the juvenile hallux valgus deformity (**a**) with a (short) Scarf osteotomy with slight rotation of the distal fragment to address the distal articular surface angle and additional Akin osteotomy distally of the phalangeal growth plate (**b**)

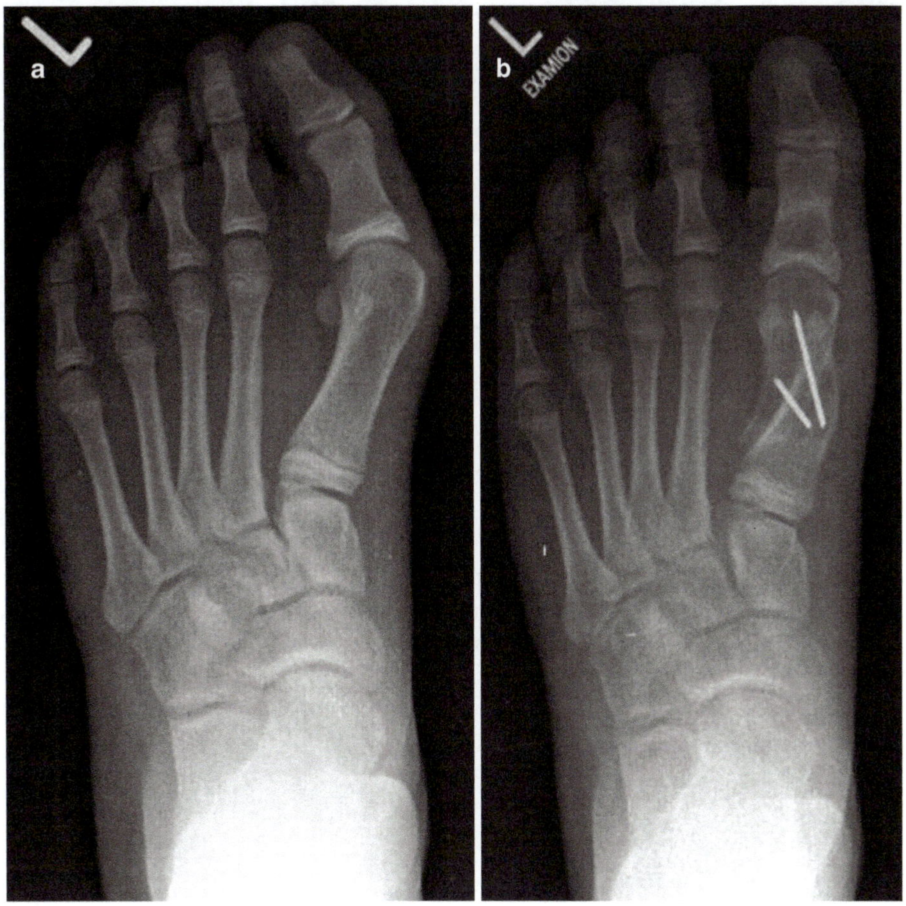

Fig. 10.3 12-Year-old girl with juvenile hallux valgus before (**a**) and after combined bony and soft tissue correction with Scarf osteotomy, soft tissue recentering, and phalangeal osteotomy (**b**)

Three treatment examples will explain this standard procedure and its effect (Figs. 10.3, 10.4, and 10.5).

10.1.1.3 Specifics of the Juvenile Hallux Valgus Correction

The treatment of the soft tissues is essential also in a juvenile hallux valgus. The transfer of the tendon of the M. adductor hallucis according to McBride (1967) was recommended in the past. As shown in Fig. 10.6, this measure is effective in the long term, but its effects are difficult to dose. On the other hand, if the soft tissues are not rebalanced sufficiently, a relapse is not uncommon (Fig. 10.7). Pronounced planovalgus deformities are also associated with an increased hallux valgus recurrence and should also be treated (Fig. 10.8). In the case of considerable connective tissue weakness—for example, in the context of Trisomy 21—a Lapidus arthrodesis can be performed after closure of the metatarsal I growth plate also in adolescents (Fig. 10.9).

An increased recurrence and overcorrection rate compared to adult hallux valgus patients is to be expected in growing age. Agrawal et al. (2015) found recurrences after Scarf and Akin osteotomy in 29.8% of cases. Coughlin (1995) reported 65 cases of surgical correction of younger patients with hallux valgus development already in childhood or adolescence. However, only seven of these cases were corrected with open growth plates. According to the author's experience, a surgical procedure with cautious indication (see above) can be justified even in growth age. There is no own experience with the lateral hemiepiphysiodesis of the metatarsal I growth plate for growth control and successive reduction of the intermetatarsal angle (Davids et al. 2007). However, this concept does not provide an ad hoc correction, and undesirable effects of growth control in the sagittal plane cannot be excluded. According to Schlickewei et al. (2018), the intermetatarsal angle could be improved by 3.6° in an average observation period of 27 months and the hallux valgus angle by 6.3°; however, an additional night splint was used.

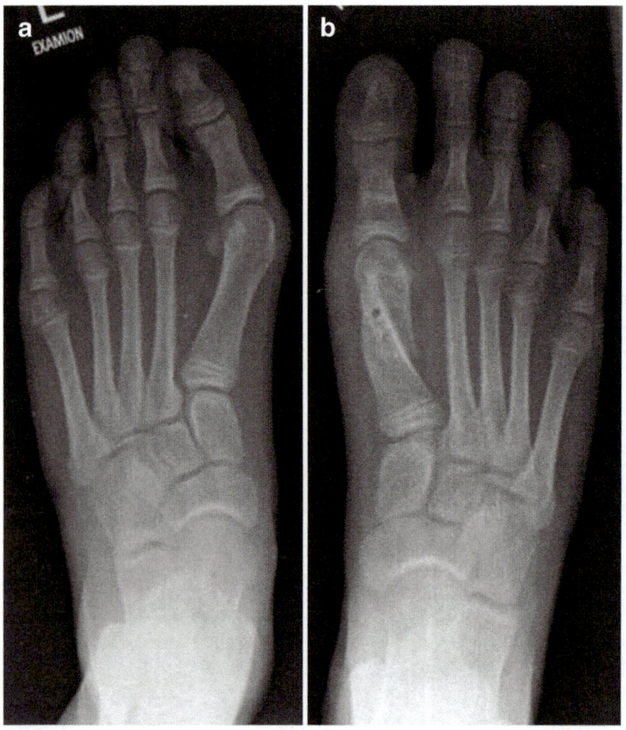

Fig. 10.4 10-Year-old girl with hallux valgus syndrome on the left (**a**) and condition after correction on the right (**b**). Here, resorbable screws could be used for the Scarf osteotomy. A characteristic feature of the juvenile hallux valgus is the slight lateral indentation of the metatarsal I head contour

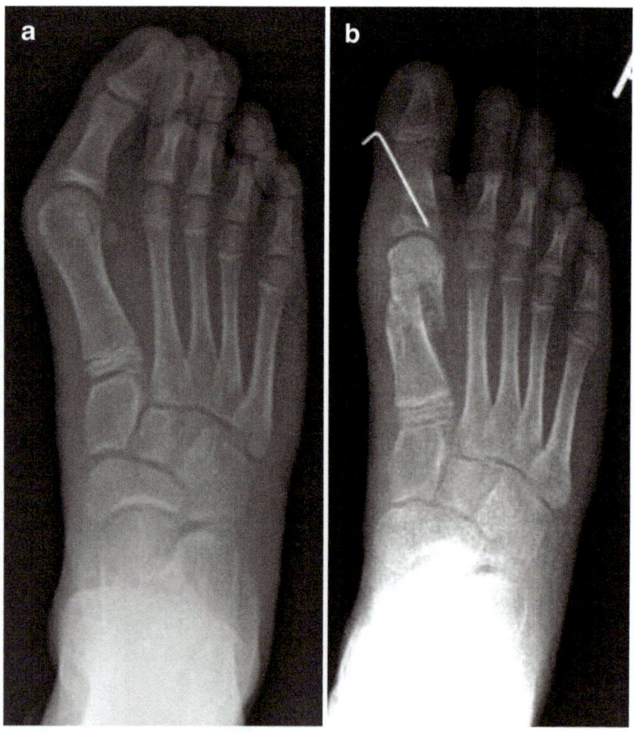

Fig. 10.5 Before (**a**) and after (**b**) short dimensioned Scarf osteotomy with soft tissue recentering and phalangeal osteotomy with attention to the growth plate in an 11-year-old girl. The metatarsal I osteotomy was fixed with resorbable screws

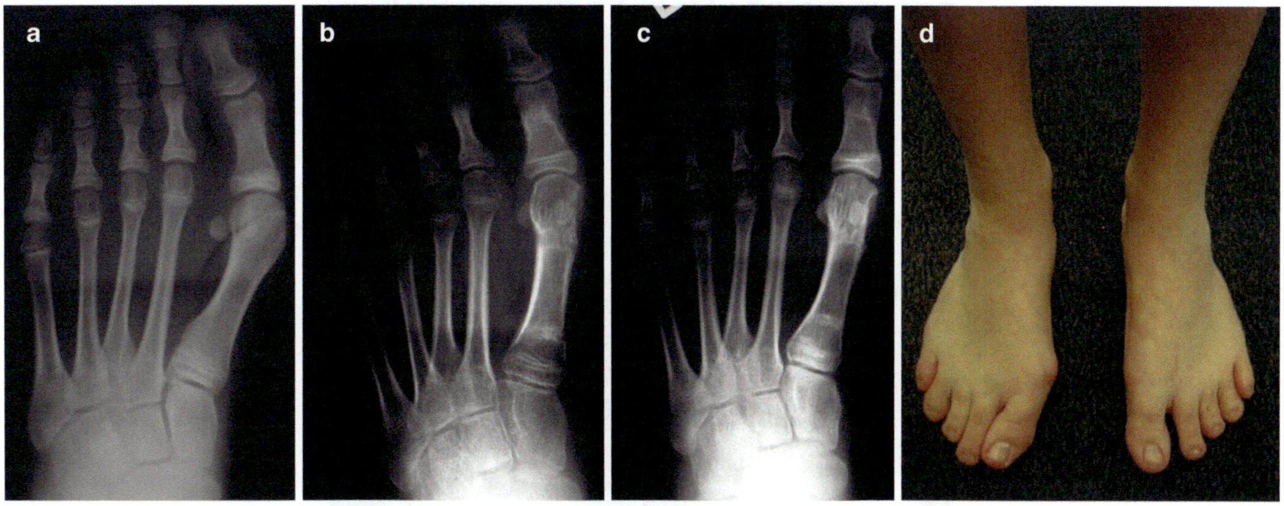

Fig. 10.6 Before (**a**), 6 weeks after (**b**) and 1 year after metatarsal I base osteotomy and McBride procedure (**c**) in a 12-year-old female patient with juvenile hallux valgus syndrome. The retrospective effect of the tendon transfer is clearly visible. In this case it resulted in a good straightening of the big toe, an overcorrection did not occur (**d**)

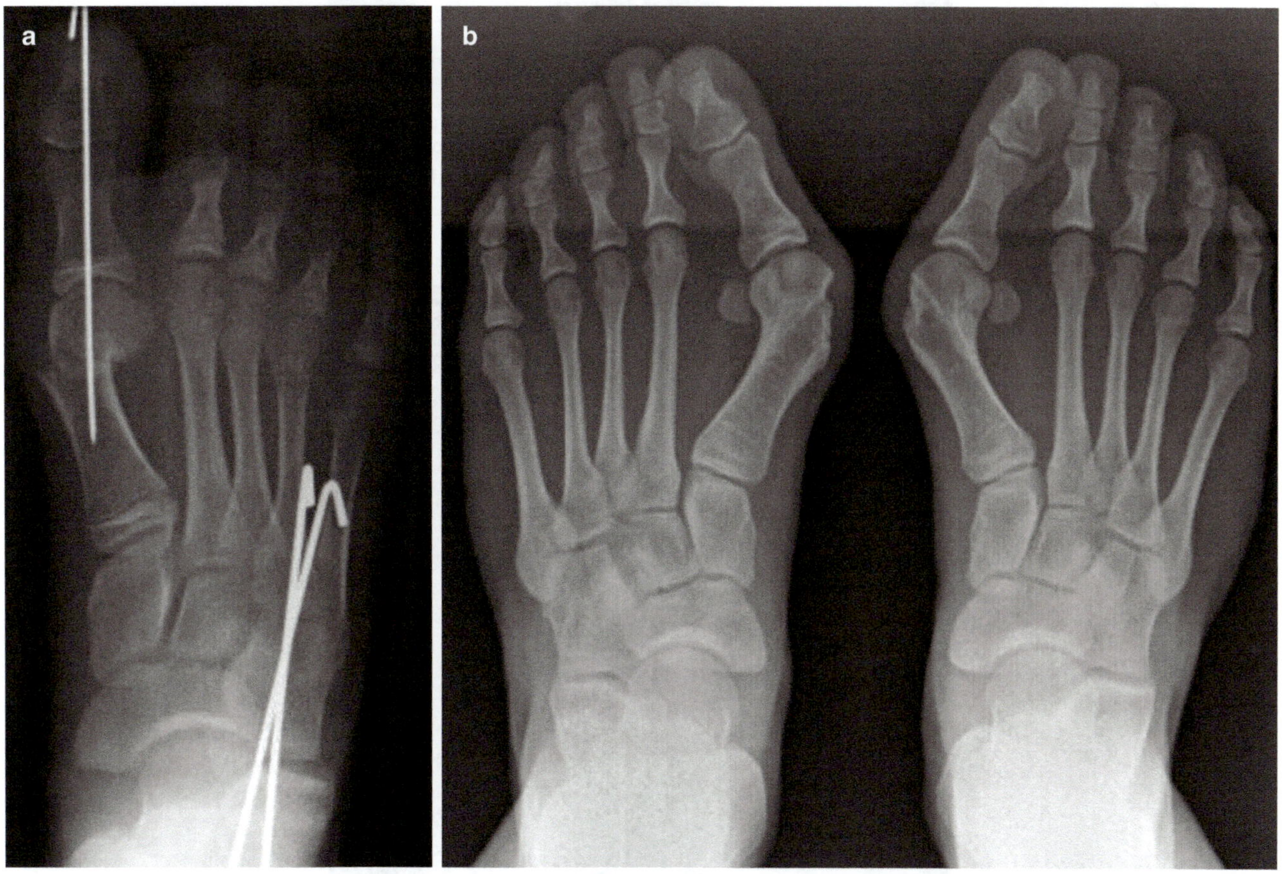

Fig. 10.7 13-Year-old girl with simultaneous hallux valgus correction and calcaneal lengthening osteotomy, performed externally (**a**). 5 Years later severe recurrence of hallux valgus syndrome on both sides (**b**). Presumably the soft tissue recentering measures were not sufficient here

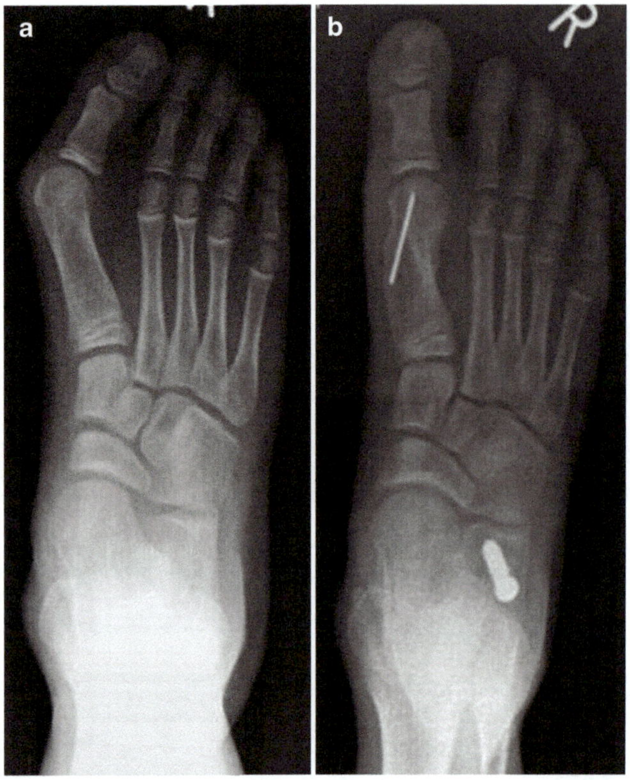

Fig. 10.8 10-Year-old boy with pronounced juvenile hallux valgus syndrome and moderate planovalgus deformity (**a**). In this case, a combined bony and soft tissue correction of the first ray was supplemented with a calcaneostop arthroereisis (Sect. 4.10.2), since the planovalgus deformity could otherwise promote a recurrence of the hallux valgus (**b**)

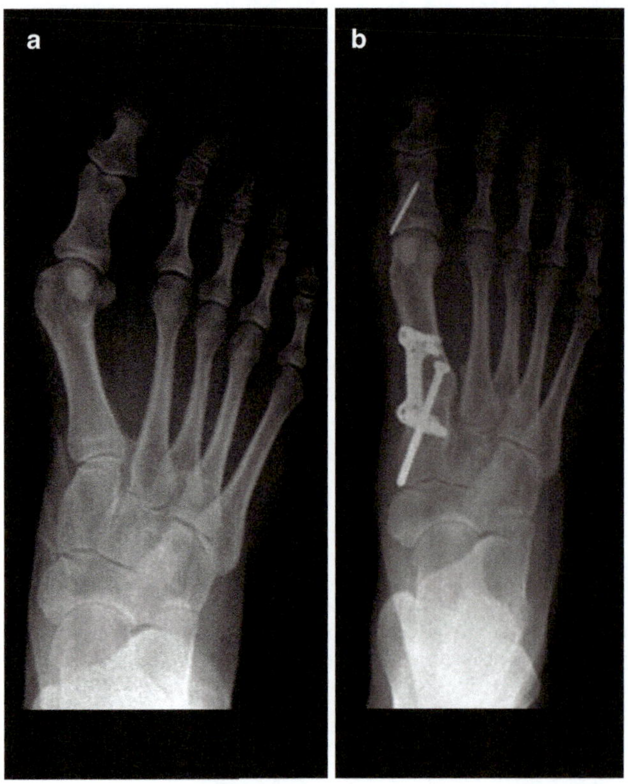

Fig. 10.9 16-Year-old female patient with Trisomy 21, hallux valgus syndrome and Os intermetatarseum before (**a**) and after Lapidus arthrodesis, resection of the Os intermetatarseum and soft tissue recentration combined with phalangeal osteotomy (**b**)

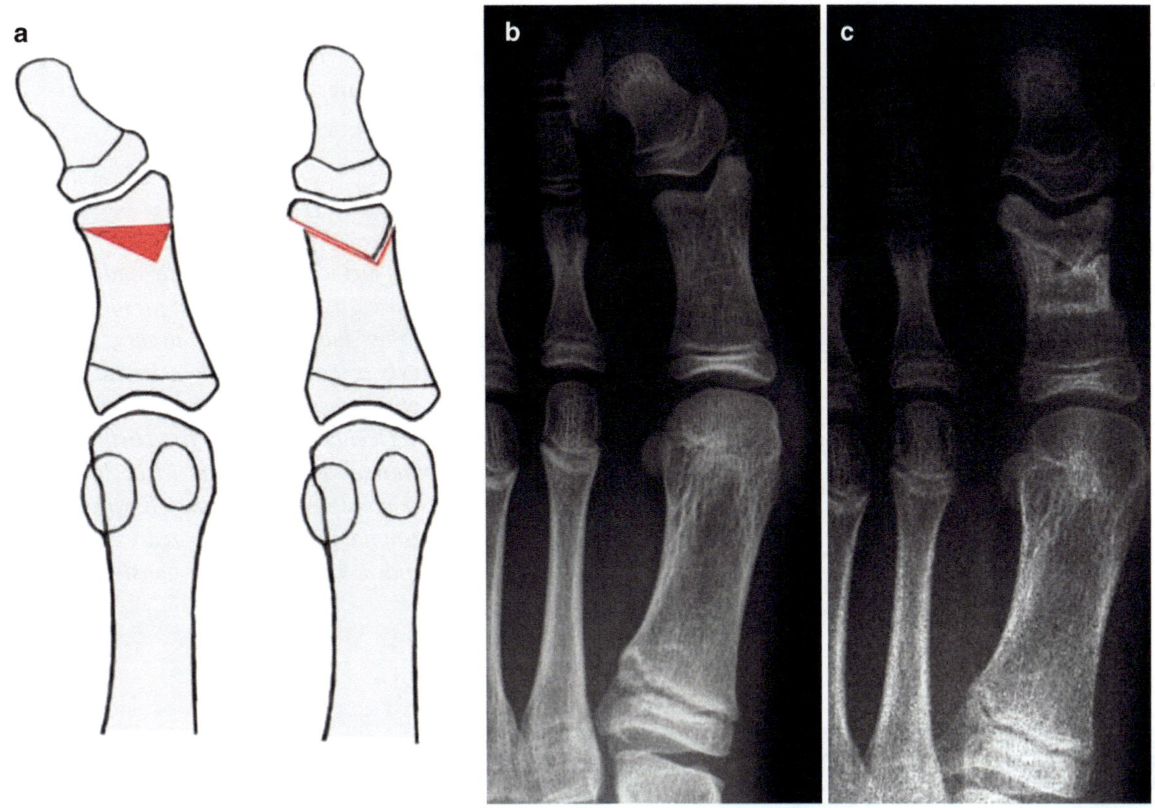

Fig. 10.10 Distal osteotomy of the proximal phalanx for hallux valgus interphalangeus correction (**a**). A groove is cut in the proximal partner of the osteotomy for the distal fragment. On the right, a clinical example (**b**, **c**)

10.1.2 Hallux Valgus Interphalangeus

This is frequently a symmetrically occurring growth disorder of the proximal phalanx of the big toe, which usually manifests itself distinctly in early school age and can cause symptoms such as a shoe conflict or chronically recurring paronychia. The valgus deviation with curvature apex in the distal part of the proximal phalanx is often combined with a flexion contracture of the interphalangeal joint. Since there are no growth zones in the distal phalanx, the deformity can be corrected at any age in pronounced cases and/or with local complaints.

A distal osteotomy of the proximal phalanx with complete dissection in accordance with the principles of CORA (center of rotation of angulation, Paley 2002) is generally capable of correcting all components of the deformity and is preferable to a closed-wedge osteotomy with purely angular effect. In the case of additional flexion contracture of the interphalangeal joint, it is also possible to correct it in the sagittal plane.

Technique

From a medial approach, the proximal phalanx is completely osteotomized distally transversely. A groove is cut in the proximal fragment while preserving the medial corticalis, into which the distal fragment is fitted with rotation and shifting to fibular (Fig. 10.10). The fixation is performed with two K-wires.

10.1.3 Hallux Varus

The deformity occurring at school age is rare and etiologically unexplained. The pathogenetic cause is a muscular imbalance of the muscles that guide the metatarsophalangeal joint. In most cases, there is also a varus position of the small toes (Figs. 2.8 and 10.11). The skew foot deformity must be differentiated from hallux varus, as well as conditions of compensatory hyperactivity of the long toe flexors in the case of severe tarsal instability (e.g., Marfan syndrome) or gastrocnemius weakness, as observed in clubfoot overcorrection. Slight malpositioning can remain as it does not represent a significant functional restriction.

In addition to an intramuscular lengthening of the abductor hallucis muscle and a medial soft-tissue release, ligamentoplasty for reinforcement of the lateral capsule of the metatarsophalangeal joint using a distally-rooted extensor hallucis brevis tendon can be performed (Fig. 10.12). Bony corrections, similar to procedures for iatrogenic overcorrection after hallux valgus surgery in adults (reversed Chevron Osteotomy), are also part of the recentering procedure.

Technique

In addition to further capsuloplastic and osseous corrective measures, as recommended for iatrogenic overcorrection after hallux valgus surgery, the extensor hallucis brevis tendon can be detached at the muscle-tendon junction, passed under the intermetatarsal ligament with a Dechamps awl and fixed to the periosteum of the metatarsal I metaphysis (drill hole or bone anchor also possible). Temporary K-wire fixation of the metatarsophalangeal joint or redressing bandages is recommended, because of the considerable risk of recurrence.

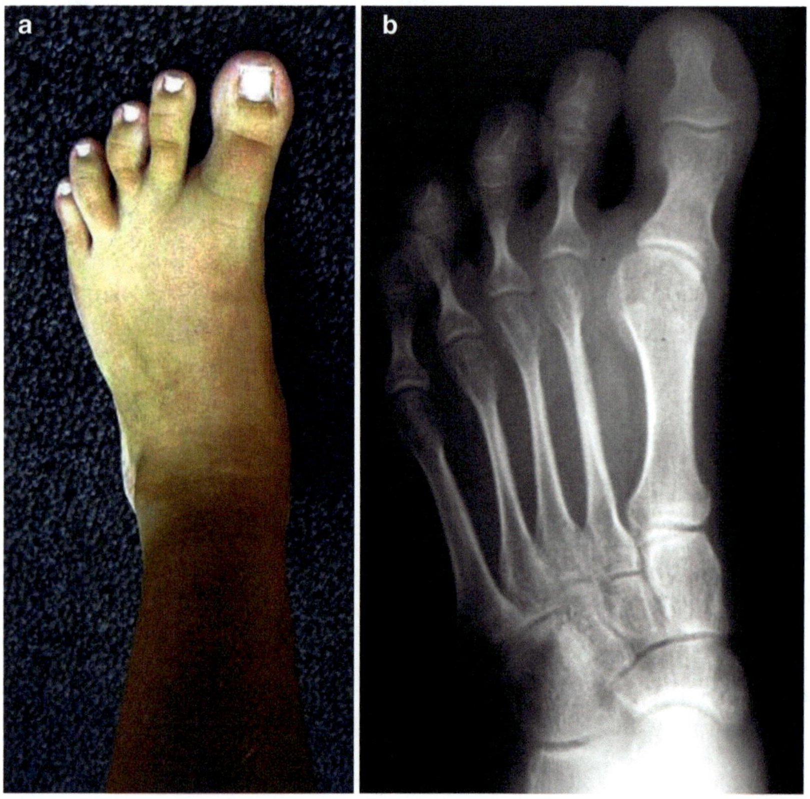

Fig. 10.11 Hallux varus in a child (**a**) with radiological findings (**b**). Note the accompanying adduction of the small toes

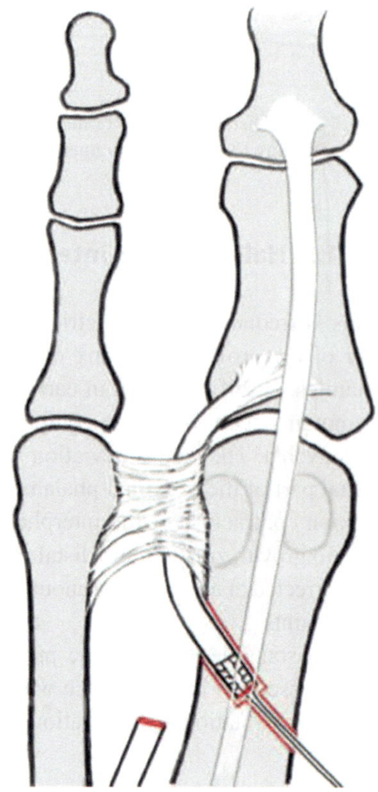

Fig. 10.12 Lateral ligamentoplasty of the metatarsophalangeal joint using the distally stemmed extensor hallucis brevis tendon

10.1.4 Hallux Varus Congenitus

The congenital form of hallux varus is characterized by varus malposition at the metatarsophalangeal and/or the interphalangeal joint region. The pathomorphology is heterogenous and shows a wide range of different phenomena, that may be observed singularly or in combination: e.g. medial tight fibrous band that has to be excised completely, shortened M. abductor hallucis, different forms of preaxial polydactylism, delta phalanx, longitudinal epiphyseal bracket at the first metatarsal. The latter may be strongly widened and shortened in the sense of a duplication (see Sect. 10.3.1), frequently with a growth plate extending far to the medial side ("longitudinal epiphyseal bracket") (Bader et al. 1999; Shim et al. 2014; Mosca 2014). Due to significant progression, a surgical correction should be planned at an early stage, to interrupt the otherwise threatening extreme longitudinal growth disorder. The non-anatomical growth plate located medially at metatarsal I must be completely resected (Figs. 10.13 and 10.14d).

In cases without longitudinal epiphyseal bracket or after closure of the LEB, favorable results have been achieved with osteotomy of the metatarsal I and one-stage lengthening by insertion of a corticospongious bone graft, e.g., from the fibula (Fig. 10.15). The growth disturbance can thereby be overcome. Elaborate soft tissue recentering measures on the metatarsophalangeal joint, abductor hallucis muscle-tendon unit, and skin plastic measures (Fig. 10.14) are additionally required, often also later subsequent interventions.

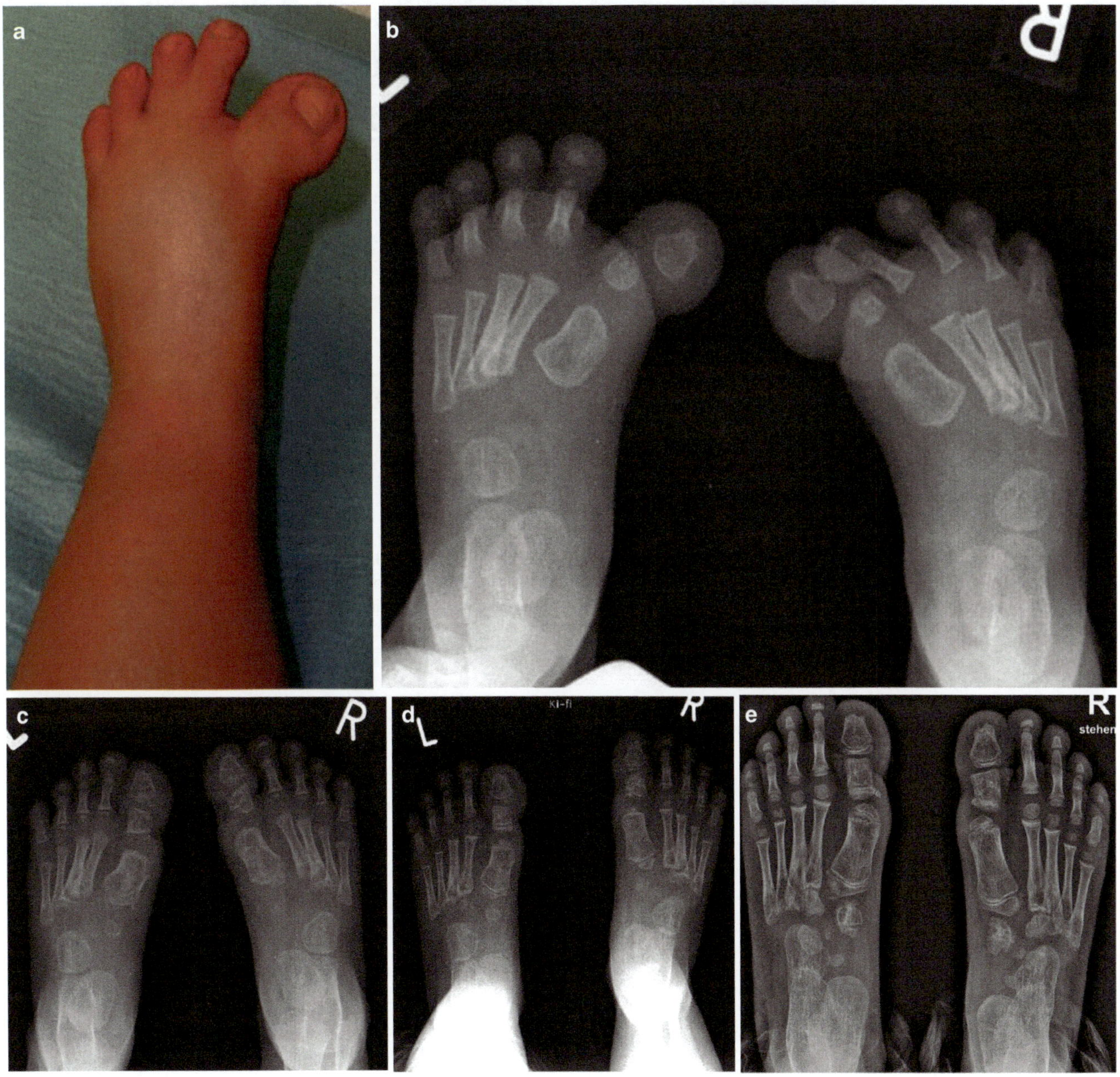

Fig. 10.13 18-Month-old boy with hallux varus congenitus (**a**) with longitudinal epiphyseal bracket at the metatarsal I and delta epiphysis at the proximal phalanx D 1 (**b**). X-ray pre- (**b**), 3 (**c**), 12 (**d**), and 36 months (**e**) postoperatively after resection of the non-anatomical epiphyses and open-wedge osteotomy of metatarsal I and proximal phalanx on both sides. In addition there is a calcaneocuboid synostosis

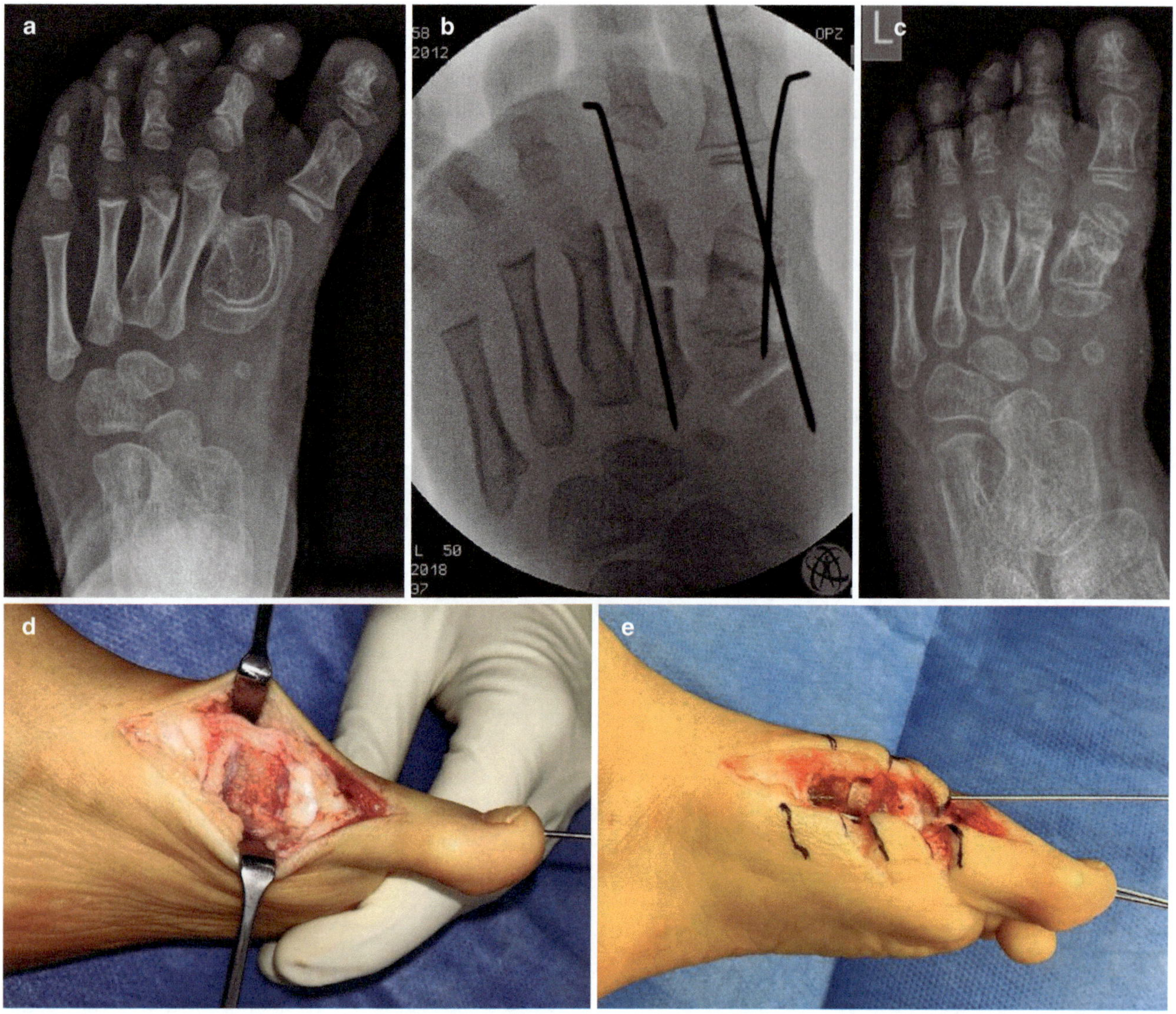

Fig. 10.14 5-Year-old boy with hallux varus congenitus and longitudinal epiphyseal bracket, metatarsal synostosis, long metatarsal II, and talonavicular synostosis (**a**). Metatarsal correction with resection of the LEB (**b**, **d**), osteotomy of the first and second metatarsal, and soft tissue release including Z-plasty of the skin (**e**) resulted in improved alignment (**c**). The resection leaves the medial wall of the first metatarsal bone without any cortical surface (**d**)

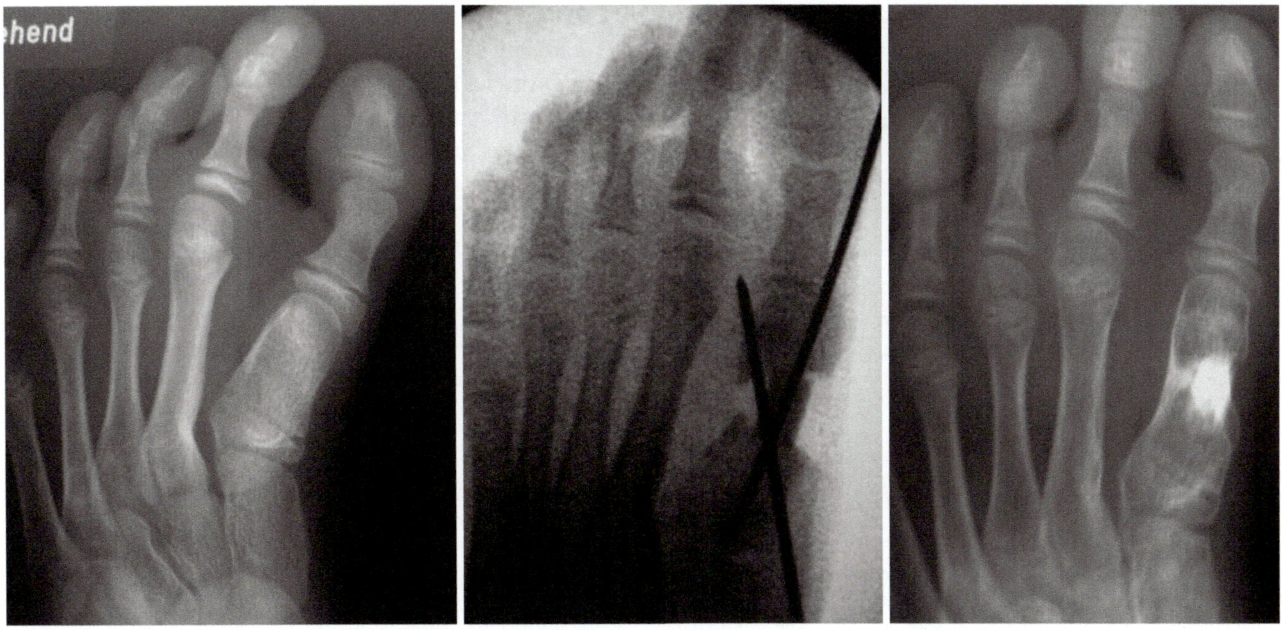

Fig. 10.15 Radiological course of a hallux varus correction by interposition of a fibula graft (the images were kindly provided by Dr. E. Lamprecht, Winterthur)

10.2 Typical Deformities of the Lesser Metatarsophalangeal Rays

10.2.1 Small Toe Flexion Contracture: "Curly Toe"

Especially on the fourth toe ray, flexion contractures are often observed already in infancy, often with additional supination of the toe. Surgical treatment is recommended at the age of about 6 years (Ricco et al. 2014). A percutaneous tenotomy of the long flexor tendon at the level of the metatarsophalangeal joint, using a sharp scalpel or a sharpened needle may be sufficient for correction. A similar procedure is used for toe flexor contractures in the context of clubfoot deformities (Mosca 2014).

10.2.2 Bunionette (Tailor's Bunion)

A widening of the lateral forefoot section with an increased intermetatarsal angle IV/V and varus position of the fifth toe causes a shoe conflict laterally above the metatarsal V-head, which may show a pseudoexostosis in correspondence to the hallux valgus syndrome. Three morphological types of the metatarsal V deformity are distinguished (Fallat and Buckholz 1980): widening of the metatarsal head, increased intermetatarsal angle, and laterally curved metatarsal V shaft. Surgical indication is given for recurrent shoe conflict above the metatarsal V-head on the lateral side in spite of wearing adequate footwear.

In analogy to the Hallux valgus syndrome, a metatarsal osteotomy—depending on the morphological type—must be performed close to the base, at the metatarsal diaphysis or retrocapital with a soft tissue intervention on the metatarsophalangeal joint V (release at the tibial side, capsular reefing at the fibular side). The distal growth plate has to be respected and Chevron or Scarf-like osteotomies have to be performed by open surgery or minimally invasive only after completion of growth.

10.2.3 Digitus Quintus Superductus

Contracted hyperextension of the metatarsophalangeal joint V with or without superductus position of the fifth toe due to additional varus component is usually already recognizable in toddlers. In infancy, successes of very consistent redression treatment (Steristrip) have been reported. In the long term, the deformity regularly leads to pressure sores over the PIP joint of the small toe. The time of correction can be postponed until the shoe conflict manifests itself.

The surgical procedure depends on the severity of the deformity. In mild cases, lengthening of the extensor tendon with release of the metatarsophalangeal joint and Z-plasty of the skin may be sufficient; in more pronounced cases, the Lapidus (1942) procedure (tenodesis with the distally stemmed extensor tendon, which is transferred plantarward around the proximal phalanx and fixed to the abductor digiti minimi muscle), is recommended. Alternatively, the Butler (Cocking 1968) procedure is suggested, in which the small toe is released from all soft tissue connections except the neurovascular bundles and reimplanted further plantar in the soft tissue mantle through a circular incision (Fig. 10.16). Only with the latter procedure is it possible to use the plantar skin excess for a dorsal skin plasty. Experience has shown that the digitus quintus superductus is often underestimated, so that residual deformities or recurrences are not uncommon, depending on the chosen procedure.

Surgical Technique (Butler-Release)

Tennis racket-like incision above the metatarsophalangeal joint of the fifth toe with a circular incision line, which unites plantar to form a short longitudinal incision here (Fig. 10.16a). While carefully preserving the neurovascular structures, the extensor tendons (resection) and dorsal capsule are mobilized to such an extent that the toe can be reimplanted further plantar in the soft tissue mantle without constraint (Fig. 10.16b). In this way, the excess of skin and soft tissue after correction is moved dorsally to where it is needed (Fig. 10.16c). Necrosis and loss of the toe is possible but can usually be avoided in children through careful preparation.

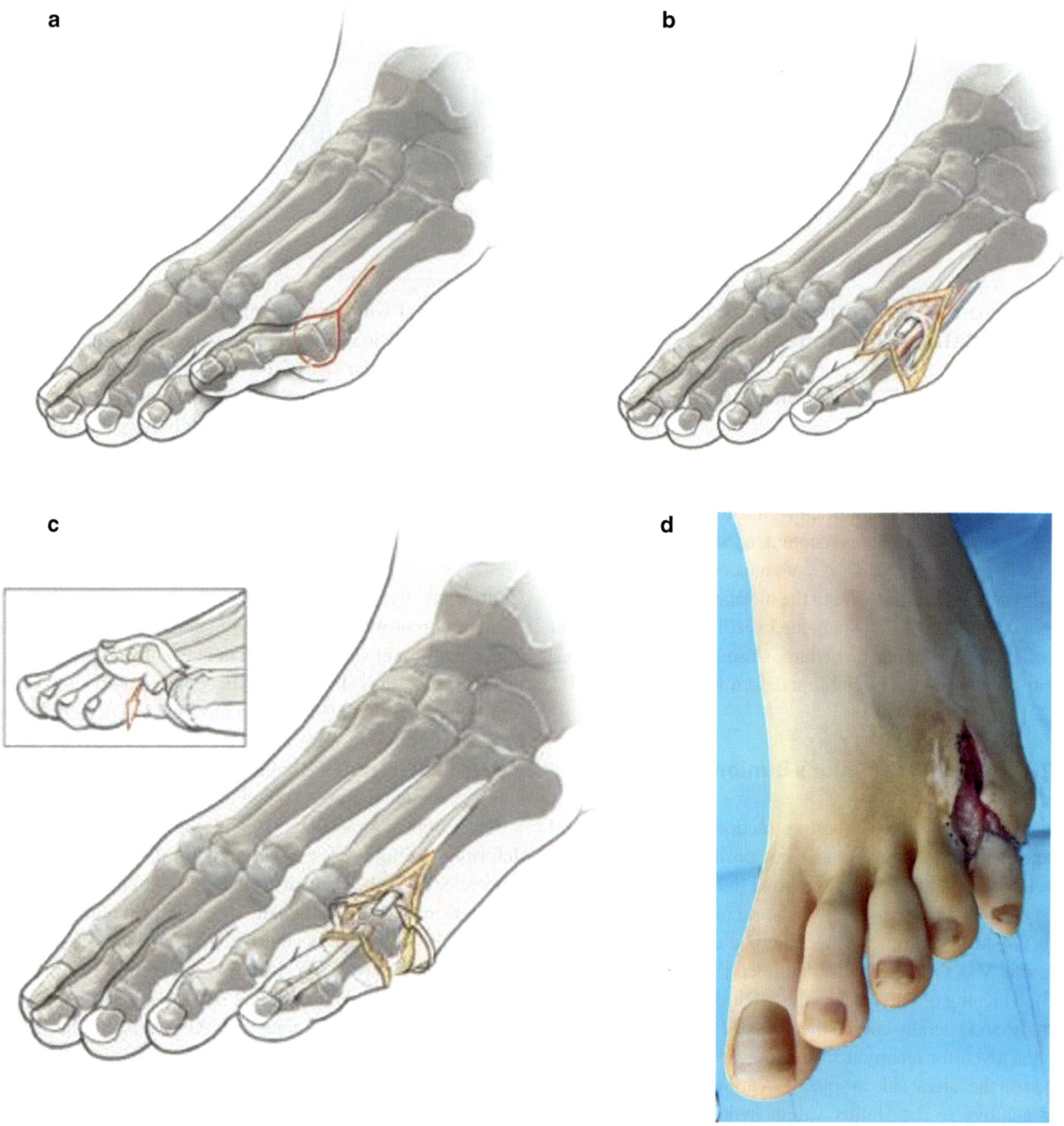

Fig. 10.16 Butler-Release for digitus quintus superductus. The metatarsophalangeal joint region of the fifth toe is circularly incised (**a**), the soft tissue structures are released including the extensor tendon with protection of the neurovascular bundles as far as possible (**b**), the skin is mobilized medial and lateral to shift plantar skin excess to the dorsal region (**c**), and the toe is reimplanted further plantar (**d**) by skin sutures

10.2.4 Morbus Köhler II

Especially in girls, osteonecrosis of the metatarsal II head (Köhler II disease, Freiberg's disease) occurs at an age peak of 13–15 years. The disease leaves a bowl-shaped defect, which is located dorsally and can extend far into the plantar region. In the acute stage, it is advisable to wait until the definite extent of osteonecrosis can be assessed. A reduction of the resulting defect is then possible by means of a wedge-shaped bony resection from the metatarsal head, with which the remaining cartilaginous parts of the head are swivelled into joint contact with the phalangeal joint surface (Fig. 10.17). This procedure is associated with a slight elevation of the head and thus with a relief, which may be desired to a certain degree. Otherwise, the procedure can be combined with a slightly plantarizing osteotomy in the metatarsal II base area (Fig. 10.18). Good functional results can be expected in most cases.

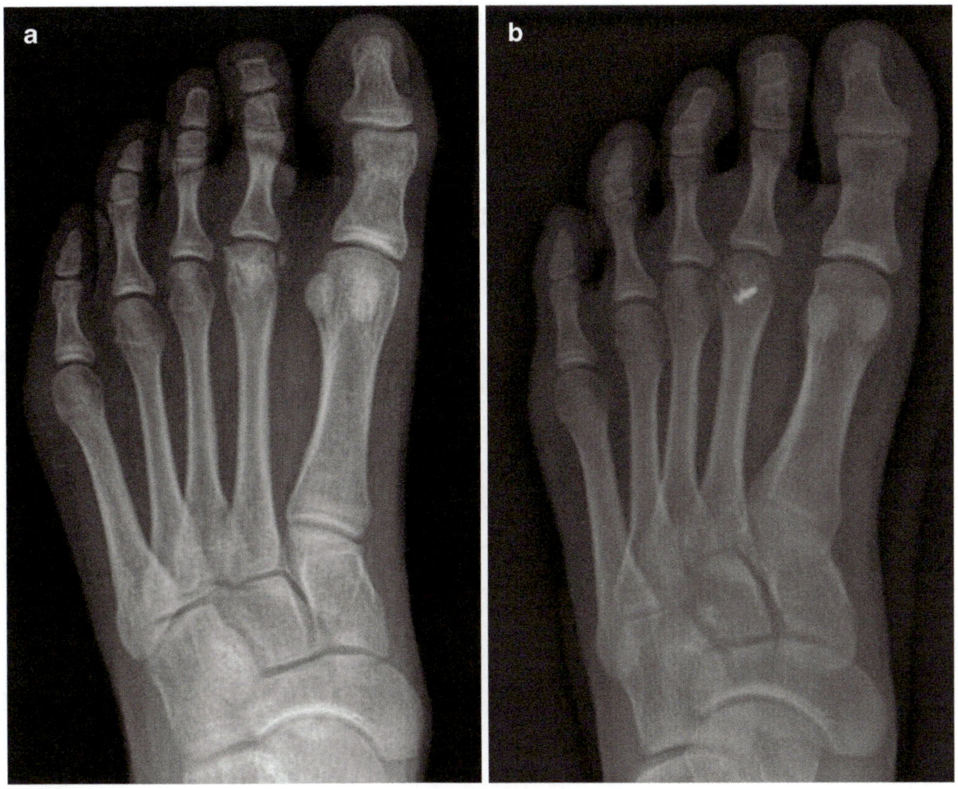

Fig. 10.17 14-Year-old female patient before (**a**) and after (**b**) wedge resection from the defect in Köhler II disease

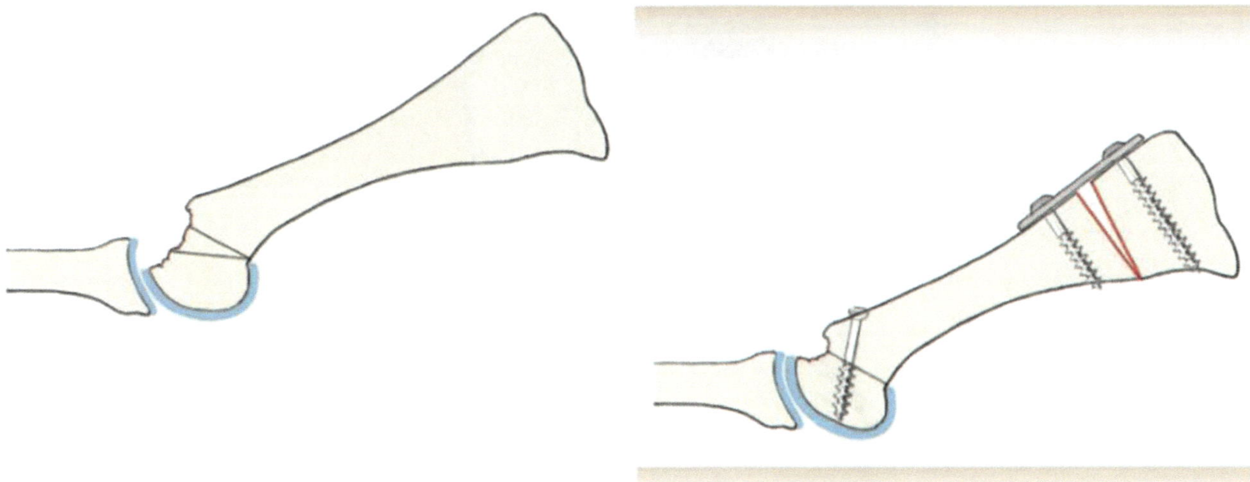

Fig. 10.18 Principle of defect reduction by wedge excision in Köhler's II disease. As a result, parts of the articular surface of the metatarsal head are swung back into the contact zone with the base of the phalanx. The resulting elevation and release of the affected metatarsal can be compensated in pronounced cases by proximal osteotomy

10.3 Disorder of Growth and Differentiation in the Child's Forefoot

10.3.1 Polydactylism

The manifestations of additional ray formations are highly diverse (Bader et al. 1999). Medial (preaxial) (Figs. 10.19 and 10.20), central and—most frequently—lateral (postaxial) manifestations (Figs. 10.21 and 10.22) at different heights (toe type, metatarsal type; classification according to Venn-Watson (1976) or Blauth and Olason (1988)) and in combination with syndactylism or synostosis (Fig. 10.23) are observed. Surgical indication is given in the case of widening of forefoot sections with (foreseeable) shoe conflict; cosmetic aspects are also often decisive for surgical correction.

Some basic rules for the very differentiated choice of procedure are, for instance:

- The hypoplastic ray should be removed (decision sometimes difficult).
- Preservation of the marginal rays 1 and 5 offers advantages.
- Special attention must be paid to the metatarsophalangeal joint (cheilotomy of the metatarsal head, tendon transfer, capsuloplasty).
- Preservation of the mobility of metatarsal rays (Fig. 10.23) (Sahin et al. 2013).

The procedure is carried out under plastic-reconstructive aspects and often goes far beyond a mere "amputation." In most cases it is advisable to wait until the first year of life or when sufficient ossification is achieved, so that the type and extent of the resection can be better planned. Today, an MRI image is also increasingly used for treatment planning (Choi 2018).

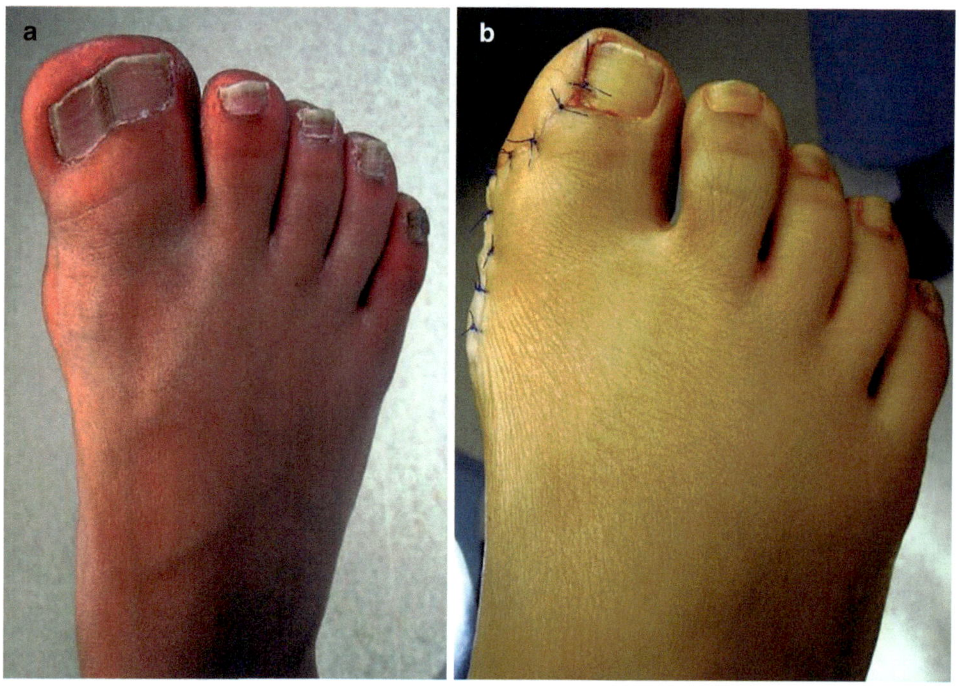

Fig. 10.19 Reduction of a big toe duplication (**a**) with central narrowing of the distal phalanx and partial nail resection (**b**)

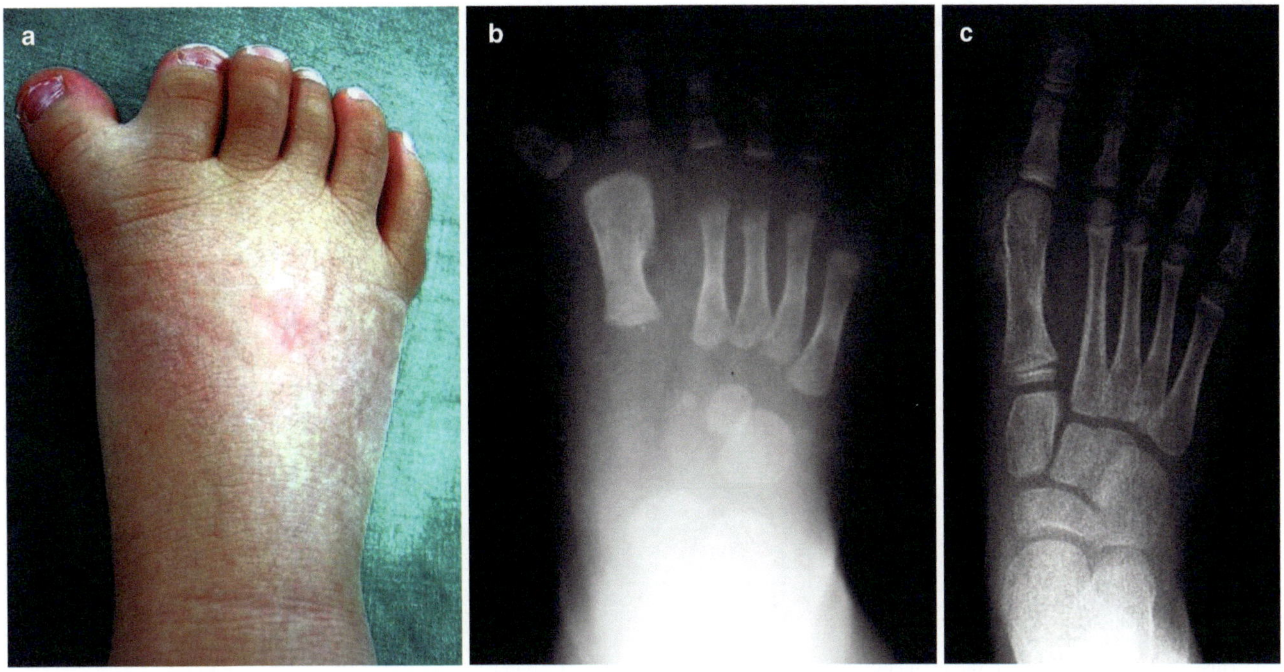

Fig. 10.20 Preaxial polydactyly of the metatarsal type (**a**, **b**). A—not quite complete—cheilotomy of the metatarsal I head with capsuloplasty and transfer of the M. abductor-hallucis tendon to the remaining ray was performed at the age of 12 months. Postoperative image 6 years after surgery (**c**)

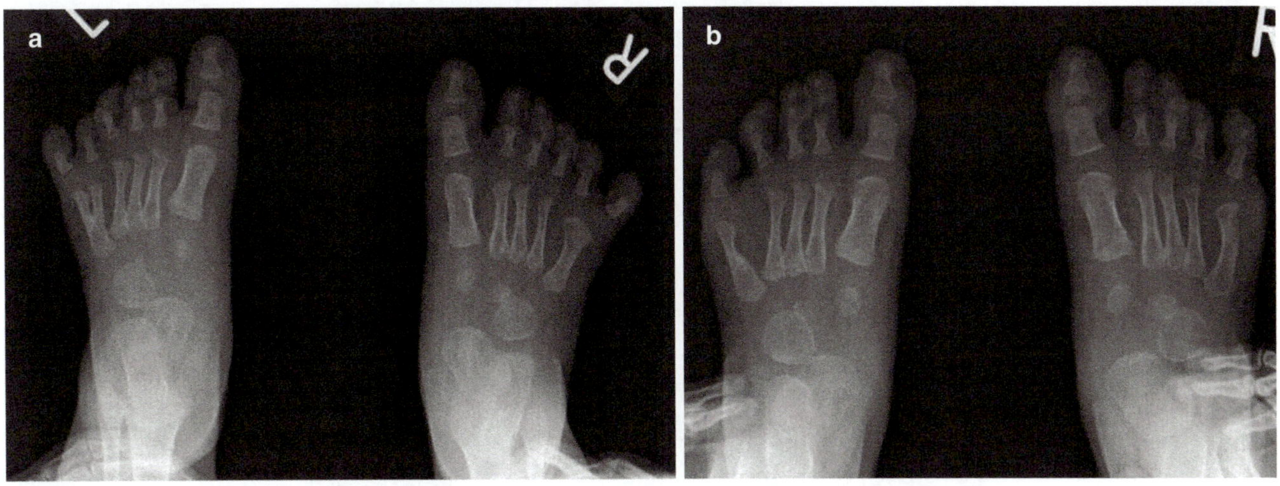

Fig. 10.21 Postaxial polydactyly of the metatarsal type before (**a**) and after surgical correction (**b**) at the age of 2.8 years. On the left, the hypoplastic fifth ray was resected, on the right the marginal ray with performance of also a cheilotomy on the metatarsal V-head

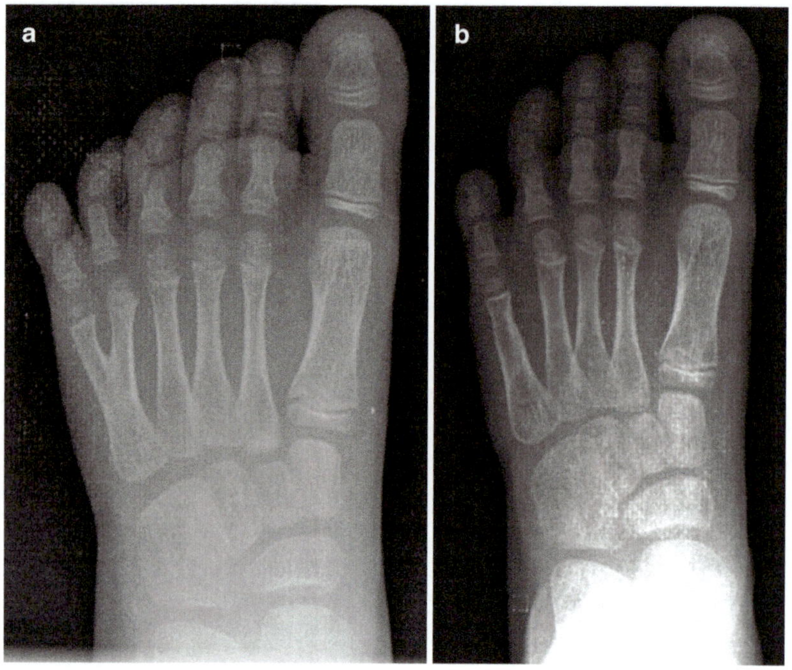

Fig. 10.22 Postaxial polydactyly at the age of 5 years (**a**), resection of the fifth ray, metatarsal osteotomy of the marginal ray, stabilization metatarsal IV/V with tendon graft (**b**)

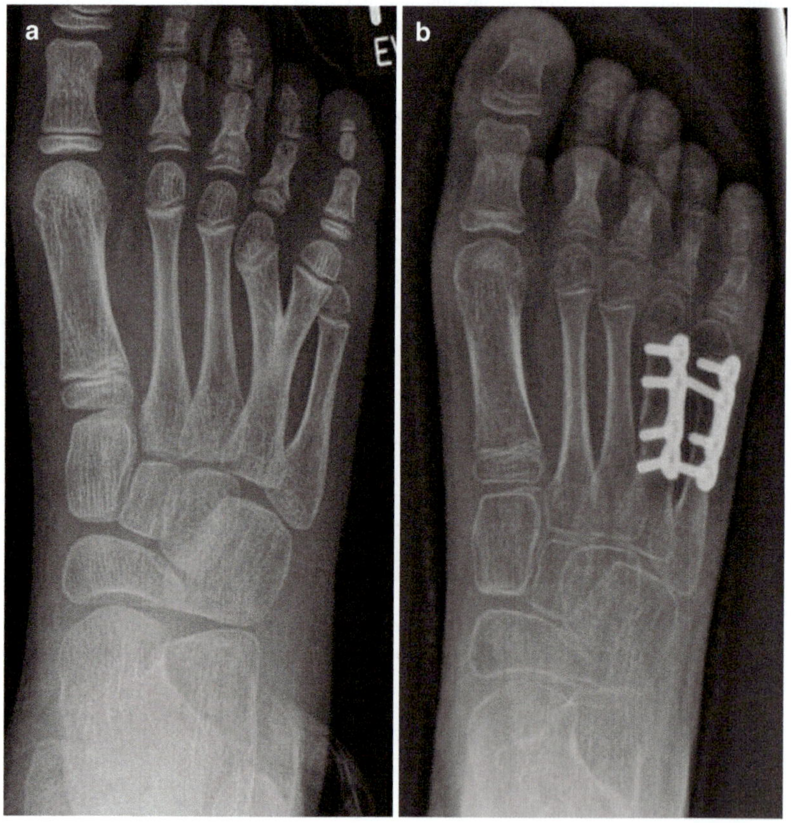

Fig. 10.23 Metatarsal transposition of the distal fifth to the sixth metatarsal with resection of the synostosis of the fourth and fifth metatarsal in a 6-ray midfoot skeleton of an 8-year-old girl (**a**). Postoperatively, the tarsometatarsal and metatarsophalangeal joints could be functionally preserved with free mobility of the metatarsal rays among each other (**b**). This is of great importance for the flexibility especially in the lateral metatarsal region

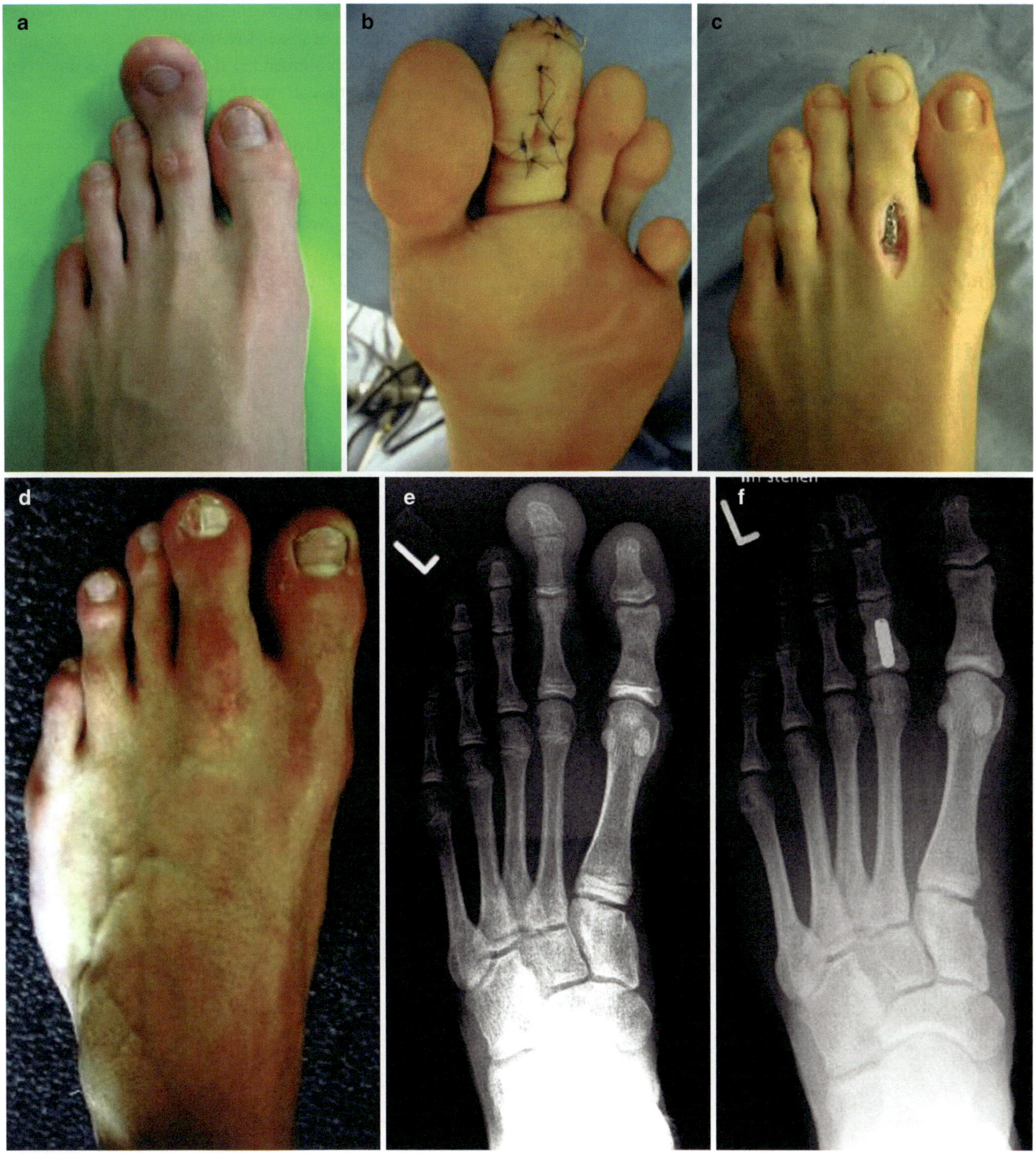

Fig. 10.24 Reduction of a macrodactyly of the second toe ray (**a**, **e**) by soft tissue reduction in combination with shortening osteotomy and phalangeal epiphysiodesis (**b**–**d**, **f**). Alternatively, ray resection including metatarsal II should be discussed

10.3.2 Macrodactylism

The excessive bone and soft tissue growth in the toe or even metatarsal area of individual rays (Fig. 10.24) occurs in connection with superordinate syndromes, but also singularly. As a rule, it represents a very difficult problem for the foot surgeon. The extent, localization, and prognostic aspects determine the indication and timing of often multiple surgical interventions. Soft tissue reduction, bony shortening or epiphysiodesis (Fig. 10.24), partial amputation or ray resection (Figs. 10.25 and 10.26) should be considered in each individual case. According to Chang et al. (2002) ray resection is superior to other procedures for most cases of lesser ray involvement, whereas multiple surgeries are recommended if the great toe is involved. The following in particular must be taken into account:

- The soft tissue part of the malformation is easily underestimated.
- Every measure that shortens the bone leads to an—undesirable—increase in circumference.
- A three- or four-ray foot after ray resection can provide a cosmetically and functionally very satisfying result.

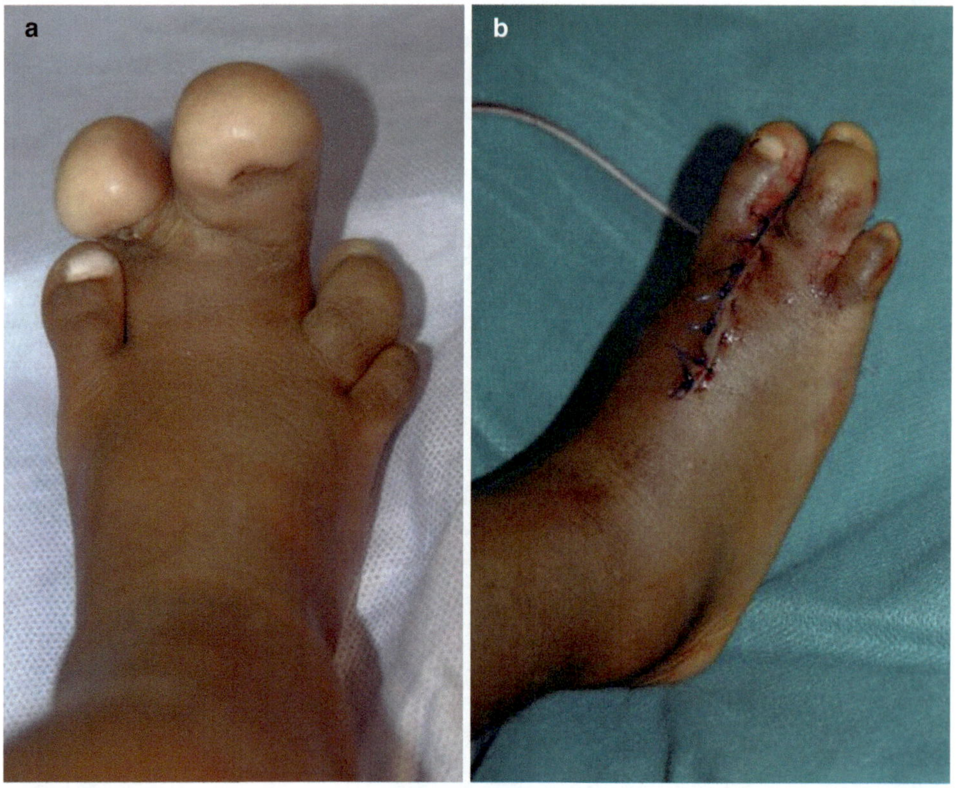

Fig. 10.25 Macrodactyly of the central mid-forefoot (**a**). Ray resection of the second and third ray. The fourth ray, which is also affected, was left in place to avoid excessive narrowing of the metatarsus (**b**)

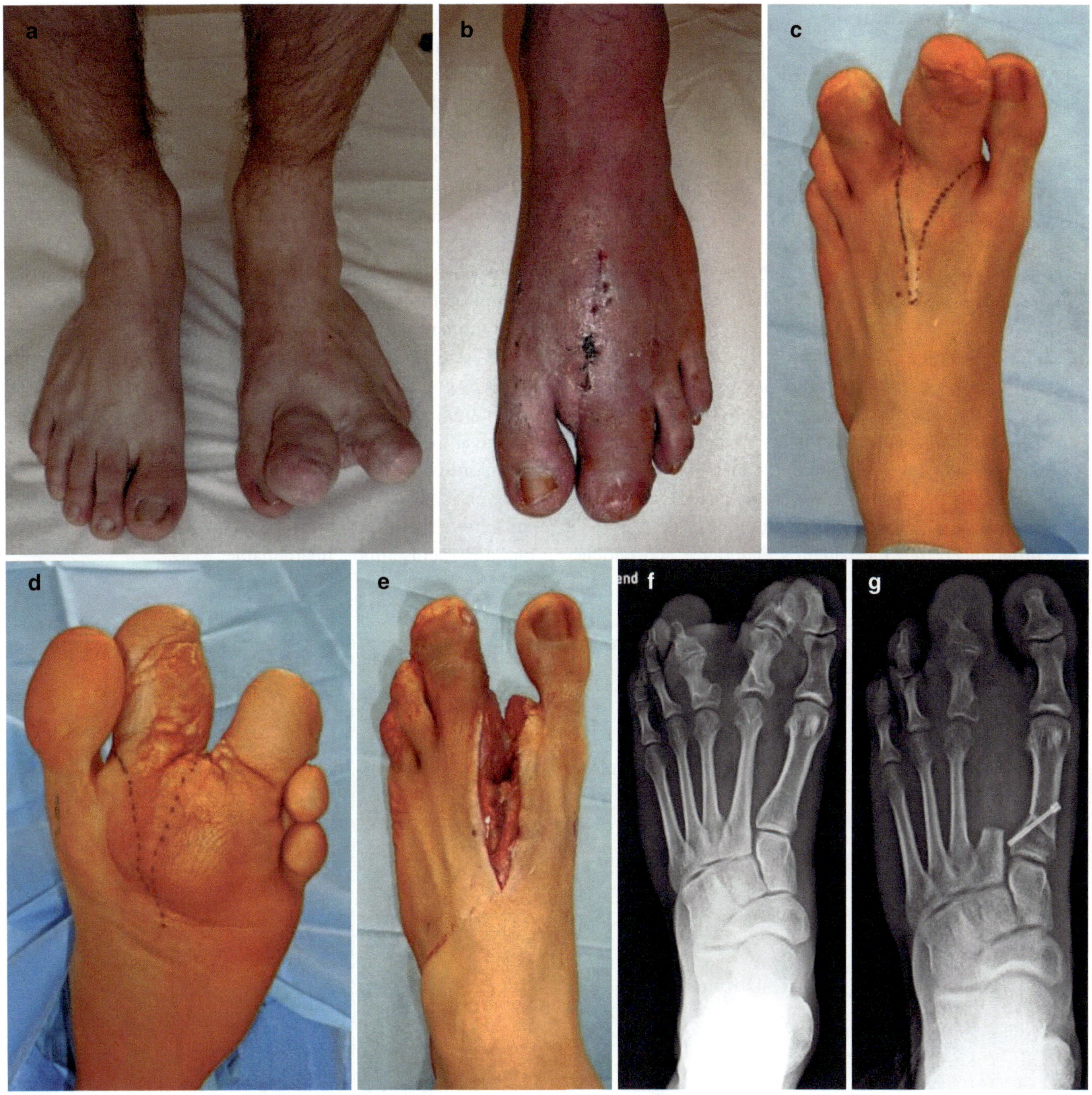

Fig. 10.26 Macrodactylism of the second and third ray and condition after previous reduction interventions in a young patient (**a**, **f**). Ray resection of the second ray with further soft tissue reduction of the third ray as well as metatarsal I base osteotomy to narrow the metatarsus gave a cosmetically and functionally satisfactory result (**b**, **g**). Intraoperative images document the resection of larger skin-soft tissue portions as part of the correction (**c**–**e**)

10.3.3 Brachymetatarsia

The longitudinal growth disorder of individual metatarsal bones—particularly common on the fourth ray—with functional restriction and deformity of the associated toe is in many cases especially a cosmetic problem. The mostly hyperextended toe or the toe that "rides" on the metatarsus and is without any function can cause a shoe conflict. In other cases there is a considerable functional disorder of the forefoot with overloading of individual metatarsal rays with—relative—excess length (Fig. 10.27).

10.3.3.1 Surgical Indication

Since corrections, especially in the case of metatarsal lengthening with callus distraction, are not easy and often lengthy, and the results are not always satisfactory and the impairment is often more of a cosmetic nature, the information provided to the child and parents must be very detailed. Especially in the peripuberty age, where the sensation of a "deformity" is very pronounced, but the patient's endurance and patience for a protracted healing process is limited, restraint should be exercised in the absence of a functional disorder. The situation is different in cases such as the one shown in Fig. 10.27 with considerable overloading of individual metatarsal rays and resulting pressure peaks with metatarsalgia.

10.3.3.2 Principle of Surgery

Single-session or continuous lengthening (Klauser and Mellerowicz 2009; Ruffer et al. 2006) of shortened metatarsal rays (bone interposition (Fig. 10.23) or callus distraction with external or better internal mini-fixators) must be combined with soft tissue release measures. Jones et al. (2015) describe in a literature review that callus distraction achieves greater lengthening distances, but the complication rate is significantly higher than with single-stage procedures. Aggravating factors are often that the neighboring toes fill the interdigital space of the affected toe and thus additional interventions are required. The regaining of load-bearing capacity of the affected metatarsal head and a true active toe function seems almost unattainable.

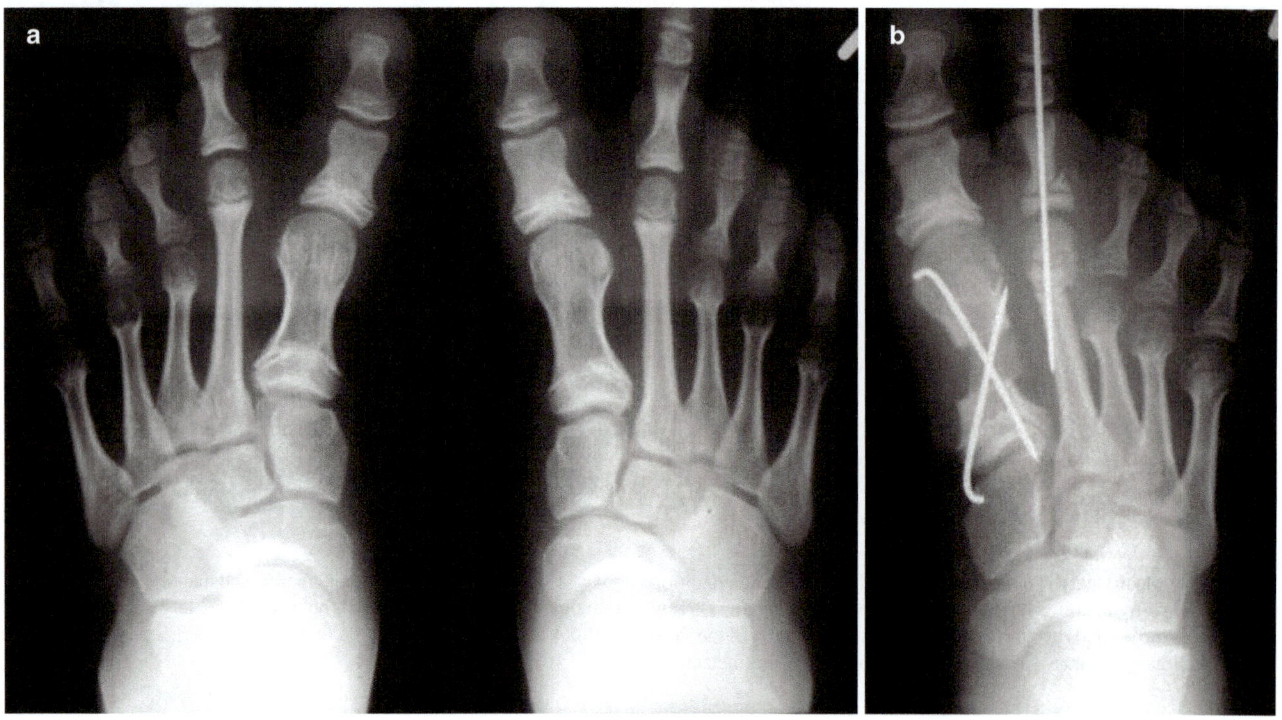

Fig. 10.27 Correction of a case with multiple ray brachymetatarsia (**a**) by single-stage lengthening osteotomy of metatarsal I and shortening at the second ray (**b**). The rays 3–5 were retained in this case

10.3.4 Metatarsal Synostoses

Synostosis of individual metatarsal bones can cause deformities and incorrect weight bearing in the forefoot area. This is particularly painful in the case of the physiologically mobile lateral metatarsal rays (Figs. 10.28 and 10.29). The indication for surgical correction must be considered individually for each case. By osteotomy and/or release of synostoses, a physiological load distribution of the forefoot should be aimed for.

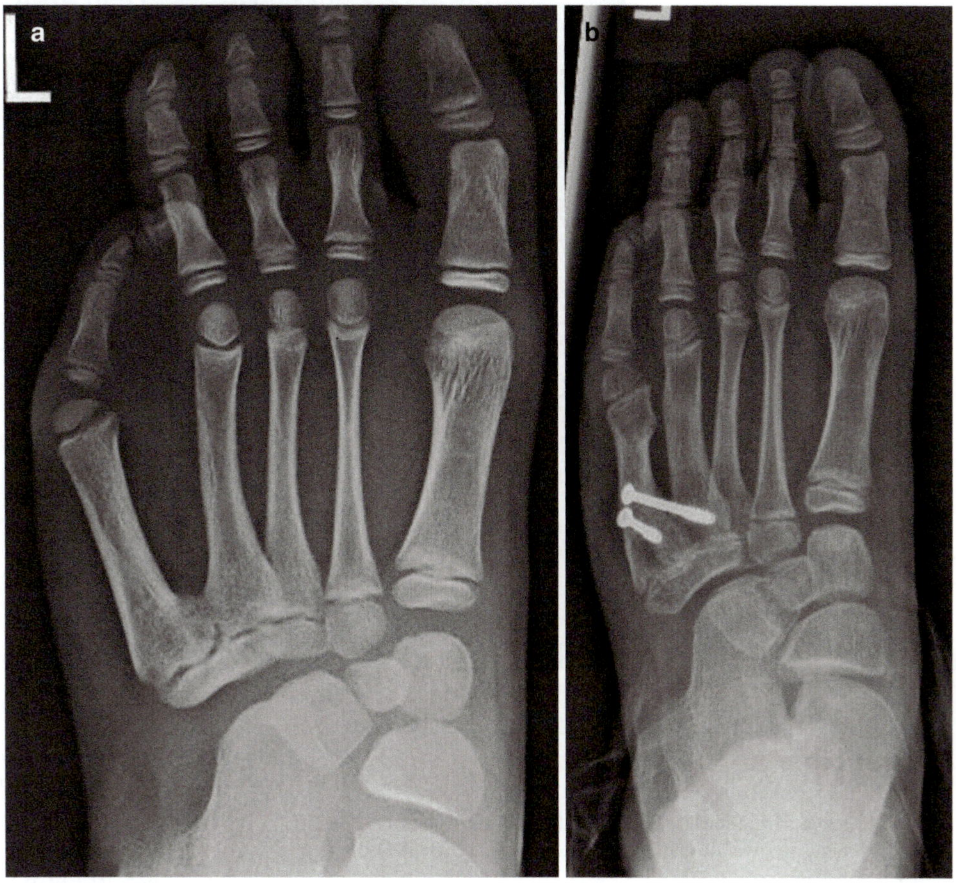

Fig. 10.28 Correction of a synostosis of the metatarsal bases four and five with strong metatarsal widening and overloading of the plantarly flexed fifth metatarsal bone (**a**), which was swivelled and elevated through osteotomy (**b**). Additionally tarsal synostoses are visible

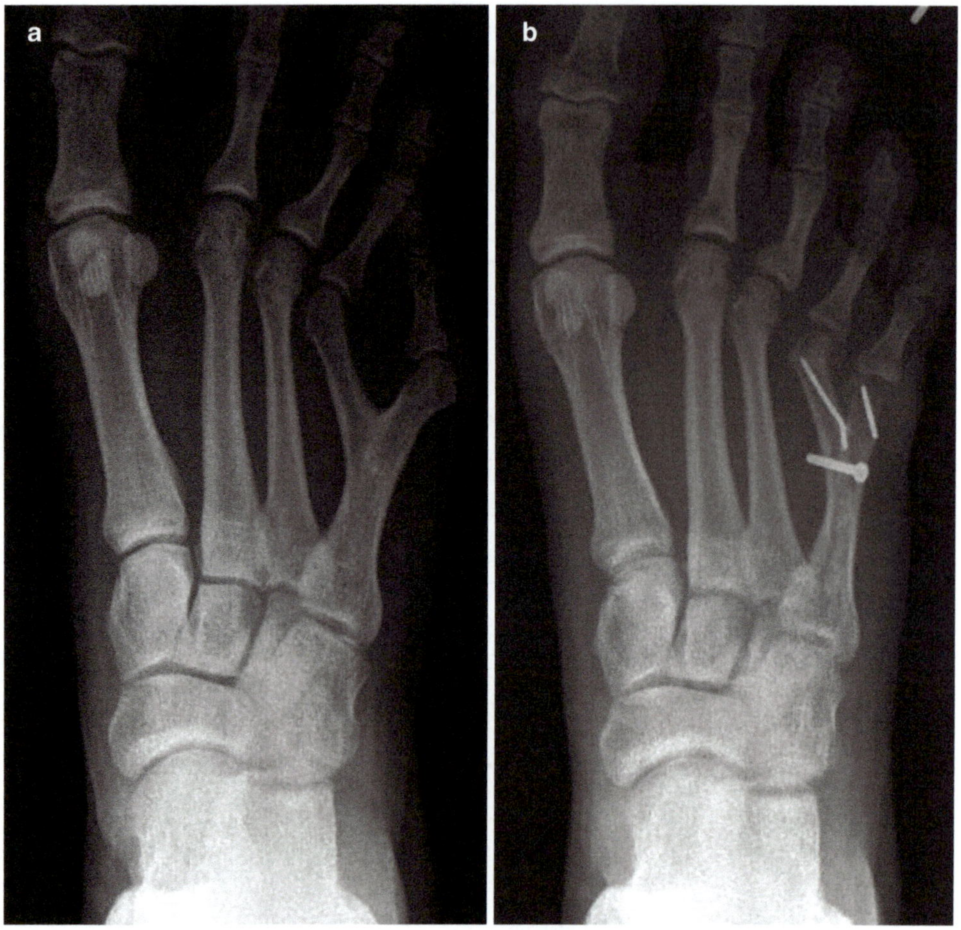

Fig. 10.29 18-Year-old patient with synostosis of metatarsals four and five and pain above the lateral midfoot (**a**). The metatarsus was narrowed by osteotomies; the metatarsophalangeal joints were recentered (**b**)

References

Agrawal Y, Bajaj SK, Flowers MJ (2015) Scarf-Akin osteotomy for hallux valgus in juvenile and adolescent patients. J Pediatr Orthop 24-B:535–540

Bader B, Grill F, Lamprecht E (1999) Die Polydactylie des Fußes. Orthopade 28:125–132

Blauth W, Olason AT (1988) Classification of polydactyly of the hand and feet. Arch Orthop Trauma Surg 107:334–344

Chang CH, Kumar SJ, Riddle EC Glutting J (2002) Macrodactyly of the foot. J Bone Joint Surg 84-A: 1189–1195

Choi JU (2018) Analysis of congenital postaxial polydactyly of the foot using magnetic resonance imaging. Poster P033 EFAS-Congress 2018, Geneva

Cocking J (1968) Butler's operation for an overriding fifth toe. J Bone Joint Surg 50-B:78–81

Coughlin MJ (1995) Juvenile hallux valgus: Etiology and treatment. Foot Ankle Int 16:682–697

Davids JR, Mc Brayer D, Blackhurst DW (2007) Juvenile hallux valgus deformity: Surgical management by lateral hemiepiphysiodesis of the great toe metatarsal. J Pediatr Orthop 27:826–830

Fallat LM, Buckholz J (1980) An analysis of the tailors's bunion by radiographic and anatomical display. J Am Podiatr Assoc 70:591–603

Fuhrmann RA (2013) Therapie des kindlichen Hallux valgus. Orthopade 42:38–44

Jones MD, Pinegar DM, Rincker SA (2015) Callus distraction versus single-stage lengthening with bone graft for treatment of brachymetatarsia: a systematic review. J Foot Ankle Surg 54:927–931

Klauser H, Mellerowicz H (2009) Die Korrektur der Brachymetatarsie mittels Minifixateur interne—ein neues Therapiekonzept. FussSprungg 7:22–30

Lapidus PC (1942) Transplantation of the extensor tendon for correction of the overlapping fifth toe. J Bone Joint Surg 24:555

McBride ED (1967) The McBride bunion hallux valgus operation. J Bone Joint Surg 49-A:1675–1683

Mosca VS (2014) Principles and management of pediatric foot and ankle deformities and malformations. Wolters Kluwer, Philadelphia

Paley D (2002) Principles of deformity correction. Springer-Verlag, Berlin

Ricco AI, Richards BS, Herring JA (2014) Chapter 23: Disorders of the foot. In: Tachdjian's pediatric orthopaedics. Elsevier Saunders, Philadelphia

Ruffer M, Heijens E, Pfeil J (2006) Kalluxdistraktion mit intramedullärer Schienung zur Verlängerung des vierten Strahles bei Brachymetatarsie. FussSprungg 4:234–239

Sahin O, Kuru I, Akgun RC, Sahin BS, Canbeyli ID, Tuncay IC (2013) Metatarsal transfer for the treatment of postaxial metatarsal-type foot synpolydactyly. Bone Joint J 95-B:929–934

Schlickewei C, Ridderbusch K, Breyer S, Spiro A, Stücker R, Rupprecht M (2018) Temporary screw epiphysiodesis of the first metatarsal for correction of juvenile hallux valgus. J Child Orthop 12:375–382

Shim JS, Lim TK, Koh KH, Lee DK (2014) Surgical treatment of congenital hallux varus. Clin Orthop Surg 6:216–222

Venn-Watson E (1976) Problems in polydactyly of the foot. Orthop Clin North Am 7:909–927

Index

J. Hamel, *Foot and Ankle Surgery in Children and Adolescents*, https://doi.org/10.1007/978-3-030-58108-4

GPSR Compliance

The European Union's (EU) General Product Safety Regulation (GPSR) is a set of rules that requires consumer products to be safe and our obligations to ensure this.

If you have any concerns about our products, you can contact us on ProductSafety@springernature.com

In case Publisher is established outside the EU, the EU authorized representative is:

Springer Nature Customer Service Center GmbH
Europaplatz 3
69115 Heidelberg, Germany

Batch number: 10731524

Printed by Printforce, the Netherlands